AF667863

Excellence in Medical Education

Volume 3

The *Excellence in Medical Education* series helps readers understand the requisite structure and programming to ensure a highly functioning and innovative medical education program across levels of educational training and medical specialties. This includes key content areas, such as program administration and teaching methodology. Each book covers basic and advanced principles to help readers meet accreditation requirements, develop clinical and didactic curricula, ensure equitable assessment and evaluation, promote learner and faculty wellness, and implement novel educational approaches.

Heather McPhillips
Patricia Poitevien
Joanna Lewis • Rebecca Blankenburg
Editors

Graduate Medical Education in Pediatrics

From Basic Processes to True Innovation

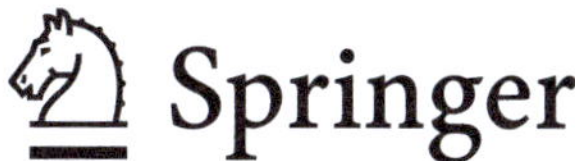

Editors
Heather McPhillips
Department of Pediatrics
UW School of Medicine
Seattle, WA, USA

Patricia Poitevien
Department of Pediatrics
Brown University
Providence, RI, USA

Joanna Lewis
Advocate Children's Hospital –
Park Ridge
Park Ridge, IL, USA

Rebecca Blankenburg
Department of Pediatrics
Stanford School of Medicine
Palo Alto, CA, USA

ISSN 2731-9148 ISSN 2731-9156 (electronic)
Excellence in Medical Education
ISBN 978-3-032-12951-2 ISBN 978-3-032-12952-9 (eBook)
https://doi.org/10.1007/978-3-032-12952-9

This Springer imprint is published by the registered company Springer Nature Switzerland AG
The registered company address is: Gewerbestrasse 11, 6330 Cham, Switzerland

Contents

Part I Foundations of Pediatric Graduate Medical Education

1 **Introduction** 3
Heather McPhillips, Rebecca Blankenburg, Joanna Lewis, and Patricia Poitevien

2 **Pediatric Organizations** 5
Heather McPhillips, Joanna Lewis, Rebecca Blankenburg, and Patricia Poitevien

3 **Funding Pediatric Education** 9
Sidney Hilker, Laura Chiel, and Debra Boyer

4 **Residency Program Accreditation** 19
Stephanie B. Dewar, Shawna Segraves Duncan, and Gabriel M. Daniels

5 **Learner Certification Through the American Board of Pediatrics** 33
Suzanne K. Woods

Part II Program Design and Development

6 **Starting a New Program** 41
Amber M. Hoffman and Heather A. Fagan

7 **Starting a New Training Track** 59
Amanda Stewart, Yael Smiley, and Olanrewaju Falusi

8 **Developing One's Residency Leadership Team** 69
Margaret (Meg) McNamara and Michelle Thompson

9 **Program Director Career Advancement and Leadership** 77
Rebecca R. Swan and Brian Lurie

Part III Recruitment and Transition to Residency

10 Recruitment ... 93
Uchenna Anani and Lahia Yemane

11 Transition from Medical School, Orientation, and Onboarding ... 109
Emma Omoruyi and Veronica M. Gonzalez

Part IV Curriculum and Educational Design

12 Curriculum Development ... 131
Sarah Gustafson, Christiana M. Zhang, and Belinda Y. Chen

13 Clinical Curriculum ... 149
Stacy Laurent and Ross E. Myers

14 Academic/Planned Curriculum ... 161
Emily Borman-Shoap, Johannah Scheurer, and Rachel Poeppelman

15 Individualized Curriculum and Career Choice ... 175
Heather Howell and Lynn Thoreson

16 Interprofessional Education ... 185
Jennifer D. Baird, Glenn Rosenbluth, and Sandrijn van Schaik

17 Advocacy ... 199
Michelle M. Barnes and Ana C. Monterrey

18 Incorporating Mental and Behavioral Health into Pediatric Training Programs ... 217
Elizabeth M. Chawla and Sue E. Poynter

19 Procedures and Simulation ... 229
Amanda J. Rogers and Adrian D. Zurca

20 Using Technology in Curriculum ... 247
Linda Waggoner-Fountain and Alan Chin

Part V Assessment and Program Evaluation

21 Competency-Based Assessment ... 265
Katherine Nowicki and David A. Turner

22 Clinical Competency Committees ... 279
Su-Ting T. Li

23 Resident Performance Challenges and Remediation ... 291
Katherine Mason and Christine Barron

24 Faculty Performance ... 305
Hayley Gans

Part VI Resident Development and Support

25 **Advising, Mentoring, and Coaching** 317
Caroline E. Rassbach and Kim Hoang

26 **Well-Being in GME: Finding Meaning in Medicine** 325
Jennifer G. Duncan and Elizabeth L. Seashore

27 **Supporting Residents with or Planning Families**............. 349
Ann E. Burke and Sabrina Ben-Zion

28 **Developing an Inclusive and Safe Learning Environment** 359
Courtney A. Gilliam and Deawodi Ladzekpo

29 **Chief Residents** 371
Jason (Jay) Homme and Kristin Sundy

Part VII Faculty and Leadership Development

30 **Faculty Development** 387
H. Barrett Fromme and Nicola Orlov

Part VIII Innovation and the Future of Pediatric Education

31 **The Future of Pediatric Education: Challenges, Opportunities and Innovation** 409
Megan E. Aylor, Aisha Barber, and Mike Weisgerber

32 **Concluding Remarks** 443
Heather McPhillips, Patricia Poitevien, Rebecca Blankenburg, and Joanna Lewis

Index... 445

Contributors

Uchenna Anani Vanderbilt University Medical Center, Nashville, TN, USA

Megan E. Aylor Oregon Health Sciences University, Portland, OR, USA

Jennifer D. Baird Children's Hospital Los Angeles, Los Angeles, CA, USA

Aisha Barber George Washington University and Children's National Hospital, Washington, DC, USA

Michelle M. Barnes University of Illinois College of Medicine at Chicago, Chicago, IL, USA

Christine Barron Warren Alpert Medical School of Brown University, Providence, RI, USA

Sabrina Ben-Zion Akron Children's Hospital, Akron, OH, USA

Rebecca Blankenburg Stanford School of Medicine, Stanford, CA, USA

Emily Borman-Shoap University of Minnesota School of Medicine, Minneapolis, MN, USA

Debra Boyer Nationwide Children's Hospital, Columbus, OH, USA

Ann E. Burke Dayton Children's Hospital/Wright State University Boonshoft School of Medicine, Dayton, OH, USA

Elizabeth M. Chawla Medstar Georgetown University Hospital, Washington, DC, USA

Belinda Y. Chen Johns Hopkins School of Medicine, Baltimore, MD, USA

Laura Chiel Boston Children's Hospital, Boston, MA, USA

Alan Chin UCLA Mattel Children's Hospital, Los Angeles, CA, USA

Gabriel M. Daniels University of Alabama at Birmingham, Department of Pediatrics, Birmingham, AL, USA

Stephanie B. Dewar University of Pittsburgh School of Medicine, Pittsburgh, PA, USA

Jennifer G. Duncan Washington University in St. Louis School of Medicine, St. Louis, MO, USA

Shawna Segraves Duncan Oklahoma State University College of Osteopathic Medicine at Cherokee Nation, Tahlequah, OK, USA

Heather A. Fagan Nemours Children's Hospital Florida (NCHFL) in Orlando, Orlando, FL, USA

Olanrewaju Falusi Children's National Hospital, George Washington University School of Medicine and Health Sciences, Washington, DC, USA

H. Barrett Fromme University of Chicago Pritzker School of Medicine, Chicago, IL, USA

Hayley Gans Stanford University, Stanford, CA, USA

Courtney A. Gilliam Department of Pediatrics, University of Cincinnati College of Medicine, Cincinnati, OH, USA

Veronica M. Gonzalez McGovern Medical School at UTHealth Houston, Houston, TX, USA

Sarah Gustafson University of California, Los Angeles, Los Angeles, CA, USA

Sidney Hilker Boston Children's Hospital, Boston, MA, USA

Kim Hoang Stanford School of Medicine, Stanford, CA, USA

Amber M. Hoffman University of Pittsburgh School of Medicine, Pittsburgh, PA, USA

Heather Howell New York University Grossman School of Medicine, New York, NY, USA

Jason (Jay) Homme Mayo Clinic, Rochester, MN, USA

Deawodi Ladzekpo Cincinnati Children's Hospital Medical Center, Cincinnati, OH, USA

Stacy Laurent University of Illinois College of Medicine at Chicago, Chicago, IL, USA

Joanna Lewis Advocate Children's Hospital, Park Ridge, IL, USA

Su-Ting T. Li University of California Davis, Davis, CA, USA

Brian Lurie Brown University Health - Hasbro Children's, Providence, RI, USA

Katherine Mason Warren Alpert Medical School of Brown University, Providence, RI, USA

Heather McPhillips University of Washington School of Medicine, Seattle, WA, USA

Margaret (Meg) McNamara University of California San Francisco, San Francisco, CA, USA

Ana C. Monterrey Baylor College of Medicine, Houston, TX, USA

Ross E. Myers Rainbow Babies and Children's Hospital and Case Western Reserve University School of Medicine, Cleveland, OH, USA

Katherine Nowicki University of Colorado School of Medicine, Aurora, CO, USA

Emma Omoruyi McGovern Medical School at UTHealth Houston, Houston, TX, USA

Nicola Orlov University of Chicago Pritzker School of Medicine, Chicago, IL, USA

Rachel Poeppelman University of Minnesota School of Medicine, Minneapolis, MN, USA

Patricia Poitevien The Warren Alpert Medical School of Brown University, Providence, RI, USA

Sue E. Poynter Cincinnati Children's Hospital Medical Center and University of Cincinnati College of Medicine, Cincinnati, OH, USA

Caroline E. Rassbach Stanford School of Medicine, Stanford, CA, USA

Amanda J. Rogers Medical College of Wisconsin and Children's Wisconsin, Milwaukee, WI, USA

Glenn Rosenbluth University of California, San Francisco, San Francisco, CA, USA

Johannah Scheurer University of Minnesota School of Medicine, Minneapolis, MN, USA

Elizabeth L. Seashore University of California, San Francisco School of Medicine, San Francisco, CA, USA

Yael Smiley Children's National Hospital, George Washington University School of Medicine and Health Sciences, Washington, DC, USA

Amanda Stewart Children's National Hospital, George Washington University School of Medicine and Health Sciences, Washington, DC, USA

Kristin Sundy University of North Carolina, Chapel Hill, NC, USA

Rebecca R. Swan Vanderbilt University Medical Center, Nashville, TN, USA

Michelle Thompson CHLA, Los Angeles, CA, USA

Lynn Thoreson Dell Medical School, The University of Texas at Austin, Austin, TX, USA

David A. Turner American Board of Pediatrics, Chapel Hill, NC, USA

Sandrijn van Schaik University of California, San Francisco, San Francisco, CA, USA

Linda Waggoner-Fountain University of Virginia School of Medicine, Charlottesville, VA, USA

Mike Weisgerber Medical College of Wisconsin – Milwaukee, Milwaukee, WI, USA

Suzanne K. Woods American Board of Pediatrics, Chapel Hill, NC, USA

Lahia Yemane Stanford University School of Medicine, Palo Alto, CA, USA

Christiana M. Zhang Johns Hopkins School of Medicine, Baltimore, MD, USA

Adrian D. Zurca Northwestern University Feinberg School of Medicine, Chicago, IL, USA

Part I

Foundations of Pediatric Graduate Medical Education

1 Introduction

Heather McPhillips, Rebecca Blankenburg,
Joanna Lewis, and Patricia Poitevien

Graduate Medical Education in Pediatrics: From Basic Processes to True Innovation is designed to meet the needs of both experienced and new pediatric residency program leaders. This is the first comprehensive resource of its kind—a definitive guide to the standard structures, best practices, and forward-looking innovations in pediatric residency education. With contributions from nationally recognized leaders in pediatric GME and editors representing diverse institutions and regions, this volume reflects the evolving priorities of our field: educational excellence, resident and faculty well-being, inclusive learning environments, and a commitment to health equity for all children.

This book is intended for a wide audience: program directors and associate program directors, chief residents, faculty educators, program administrators and coordinators, hospital and clinic leadership, and residents and fellows considering a career in medical education. Each chapter aims to be practical, evidence-informed, and responsive to the needs of real-world residency programs.

In addition to providing guidance for achieving and maintaining program accreditation, this book offers strategies to improve clinical and didactic training, support resident development, and implement practices that promote wellness, diversity, and belonging. We also highlight innovations—such as novel curricular structures like the X + Y model and successful diversity, equity and inclusion initiatives—that are reshaping pediatric residency education nationwide.

With nearly 3000 new pediatric residents entering training each year and hundreds of fellowship programs depending on well-prepared graduates, the impact of pediatric residency education is profound. We hope this volume serves as both a foundational reference and a source of inspiration for program leaders striving to meet the evolving needs of today's learners and tomorrow's pediatricians.

H. McPhillips (✉)
University of Washington School of Medicine, Seattle, WA, USA
e-mail: hmcphil@uw.edu

R. Blankenburg
Stanford School of Medicine, Stanford, CA, USA

J. Lewis
Advocate Children's Hospital, Park Ridge, IL, USA

P. Poitevien
The Warren Alpert Medical School of Brown University, Providence, RI, USA

H. McPhillips et al. (eds.), *Graduate Medical Education in Pediatrics*, Excellence in Medical Education 3, https://doi.org/10.1007/978-3-032-12952-9_1

Pediatric Organizations

2

Heather McPhillips, Joanna Lewis,
Rebecca Blankenburg, and Patricia Poitevien

Program Accreditation Versus Learner Certification

One of the important roles of residency program leadership is to ensure that residents meet the requirements of certification. Pediatricians become board certified through two organizations: the American Board of Pediatrics (ABP) and the American Board of Osteopathic Pediatrics (AOBP). Established in 1933, the ABP is one of 24 member boards of the American Board of Medical Specialties (ABMS), which oversees the certification of physician specialists in the United States [1]. Established in 1941, the AOBP is one of 18 member boards approved by the American Osteopathic Association (AOA) Bureau of Osteopathic Specialists [2].

An area of frequent confusion for new program leadership is how the Accreditation Council of Graduate Medical Education (ACGME) and the ABP or AOBP work together to graduate residents eligible for specialty certification. The ACGME accredits pediatric training programs that meet standards set by the Review Committee (RC) for Pediatrics [3]. In 2020, a single accreditation system for graduate medical education programs was implemented; so, all residency programs in the United States, including those for osteopathic physicians, are accredited by the ACGME [4]. The ACGME Pediatric RC does not certify individual residents or fellows.

To be board certified, the individual resident or fellow must graduate from an accredited training program and pass an initial certifying examination. The ABP and the AOBP certify individual residents for the practice of general pediatrics through an initial certification examination. To take the ABP General Pediatrics initial certifying exam, applicants must satisfactorily complete and graduate from a pediatric residency program accredited by the ACGME or a program in Canada accredited by the RCPSC and must satisfactorily complete and receive credit for the full three-year residency [1]. To be eligible to take the AOA/AOBP initial certifying exam, residents must complete a three-year osteopathic or allopathic ACGME-accredited pediatric residency training program. Residents in their third year may apply to take the AOA/AOBP exam prior to completing residency but must have completed at least 30 months of residency or 80% of the total program rotations by the exam date and upon passing, will not be submitted for certification

H. McPhillips (✉)
University of Washington School of Medicine, Seattle, WA, USA
e-mail: hmcphil@uw.edu

J. Lewis
Advocate Children's Hospital, Park Ridge, IL, USA

R. Blankenburg
Stanford School of Medicine, Stanford, CA, USA

P. Poitevien
The Warren Alpert Medical School of Brown University, Providence, RI, USA

H. McPhillips et al. (eds.), *Graduate Medical Education in Pediatrics*, Excellence in Medical Education 3, https://doi.org/10.1007/978-3-032-12952-9_2

until their training status is complete and verified by AOA Postdoctoral Education [2]. In order to take either the ABP or the AOA/AOBP certifying exam, the resident's program director must attest that the resident is eligible for certification by meeting the requirements of the training program and achieving the competencies set by the individual board. It is critically important that program leadership familiarize themselves with both the training program requirements set by the ACGME for Pediatrics and certification requirements for the individual trainee as set by the specialty board(s).

Organizations Involved in Graduate Medical Education

Name	Description	Link
Accreditation Council for Graduate Medical Education (ACGME) [5]	Sets accreditation standards and oversees program compliance for all GME programs.	https://www.acgme.org
ACGME Pediatric Review Committee [3]	Ensures the quality and integrity of pediatric GME by accrediting programs, defining educational requirements, monitoring outcomes, and promoting continuous improvement.	https://www.acgme.org/specialties/pediatrics/overview
American Board of Pediatrics (ABP) [1]	Certifies pediatricians who meet established standards of excellence and who demonstrate commitment to life-long learning and improvement.	https://www.abp.org
American Osteopathic Association (AOA) [6]	Promotes excellence in osteopathic medical education, research, and practice. Is the final approving body for osteopathic board certification following receipt of a recommendation from the specialty certifying board.	https://certification.osteopathic.org/
American Osteopathic Board of Pediatrics (AOBP) [7]	Administers the certifying exam for pediatrics and appropriately recommends osteopathic certification to the AOA.	https://certification.osteopathic.org/pediatrics
Association of American Medical Colleges (AAMC) [8]	Administers the Electronic Residency Application Service (ERAS) as a platform for managing residency applications. Advocates for public policies that support medical research, education, and access to care.	https://www.aamc.org https://www.aamc.org/services/eras
Association of Pediatric Program Directors (APPD) [9]	Central hub for pediatric residency education leaders, resources, mentorship, and innovation.	https://www.appd.org
National Resident Matching Program (NRMP) [10]	Administers the Main Residency Match and provides match data insights.	https://www.nrmp.org

Pediatric Partner Organizations

Name	Description	Link
Academic Pediatric Association (APA) [11]	Advances academic pediatrics through faculty development, scholarship, and advocacy.	https://www.academicpeds.org
American Academy of Pediatrics (AAP) [12]	Professional organization supporting pediatric advocacy, education, and resident development.	http://www.aap.org
Association of Medical School Pediatric Department Chairs (AMSPDC) [13]	Supports leadership and advancement of academic pediatric departments. Leads the Pediatric Workforce Initiative.	https://www.amspdc.org
Council of Pediatric Subspecialties (CoPS) [14]	Provides a unified voice for pediatric subspecialties and promotes excellence in pediatric subspecialty education and training.	http://www.pedsubs.org
Council on Medical Student Education in Pediatrics (COMSEP) [15]	Focuses on pediatric undergraduate medical education, curriculum, and transitions.	https://www.comsep.org
Federation of Pediatric Organizations (FOPO) [16]	Umbrella organization that unites major pediatric societies to promote optimal health for children.	https://www.fopo.org

References

1. American Board of Pediatrics (ABP): About the ABP. https://www.abp.org/content/about-us. Accessed 13 September 2025.
2. https://osteopathic.org/index.php?aam-media=/wp-content/uploads/past-resolutions/H214-A2024-AOA-Recognition-of-the-ACOP-and-AOBP-Pediatricians-wAction.pdf. Accessed 13 September 2025.
3. Accreditation Council for Graduate Medical Education (ACGME): Pediatrics Program Requirements & FAQs; 2025. https://www.acgme.org/specialties/pediatrics/program-requirements-and-faqs-and-applications/. Accessed 13 September 2025.
4. Accreditation Council for Graduate Medical Education (ACGME): Single Graduate Medical Education (GME) Accreditation System—History and Overview. https://www.acgme.org/about/transition-to-a-single-gme-accreditation-system-history/. Accessed 13 September 2025.
5. Accreditation Council for Graduate Medical Education (ACGME): https://www.acgme.org. Accessed 13 September 2025.
6. American Osteopathic Association (AOA), Bureau of Osteopathic Specialists (BOS): About the BOS; 2025. https://certification.osteopathic.org/. Accessed 13 September 2025.
7. American Osteopathic Board of Pediatrics (AOBP): Certification in Pediatrics—Eligibility & Process; 2025. https://certification.osteopathic.org/pediatrics/. Accessed 13 September 2025.
8. Association of American Medical Colleges (AAMC): Electronic Residency Application Service (ERAS®)—Overview; 2025. https://www.aamc.org. Accessed 13 September 2025.
9. Association of Pediatric Program Directors (APPD): About APPD—Mission, Vision, and Programs; 2025. https://www.appd.org. Accessed 13 September 2025.
10. National Resident Matching Program (NRMP): Results and Data—2025 Main Residency Match®; 2025. https://www.nrmp.org/match-data-analytics/. Accessed 13 September 2025.
11. Academic Pediatric Association (APA): About the APA—Mission & Strategic Priorities; 2025. https://www.academicpeds.org. Accessed 13 September 2025.
12. American Academy of Pediatrics (AAP): About the AAP—Mission and Strategic Plan; 2025. https://www.aap.org. Accessed 13 September 2025.
13. Association of Medical School Pediatric Department Chairs (AMSPDC): About AMSPDC; 2025. https://www.amspdc.org/. Accessed 13 September 2025.
14. Council of Pediatric Subspecialties (CoPS): About CoPS—Mission & Activities; 2025. https://www.pedsubs.org. Accessed 13 September 2025.
15. Council on Medical Student Education in Pediatrics (COMSEP): About COMSEP—Organization and Strategic Priorities; 2025. https://www.comsep.org. Accessed 13 September 2025.
16. Federation of Pediatric Organizations (FOPO): About FOPO—Purpose and Member Organizations; 2025. https://www.fopo.org. Accessed 13 September 2025.

Funding Pediatric Education

3

Sidney Hilker, Laura Chiel, and Debra Boyer

Introduction

In considering individual trainees, the Association of American Medical Colleges reported that in 2023, 70% of medical school graduates had education debt, with a median education debt of $200,000 [1]. More than one in three pediatric trainees identifying as Black/African American reported having at least $300,000 in education debt [2]. Understanding how resident salaries are determined represents a key step in being able to advocate for fair compensation. Beyond salary, certain educational experiences, such as conference attendance, membership to professional societies, and advanced educational experiences, are tied to what funding programs can offer [3]. Thus, although the ACGME standardizes clinical experiences across programs, the professional affordances a program may or may not grant to a trainee can differ widely based on funding.

At the program level, Medicare GME funding is allocated to hospitals, rather than sponsoring GME institutions, and the creation of training positions may be divorced from the needs of patients in that community, with little incentive to support general pediatrics training positions over those in whichever specialty the hospital deems more profitable [4, 5]. Thus, the size of a training program may be limited by funding [3], which is of particular concern in light of shortages of pediatricians in certain specialties and in particular geographic locations [6, 7]. Furthermore, while the majority of GME funding is through Medicare and supplemented by Medicaid, free-standing children's hospitals are not eligible for significant Medicare funding [5, 8]. With the lens that a solid understanding of GME funding has meaningful implications, we begin with a detailed description of governmental GME funding, both for residents at general hospitals and at free-standing children's hospitals, and expand upon the considerations unique to pediatric program leaders.

GME Funding Mechanisms

Federal Medicaid and Children's Hospital Funding

Funding for GME in the United States is complicated and differs for free-standing children's hospital programs versus those that are part of adult hospitals. Free-standing children's hospitals are defined as those that primarily serve patients under 18, have an accredited pediatric training program, and do not receive Medicare GME funding [9]. The majority of governmental funding, approximately 60%, is provided through

S. Hilker · L. Chiel
Boston Children's Hospital, Boston, MA, USA

D. Boyer (✉)
Nationwide Children's Hospital,
Columbus, OH, USA
e-mail: Debra.Boyer@nationwidechildrens.org

H. McPhillips et al. (eds.), *Graduate Medical Education in Pediatrics*, Excellence in Medical Education 3, https://doi.org/10.1007/978-3-032-12952-9_3

Medicare from the Centers for Medicare and Medicaid Services (CMS). A smaller proportion of government funding comes from the Health Resources and Services Administration (HRSA), providing payments to free-standing children's hospitals (CHGME) and teaching health centers, as well as funding from the US Department of Veterans Affairs (VA), the Department of Defense, and other federal agencies.

Pediatric residency programs that are part of a teaching hospital treating adults on Medicare are eligible for CMS payments. This Medicare funding mechanism was created in 1965 and is currently a mandatory program, which grows yearly in proportion to increases in its funding. The mean per resident amount for this GME Medicare funding was $177,323 in 2020 and increased from $138,938 in 2015 [10]. This funding is divided into direct GME (DGME) and indirect medical education (IME), which are paid directly to hospitals, not specific GME programs. DGME funding helps to overcome the added costs involved in training residents, such as salaries, benefits, GME infrastructure, and other administrative costs. Importantly, this DGME amount is based on a previously established, institution-specific, per resident amount (PRA), the teaching hospital's approved FTE count, and the total number of inpatient Medicare days. Two important components of the DGME funding are the cap and the initial residency period (IRP). A cap was established, limiting the number of reimbursable residents to the number of FTEs the hospital had in 1996. The IRP reflects trainees in their initial residency period. Any trainees past their IRP only count as 50% of an FTE. Practically, this results in all pediatric subspecialty fellows only adding 0.5 FTE to federal reimbursement. IME payments reflect the indirect costs that occur while training residents and fellows related to learner inefficiencies [11].

The children's hospitals GME (CHGME) program was created as a discretionary program in 1999 and requires reauthorization by Congress every 5 years, as well as annual appropriations. CHGME is funded through the Health Resources and Services Administration (HRSA). In 2020, the final appropriation for CHGME was $340,000,000 compared to $16.2 billion for CMS Medicare payments [12]. Critically, CHGME is less than 2.5% of the total federal funding for all of GME, and reimbursement for CHGME per resident FTE is less than half of the amount allocated to the Medicare GME program.

There are 59 children's hospitals that currently receive CHGME funds, and these institutions are part of the Children's Hospital Association (CHA). In 2021, these hospitals trained approximately 15,000 residents, and more than 50% of pediatricians and pediatric subspecialists are educated at these CHGME-funded hospitals. The individuals trained under CHGME are broad and include general pediatricians, pediatric subspecialists, child and adolescent psychiatrists, pediatric dentists, pediatric podiatrists and family medicine/adult specialists doing pediatric rotations at a CHGME institution [13]. The same cap established in 1996 for Medicare supported payments applies to CHGME reimbursement and these freestanding children's hospitals are capped by the number of residents they had in 1996 to determine their FTE counts. The amount of CHGME funding is set with each appropriation; therefore, if new programs or children's hospitals are created, the result will be a decrease in the per resident amount received for each trainee. This is in direct contrast to CMS-funded adult institutions, where the per resident amount received each year can increase with inflation and the number of residents.

Most programs are funded predominantly through CMS and CHGME; however, there are additional funding sources from the NIH, philanthropists, industry, and hospitals that can be used to support pediatric trainees.

Stimulating Access to Research in Residency (StARR) (R38)

The StARR (R38) program is run by the National Institute of Health with the aim to "provide clinicians with in-depth research experiences early in their careers, in order to recruit, retain and accelerate independence of a pool of clinician-investigators with both clinical and research experience necessary to perform basic, clinical and/or translational research." [14] This award supports residents to perform research, including 80% of their salaries and funding for research and professional development support for 1–2 years during residency. Institutions apply for the award. The number of awards granted depends on NIH funding and the quality of applications.

Philanthropy

Reviews of many pediatric residency websites reveal the opportunity to donate to support resident education. Some residency programs have established alumni councils as a way for alumni to provide support. While many donations are intended to defray the cost of operations or to contribute to program enhancements (such as well-being initiatives), some programs benefit from more substantial donations. For example, in 2023, the E.L. Wiegand Foundation donated $500,000 to a new pediatric residency program at the University of Nevada, Reno School of Medicine and Renown Health [15]. The donation was intended for the startup of operations and salaries.

Industry

Private funding is another mechanism through which to support residency positions. Private insurers provide support through GME by paying higher rates to teaching hospitals [16]. Both the ACGME [17] and AAMC [18] have given specific guidance regarding the interplay between medical education and industry, although how often programs rely on industry to support residency pediatric positions is not clear. The AAMC outlines that "Academic medical centers should establish and implement policies requiring that: 1. All scholarships or other educational funds from industry must be given centrally to the administration of the academic medical center; 2. No *quid pro quo* be involved in any way; and 3. The evaluation and selection of recipients of such funds must be the sole responsibility of the academic medical center or of a nonprofit granting entity, with no involvement by the donor industry." [18]

Department and Hospital Funding

Department and hospital funding is another important source of residency funding, although the extent to which this is relied upon is uncertain. At the fellowship level, a recent survey of fellowship directors revealed that department and subspecialty division funding was significant [3].

ACGME Requirements and How They Impact Budgets

Financial Impact of ACGME Changes

The Accreditation Council for Graduate Medical Education (ACGME) specifies residency program requirements and updates these requirements on a 10-year cycle. As of July 1, 2025, pediatric residency requirements changed to align with updated workforce demands. Overall, the changes may increase costs for pediatric residency programs and reduce the revenue many hospitals make from having a predominantly inpatient resident workforce.

Changes included increasing the amount of time residents spend on individualized curricula and in the ambulatory setting [19]. While residency is primarily intended to train new physicians, resident physicians can enable a hospital to see more patients and, in some cases, increase hospital revenue. Shifting residents to more outpatient settings may have financial implications for hospitals and residency programs. Small studies on the impact of having residents in outpatient settings suggest that residents can enable a clinic to see more patients on average than a clinic staffed with attending physicians alone. It is also possible to increase the revenue per faculty member using resident clinics compared to non-resident clinics. However, resident clinics are associated with higher costs due to the need for additional exam rooms, medical assistants, and precepting faculty. This can result in lower operating margins for resident clinics compared to non-resident clinics [20]. Therefore, as many residency programs shift to support increased ambulatory time for residents, pediatric programs may feel pressure to consider creative models that allow residents to have educational experiences while also maintaining operating margins for the hospital.

In addition to the costs associated with adding residents to outpatient clinics, there can be financial losses associated with decreasing resident coverage of inpatient services. Programs that rely on residents to cover general pediatrics and subspecialty inpatient teams will likely need to hire advanced practice practitioners (APPs) and hospitalists. This process can also be costly, particularly given that residents are permitted to work up to 80 hours per week while a typical full-time employee is scheduled for 36–40 hours of clinical time. Studies comparing costs of residents and APPs are primarily from surgical specialties. One study found that replacing 30 general surgery residents with APPs would cost $4.5 million based on a 1 resident to 3 APP replacement ratio [21]. A similar study of anesthesiology residents estimated that replacing one resident costs about $153,000 over 3 years of training [22]. It is worthwhile for a program to consider where it is most educationally and financially beneficial to have residents versus APPs or hospitalists provide care.

Given that government funding is linked to the number of patients with received Medicare at a teaching hospital, there may be financial incentives to limit the time trainees spend in non-hospital clinics (e.g., public health clinics, global health experiences, private practices) and research pursuits in an effort to increase the number of patients seen within a hospital [5]. Ultimately, more studies are needed to understand the financial implications of the 2025 ACGME requirements.

Program Leadership and Administrative Support

ACGME requirements continue to mandate that every residency program has a program director, and that the aggregate program leadership FTE increase with the number of residents in the program. For example, a program with fewer than 7 residents must have at least 0.2 FTE of program leadership time and a program with 100 residents must have a minimum of 2.2 FTE of program leadership time. A residency program coordinator is also required with a program of fewer than 7 residents having at least 0.5 FTE and a program of 100 residents requiring at least 2.5 FTE [19]. While minimum FTE required increases with the number of residents, smaller programs are likely to incur higher per resident costs. For example, even a program with six residents needs someone to oversee scheduling, education, resident recruitment, and professional development, which requires significant investment.

Core Faculty Time

New residency ACGME requirements in July 2025 specified subspecialty rotations that must have pediatric subspecialty faculty members who have certification in their subspecialty. One core faculty member is required for every five residents in a program. Programs must provide at least 0.1 FTE in aggregate per core faculty member of protected time for educational and administrative responsibilities related to the residency [19]. Dedicated faculty time will help ensure that residents have robust educational experiences, particularly during individualized time when residents may need more one-on-one guidance to meet their learning goals, but this requirement will also increase the costs associated with hosting a residency program.

Residency Budget Considerations

A sample residency proforma, including revenue, expenses, operational margins, and capital cost/expenses, was recently published by Monks and colleagues in the *Journal of Graduate Medical Education* [23]. The authors cite the following as key revenue considerations: direct medical education funding, indirect medical education funding, state grants, philanthropy/foundation, and clinical earning. In terms of expenses, the authors cite resident expenses, with examples including: annual stipend by PGY level; fringe/FICA, benefits (such as dental, vision, and health), liability insurance, professional society membership dues, lab coats, and in-training exams. They also cite program expenses, such as accreditation fees, catering/food services, office supplies, rent, program coordinator salary, and recruitment. Faculty expenses include program director and associate program director compensation, and faculty development, as well as clinical expenses for "additional cost for expanded or new clinical services including staff." Capital costs/expenses include physical work space, computers, conference space, etc. The specifics of every residency program's proforma will differ, and program leaders should consider comparing what items appear in your residency program's budget with those from other programs.

Influence of Resident Unions

As of 2024, about 1 in 7 residents was represented by a union. The number of resident unions is increasing, with at least seven programs unionizing in 2023 alone [24]. The salary for a first-year resident averaged $63,800 in 2023 [25]. Residents are training in a time when other professions requiring a similar level of education often have higher salaries [26], coming out of graduate school with more flexible working environments, including options to work from home with unlimited vacation and additional benefits, such as free in-office meals, childcare, and gyms. All of this has coincided with a rise in resident unions as more trainees look for ways to have their voices heard with respect to their compensation and benefits.

It remains unclear whether unions have had a substantial impact on resident compensation and wellness to date. A 2021 study of surgical programs with and without unions found that unionized programs offered more vacation and were more likely to provide a housing stipend, but there was no significant change in salary or burnout [27]. With more unionized programs emerging, further research is needed to better understand the impact of unions on residency programs and their trainees.

For program leadership, it is important to consider the impact of unions on both the financials of their program as well as the resident-leadership dynamics [28]. Unionized programs used a structured negotiation process that all labor unions follow. Changes to salary and benefits are decided through formal negotiations rather than ad hoc. The financial decision-making of a residency program looks different for a unionized program compared to a non-unionized program. These dynamics are important to take into consideration when considering program funding.

Impact of Finances on the Pediatric Workforce

Pediatrics is seeing a decline in applicants and an increase in the number of open resident, subspecialty, and primary care positions. Between 2015 and 2020, there was an 8% decline in the number of matched pediatric residents while almost all other specialties saw an increase [29]. In 2023, fewer than 70% of pediatric subspecialty fellowship programs filled their programs with less than half of positions filled in child abuse, developmental and behavioral pediatrics, endocrinology, infectious diseases, nephrology, and pulmonology [30].

Demand for Primary Care Pediatricians

Primary care pediatricians are also in demand, particularly in rural areas. Between 2010 and 2020, the percentage of counties without any pediatric trained physicians increased by over 10% [31]. Of the $16 billion of federal GME funding, very little is dedicated to primary care and other specialties with workforce shortages [32]. Some have argued that the structure of GME funding, particularly the 1996 national cap on the number of residents eligible for federal funding, has contributed to the shortage of primary care physicians.

Large residency programs often account for most residency slots available, leaving other programs with little room to expand their residency. Based on the number of residency spots at large and established residencies in 1996, New York alone received about 20% of GME funding, leaving other states with little [33]. New programs can apply for additional GME funding, but expanding programs to meet primary care demands is more difficult to fund for this reason. Hospitals often fund additional residents without additional GME funding, instead spending dollars from their hospital budgets. Despite a lack of federal funding for new residency positions, more than 15,000 residency positions have been created since 2003, including over 1700 pediatric residency positions [34, 35]. However, many of these residents are training in procedure-based specialties that are generally more lucrative for the hospital [36] which makes it easier for hospitals to justify spending more money in these areas.

Congress has enacted legislation, including the *Primary Care Residency Expansion, Teaching Health Center Graduate Medical Education, and the Title VII Health Care Workforce Act,* to bolster the primary care workforce. However, each of these laws has been limited to 5 years or fewer of funding, and there has not been a significant change in the number of primary care physicians, particularly primary care pediatricians [33].

States are getting involved to support local workforce demands and recognize that residents often stay in the state where they trained. For example, Georgia provides funding for new GME programs in key specialties, including family medicine and child psychiatry, with the aim of opening 27 programs and adding 613 residency positions by 2025 [37]. New Mexico created a Primary Care Training Consortium in 2013 that funds residency training at Federally Qualified Health Centers (FQHCs) and allows for the expansion of existing residency programs [38]. Texas allocated about $183 million for new GME programs and expansions and successfully increased the number of residency positions in the state to be more than one for each of the state's medical school graduates. Finally, California also dedicated funds to primary care GME programs with a focus on underserved areas [32]. Initial funding for program startup may also come from the sponsoring institution, grant funding, philanthropy, and loan repayment programs in underserved areas [39]. Establishing new GME programs may be one way to expand patient care and help address physician shortage issues while avoiding federal funding caps, which limit the expansion of existing programs [39]. It is important to note that as new programs are added to institutions receiving CHGME or Medicare funding, these institutions will likely not receive additional funding if they are at their cap. Specifically, if a program is started at an institution not previously receiving this funding, the "cap" will be determined by the number of residents at that hospital at the end of 5 years. Importantly, if residents from other programs have rotated at some point at your institution, that might have already started the clock towards determining the cap.

Volatile Pediatric Funding and Pediatric Hospital Closures

Pediatrics funding is particularly volatile, given that each year it is subject to discretionary appropriations (the government must re-approve CHGME funds each year). Even with these funds, only about 40% of CHGME funds go to general pediatric trainees, which further limits the funds going to residents pursuing pediatric primary care. The remainder of the funds go to pediatric subspecialties, dental training, and other specialties such as family medicine and surgery who have residents rotating through qualified children's hospitals [40]. In addition to unreliable pediatric GME funding, there is a concerning trend of pediatric inpatient unit closures. In 2022, pediatric units in Richmond, VA; Boston, MA; Colorado Springs, CO; Raleigh, NC; and Doylestown, PA, all closed, citing a lack of revenue from pediatric services [41]. Closure of pediatric inpatient units limits access to care for patients but also eliminates opportunities for residents to train in these smaller access hospitals.

Drivers of the Decline in Pediatric Interest

Ultimately, the decline in pediatric trainees is multifactorial. The structure of GME funding may exacerbate workforce shortages by failing to reward trainees who enter high-demand fields of medicine. However, pediatrician salaries are also significantly lower than other medical specialties, and many find it difficult to choose a lower-paying specialty given that the average debt of pediatric residents in 2020 was $264,000 [42]. Adult subspecialists earn about 25% more than their pediatric subspecialist counterparts [6]. Given that higher earning subspecialties have higher fill rates, trainees seem less likely to pursue lower-paid specialties. Salaries are primarily driven by insurance reimbursement, with more procedural subspecialties receiving higher reimbursement, which explains challenges filling subspecialties such as child abuse, developmental and behavioral pediatrics, and infectious diseases that typically do not perform procedures. Pediatric programs will need to consider how to continue recruiting and retaining trainees across subspecialties in the setting of these growing compensation gaps.

Funding Advocacy

As discussed above, funding for pediatric-focused training is unstable and advocacy is essential to ensure the stability of our pediatric programs. Organizations such as the Association of Medical School Pediatric Department Chairs (AMSPDC), AAP, and CHA are involved in advocacy efforts regarding GME funding. A critical element of advocacy efforts is seeking parity with Medicare funding to equate the CHGME per resident amount with that provided with Medicare CMS funding for GME. Equally important are efforts to change CHGME funding from a discretionary program requiring reauthorization to a mandatory program like Medicare funding. While these efforts are led by these organizations, it is essential that all pediatric GME leaders join these efforts to prioritize GME funding. Similarly, AMSPDC, AAP, and CHA are also advocating for improvements in reimbursement for pediatric care to levels equal to adult care. This, in turn, would allow institutions to increase salaries for general pediatricians and pediatric subspecialists and therefore improve workforce gaps.

References

1. Medical student education: debt, costs, and loan repayment fact card for the class of 2023. Accessed 2 July 2024. https://students-residents.aamc.org/media/12846/download.
2. Orr CJ, Turner AL, Ritter VS, Gutierrez-Wu J, Leslie LK. Pursuing a career in pediatrics: intersection of educational debt and race/ethnicity. J Pediatr. 2023;252:162–70. https://doi.org/10.1016/j.jpeds.2022.08.014.
3. Weiss P, Myers A, McGann K, et al. Funding sources and perceived financial insecurity.
4. Chen C, Xierali I, Piwnica-Worms K, Phillips R. The redistribution of graduate medical education positions in 2005 failed to boost primary care or rural training. Health Aff (Millwood). 2013;32(1):102–10. https://doi.org/10.1377/hlthaff.2012.0032.
5. Committee on Pediatric Workforce. Financing graduate medical education to meet the needs of children and the future pediatrician workforce.

Pediatrics. 2016;137(4). https://doi.org/10.1542/peds.2016-0211.
6. Leslie LK, Orr CJ, Turner AL, et al. Child health and the US pediatric subspecialty workforce: planning for the future. Pediatrics. 2024;153(Suppl 2). https://doi.org/10.1542/peds.2023-063678B.
7. Shah S, Cheng TL. Optimizing the children's hospitals graduate medical education payment program at a time of pediatric workforce challenges and health need. J Pediatr. 2022;245:4–6.e2. https://doi.org/10.1016/j.jpeds.2021.11.017.
8. Comparative Analysis of GME Funding Programs for Children's Hospitals and General Acute Care Teaching Hospitals.
9. Children's Hospital Association. Everything you need to know about CHGME. Accessed 18 Mar 2025. https://www.childrenshospitals.org/content/public-policy/fact-sheet/everything-you-need-to-know-about-chgme.
10. Chen C, Chung Y, Petterson S, Bazemore A. Changes and variation in Medicare graduate medical education payments. JAMA Intern Med. 2020;180(1):148–50. https://doi.org/10.1001/jamainternmed.2019.4429.
11. Federal Support for Graduate Medical Education: an Overview.
12. https://www.ama-assn.org/system/files/2023-gme-compendium-report.pdf. Accessed 5 Oct 2024. https://www.ama-assn.org/system/files/2023-gme-compendium-report.pdf.
13. https://www.childrenshospitals.org/-/media/files/public-policy/chgme_workforce/fact_sheets/cha-chgme-fact-sheet.pdf. Accessed 5 Oct 2024. https://www.childrenshospitals.org/-/media/files/public-policy/chgme_workforce/fact_sheets/cha-chgme-fact-sheet.pdf.
14. Stimulating Access to Research in Residency (StARR) (R38). Accessed 3 July 2024. https://grants.nih.gov/grants/guide/rfa-files/RFA-HL-18-023.html.
15. E. L. Wiegand Foundation donates $500,000 to new Pediatric Residency Program. Accessed 5 July 2024. https://www.unr.edu/nevada-today/news/2023/wiegand-peds-donation.
16. Committee on the Governance and Financing of Graduate Medical Education, Board on Health Care Services, Institute of Medicine. In: Eden J, Berwick D, Wilensky G, editors. Graduate medical education that meets the nation's health needs. National Academies Press; 2014. https://doi.org/10.17226/18754.
17. Principles to guide the relationship between Graduate Medical Education, Industry, and Other Funding Sources for Programs and Sponsoring Institutions Accredited by the ACGME. https://www.acgme.org/globalassets/pfassets/publicationspapers/gme-funding-industry-other-sources.pdf.
18. Industry Funding of Medical Education: report of an AAMC Task Force.
19. ACGME Program Requirements for Graduate Medical Education in Pediatrics. ACGME. February 4, 2024. Accessed 2 July 2024. https://acgme.org/globalassets/pfassets/programrequirements/2025-prs/320_pediatrics_2025.pdf.
20. Stipelman CH, Poss B, Stetson LA, et al. Financial analysis of pediatric resident physician primary care longitudinal outpatient experience. Acad Pediatr. 2018;18(7):837–42. https://doi.org/10.1016/j.acap.2018.05.001.
21. Mrdutt MM, Weber RA, Burke LM, Thomas JS, Papaconstantinou HT, Cable CT. Financial value analysis of surgical residency programs: an argument against replacement. J Surg Educ. 2018;75(6):e150–5. https://doi.org/10.1016/j.jsurg.2018.07.004.
22. Pisetsky MA, Lubarsky DA, Capehart BP, Lineberger CK, Reves JG. Valuing the work performed by anesthesiology residents and the financial impact on teaching hospitals in the United States of a reduced anesthesia residency program size. Anesth Analg. 1998;87(2):245–54. https://doi.org/10.1097/00000539-199808000-00003.
23. Monks SR, Bidwell JL, Wagner MJ. Making a business case for investing in graduate medical education. J Grad Med Educ. 2024;16(2):227–8. https://doi.org/10.4300/JGME-D-24-00149.1.
24. Zeitouni F, Attaluri PK, Wirth PJ, Shaffrey EC, Rao V. State of physician unionization. J Surg Educ. 2024;81(7):929–37. https://doi.org/10.1016/j.jsurg.2024.04.002.
25. AAMC Survey of Resident/Fellow Stipends and Benefits | AAMC. Accessed 15 July 2024. https://www.aamc.org/data-reports/students-residents/report/aamc-survey-resident/fellow-stipends-and-benefits.
26. US Bureau of Labor Statistics. May 2023 National Occupational Employment and Wage Estimates. Occupational Employment and Wage Statistics. May 2023. Accessed 15 July 2024. https://www.bls.gov/oes/current/oes_nat.htm.
27. Brajcich BC, Chung JW, Wood DE, et al. National evaluation of the association between resident labor union participation and surgical resident well-being. JAMA Netw Open. 2021;4(9):e2123412. https://doi.org/10.1001/jamanetworkopen.2021.23412.
28. Krzyzaniak SM, Sebok-Syer SS, Akhtar S, Gallahue F. Exploring how house staff unions impact the program director-resident educational alliance. Acad Med. 2024; https://doi.org/10.1097/ACM.0000000000005649.
29. Vinci RJ. The pediatric workforce: recent data trends, questions, and challenges for the future. Pediatrics. 2021;147(6). https://doi.org/10.1542/peds.2020-013292.
30. The MATCH. Match Results Statistics: Medicine and Pediatric Specialities - 2023. National Resident Matching Program. November 29, 2023. Accessed 6 July 2024. https://www.nrmp.org/wp-content/uploads/2023/11/2023-MPSM-Match-Results-Statistics-Report.pdf.
31. Ramesh T, Yu H. US pediatric primary care physician workforce in rural areas, 2010 to 2020. JAMA Netw Open. 2023;6(9):e2333467. https://doi.org/10.1001/jamanetworkopen.2023.33467.

32. Rittenhouse DR, Ament AS, Grumbach K. Sponsoring institution interests, not national plans, shape physician workforce in the United States. Fam Med. 2020;52(8):551–6. https://doi.org/10.22454/FamMed.2020.507727.
33. Amezquita L, George P, Adashi EY. Clogs in the pipeline: how GME funding contributes to the primary care shortage. Am J Med. 2020;133(9):e455–6. https://doi.org/10.1016/j.amjmed.2020.02.049.
34. Grischkan JA, Friedman AB, Chandra A. Moving the financing of graduate medical education into the 21st century. JAMA. 2020;324(11):1035–6. https://doi.org/10.1001/jama.2020.15480.
35. Yearly Growth in General Pediatrics Residents by Demographics and Program Characteristics | The American Board of Pediatrics. Accessed 18 Mar 2025. https://www.abp.org/dashboards/yearly-growth-general-pediatrics-residents-demographics-and-program-characteristics.
36. Royce TJ. Financing of US graduate medical education. JAMA. 2021;325(6):585–6. https://doi.org/10.1001/jama.2020.23979.
37. Nuss MA, Buckley PF. Georgia's innovative response to GME expansion. J Med Assoc Ga. 2015;104(1):10–1.
38. Henderson TM. How accountable to the public is funding for graduate medical education? The case for state medicaid GME payments. Am J Public Health. 2021;111(7):1216–9. https://doi.org/10.2105/AJPH.2021.306246.
39. Barajaz M, Turner T. Starting a new residency program: a step by step guide for institutions, hospitals, and program directors. Med Educ Online. 2016;21:32271. https://doi.org/10.3402/meo.v21.32271.
40. HRSA Health Workforce. Children's Hospital Graduate Medical Education Program. Bureau of Healthcare Workforce. Accessed 7 July 2024. https://bhw.hrsa.gov/sites/default/files/bureau-health-workforce/data-research/childrens-hospital-graduate-medical-education-annual-report-2021-2022.pdf.
41. As Hospitals Close Children's Units, Where Does That Leave Lachlan? - The New York Times. Accessed 7 July 2024. https://www.nytimes.com/2022/10/11/health/pediatric-closures-hospitals.html.
42. Opinion | Why It's So Hard to Find a Pediatrician - The New York Times. Accessed 4 Aug 2024. https://www.nytimes.com/2024/07/01/opinion/pediatrician-shortage.html.

Residency Program Accreditation

4

Stephanie B. Dewar, Shawna Segraves Duncan, and Gabriel M. Daniels

Introduction to Residency Program Accreditation

Residency and fellowship training programs require significant time and effort on both the part of administrators and learners. Accreditation represents a process by which this time and effort is guided and recognized for all stakeholders in medical education. This section discusses what accreditation is, how it is conferred, and its overall purpose and significance.

Definition of Accreditation and Overview of Process

Accreditation Council for Graduate Medical Education (ACGME) accreditation of residency and fellowship programs is a voluntary, non-government-directed, peer-reviewed process whereby the ACGME's accreditation-related subcommittees evaluate programs for compliance with common and specialty-specific program requirements. Programs accredited by the ACGME are known to be in substantial compliance with the professional standards set forth by the ACGME in conjunction with specialty professional societies, the public, and other stakeholders in medical education and healthcare delivery. ACGME structure is discussed further in the next section.

The ACGME accreditation process occurs in annual cycles. That is, every ACGME-accredited program is reviewed once per year to determine compliance with standards. Data facilitating these annual reviews include ACGME Resident/Fellow and Faculty Surveys completed every spring, the Accreditation Data System (ADS) Annual Update (including responses to survey data) completed by programs every summer, and board certification information, including trainee initial certification rates produced by each specialty's board. Accreditation is also at times influenced by site visits and comments/complaints received through the ACGME outside of the aforementioned methods. As programs are assessed for compliance with requirements for training, areas for improvement and citations are used to indicate concerns or non-compliance. Each program is conferred an accreditation decision based on the degree to which it upholds the expectations set forth for ACGME accreditation. Decisions are made before each new academic year begins in July. For those programs on

S. B. Dewar (✉)
University of Pittsburgh School of Medicine, Pittsburgh, PA, USA
e-mail: sbd12@pitt.edu

S. S. Duncan
Oklahoma State University College of Osteopathic Medicine at Cherokee Nation, Tahlequah, OK, USA

G. M. Daniels
University of Alabama at Birmingham, Department of Pediatrics, Birmingham, AL, USA

H. McPhillips et al. (eds.), *Graduate Medical Education in Pediatrics*, Excellence in Medical Education 3, https://doi.org/10.1007/978-3-032-12952-9_4

probation or whose accreditation has been withdrawn, these accreditation decisions must be made known to trainees within and applying for matriculation into the program.

Overview of Accrediting Body (ACGME)

Residency and fellowship program accreditation within the United States is overseen by the ACGME, a not-for-profit organization grounded in the mission to "improve health care and population health by assessing and enhancing the quality of resident and fellow physicians' education through advancements in accreditation and education." [1] The ACGME seeks to impact graduate medical education and actualize a quadruple aim that "simultaneously improves patient experience of care, population health, and health care practitioner work life, while lowering per capita cost."

The ACGME, like other organizations, has a Board of Directors and multiple subcommittees tasked with carrying out its functions. Many of the internal functions are conducted by employed staff members. The ACGME Review Committees—which include specialty Review Committees, a Transitional Year Review Committee, and an Institutional Review Committee—govern the accreditation within their respective domains through the establishment of accreditation standards, assessment of program compliance with said standards, and conferring of an accreditation status on each program [2]. Given this important function, the Review Committees are composed of volunteer members with expertise in the specialty area and active participation in ACGME-accredited graduate medical education. Said members are nominated by committee-specific nominating organizations and confirmed by the ACGME Board of Directors. Each Review Committee also has one resident/fellow representative and one public member. The trainee representative does not have to be a part of a nominating organization but is expected to be in training within an ACGME-accredited program at the time of selection for service on the Review Committee. Recruitment occurs both through the ACGME's regular *e-Communication* and letters to the specialty-specific professional organizations with trainee groups. The public member is recruited at large and expected to have experience in professional/educational settings, with committee/board working groups, and with the United States healthcare system.

The composition and accreditation decisions of the RCs are reviewed by the ACGME Monitoring Committee; meanwhile, the accreditation standards developed by the RCs are reviewed by the ACGME Committee on Requirements. Review Committee decisions that involve adverse actions (probation, withholding, or withdrawal of accreditation) can be appealed by programs/institutions and are accordingly reviewed by the ACGME Appeals Committee and presented before the ACGME Board of Directors for final ruling. These checks and balances serve to ensure high quality and fair accreditation standards, decisions, and processes.

Structure and the Role of Review Committee for Pediatrics

The Review Committee for Pediatrics is one specialty Review Committee among the nearly 30 Review Committees within the ACGME. Members of the Review Committee for Pediatrics are nominated by the American Board of Pediatrics, the American Osteopathic Board of Pediatrics, the American Academy of Pediatrics, and the American Medical Association. The Review Committee for Pediatrics, as with all Review Committees, has a Resident Member and Public Member. The Review Committee for Pediatrics also has four ex-officio members representing each of these nominating organizations.

The Review Committee for Pediatrics meets three times annually, typically in September, January, and April. The Review Committee for

Pediatrics uses information available at the time of its meetings to determine accreditation decisions for all Pediatric residency and fellowship programs, including some multispecialty subspecialties with pediatric trainees (e.g., adolescent medicine, which could have Pediatric, Internal Medicine, Internal Medicine-Pediatrics, and Family Medicine trainees). Given the timing of meetings, the Review Committee will have annual program updates to ADS and trainee/faculty survey results to guide decisions.

The Review Committee for Pediatrics also accredits new program applications, approves pediatrics residency/fellowship complement and program director changes, and reviews submitted complaints and other matters of accreditation specific to pediatrics training.

Purpose of Accreditation Standards

Accreditation by the ACGME serves multiple purposes as outlined in "The Accreditation Council for Graduate Medical Education Policies and Procedures, effective June 7, 2025, page 11." [3] First and foremost, accreditation ensures the public that training programs graduate competent and professional physicians while upholding that the training process does not diminish the quality or safety of patient care. Accreditation also protects trainee interests by standardizing educational expectations, working conditions, and well-being requirements. This includes expectations for higher "quality of teaching, learning, research, and professional practice." Accreditation further serves all stakeholders in medical education by requiring certain expectations of training programs and their trainees through publicly available standards.

More globally, and discussed further in section on "Understanding Accreditation Standards," the accreditation standards serve an important purpose in ensuring that all graduates of ACGME-accredited programs attain certain minimum standard experiences, curricula, and education opportunities to ensure adequate training to qualify for licensure and independent practice.

Importance of Accreditation for Pediatric Residency Programs

ACGME accreditation provides numerous benefits to each of its stakeholders, which includes the programs themselves. With well-defined expectations and policies, the accreditation standards offer meaningful guidance for program direction and administration. Further, where expectations are not being met, the opportunity for ACGME accreditation provides program leaders with leverage in approaching hospital administrators and other stakeholders for support in meeting standards. ACGME-accredited programs also receive funding from CMS through Medicare for Direct Graduate Medical Education and Indirect Medical Education. Thus, ACGME accreditation also unlocks financial benefits for programs.

Finally, ACGME accreditation is invaluable for programs' relationship with trainees and the public. As mentioned before, the standards associated with ACGME-accredited programs appeal to both trainee and public interests by protecting both the quality of patient care and education delivery. Beyond the promise of standardized, high-quality education, ACGME-accredited program completion is also a pathway for certification eligibility by ABP/ABOP, which makes ACGME-accredited programs more appealing places for trainees to matriculate.

Thus, ACGME accreditation serves pediatric residency programs by guiding and providing leverage for program administration, securing funding, and recruiting and protecting trainees and patients.

Understanding Accreditation Standards

Equally valuable as recognizing the origin and importance of accreditation standards is understanding their meaning and uses. The following section will explain the accreditation standards established by the ACGME for all training programs and trainees, the different types of standards, the specialty-specific requirements for

Pediatrics, and how these standards beget outcomes. Further details are also available in the "Guide to the Common Program Requirements (Residency)." [4]

Common Program Requirements

The Common Program Requirements are a set of standards created by the ACGME for the training of residents and fellows. These requirements are meant to guide programs in creating a clinical learning environment in which trainees can develop the "skills, knowledge, and attitudes necessary to take personal responsibility for the individual care of patients." [4] The Common Program Requirements were first established in 2003 as a unifying refinement of the previously separate general requirements for programs/sponsoring institutions and special requirements for subspecialties.

The Common Program Requirements include a standardized overview of graduate medical education along with a common language that grounds training in every specialty, including trainee oversight, program personnel, trainee appointment and educational curriculum, evaluations, and the clinical learning environment. Within the educational program requirements, the ACGME also specifies the need for trainee development in six Core Competency areas, including Professionalism, Medical Knowledge, Practice-Based Learning and Improvement, Interpersonal and Communication Skills, and Systems-Based Practice.

Since their inception, the Common Program Requirements have been adapted for use in fellowships, single-year fellowships, and other medical or medicine-related post-doctoral educational programs. The Common Program Requirements have also undergone both minor (approximately every 3 years) and major (approximately every 10 years) revisions to ensure requirements continue to serve the ACGME Mission with updated context and priorities. The first major revision to the Common Program Requirements, which went into effect in 2016, occurred in two phases—the first involving only Section 6, and the second revising Sections 1–5. Along with wording and formatting changes, this major revision created new standards around well-being, quality and safety, mistreatment, diverse recruitment and retention, program leadership time, faculty development and scholarly activity, and board pass rate. The minor revisions have also gradually adapted the Common Program Requirements around duty hours, resident eligibility criteria, clinical competency committees, and dedicated program leadership time. The Common Program Requirements also underwent a minor revision in 2023 that sought only to reduce redundancy and overall requirement counts. At the time of this textbook's publication, the Common Program Requirements are set to undergo a multi-year major revision process beginning in the spring of 2025.

Taken together, these Common Program Requirements facilitate uniformity in the standard of graduate medical education training throughout the United States while allowing flexibility for innovation and meeting the needs of the local patient populations.

Types of Requirements

The Common Program Requirements are delineated into core, detail, and outcome statements that contribute further to defining areas of required uniformity, innovation, and measurable standards. Throughout the ACGME requirements, these delineations are made known through parenthetical notation at the end of each statement.

Core Requirements

The core requirements are meant to define structures, resources, and/or process elements that are essential to every graduate medical education program. Compliance with core requirements must be demonstrated at the time of initial application and maintained throughout the duration of a program's ACGME accreditation. Some examples of core requirements within the Common Program Requirements include the following:

1. Structure example: "The program must be sponsored by one ACGME-accredited Sponsoring Institution."
2. Resource example: "The program, in partnership with its Sponsoring Institution, must ensure the availability of adequate resources for resident education."
3. Process example: "Core faculty members must complete the annual ACGME Faculty Survey."

Detail Requirements

The detailed requirements convey specific structures, resources, or processes that could be utilized to achieve a core requirement. At the time of initial accreditation, a program must demonstrate compliance with all core and detail requirements. Once Continued Accreditation status has been achieved, programs can innovate on detailed requirements to create alternate structures, resources, and processes that ensure continued achievement of the core statement through different means. Examples of detailed requirements in the Common Program Requirements include the following:

Core requirements: "Faculty members must pursue faculty development designed to enhance their skills at least annually."

Detail requirements: "as educators and evaluators; in quality improvement, eliminating health inequities, and patient safety; in fostering their own and their residents' well-being; and, in patient care based on their practice-based learning and improvement efforts."

Outcome Requirements

The outcome requirements indicate requirements tied to a measurable or observable attribute of every graduate. As noted earlier, the Common Program Requirements guide programs in creating environments where trainees develop the "skills, knowledge, and attitudes necessary to take personal responsibility for the individual care of patients" [4] and the outcome requirements further delineate measurable ways in which this is occurring. Outcome requirements are typically tied to data reported in the Accreditation Data System (ADS) and annual program updates. Examples of Common Program Requirement outcome requirements include the following:

> The program must demonstrate dissemination of scholarly activity within and external to the program by the following methods: faculty participation in grand rounds, posters, workshops, quality improvement presentations, podium presentations, grant leadership, non-peer-reviewed print/electronic resources, articles or publications, book chapters, textbooks, webinars, service on professional committees, or serving as a journal reviewer, journal editorial board member, or editor; peer-reviewed publication. [4]
>
> Programs must ensure that residents are competent in communicating with team members in the hand-off process. [4]

Specialty-Specific Requirements for Pediatric Residency Programs

The Common Program Requirements serve as a foundational template upon which every specialty further specifies standards unique to its trainees. In this way, the ACGME Program Requirements for Graduate Medical Education in Pediatrics represents the universal standards for training pediatric residents under ACGME accreditation. Throughout the document, the plain text (unbolded) statements are specialty-specific expansions to the (bolded) Common Program Requirements. As with statements in the Common Program Requirements, the specialty-specific statements are also delineated into core, detail, and outcome requirements.

Importantly, specialty-specific requirements can add additional requirements to the Common Program Requirements but cannot grant a specialty exemption from existing Common Program Requirements. As an example, the Pediatric specialty-specific language around in-house night float adds that "Night experiences should be of educational value." [5]. That said, specialty-specific language could not undo the existing language stating that "night float must occur within the context of the 80-hour and one-day-off-in-seven requirements."

The Pediatric specialty-specific language primarily expands on the Common Program Requirements through definition of the specialty and ideal Pediatrician, length of training, necessary resources such as patient volumes and program director/coordinator/core faculty dedicated education time and qualifications, education unique to pediatrics, and the standardized training experiences required to attain said education [5].

Exploring ACGME Outcomes-Based Accreditation

From the early 1900s to the early 2000s, the Flexner Report and publications from the National Academy of Medicine (among others) raised concerns regarding the unequal standards of medical education training, with resulting quality and safety impacts for patient care [6]. As a result, the ACGME launched the Outcome Project in 2001, which led to the creation of the six clinical competencies that are integrated into the Common Program Requirements. The ACGME has since also gradually developed specialty-specific Milestones and Entrustable Professional Activities (EPAs) as checkpoints and achievable tasks/responsibilities, respectively, that could be used to measure a trainee's progression towards competence in the six competencies. Various boards have started to explore the use of these progression frameworks as ways to determine eligibility for testing and ultimately independent practice, with the American Board of Surgery being the first to require the use of EPAs for this purpose.

In Pediatrics, both Milestones and EPAs have been developed through collaborative work between professional associations, patients/caregivers, and other stakeholders in pediatric care. The 2025 revision of the ACGME Program Requirements for Graduate Medical Education in Pediatrics integrates the language of all pediatric Milestones and EPAs into the requirements, thereby standardizing the use of measurable outcomes-based requirements for pediatric training. As the medical education community continues to explore progression towards competency-based medical education as opposed to process-based models (e.g., time- and experience-fixed), this intentional inclusion sets the stage for pediatric education to be individualized for each learner's development of competence for independent practice [6, 7].

Preparing for Accreditation Site Visits

Timeline for Accreditation Cycle

Preparing for an accreditation site visit begins with understanding the timeline of the accreditation cycle and the types of site visits. It involves several stages, beginning with submission of a program application and ending with site visits and reviews. There are several types of site visits: new application site visit, new program site visit at the end of the Initial Accreditation period, existing program site visit prompted by review of annual data or randomized selection, and site visit for programs on probation.[8] Programs that are found not to be in significant compliance with the requirements based on Review Committee review of ACGME Accreditation Data System (ADS), including resident and faculty survey results, or complaints submitted to the ACGME, may have a site visit in order to better clarify the training environment. This site visit is necessary in order for the Review Committee to render an annual accreditation decision.

The preparation needed will depend on the type of site visit the program is undergoing. In general, key preparation milestones include the following: initial planning meetings, development and submission of required documents, periodic internal reviews, and pre-site visit stakeholder meetings. Regardless of the type of visit, the program will receive notification from ACGME prior to the site visit. This notification will include the format, in person or remote, and a request for dates to avoid the scheduling of the visit (blackout dates). The program will receive advanced notice of the date of the site visit. This will generally occur approximately 30 days prior to the visit, but may be less if required to meet the Review Committee's deadline or for other extenuating circumstances. In general, establishing a detailed timeline for the site visit type will ensure that all necessary preparations are completed on schedule, allowing for time to address any potential issues that may arise. Adherence to the timeline is crucial to ensuring a smooth and successful accreditation process.

The timeline for preparing for an initial site visit begins long before the program receives the 30-day notice of the site visit date. The Sponsoring Institution wishing to obtain ACGME accreditation for a program must prepare and submit a program application [9]. This process typically takes 6–12 months to gather the necessary information and complete the program application. After the submission of the application, it may take 4–12 months for the Review Committee to make an accreditation decision. It is important to be aware of the Review Committee's agenda closing and meeting dates when you are considering submitting an application for accreditation. These dates are published on the specialty section of the ACGME website, but you may contact the Review Committee Staff members to confirm when an application for accreditation would need to be submitted.

Documentation and Data Collection

Documentation and data collection are crucial components of the accreditation process. Programs must gather and maintain comprehensive records of educational outcomes, academic records, faculty qualifications, resident evaluations, and annual program evaluations, and any other documents needed to complete the application for accreditation or to maintain an updated and accurate ACGME Accreditation Data System (ADS), which serves as a central repository for all accreditation-related data. Reviewing the program requirements and collecting the necessary policies and documents needed to show compliance with each requirement can be a guide for deciding if any additional documents and data need to be collected. Accurate and up-to-date documentation is essential for demonstrating compliance with ACGME requirements and facilitating a smooth site visit and accreditation process.

Further information about documentation and preparation for site visits can be found on the ACGME website under site visits [8].

Strategies for Organizing Site Visit Logistics

Organizing the logistics for an accreditation site visit involves meticulous planning and coordination. Key strategies include establishing a dedicated site visit committee, creating detailed schedules, and ensuring that all logistical arrangements are in place. This includes preparing meeting spaces and arranging for technology and materials needed during the visit. Clear communication with all stakeholders is vital to ensure that everyone is aware of their roles and responsibilities. Providing comprehensive briefings and training for faculty, residents, and program coordinators can help them prepare for their interactions with the site visit team. It is critical that stakeholders are aware of how the program meets the program requirements and are familiar with the policies and procedures of the program. Having multiple stakeholders review and edit all documents to be submitted ensures that documents are free of errors and clearly reflect how the program meets requirements. Additionally, conducting mock site visits or rehearsals can help identify and address any potential issues in advance, ensuring a smooth and successful visit.

Developing a Self-Study Report

Developing a self-study report is essential (or can be helpful) to preparing for an ACGME site visit for programs with Continued Accreditation status [10]. The self-study is the program's guide to continuous improvement but is not reviewed during the site visit. This document provides an in-depth evaluation of the program, highlighting its strengths, identifying areas for improvement, and outlining plans for addressing areas of deficiency. The self-study process involves collecting feedback from faculty, residents, and other stakeholders, and analyzing program performance data. The report should be accurate, thorough, and reflective of the program's commitment to continuous improvement [10].

Addressing Common Challenges in Accreditation

Information gathered during the annual ACGME Resident/Fellow and Faculty Surveys, annual program summary information submitted through ADS, and data collected at site visits are used by the RC to make annual accreditation decisions for each program.

Prior to the ACGME Program Requirements for Graduate Medical Education in Pediatrics that went into effect July 2025, the program requirements that resulted in the most frequent citations in pediatric programs were as follows. (This information can be found on the ACGME.org website. Each year, there is an annual summary for each specialty. The language about each of these areas comes from the ACGME Program Requirements for Graduate Medical Education in Pediatrics and is either specialty-specific or common program requirement language.) [11].

Faculty Qualifications

All faculty members, including the program director, must be certified in pediatrics and meet the requirements for either Maintenance of Certification in pediatrics or a subspecialty of pediatrics through the ABP or Osteopathic Continuous Certification through the AOBP or possess qualifications judged acceptable to the Review Committee. For categorical programs, there must be ABP- or AOBP-certified subspecialty physician faculty available to teach and supervise pediatrics residents, including subspecialty faculty in adolescent medicine, developmental-behavioral pediatrics, neonatal-perinatal medicine, pediatric critical care medicine, pediatric emergency medicine and in each available subspecialty rotation or they must possess qualifications judged acceptable to the Review Committee. Faculty members who recently graduated from an ACGME-accredited or AOA-approved pediatrics program must take and pass the next available ABP or AOBP pediatrics certifying examination. An explanation is to be provided for any faculty member unable to take the next administration of the certifying examination.

Culture of Professional Responsibilities

The curriculum must be structured to optimize resident educational experiences, the length of the experiences, and the supervisory continuity. These educational experiences include an appropriate blend of supervised patient care responsibilities, clinical teaching, and didactic educational events. Assignment of rotations must be structured to minimize the frequency of rotational transitions, and rotations must be of sufficient length to provide a quality educational experience, defined by continuity of patient care, ongoing supervision, longitudinal relationships with faculty members, and meaningful assessment and feedback.

Clinical experiences should be structured to facilitate learning in a manner that allows residents to function as part of an effective interprofessional team that works together longitudinally with shared goals of patient safety and quality improvement. Frequent rotational transitions, inadequate continuity of faculty member supervision, and dispersed patient locations within the hospital have adversely affected optimal resident education and effective team-based care.

The learning objectives of the program must be accomplished without excessive reliance on residents to fulfill non-physician service obligations. Routine reliance on residents to fulfill non-physician obligations increases work compression for residents and does not provide an optimal educational experience. Nonphysician obligations are duties that are mostly performed by nursing and allied health professionals, transport services, or clerical staff. Examples of such obligations include transport of patients from the wards or units for procedures elsewhere in the hospital; routine blood drawing for laboratory tests; routine monitoring of patients when off the ward; and clerical duties, such as scheduling. While it is understood that residents may be expected to do any of these things on occasion when the need arises, these activities should not be performed by residents routinely and must be kept to a minimum to optimize resident education.

Evaluations

Timely faculty feedback may be found to be infrequent or not formative. Feedback is ongoing information provided regarding aspects of one's performance, knowledge, or understanding. The faculty empowers residents to provide much of that feedback themselves in a spirit of continuous learning and self-reflection. Feedback from faculty members in the context of routine clinical care should be frequent and need not always be formally documented.

However, trainees must also receive timely end-of-rotation evaluations. Evaluation must be documented at the completion of the assignment. For block rotations of greater than three months in duration, evaluation must be documented at least every three months. Longitudinal experiences, such as continuity clinic in the context of other clinical responsibilities, must be evaluated at least every three months and at completion.

At least annually, there must be a summative evaluation of each resident that includes their readiness to progress to the next year of the program. The required language of readiness to progress to the next year must be included in the summative evaluation. At the end of training, there must be an attestation that the resident has demonstrated the knowledge, skills, and behaviors necessary to enter autonomous practice.

Responsibilities of the Faculty

Faculty members must be role models of professionalism. Residents report unprofessional behavior such as favoritism, verbal abuse, racism, and sexism by faculty.

Faculty members must demonstrate a strong interest in the education of residents, including devoting sufficient time to the educational program to fulfill their supervisory and teaching responsibilities. Trainees are dependent on the tone and motivation of the faculty members in order to grow in the specialty. Faculty who have an inordinate amount of clinical and/or research responsibility may not provide adequate observation, feedback, and modeling for trainees.

Curricular Development

There must be a longitudinal general pediatric outpatient experience in a setting that provides a medical home for the spectrum of pediatric patients, allowing residents to develop a continuous, long-term therapeutic relationship with a panel of pediatric patients which is in addition to the other required 40 weeks of ambulatory experiences. There may be challenges in assuring that there is a group of patients that identify the resident as their doctor. There must be a longitudinal working experience between each resident and a single or core group of faculty members with expertise in primary care pediatrics and the principles of the medical home.

Quality Improvement and Accreditation Strategies for Program Enhancement

Maintaining accreditation and program excellence is a dynamic and ongoing process that can be addressed strategically using quality improvement methodology to enhance the program. Programs must continuously assess and refine their educational practices to maintain accreditation and to provide quality training for residents.

Implementing Program Quality Improvement Projects Using Faculty and Resident Survey

Achieving effective quality improvement (QI) in graduate medical education (GME) relies on the active participation of both faculty and residents. Faculty and resident surveys can play a crucial role in identifying areas for improvement and gauging the effectiveness of current strategies and practices. By leveraging survey data, programs can implement targeted QI projects to address specific weaknesses and enhance overall educational outcomes. The mandatory annual ACGME Resident/Fellow and Faculty Surveys are critical to providing feedback on program compliance and performance. In addition to using the ACGME survey data to identify areas of improvement, programs can also utilize information from internal anonymous program evaluations, resident town halls, which may be led by either chief residents or non-pediatric GME faculty, which may yield additional data to assist in addressing areas of concern. Utilization of these tools helps identify trends and areas needing intervention, thereby guiding the development of QI initiatives. Engaging faculty and residents in the QI process through regular feedback sessions ensures that projects align with educational goals and clinical needs [12, 13].

Demonstrating Continuous Improvement in Program Outcomes

Continuous improvement in program outcomes is essential for maintaining high standards in GME. Programs should adopt a systematic approach to monitor and enhance performance, using metrics derived from resident performance, faculty evaluations, and patient care outcomes. The ACGME emphasizes the use of the Milestones as a framework for assessing resident progress across various competencies, which facilitates ongoing program evaluation and adjustment. By regularly reviewing these metrics and implementing iterative improvements through Plan-Do-Study-Act (PDSA) cycles, programs can demonstrate a commitment to excellence and adaptability [13]. Successful QI projects often culminate in presentations at institutional meetings or academic conferences, highlighting the program's achievements and fostering a culture of continuous improvement.

Utilizing Feedback mechanisms for Program Enhancement

Feedback mechanisms are pivotal in the continuous enhancement of GME programs. Regular and structured feedback from residents and faculty provides actionable insights into the strengths and weaknesses of the educational environment. Implementing changes based on this feedback can significantly improve program quality. For instance, Resident/Fellow and Faculty Surveys administered by the ACGME are designed to capture comprehensive feedback on various aspects of the program, from clinical experience to educational support. Programs that actively use this feedback to make data-driven decisions often see marked improvements in resident satisfaction and educational outcomes [14]. Additionally, celebrating successes and making QI efforts visible, such as through QI symposiums and grand rounds, can reinforce the importance of feedback in driving program enhancement [12].

Utilizing Accreditation feedback for Program Improvement

Accreditation feedback provides a critical external perspective on program performance. The ACGME's Site Visit Reports and accreditation decisions often include specific recommendations for improvement, which programs can use to refine their practices. By systematically addressing these recommendations, programs can not only correct deficiencies but also proactively enhance areas of strength. Engaging with accreditation feedback involves a thorough review of site visit reports, prioritizing actions based on the urgency and impact of the feedback and involving stakeholders in the implementation process. Continuous monitoring and reassessment ensure that the changes are effective and sustainable.

Addressing areas of concern identified during accreditation requires a strategic and proactive approach. Programs should develop action plans that outline specific steps to rectify identified issues, assign responsibilities, and set timelines for completion. This process involves detailed analysis of the accreditation report, stakeholder engagement, and regular progress reviews. Effective communication with the accrediting body during this phase can also provide clarity and ensure that corrective actions meet the required standards. By systematically addressing these concerns, programs can mitigate risks of future non-compliance and demonstrate their commitment to continuous improvement and educational excellence.

Long-Term Planning for Sustaining Accreditation Excellence

Long-term planning is crucial for sustaining accreditation excellence in GME programs. This involves developing a comprehensive strategy that aligns with the program's mission and goals, ensuring ongoing compliance with accreditation standards, and fostering a culture of continuous improvement. Programs should establish robust monitoring systems to track key performance indicators, engage in regular self-assessment, and remain adaptable to changes in accreditation requirements. Investing in faculty development, enhancing resident training, and integrating innovative educational practices are also vital components of long-term planning. By maintaining a forward-thinking approach and leveraging feedback mechanisms, programs can achieve and sustain high standards of educational quality and accreditation success.

By utilizing these strategies, GME programs can not only meet accreditation requirements but also significantly enhance their educational quality and outcomes.

Leveraging Available Resources to Assist with the Accreditation Process

ACGME Resources

The ACGME provides a wide array of resources on its website [15].

The vast majority of requirements in pediatric training are actually Common Program Requirements which apply across specialties. The ACGME has robust resources for both residency and fellowship training that are helpful for not only program directors but also coordinators, chief residents, faculty, and trainees [16].

The block diagram is reviewed by the Review Committee and can be extremely helpful to clarify the resident experience in your program. There is a wide variability in the way that programs present information and at times may not clarify all of the questions that the Review Committee has about the educational program. For that reason, there are guidelines available on the ACGME website to assist in presenting your schedule in a way that will facilitate review by the Review Committee. These can be found under The Guide to Construction of a Block Diagram tab [17, 18].

Each year, the ACGME presents an Annual Educational Conference. Highlights of this conference include a Full-Day Course designed for program directors and coordinators to experience the ACGME processes that affect accreditation of their program, annual specialty updates for each specialty, breakout sessions to assist program directors, program coordinators, chief residents, and trainees to understand and discuss requirements and approaches to compliance in their respective programs. There is ample opportunity for questions and also networking across your specialty and with ACGME personnel [19].

Learn at ACGME is an additional resource available through the ACGME [20]. There you will find online modules to enhance your expertise in accreditation, faculty development, and well-being, among other areas. These resources are organized by the roles in GME: coordinator,

DIO, faculty, program director, residents, and fellows. There is additional information about Trending Topics and ACGME initiatives, such as *Back to Bedside*, the Milestones, and Well-Being. There are also resources about faculty development, events and conferences, and continuing education. A free account is required to access the majority of the content housed in the platform.

Other Resources

Each sponsoring institution is supported by a graduate education committee (GMEC), which is responsible for assuring institutional compliance with ACGME Institutional Requirements. A copy of these institutional requirements can be found on the ACGME website [21]. This committee is responsible not only for the institutional requirements but also for ensuring that all training programs are in compliance with their requirements. The GMEC at your sponsoring institution can provide structure and feedback about ADS Annual Updates, new applications, annual Resident/Fellow and Faculty Survey results, and work hour logging and compliance. The designated institutional official (DIO) is the individual responsible for GMEC oversight at each Sponsoring Institution. The DIO approves program letters of agreement (PLAs), oversees submissions of the Annual Update for each program and the Sponsoring Institution to the ACGME; and, oversees the submission of applications for ACGME accreditation and recognition, requests for Voluntary Withdrawal of Accreditation or Recognition, and requests for changes in residency and fellowship program complements.

The Association of Pediatric Program Directors (APPD) [22] is a national organization whose mission is to ensure the health and well-being of all children by leading the advancement of pediatric medical education, the development of a sustainable and diverse workforce, the cultivation of an inclusive learning environment, and the promotion of educational innovation. The APPD is an invaluable source of information and support for program directors. The organization sponsors in-person meetings, educational collaboration, leadership training, special interest groups, educational curricula, and professional development for program directors, faculty, coordinators, and chief residents. In addition to established programming, the APPD brings together program directors with various levels of experience.

Conclusion

Accreditation of pediatric residency programs is a critical process that ensures uniform, high-quality medical education and trainee experience. Successful program accreditation depends on program leaders and is supported by institutions, professional organizations, and the ACGME, which offer invaluable guiding resources. Program commitment to continuous improvement, innovation, and excellence in residency training programs is crucial to maintaining accreditation of pediatric residency programs. The accreditation process ensures quality training and that future pediatricians are ready to deliver exceptional care to patients and families.

References

1. https://www.acgme.org/about/overview/mission-vision-and-values/
2. https://www.acgme.org/about/committees-and-members-selection-process/
3. https://www.acgme.org/globalassets/ab_acgmepoliciesprocedures.pdf
4. https://www.acgme.org/programs-and-institutions/programs/common-program-requirements/
5. https://www.acgme.org/specialties/pediatrics/program-requirements-and-faqs-and-applications/
6. https://meridian.allenpress.com/jgme/article/15/5/617/496160
7. https://www.acgme.org/milestones/resources
8. Site Visit (acgme.org)
9. Program Application Information (acgme.org)
10. https://www.acgme.org/programs-and-institutions/programs/self-study/
11. https://www.acgme.org/globalassets/pfassets/presentations/2025-specialty-updates/pediatrics-update-2025.pdf

12. BMC Medical Education. Engaging faculty and residents in quality improvement projects. 2023. Available from: BMC Medical Education.
13. American College of Surgeons (ACS). Six steps to engage residents in quality improvement education. 2023. Available from: American College of Surgeons.
14. Resident/Fellow and Faculty Surveys (acgme.org) www.acgme.org/data-systems-technical-suppport/resident-fellow-and-faculty-surveys
15. ACGME website: acgme.org
16. https://www.acgme.org/education-and-resources/program-directors-guide-to-the-common-program-requirements/
17. https://www.acgme.org/globalassets/PDFs/Guide_to_the_Construction_of_the_Block_Diagram_3.30.17.pdf
18. https://www.acgme.org/globalassets/pfassets/programresources/blockdiagraminstructions_pediatrics.pdf
19. www.acgme.org/newsroom/cat/annual-educational-conference
20. https://dl.acgme.org/
21. https://www.acgme.org/globalassets/pfassets/programrequirements/800_institutionalrequirements2022.pdf
22. www.appd.org

Learner Certification Through the American Board of Pediatrics

5

Suzanne K. Woods

Background

Accrediting and certifying bodies work together to uphold the integrity of pediatric graduate medical education and practice. Accreditation of pediatric residency programs is conducted by the Accreditation Council for Graduate Medical Education (ACGME). The ABP certifies individual physicians for the practice of general pediatrics through an initial certification examination after residency training and, thereafter, through maintenance of the certification process throughout the lifetime of one's practice [1]. Program directors serve a vital role in training oversight, educational planning, and final attestation of residents' readiness to independently practice pediatrics.

Residency training must meet national standards of competence across six core domains: patient care and procedural skills, medical knowledge, practice-based learning and improvement, interpersonal and communication skills, professionalism, and systems-based practice. These competencies serve as the foundation for both accreditation and certification decisions. The program director must ensure that each resident demonstrates proficiency in these areas before completing training, as the submission of an evaluation will be used for board eligibility.

Training Pathways

Certification eligibility may be achieved through multiple training pathways [2]:

- The standard three-year pediatric residency in an ACGME-accredited program
- Combined training programs integrating pediatrics with another specialty
- Structured research pathways that support physician-scientists
- Sequential training programs that combine pediatrics with a second specialty
- Shortened pathways for specialties, including child neurology and neurodevelopmental disabilities

Each pathway has specific curricular requirements and timeframes. Generally, residents must complete a minimum of 36 months of pediatric training unless otherwise specified by combined or research program requirements. Time away from training due to leave is limited and must be accounted for in the final verification of training.

Combined residency programs allow for an integrated approach to board eligibility in two disciplines, such as Medicine-Pediatrics or Pediatrics-Medical Genetics. These programs

S. K. Woods (✉)
American Board of Pediatrics, Chapel Hill, NC, USA
e-mail: SWoods@abpeds.org

H. McPhillips et al. (eds.), *Graduate Medical Education in Pediatrics*, Excellence in Medical Education 3, https://doi.org/10.1007/978-3-032-12952-9_5

must be approved by the ACGME effective July 2025. Research pathways offer additional time for research during residency and require early identification and careful monitoring of clinical competence.

The training program must ensure residents complete 12 months of training at each level, meet curricular expectations, and demonstrate progressive responsibility. Any deviation due to extended leave or remediation must be documented and addressed. Out of the 36 months, four weeks annually is allowed for time out of training due to vacation, medical leave, parental leave, or caregiver leave. The ABP has a detailed policy on absences from training for further information [3].

Prerequisites for Certification

The ABP publishes the prerequisites for initial certification, and the updated guide is available each year before the general pediatrics application period opens in January. The ABP offers certification in general pediatrics, 15 core pediatric subspecialties, and cosponsors certificates in five other disciplines.

To be eligible for initial certification, candidates must:

- Graduate from an accredited medical school
- Hold a valid, unrestricted license to practice medicine in the United States or Canada
- Successfully complete a full pediatric residency in an accredited program
- Receive confirmation from their program director that all required competencies have been met

Applicants must successfully complete three years of general pediatric training, or the training required in other available pathways for graduates to take the general pediatrics initial certifying exam. All pediatric training must take place in programs accredited by the ACGME or in programs in Canada accredited by the Royal College of Physicians and Surgeons of Canada (RCPSC) [4].

The ABP recognizes and defines the three levels of general pediatrics residency (R-1 through R-3) as follows:

1. R-1: The first postgraduate year in general comprehensive pediatric training in an accredited program.
2. R-2: The second postgraduate year, following R-1, in general comprehensive pediatric training in an accredited program, but with increased responsibility for patient care and the supervision of junior house staff and medical students.
3. R-3: The third postgraduate year, following R-2, in general comprehensive pediatric training in an accredited program, but with increasing responsibility for patient care and supervision of junior house staff and medical students.

Effective January 2025, applicants who trained in a Canadian program accredited by the RCPSC must have successfully completed the whole duration of training in the program to meet the training requirements to take the General Pediatrics Certifying Exam.

Training curricula must align with ACGME program requirements [5]. Trainees are expected to assume progressive responsibility for the care of patients and satisfactorily complete at least 12 months at each training level. Trainees are expected to participate fully in inpatient and outpatient care and demonstrate increasing independence and supervisory experience over the course of training. Certification examination eligibility is contingent on completion of all training prior to the exam month. The ABP requires program directors to verify satisfactory completion of training and to evaluate the acceptability of applicants as a practitioner of pediatrics.

Training completed in ACGME International (ACGME-I) programs does not count as credit toward ABP certification.

Program Director Responsibilities

Program directors (PD) are responsible for overseeing training and verifying competence. This includes regular assessment and documentation of resident performance across all competency domains. Both PDs and faculty play critical roles in the certification process, serving as key decision-makers in determining which applicants are ready for the certifying exam. Assessments should rely on direct observation, multisource evaluations, and clinical performance data. Clinical Competency Committees contribute to milestone evaluations, progression decisions, and entrustment decisions.

PDs are required to annually assess and report whether each resident's or fellow's performance is satisfactory, marginal, or unsatisfactory in overall clinical competence, and whether their professionalism meets the required standards. The PD's role in certification should be taken very seriously because, other than the possession of a valid and unrestricted state medical license, the program director's verification is the only way that the ABP can judge the applicant's qualification to take the certifying examination. By verifying the applicant's qualification as a candidate for the certifying examination, the PD confirms that the applicant has successfully completed a training curriculum compliant with the requirements for accredited training.

The evaluation process calls for multiple methods of assessment. The basis of these assessments should be grounded in direct observation of the residents in a variety of settings, which can include simulation or telemedicine, performing a variety of patient care tasks, including demonstration of evidence to support procedural competence. There are many resources available on which to rely for principles of assessment, as well as tools to carry out the necessary observations. The ABP has guides for program directors, which include Assessment in Graduate Medical Education: A Primer for Pediatric Program Directors and Teaching, Promoting, and Assessing Professionalism Across the Curriculum: A Medical Educator's Guide, and the Professionalism Guide available on its website [6]. In addition, the Association of Pediatric Program Directors (APPD), ACGME, and Academic Pediatric Association (APA) have resources as well.

The ABP embraces Competency-Based Medical Education (CBME) and will require reporting of data on Entrustable Professional Activities (EPAs) prior to being eligible to meet the training requirements for the ABP certifying examinations beginning in 2028. This information will be communicated to programs in advance.

The ABP Program Portal is used for the submission of roster information for all trainees, including demographic information and training dates for each academic year. The ability to track trainees and submit assessments online has streamlined the completion of required documentation for programs and enhanced the timely submission of information to the ABP. The communication feature allows for two-way exchange of information between programs and ABP staff. It is essential that program directors and coordinators are well-versed in the features and use of the Program Portal. The ABP has created guides and videos to assist programs with the system [6].

Trainee Responsibilities

Residents are expected to take ownership of their education and develop lifelong learning habits. Active engagement in self-assessment, feedback processes, and individualized learning plans is essential to success in training and future certification maintenance.

Certification Assessments

Initial certification examinations and in-training examinations (ITE) are based on standardized content outlines developed by subject matter experts. Exams assess core pediatric knowledge and clinical reasoning through multiple-choice questions that reflect real-world scenarios. In-training exams help identify learning needs and benchmark resident progress; however, they are not used for fellowship application decisions.

Passing the initial certification exam requires meeting a defined passing standard, which is set and maintained across exam versions using statistical methods. Results are reported on a scaled score to ensure fairness.

General Pediatrics In-Training Examination

The ITE is a three-hour exam consisting of approximately 150 multiple-choice questions and is administered on designated days in July [7]. The purpose of the ITE is:

1. To enable residents to assess strengths and gaps in general pediatric knowledge at the time of the exam
2. To assess progress from year to year
3. To compare performance with national peer groups

In addition, PDs can use ITE results to provide counseling and remediation to residents and in the creation of specific goals in an Individualized Learning Plan (ILP). They can also gather and analyze results over multiple years to assess the overall quality of training their program has delivered.

Because the ITE is designed as an abbreviated version of a certifying exam and is based on the same content outline, it allows residents to familiarize themselves with ABP exams and, to some extent, predict their performance on a subsequent certifying exam. Program directors should not use the ITE as the sole means of determining if a resident has satisfactorily completed a year of training. Also, the ABP strongly discourages program directors and residents from providing ITE test results as part of the fellowship application process. Using the exam for purposes other than self-assessment (either individual or program) constitutes a misuse of the scores and compromises the validity and meaningfulness of the results. It is recommended that program directors explain this philosophy and the proposed use of ITE results to residents who will take the ITE.

General Pediatrics Initial Certification Examination

General pediatric initial certifying exams come in several versions, but a strict scoring process maintains a uniform passing standard that all candidates are held to. After the exam is administered, statistical analyses are performed, and a few questions may be removed if they do not meet the standards for statistical and psychometric validity. These deleted questions are not included in the final score calculation. Once invalid questions are removed, the total score is calculated based on the number of correct answers. Incorrect answers do not result in point deductions, and all questions are weighted equally.

Although the total score reflects the number of correct answers, results are reported on a 1–300 scale, with 180 as the passing mark. This conversion accounts for the fact that different versions of the exam may vary slightly in difficulty due to differing questions. To ensure fairness, a statistical process known as equating is applied to hold all candidates to the same passing standard. Thus, a score of 180 represents the minimum level of knowledge required to pass and does not directly correlate with the percentage of questions answered correctly [8].

Time-Limited Eligibility

The ABP requires that applicants complete their training for initial certification in general pediatrics within the preceding seven years (e.g., for exams in 2025, training must have been completed in 2018 or later). The Time-Limited Eligibility Policy states that if the required training was not completed within the previous seven years, the applicant must undergo at least six months of supervised practice in an accredited training program or observation in a preceptor pathway to establish a second period of time-limited eligibility for general pediatrics. This requirement allows the ABP to collect a current assessment of the individual's competence to practice pediatrics unsupervised [9].

Maintenance of Certification

After initial certification, pediatricians enter a maintenance of certification process, which includes the following:

- Lifelong learning and self-assessment.
- Engagement in quality improvement activities.
- Regular assessments of knowledge and practice.
- Trainees may begin participating in maintenance activities during residency and apply earned credit toward future certification cycles.

Conclusion

Certification ensures that pediatricians meet high standards of knowledge, skill, and professionalism. Training programs, faculty, and program directors play essential roles in preparing residents for certification and lifelong practice. Ongoing collaboration and adherence to national standards support the development of competent, compassionate, and accountable pediatricians.

References

1. ABP – About Us. https://www.abp.org/content/about-us. Accessed 16 Sept 2025.
2. ABP – Non-Standard Pathways and Combined Programs. https://www.abp.org/content/non-standard-pathways-and-combined-programs. Accessed 23 Oct 2025.
3. ABP – Absences from Training. https://www.abp.org/content/absences-general-pediatrics-training. Accessed 19 Sept 2025.
4. ABP – General Pediatrics-Admission Requirements. https://www.abp.org/become-certified/general-pediatrics/admission-requirements. Accessed 16 Sept 2025.
5. ACGME – Program Requirements. https://www.acgme.org/specialties/pediatrics/program-requirements-and-faqs-and-applications/. Accessed 19 Sept 2025.
6. ABP – Program Directors. https://www.abp.org/content/program-directors. Accessed 16 Sept 2025.
7. ABP – General Pediatrics In-Training Examination. https://www.abp.org/content/general-pediatrics-training-examination. Accessed 23 Oct 2025.
8. ABP – Scoring. https://www.abp.org/content/scoring. Accessed 23 Oct 2025.
9. ABP – Time-Limited Eligibility for General Pediatrics. https://www.abp.org/content/scoring. Accessed 23 Oct 2025.

Part II

Program Design and Development

Starting a New Program

6

Amber M. Hoffman and Heather A. Fagan

Establishing a New Accreditation Council for Graduate Medical Education (ACGME) Sponsoring Institution (SI) and Pediatric Residency Program Versus Initiation of a Pediatric Residency Program with an Established SI

One of the first imperatives is whether the pediatric residency program will be sponsored by a new ACGME Sponsoring Institution (SI) or if it will join a pre-existing ACGME SI. Creating a new SI and Graduate Medical Education (GME) infrastructure to sponsor the new pediatric residency program, and subsequently other residency and fellowship programs as applicable, requires a different starting point, enhanced institutional resource allocation, and an extended time frame for program accreditation. Although work in both areas can occur simultaneously, the successful accreditation of the new ACGME SI is foundational and necessary prior to a residency program application. Accreditation of a new SI requires a skilled visionary to assist hospital administrators and/or a medical school dean to understand the requirements from an infrastructure perspective, including recruitment of physician faculty, engagement of GME administrative team members, and formalized GME processes and procedures. There is a demand for significant resource allocation, a requirement for space and technology, as well as the potential requirement for new collaborations with other clinical sites or health care systems to ensure adequate clinical exposure and faculty expertise to qualify as an ACGME-accredited SI. This vision is one that requires a growth mindset of all staff members, including physicians and allied health professionals. An institutional transition from one focused solely on clinical care to one that will support the educational development of learners may not be embraced by those experiencing changes in care delivery. Educational initiatives that clearly explain the benefits and rationale behind launching a teaching program—as well as ongoing education before and after trainees arrive—are essential. A leader who can effectively communicate the significant upfront costs and resource investments, while also emphasizing the long-term institutional benefits in terms of reputation, clinical excellence, quality and safety infrastructure, and faculty recruitment, is paramount. At a

A. M. Hoffman (✉)
University of Pittsburgh School of Medicine, Pittsburgh, PA, USA
e-mail: hoffmana13@upmc.edu

H. A. Fagan
Nemours Children's Hospital Florida (NCHFL) in Orlando, Orlando, FL, USA

H. McPhillips et al. (eds.), *Graduate Medical Education in Pediatrics*, Excellence in Medical Education 3, https://doi.org/10.1007/978-3-032-12952-9_6

minimum, this will require a 10-year investment of resources, infrastructure and faculty time to see the fruits of the labor recognized in the form of successful program accreditations, state and federal funding streams and ultimately with the graduation of residents and fellows that will change the landscape of the local healthcare arena and environment of care.

Joining an already established GME infrastructure and accredited SI ensures that there is a foundational framework, GME policies and procedures, and a known appreciation of the many requirements for an accredited ACGME residency program. The burden of a completely novel GME build is lessened with leaders, including a DIO, GME infrastructure, and resource allocation that is familiar and anticipated. This framework allows for more rapid implementation and program accreditation. However, the degree of innovation, visionary strategic leadership, and tangible institutional impact may be muted in a system that has predefined educational culture, process, and expectations for GME.

Mission Alignment with the Sponsoring Institution, C-Suite or Medical School, and Department of Pediatrics (If Applicable) for Resource Allocation and Philanthropy

It is highly recommended that the new residency program be aligned with the mission and vision of the sponsoring institution. This allows for more collaboration between the residency program and current/future projects of the SI, as well as having singular messaging regarding the residency program. For example, a community-based hospital with strong relationships with rural primary care providers would be an ideal SI for faculty and trainees interested in rural primary care. Mission alignment also allows for both the SI and the residency program to collaborate more effectively with philanthropy, the medical school or executive leadership at the hospital, and the Department of Pediatrics, if applicable, for resource allocation.

Capacity Building (SI Without Previous Resident Educational Opportunities)

Although capacity building (cap building) is discussed in another chapter, it is imperative that a new SI be on high alert during the building of the core residency program(s). Engagement of any resident or fellow trainee in the SI for educational rotations or experiences could significantly limit funding under current legislation, as the capacity-building funding mechanism is enacted on the first day any resident trainee enters the building for an educational experience. Many faculty and staff will be excited about the new residency program starting and may, inadvertently with this exuberance, welcome an alternate trainee into the institution for a rotation. This invited resident may trigger the capacity building phase, before the inaugural core program(s) welcome trainees, and therefore may prematurely end the capacity building phase intended by the SI. It is highly recommended that there be a strict approval process in place for any visiting resident/fellow to safeguard the new SI/GME department's long-term funding potential. This includes residents or fellows from pediatric and non-pediatric programs, i.e., surgery, anesthesia, radiology, neurology, emergency medicine, family practice, etc. If a trainee comes from a program that is currently in its capacity-building phase, or accredited after 1995, the new SI will potentially lose millions of dollars of educational funding with the premature closure of the capacity-building phase.

For example, if the visiting trainee is in a program that is 4.9 years into their 5 year capacity-building phase and they spend a month at the new SI for an educational experience, the new SI/GME program automatically defaults to having a start date for their capacity building aligned with the visiting trainee's program start and would only have 0.1 years' worth of capacity building time left to help fund future trainees at the institution rather than the full 5 years. However, there may be times when having the shortened capacity building may be beneficial and strategic. This could be the case if a collaboration with an alternate SI will result in an influx of multiple visiting residents, with full-time equivalents (FTE's) so significant to the capacity building that the shortened capacity-building window is desirable as the overall benefit outweighs the risk. A new pediatric residency program with 12 residents per year would achieve a complement of 36 residents over a 3-year period and additional capacity for any fellowships initiated during the 5 year window. However, this capacity could be substantially increased if the SI joined with a system that was 1 year into their 5-year capacity-building phase but had fifty trainees that needed 1–3 months of experience at the new institution for accreditation purposes. Although the capacity for the new program may close in four instead of 5 years, the number of trainees funded in the future would be significantly greater due to the influx of the visiting residents and fellows and their contribution to the overall full-time equivalent (FTE) of trainees at the institution for federal funding purposes.

Media Engagement

Starting a new pediatric program is an exciting opportunity to interact with the local media and simultaneously promote children's health. Intentional media engagement allows promotion of the program prior to matriculation of the first class, creating a sense of excitement and pride in the program launch. In addition, it may serve to attract future applicants interested in a new program where their impact is tangible. The mission and vision of the program can be shared prior to the inaugural day, and the media can then be engaged throughout many of the program's firsts; first match, first class, first day, first graduation, first fellowships, etc. As the residents embark on treating acutely ill children, creating new educational programs for their patients and community, volunteering, pursuing grants, and disseminating novel scholarship, the media can be welcomed back to hear their stories and share in the promotion of their scholarly work, highlighting both the institutional and community impact. Ultimately, there is recognition of the hospital or department's strategic focus and a lens on new and innovative programs in service to the community and scientific arena.

Considerations Regarding Size and Matriculation of Trainees to the Program

The optimal size of the new residency program depends on many factors, including institutional support and resources, patient volume, clinical acuity and complexity, and faculty expertise and scholarship. The accreditation application will require detailed information regarding each of these metrics. The ACGME requires a significant amount of deidentified patient data to demonstrate not only adequate volume but also depth and breadth of pathology and exposure for the trainees. For example, in the initial ACGME accreditation application, you will provide several lists of consecutive patients admitted to the hospital for the pediatric residency review committee to discern if the volume and diversity of the patient pathology will promote an adequate learning environment. If there are noted gaps in any of the required submission areas, they will require explanation in the submission paperwork, including a robust plan, that must be executed well in advance of the continued accreditation site visit after approximately 2 years of initial accreditation. The planning and implementation of any notable deficits will be mandatory to ensure that the specific patient experience will be supplemented or augmented.

Although filling most of the approved residency positions at the outset of the program accreditation may be lucrative from a capacity-building standpoint for a new sponsoring institution, there are important considerations to this approach. For any program director who has taken on a resident transfer during the postgraduate year (PGY) 2 or 3, they appreciate that each transfer can require a significant investment to ensure the resident transitions well, and has the opportunity to navigate any knowledge or performance deficits requiring attention before successful completion of the training program with appropriate competence to practice autonomously. Each upper-level resident who is requesting transfer has a unique circumstance or situation that will impact the receiving, and in this case, new, residency program. There may be an opportunity to capitalize on multiple senior residents needing placement if a program is closing, but that is not something that occurs frequently and is certainly not predictable. Although there may be highly qualified and outstanding resident physicians looking to change into a different program for personal reasons related to family, location, finances, or fit, there are others who quit or were dismissed from their former programs. Depending on the mission and vision of the new program, these displaced resident trainees may not benefit from a new program where the culture is being created and nurtured. Resident remediation is challenging for well-established programs; absorbing multiple residents who are likely to need additional support may overwhelm a naive program. Therefore, matriculation of 1 year of the resident complement through the National Resident Matching Program (NMRP) allows for deliberate recruitment of the new trainees with the opportunity for them to be the inaugural face of the program and mature to lead the successive classes as they matriculate on an annual basis. Although challenging to engage only interns in the clinical space, the faculty have a unique opportunity for mentorship and guidance in this model while directly helping to engage and sow the seeds of culture that will be critical to successful continued accreditation and future recruitment of resident and faculty physicians to this greenfield space. Therefore, alignment between the program leadership and core faculty is critical during recruitment for a new program. The applicants need a coherent and uniform message and vision.

Finally, although all residency programs share the common goal of creating knowledgeable and well-rounded general pediatricians, each program may have its own areas of focus that will impact recruitment. For example, some programs may recruit residents who are more likely to enter practice in rural regions based on their geography and community needs. Another program may focus on political advocacy due to its location or policy priorities, with a vision to improve healthcare legislation for children.

Program Leadership Requirements and FTE Allocation

The minimum full-time equivalent (FTE) for the program director (PD) and associate program director(s) or other physician leadership is dictated by the ACGME based on approved resident positions for the program. The program director must be a single faculty member with ultimate accountability for the residency program who holds current pediatric board certification in their specialty and maintains ongoing clinical activity. The program coordinator (PC) is another essential member of the program leadership team, responsible for daily program operations and engagement with the trainees, faculty, and the ACGME. The amount of PC FTE support is also dictated by the ACGME guidelines based on the approved resident complement. In addition to the program director, program coordinator, and the program leadership team, the residency program must identify core faculty who will have a significant role in the education, supervision, and evaluation of the resident physicians. In the most recent ACGME guidelines, there must be a minimum of one core faculty for every five approved resident positions. These core faculty members must be provided with support averaging 0.1 FTE for their educational and administrative responsibilities distinct from patient care activities. At the outset, a program may choose to hire a program liaison, or chief resident, who is a new graduate from an alternate program. This affords the candidate the opportunity to engage in medical education and lead the residents in a unique way as compared to the faculty physicians. Some resident graduates may be looking to pursue a fellowship during the next recruitment cycle or may be aiming to align with a significant other's projected residency graduation. These graduates who are hired to serve in the traditional chief resident role will need coaching from the residency program leadership team as they work to guide new intern trainees through a program that they themselves did not train in or experience in the same capacity. Near daily check-ins with the PD would be recommended during the implementation of the program to ensure a unified approach and ensure aligned culture building with the mission and vision of the program. The opportunity for the chief resident to participate in this type of new educational adventure can be quite appealing to physicians interested in pursuing graduate medical education or administration in the future. If the pediatric residency program chooses to employ a Chief Resident, they may be counted as core faculty in their respective leadership role.

The planning and eventual implementation of a new residency program requires significant administrative work and resource allocation. Identifying the program director, program leadership team including the program coordinator, and the core faculty is critical. Each of them will contribute to the educational portfolio that will transform the ACGME application into a tangible curriculum that will engage trainees toward the expert practice of pediatric medicine. Each of the named positions should be appropriately funded, as required by the program requirements for the anticipated number of approved resident physicians during the application and accreditation process. A successful ACGME application and site visit is a team sport. Significant expertise and collaboration will be needed to ensure adequate preparation of the accreditation package. An ACGME site visit will be required prior to successful initial accreditation. During this visit, the program leadership and core faculty will be asked detailed questions about the proposed curriculum, teaching modalities, didactic conferences, diversity and well-being initiatives, opportunities for resident scholarship, trainee schedules, work hours, and the sponsoring institution's support of the residency leadership team. Failure to have exceptional engagement in this process is detrimental to success in the accreditation process and ultimately the ability to lead the next generation of pediatricians.

Pediatric Residency Curriculum, Rotations, and Evaluations

Creating a 3-year curriculum for a new residency program is both exciting and an opportunity to focus on the education of the resident rather than the service needs of the hospital or department. Programs that existed prior to the implementation of the 80-hour work week were challenged to provide adequate coverage of clinical services that were historically covered by residents. With additional restrictions put into place to provide residents with more autonomy in their curriculum, including individualized educational units, this squeeze became even tighter in some facilities. With a new program overlaying currently existing patient coverage, the program director can maximize those rotations that would best train a general pediatrician and eliminate those that may be better suited for fellows or advanced practice provider coverage. For example, a bone marrow transplant service may be an elective opportunity for a resident thinking about pursuing a hematology oncology fellowship. However, it may not be a service that warrants 24-hour coverage by pediatric residents. The core pediatric subspecialties should be comprised of both inpatient and outpatient experiences to best represent the general practice of that specialty. Many programs have traditionally favored heavy inpatient coverage of these services, not adequately representing the subspecialty. ACGME expectations for these subspecialty rotations can now be utilized to enhance the resident's education in these disciplines, with appropriate exposure to both inpatient and outpatient medicine aligned with the subspecialty faculty practice.

Creating a 13-block academic year (4 weeks per block) over the traditional 12-month calendar year can offer more opportunities to provide additional experiences. It can be challenged by tight schedules in which minimum requirements of a rotation may not be met if there are unforeseen circumstances such as illness or holidays that result in an outpatient clinic closure. Holiday schedules for Thanksgiving, Christmas, New Year, and/or high holidays for Christian, Judaism, Islamic, or other religions will also impact coverage and clinical experience, but having some type of additional holiday or religious leave schedule in addition to regular vacation time is often greatly appreciated by residents.

It is mandatory during the creation of the 3-year training curriculum that the residency program meets the current ACGME requirements for inpatient, outpatient, subspecialty, supervisory, NICU, PICU, adolescent medicine, developmental behavioral pediatrics, newborn nursery, and individualized educational units. Thus, it is important not to commit to coverage of services until this 3-year curriculum with proposed resident schedules is completed. Covering a service for an entire year takes more than one resident. Working 12-hour shifts, 6/7 days a week to stay under the 80-hour per week limit, and assuming 4 weeks off per year for vacation and other miscellaneous days (In Training Exam, renewing BLS, illness) with a minimum of 36 half days of a longitudinal continuity clinic, the service would need approximately 1.8 residents to provide 24/7 coverage of 1 position for 1 year. Therefore, coverage by faculty physicians or advanced practice providers (APPs) may be necessary. Coverage by faculty physicans or APPs who work between 36 and 50 hours per week is much more expensive than the average resident physician who works up to 80 hours per week. In general, a faculty physician or advanced practice provider would need a minimum of 2.4 FTEs for 24/7 coverage of a single position.

When the 3-year curriculum is completed, it is time to create level-specific goals and objectives for each of the experiences. Appointing a faculty preceptor for each of the electives is important for the administration and scheduling of the experience. The preceptor title will provide the faculty member with a role that can be included on their curriculum vitae that may help with promotion or by meeting academic criteria set up by the administrative body or medical school. The faculty preceptor can create goals and objectives with guidance from the program leadership. Providing a template and an example of what you are looking for is highly recommended. It is additionally advisable to include which procedures may be expected to be performed, if any, during that experience; so, it is clear to the faculty and team that residents should participate in those opportunities when available. It is also important for there to be clear instructions on where the resident is to report on their first day and any additional valuable information for the rotation, such as educational resources. Having rotation goals and objectives as well as any other important introductory material sent in advance of the educational experience by the residency management software is helpful in confirming receipt of this information and can decrease the burden on the residency administration team, particularly when the residency is large.

Challenging ACGME Rotation Requirements (Adolescent Medicine, Developmental and Behavioral Pediatrics, Adequate Pediatric Subspecialty Disciplines, Mental Health, and Resident Continuity Clinic)

The ACGME requirements are the best reference for DIOs and Program Directors (PDs) to utilize in engaging with departmental or executive leadership regarding faculty requirements necessary for initial accreditation of a residency program. These requirements can be used to gain a mutual understanding of the personnel, equipment, and space, all three of which are extremely expensive in the healthcare environment. Some particularly challenging requirements will be addressed in this section. Adolescent medicine and developmental and behavioral pediatrics are two mandatory block experiences that are highly relevant and required for the training of pediatricians. Both can be challenging to provide based on the smaller number of faculty currently practicing in these fields in the United States, as compared to other subspecialties with lower reimbursement models and a high level of face-to-face time required for patient encounters. Recruitment of these faculty members can be exceedingly difficult, time consuming, and challenging to gain approval from the institution due to the financial realities of these disciplines. The trainees will be required to have these experiences at their own institutions or have a program letter of agreement (PLA) for the rotational experience to occur at another SI or in a private practice setting. Any external rotation may require the program to pay for this mandatory educational experience for its trainees.

In addition to these two pediatric subspecialties, the ACGME program requirements necessitate multiple subspecialty physicians across various disciplines. Although many of these subspecialties are more common than adolescent medicine and developmental and behavioral pediatrics, the requisite number to fulfill the minimum requirements for the ACGME must be noted at the outset of program planning. It is critical for the SI to understand this need for faculty expertise, or be willing to engage external groups of faculty, potentially at a cost, to train the resident physicians. It is imperative that the ACGME requirements are met, but more importantly that the residents have access to foundational knowledge required to ensure competence as a general pediatrician at the conclusion of the training program. Finally, experience with mental health care has become mandatory for the next generation of physicians due to the high prevalence of mental health afflictions in our pediatric population. Again, this experience must be developed at the SI or be scheduled at an external facility or practice to satisfy the ACGME requirements fully.

The mandatory resident continuity clinic longitudinal experience can pose an additional challenge to the new program. The continuity clinic experience can be organized and delivered in several ways, requiring careful planning and execution. When starting a new program, it is important to understand the requirements of this experience across the 3 years of training, and the mandates of clinics annually and within the academic year, as noted by the ACGME requirements. The residents must have their own panel of patients with evidence of continuity among these patients. The clinic must function as a medical home caring for children from birth through adolescence, inclusive of children with medical and/or social complexity. The barriers to starting a new resident continuity clinic experience depend on the model. Embedding residents into already established general pediatric practices can initially impart monetary loss for faculty members who work exclusively in an RVU (relative value unit) generation-based model, as the residents take time to build their clinical skills and efficiency. There are teaching faculty rules in the Centers for Medicare and Medicaid Services (CMS) language that prohibit teaching faculty from seeing their own panel of patients simultaneously, depending on the number of trainees being supervised. In addition, residents require instructional time that is not patient facing, and therefore not revenue generating. Clinical practice variation among faculty providers can create a heterogeneous experience for the residents such that they will benefit from a strong core curriculum for the resident continuity clinic experience to ensure understanding of current general pediatric guidelines and standard of care. Establishing a new ambulatory environment for the resident continuity clinic with expert teaching faculty is a significant up-front investment that may be prohibitively expensive. However, this design can readily meet the ACGME requirements and educational needs of the program founded with these principles from the outset, with dedicated teaching faculty committed to appropriate supervision towards autonomous practice. Finally, the financial burden of the resident continuity clinic may be alleviated to some degree if the program leverages an existing Federally Qualified Health Center (FQHC); the payment structure for the patients and clinic in this arena is predetermined. The local FQHC may have many of the same concerns around the number of patients seen per clinical session as well as educational versus clinical time as the private practice model or novel continuity ambulatory space.

Residency Program Tracks

Residency programs can offer non-standard pathways and combined programs that are recognized by the American Board of Pediatrics (ABP). There can be clinical tracks, including primary care, rural health, and critical care tracks. In addition, there can be tracks for physician scientists, advocates, medical educators, quality improvement leaders, and global health leaders.

The opportunity to create novel tracks and experiences within the residency program that engage focus on individualized curriculum elective opportunities can highlight strengths for a new residency program in the recruitment process. Examples of these tracks may include a Primary Care Track, Global Health Track, or Public Policy Track. A Primary Care track may have additional individualized electives in ambulatory care, urgent care, lactation, behavioral health or psychiatry, adolescent medicine, and time in a federally qualified health center. A Global Health track may include away rotation(s) to another country with faculty mentors and electives in medical Spanish, infectious disease, and advocacy. A Public Policy track may engage numerous electives promoting child advocacy and population health, including legislative advocacy opportunities engaged with the SI government relations team.

Physician-scientist tracks encourage the development of physician-scientists while ensuring that the trainees receive adequate instruction and develop the ability to become competent pediatricians. These programs are for MD/PhDs, DO/PhDs, or those with comparable research experience and must be approved by the ABP during the first 9 months of the intern year. Two examples of these programs are the Accelerated Research Pathway (ARP) and the Integrated Research Pathway (IRP). These would likely be very challenging to establish for a new residency program and may be better suited when the program has been approved for continued accreditation.

Procedural Competency

Procedural competency is challenging, even for well-established programs. One reason residents struggle to gain firsthand experience with procedures is due to changes in clinical practice. There are fewer lumbar punctures being performed compared to a decade ago due to evidence-based practice. Additionally, many hospitals have developed specialty services to perform procedures routinely performed by residents in the past, such as IV access teams or suture medics in the emergency department. The core required procedures have been decreased to just a few at this point: PALS, neonatal resuscitation including bag-mask ventilation, IV placement, and lumbar puncture. Programs still need to provide opportunities for residents to perform procedures, and, when deemed by the program and resident to be essential for their future practice, the opportunity for exposure to those procedures or supplementation through simulation. Providing simulation opportunities for residents that involve procedures, as well as providing direct clinical experience during core rotations and electives with procedure frequency in their routine practice, is highly recommended. The ultimate practice specialty of the resident is discerned later in training, making procedural exposure throughout residency imperative to avoid a rush near the end of the training program to gain skills important for future practice.

Research and Scholarly Activity

All residency programs are required to have resident scholarship activities. Successful scholarship is best tied to the mission and vision of the residency program and concentrated in areas that are more likely to receive resources or support from the sponsoring institution or hospital. Mirroring areas of faculty expertise can also increase the opportunity for faculty mentorship and potential funding of novel work. This is most critical for residents who participate in basic, clinical, or translational science. However, many residents will focus their scholarship on patient safety, quality improvement, medical education, or population health. These residents will also benefit immensely from faculty mentorship and expertise. It is advisable to teach all residents, regardless of their area of scholarship or future practice, the basic skills of critically appraising medical literature. This is essential to ensure skills to discern robust evidence with academic rigor to inform and potentially change their future practice. With more of the population accessing online information to inform their medical decision-making, it is important for today's clinicians to understand how to quickly appraise articles and information presented to them. It is imperative that they use evidence-based information to provide treatment plans and counsel to patients they serve during training and in their future practice.

Advocacy

Advocacy efforts and education have significantly expanded in recent years, aligning with the values and direction of the American Academy of Pediatrics. These initiatives have also provided trainees with opportunities and positions within the Section on Pediatric Trainees. There is a desire by current pediatric trainees to have robust opportunities for advocacy during their training, and advocacy training is explicitly delineated in the residency program requirements. In addition to ensuring that advocacy education is incorporated into the ambulatory care experiences as per the guidelines, an advocacy elective is a unique opportunity for education and growth of the trainee, as well as an introduction to their integration into the community. Of note, this type of rotation experience will require PLAs to be completed and executed prior to a resident rotation. Education could be arranged for all residents to have the same experience, or, alternatively, they could be resident created and driven. A resident passionate about breastfeeding may have an advocacy elective in which they earn a lactation certification, spend time at a milk bank, and work with lactation consultants and doulas. A resident interested in primary care may develop a curriculum for expectant parents to learn what to anticipate prior to delivery of their child and offer that education as a class at a local hospital or in an underserved area at a community center. An advocacy rotation may involve working with the hospital's government relations team and attending the yearly state legislative session to speak with legislative leaders and inform policy decisions. The opportunities for child advocacy are numerous and may be individually tailored to create a meaningful experience for each resident physician selected from a robust portfolio of opportunities available to engage the trainees of today to care for the children of tomorrow.

Quality Improvement and Patient Safety

The quality improvement and patient safety departments of the hospital or institution can partner with the GME infrastructure and residency program to meet the ACGME requirements in this arena while simultaneously providing important education for current and future practice. A culture of safety must be present in all training locations, and the residents must be aware and report patient safety events, including near misses. They must also participate in activities such as critical event reviews or root cause analyses that provide opportunities for reflection and action plan creation for areas of safety concern. Per ACGME guidelines, residents must receive their own quality metrics related to patient care or patient populations. Examples of this may include the number of vaccine-eligible patients in their continuity clinic who received the seasonal influenza vaccine, or the number of inpatients diagnosed with status asthmaticus who were discharged home with a short or long-acting beta-agonist. Quality improvement is currently a part of the American Board of Pediatrics maintenance of certification, and developing skills in these areas will help the resident with this requirement in the long term. Residency programs can additionally capitalize on utilizing current web training opportunities such as the Institute for Healthcare Improvement (IHI) open school that has free courses for residents to obtain an IHI Open School Basic Certificate.

Space and Technology Needs

Space and technology needs for a new residency program include the following:

(a) Resident education suite: lounge/wellness space/lactation space
(b) Call rooms

(c) Hospital and ambulatory workspace (clinical workspace)
(d) Conference room(s) for residents
(e) Residency management software

No matter what the size of the residency program, there will be a need for resident educational and well-being space. If there is an opportunity to build the space, build it with the thought in mind of what is critical to have, assuming that no other institutional space will be designated over the next 10 years of growth for the program(s). For example, if the pediatric program is the inaugural program at an SI, but there is a plan for subspecialty fellowships, those trainees should be included in the planning of a novel residency education suite. The residents will need a place they view as their private refuge where they can congregate without other staff or faculty presence or interference. The resident lounge can contain workspaces to allow the residents to continue to monitor results, enter orders, or document in the Electronic Health Record (EHR). It is beneficial to have this space house a refrigerator, microwaves, coffee/tea/water, and ice machines, eating areas, and resting areas that they can use for their retreat. The call rooms may be incorporated in this area if there are no other designated call rooms for their use in the remainder of the facility. If the residents are on 24-hour shifts at the hospital, a separate and quieter space may be more beneficial. Even if the residents will not be sleeping on an overnight shift, they still have a requirement that they have a private space in which they can rest to mitigate fatigue. In greater support of lactating residents, ACMGE requirements for lactation spaces readily accessible by the trainees have become mandatory. These spaces are best situated near conference areas and/or within the residency lounge so that the residents will have easy access to them. In addition, a suitable conference space is imperative for high-caliber resident education. This space must have appropriate technology for learning both in person and via virtual means. If building the resident education suite de novo, inclusion of this conference space into the resident area ensures residency priority to the area and safeguards the technology that is imperative for exceptional education in the current environment. Many hospitals have centralized scheduling of conference rooms; so, if possible, the resident conference space should be permanently reserved for resident activities, and scheduling of other events in the space requires pre-approval by the GME staff.

Residency Management Software (RMS) has high upfront and ongoing cost, but it is a tool that allows for the most efficient and effective administration of the residency program. RMS allows for the dissemination of schedules, goals and objectives, faculty, and resident evaluations. It maintains information related to important documentation such as licensure, resident contracts, annual summative evaluations, and final summative evaluations. Finally, it is robust for duty hour tracking, and other requirements set forth by the ACGME that must be closely monitored by the program leadership. The RMS ultimately allows for the collation of all resident data for ACGME milestone submission, semi-annual reviews, and residency clinical competency committee review, and is critical to maintain continued accreditation. It is important for the RMS to offer training and support to the program. There may be a limited number of superusers who can be trained, and only one or two with unrestricted access. It is advisable to select members of the program administration who will be most likely to be present in the program for a long time and with a desire or pre-existing experience with this type of technology. Staff turnover can be incredibly challenging if there is short notice and an inability to have another staff member receive training. An effective relationship with the vendor is critical to ensure sustainability and appropriate maintenance.

Financial Benefits and Stipends (i.e., Health Care Benefits, Vacation and Leave, Licensure Cost, Educational Stipends, Meal Cards/Stipends, etc.)

In an ACGME-accredited SI, all salaries for a specific level of training are uniform and voted on by the Graduate Medical Education Committee

(GMEC). There is no opportunity for an individual program to offer a salary line that is different or altered, as compared to the institution. In addition, health care benefits are generally provided by the SI or health care system. It is important to understand these benefits and the cost to the trainee if different or unique from the faculty or other employees. Items that are frequently inquired about by residents, and in some cases may require specific GME policies due to current ACGME requirements, include parental and caregiver leave and benefits, vacation time in the academic year, fertility treatment, dental and vision coverage, mental health and well-being platforms or services, and items that may be specific to their individual family needs such as coverage of autism services. It is wise to ensure that you have partners across the institution representing benefits, leave administration, and human resources who are well acquainted with the ACGME guidelines and requirements to collaborate with GME leadership.

Highly qualified resident applicants may enage more with a new training program that reimburses them for the cost of their training license at matriculation, and potentially their unrestricted license and Drug Enforcement Agency (DEA) numbers later in their training. In addition, reimbursing residents for the United States Medical Licensing Examination (USMLE) Step 3, or equivalent Osteopathic exams, as well as for the American Board of Pediatrics (ABP) licensing exam at completion of training, are other opportunities to renumerate residents outside of their salary and benefits package with the institution. It is best to have some considerations and guardrails around these expensive benefits for residents. Establishing that there will only be one reimbursement per exam per resident, and/or that the exam must be taken within a particular time frame such as prior to the end of the PGY 1 year for the Step 3 USMLE examination can ensure that the resident is clear on the funding mechanism opportunity and engages a personal responsibility for success in these arenas. If the program is not able to establish a reimbursement benefit, it would be advisable that they consider allowing residents to roll over the annual educational stipend to allow it to be used toward the cost of the ABP licensing examination at the end of training. The fee for this examination comes at a time during which many trainees are preparing to move for fellowship, or initiate their careers, and the expense is significant.

Most residency programs provide annual educational stipends for their residents, and many also provide meals, meal tickets, or stipends for food. Creating a list of approved items to purchase with the educational funds is advisable to prevent valuable funds from being spent on extraneous items. Examples include board preparation materials, educational conferences, medical books, and medical equipment such as stethoscopes. Allowing the funds to be utilized for the purchase of a personal computer is also something to be considered if the function will aid in patient care, education, academic, or scholarly pursuits during the training program. It must be decided at the outset whether these funds will need to be used yearly for budgeting purposes, or if the program will allow the funds to roll over year to year to ensure monies for expensive pursuits by the residents, i.e., an important educational conference for networking as they approach fellowship applications or the ABP licensing examination, will be covered.

Providing breakfast or lunch, particularly when an educational conference is mandated, helps the residents to avoid standing in cafeteria lines or heating food. It can be an efficient way to feed large numbers of people but is often met with complaints related to the food quality, diversity, or availability of gluten-free, vegan, kosher, or Halal options. Paper meal vouchers can be tedious and inefficient to distribute each month to residents and are unable to be replaced if lost, whereas electronic meal card options are beneficial for reloading opportunities and potential loss but prone to technology or vendor issues outside of the SI control. Providing a meal or food stipend to the resident ensures extra funds for the trainee but does not aid in acquiring food before a noon conference or early meeting. In addition, when directly deposited and part of the resident paycheck, it is taxable income that is not earmarked for nutrition.

For residency programs that value academic productivity, it is imperative to have a plan to reimburse or pay for resident presentations at academic conferences. It is advisable that the cost of the resident registration, poster, travel, and lodging should be reimbursed from sources outside of the resident educational fund. The department chairs or division chiefs may agree to supplement the resident costs for presenting at conferences when the work was completed with faculty mentors in their divisions or departments. This is also an excellent opportunity to use funds raised with philanthropy for academic pursuits outside of the traditional ACGME programming. Alternate funding sources can lessen the financial burden on the residency program while promoting academic productivity in the trainees, augmenting their fellowship applications and job searches post-residency.

Psychological Supports and Well-Being Initiatives

It is now required that all residents have access to "confidential, affordable mental health assessment, counseling, and treatment, including access to urgent and emergent care 24 hours a day, seven days a week." [1] This access can be expensive and may need to be supplemented depending on the accessibility of appropriate mental health care providers who accept the resident's insurance. A new program may need to contract with a practice or program for the provision of these services to ensure that the regulations are met and that the residents have appropriate psychological support available.

In addition, residents must be provided with tools for self-screening and training to recognize symptoms of depression and burnout in themselves and others. Pediatric resident burnout was already at an elevated level prior to the pandemic. In a 2019 Pediatric Resident Burnout-Resilience Consortium study of 1956 residents from 46 different pediatric programs, 45% reported burnout symptoms at least weekly or more and 33% reported some form of mistreatment. This mistreatment was either bullying, discrimination, sexual harassment, or physical abuse. Clinical staff perpetrated the mistreatment 60% of the time, families 54% and faculty 43%. Women were more likely to report mistreatment than men [2]. Since the pandemic, and with changing societal norms, there are more complaints about mistreatment and burnout among health care professionals, and mistreatment can cause increased resident burnout and mental health concerns.

Current recommendations for reducing mistreatment include more than just mindfulness-based activities and the availability of therapy. They include administrative and policy-driven expectations, as well as consequences for poor behavior among faculty, staff, and patients/caregivers. Creating and implementing policies or codes of conduct at the institution can lead to a culture of trust and accountability. Training and strategies to help bystanders or second victims to speak up or report mistreatment can empower those who have been mistreated or marginalized, again promoting a culture of mutual respect and dignity. Implicit bias training or microaggression trainings encourage education and self-reflection [3].

ACGME requirements now ensure that residents have available to them the opportunity to receive their own health care during regularly scheduled work hours [1]. It is advised that the residents notify the chief residents or program leadership to approve these absences in advance so that the resident is not subject to the whim of the faculty member or service needs of the day.

Finally, some institutions have engaged well-being stipends for the trainees. They recognize that wellness is not uniform among trainees, and the stipend provides the trainee freedom to choose activities which promote their individual joy, rejuvenation, and reflection. The well-being chapter in this book will explore this important topic in a more comprehensive manner.

Faculty Development

A new residency program brings excitement for faculty, particularly those recruited with the expectation of successful program accreditation. The new residency program application will require robust engagement with the faculty, as rotation experiences, patient volume and complexity, goals and objectives, educational initiatives, and faculty scholarship are critical to a successful application. It is highly recommended that there be multiple faculty development and informational meetings during the program application, which continue throughout the recruitment of the inaugural residents to ensure understanding of the 3-year program curriculum and current ACGME requirements. A shared mental model for the training infrastructure and the importance of the faculty in the success of the program cannot be underestimated.

The ACGME requires mandatory annual faculty development, "for the purpose of enhancing transference of knowledge, skill, and behavior from the educator to the learner." [1] This can be achieved through a variety of lectures, workshops, or web-based training modules. Areas of focus for mandatory education include evaluation, quality improvement, health care inequities, patient safety, well-being, and practice-based learning and improvement.

There are requirements for faculty to receive education in fatigue mitigation, identifying burnout, depression, suicidal ideation and substance abuse disorders in trainees or their colleagues. Mitigating workplace violence or the potential for violence has also been included in this required education. Program faculty should be equipped with knowledge and resources to seek help for trainees or colleagues with these conditions and must feel institutionally supported in this work.

Professional Development for Interprofessional Team Members

When starting a new residency program, it is critical to engage other stakeholders to discuss the plans for the educational program. Do not underestimate the knowledge gap regarding current resident training requirements, resident capabilities such as order entry and prescriptive authority, supervision policies, and evaluations of the trainees when it comes to the interprofessional health care team. The non-physician team may not understand the differences between a medical student, an intern, a resident or fellow, and their interface in the healthcare environment. Likewise, they may not understand how they differ from physician faculty members other than in years of experience. Partnering with leaders in nursing, advanced practice, pharmacy, respiratory therapy, rehabilitation services, and care coordination is critical. For example, with the matriculation of residents, the nursing team will be asked to engage the resident physicians as the first call for patient care questions. The nursing team will need reassurance that the faculty physicians are still engaged and supervising the trainees, and the residents must respond diligently by addressing the nursing questions or escalating for additional help as indicated. This will be a change in process that coincides with the addition of the resident learners. From the hospital and staff perspective, it will literally be an overnight change. Initially, the interprofessional team may not recognize their role in resident education or appreciate that the addition of the residents will ultimately enhance patient safety and the quality of care provided in the institution. It is also imperative that when APPs and residents work together on a service there is an emphasis on robust collaboration with clear lines of supervision and communication with the supervising faculty member to discern roles and expectations of the delivery of care.

Policies and Procedures

The policies and procedures of a new program must be aligned with the sponsoring institution's GME policies, whether it be a university, medical school, hospital, or health care system. However, there will be some overarching institutional or hospital policies that are non-applicable to the resident trainee and may even be counterproductive to the requirements set forth by the ACGME. These policies should be highlighted, and graduate medical education or residency-specific policies should be implemented as needed. Examples of these types of policies include salary, benefits and annual salary increases, vacation and paid time off, parental or caregiver leave, and salary during this time, as well as payout of non-utilized paid time off (PTO). For example, faculty may have PTO that accrues over time whereas residents have a block of vacation that will be used in collaboration with the residency program and in alignment with the resident's clinical schedule. A new resident physician may require a 2-week block of vacation immediately in August after their matriculation. In standard hospital policy, the resident would not have accrued adequate time off to have this scheduled vacation at this point in their employment. On the other hand, policies and procedures related to the Americans with Disabilities Act (ADA) and Drug and Alcohol offenses are best aligned with the overarching institution or health care system, rather than specific GME SI policies, and can be referred to by the program in their application as they are existing organizational policies. Finally, it is advisable to create a job description for the requirements of a resident as an employee so that if issues related to ADA laws come into play for accommodations, there is an existing job description that can be referenced for expectations of the role of resident physician.

Program-specific guidelines, policies, and procedures may be best suited for items like educational stipends and how they may be spent, at which point the residents must pass the Step 3 licensing board, how absences will be covered, and any other program-specific requirements, such as mandatory scholarly productivity during training. It is important that residents know, understand, and can locate the policies and procedures that they will be held accountable for. These are best housed online in a secure location, such as the residency management software, so that all residents can freely access these documents. It is important for key policies and procedures to be acknowledged as reviewed through signature at a minimum at the outset of their matriculation into the program. It may seem perfunctory at the time, but when violations occur, it is key that there is documentation of resident acknowledgement should legal action be required.

Program Letters of Agreement

If the pediatric residents are required to spend educational time at a location that is not under the purview of the SI, a program letter of agreement (PLA) will be needed. These documents serve as an agreement between the SI residency program and the participating site where a resident will rotate for an educational experience. Ultimately, they must be signed by the residency program director and the DIO of the SI, as well as the site director for the external experience and DIO or executive leadership at the participating institution or organization. These agreements may be for required educational blocks that are not available at the sponsoring institution, or for experiences that add value to the educational curriculum within the community, or at a site distinct from the hospital or medical center. The PLA may take months to complete; so, it is advisable to start early and make sure that it is renewed as outlined by the ACGME requirements. Examples may include community rotation sites like the county health department or an advocacy organization in the community. In a free-standing children's hospital without a delivery center, an alternate newborn nursery experience is required and would necessitate a PLA with a delivery center. These PLAs tend to be utilized more often during adolescent medicine, developmental and behavioral pediatrics, newborn nursery, and advocacy rotations. They are also used frequently for elective rotations or audition rotations for residents interested in subspecialty fellowships for disciplines that are not well represented at the sponsoring institution and for global health electives. It is crucial that the program director and administrative team clearly document the time spent under the purview of the SI versus the time spent at an alternate hospital or medical center. Accuracy is critical for state and federal funding, and the resident full-time equivalent (FTE) data from the sponsoring institution and participating site must not be in conflict.

Data Requirements for New Program

It is highly recommended that those seeking to create a new program review the program application information and the available information regarding program accreditation material available on the ACGME's website. These provide a wealth of information that are critical to review and will allow the program leadership to begin to understand the financial investment required from the SI and/or hospital administration. Additionally, it is advisable to review the current program requirements and any pending or proposed requirements that may be active by the time of submission or matriculation of resident physicians. The wording of some requirements might say that a program, "may" require something that in a revision then becomes a "must." Planning for a "may" that will likely transform to a "must" can enhance the program's success with the eventual site visit and demonstrate a commitment to not just meet, but exceed, current requirements.

There are significant data collection requirements for the initial accreditation application submission, ongoing ACGME annual data requests, as well as robust data requirements for the continued accreditation submission and site visit. Data extraction and tabulation take time, and someone dedicated to creating reports or dashboards to contain accurate and detailed information is required. In addition to a program lead, dedicated personnel from the SI or hospital information technology (IT) or finance team are critical in obtaining accurate and timely information related to clinical volume and diagnoses. The number of pediatric patients admitted each year to each site, average daily census, and average length of stay are required. If working with multiple sites with different EMRs, there will be a need for collaboration among multiple IT personnel from different institutions to ensure the complete submission of data requirements.

Some of the more challenging data to acquire are the consecutive patient lists required for inpatient rotations, as well as the total number of patients seen by the general pediatricians and subspecialty pediatricians at the institution. A new program will need to provide two separate lists of one hundred consecutive final discharge diagnoses for patients 20 years of age and under who were admitted to the pediatric inpatient teaching service, excluding the Pediatric Intensive Care Unit (PICU), Neonatal Intensive Care Unit (NICU), and well-baby nursery. A secondary diagnosis can be included and is recommended to help show the depth and breadth of the pediatric pathology available to the residents for educational purposes. These lists must come from two separate periods within the most recent 12-month period prior to submission. Each individual patient on this list will need to have their age listed along with an ID number that could be utilized for patient verification, if required, by the site visitor. Choosing these patient portfolios from different seasons and during periods of time where the census was elevated will increase the diversity of the pediatric disease and complexity represented. The average length of stay for the represented population needs to be included with the submission of each list. Each list must then be divided into specialty diagnoses currently designated as allergy and immunology, cardiology, endocrinology, gastroenterology, genetics, hematology/oncology, infectious diseases, nephrology, neurology, psychiatry, developmental and behavioral pediatrics, pulmonology, rheumatology, surgery, trauma, and so on. In areas that are deficient, there is an opportunity to explain the deficiency and how the program will supplement education for the resident physicians.

The NICU level designation, annual number of admissions, total number of NICU beds, average daily census, length of stay, annual admissions less than 1500 grams, and annual number of deaths are required. The PICU admission, number of beds, average daily census, length of stay, and number of deaths per year are needed, along with whether surgical and post-operative cardiac patients are admitted to this unit.

There are additional initial accreditation data needs for the emergency department experiences and newborn nursery. The sites that will be used for the resident continuity clinic experience must be listed along with the number of residents and at which postgraduate training level will be assigned to each site, the faculty-to-resident ratio, and the total number of pediatric visits per year. Once the residents start their continuity clinic experience, there will need to be a way to record the number of patients seen per resident per half-day clinic session, to demonstrate continuity of care with the individual resident physician through repeated visits with a specific patient, as well as a demonstration that the resident is caring for children with medical complexity. If there is one clinic site for the residents, this data may be easier to pull, but if there are separate sites with different EHR systems from the SI, it may be easier to have the individual residents submit a patient log through the residency management system for this record keeping.

Resident Documentation and Requirements for ACGME, Joint Commission, Agency for Health Care Administration (AHCA), etc.

The necessary components of the resident file from the standpoint of the Sponsoring Institution and ACGME includes, but is not limited to, the residents' medical school graduating certificate, background screening and employment verification, Education Commission of Foreign Graduate Medical Education (ECFMG) certification if applicable, GME employment contracts, medical licensure, trainings as required including BLS, PALS, and NRP for pediatrics, rotation schedules, evaluations, semi-annual reviews, procedural data record, documentation of scholarly activity and quality improvement projects with copies of the posters, presentations, or publications, records of any disciplinary actions or performance improvement/remediation plans, and any other content required as determined by the SI, DIO and the program director. Ultimately, copies of the In-Training Examinations (ITE) and an official USMLE copy with documentation of successful passage of the Step 3 examination are required. Annually, the annual summative evaluation is required, and at completion of the program, the final summative document must be included. This is critical for future employment verifications of the graduated trainee, as residency program verification is required for medical staff credentialing and privileging.

The Joint Commission may ask to review a resident file during a site visit with a focus on licensure and training, resident evaluations, supervision policies as they relate the resident rotations, residency policies and procedures as well as current areas of priority for the Joint Commission. For example, they may ask a nurse how he/she would know if a resident was competent to perform a procedure and whether that resident needed direct or indirect supervision when performing the stated procedure. Additionally, they may review a patient encounter in the electronic medical record for a family with a primary language other than English and ensure documentation that an interpreter was utilized or offered and declined, particularly those involving consent. The residents are regarded as essential members of the health care team and are open to questioning and evaluation identical to any other employee at the institution during a Joint Commission site visit.

The Agency for Health Care Administration, Medical Assistance Programs, or other similar state agencies tend to focus on areas of complaint raised by patients and families regarding their care, state-mandated opioid policies and procedures, state-mandated reporter procedures, and state Medicaid or managed care programs. Educating residents on the state-specific rules and regulations is important to increase compliance and success with meeting these requirements. The use of restraints in the hospital setting has been a key area of focus for these agencies and the Joint Commission in recent years. The hospital policy for how restraints, chemical and physical, are initiated, ordered, documented, and discontinued is critical to follow to ensure patient rights. Resident physicians have a role in these processes and procedures and must be well informed and held accountable for competent practice and documentation.

Preparation for Accreditation Site Visits

The ACGME website contains many vital details regarding how to best prepare for an ACGME site visit. There is a minimum of approximately 30 days' notice for the site visit, and the program director, program coordinator(s), Director of Education and/or Chair of the Department, faculty members, and residents must be present. The request is for on-duty residents to be present, but for small programs, or programs in initial accreditation it is recommended that all residents be freed from their clinical responsibilities to attend unless on a scheduled vacation block. Large programs will require that peer-elected representatives should be present for each class. Associate program directors, if applicable, will participate and will be included as core faculty for the residency program.

The expectations regarding required paperwork and forms for the ACGME initial accreditation site visit and assessment for ongoing accreditation are clear. It takes considerable time to create these documents and to gather the appropriate data. This includes, but is not limited to, examples of goals and objectives, evaluation forms, the 3-year curriculum in block diagram format, estimated patients covered by time of day per resident, policies and procedures for the residency program, and a detailed outline of the required educational series for the residents. This includes the description of the educational activities and a mock lecture schedule over several months. For example, if the residents have a monthly quality improvement lecture, there should be a QI lecture on the mock schedule each month.

Having the application reviewed multiple times by multiple people with expertise, including the DIO, is critical to success. The document must represent the depth and breadth of educational programming and accurately reflect the program's mission and vision. In addition to the content, the document must be carefully assessed for typos, font changes, and grammatical errors, which should be eliminated prior to submission. When data are pulled for the diagnosis sections, the data must be typed into the charts provided in the ACGME application. Provide both primary and secondary diagnoses whenever possible to demonstrate the acuity and complexity of disease burden for educational purposes. The original data pull, which may be in Excel format, should be saved and clearly labeled for cross-reference if requested for review by the site visitor. Site visitors notice when there are multiple errors in an application or a sloppy appearance of scanned forms, evaluations, or goals and objectives.

On the day of the site visit, be prepared to produce documents or files for any resident in the program when the continuing accreditation site visitor comes. In addition to reviewing resident(s) from each year of the program, they may focus on residents who have transitioned into the program from other programs, have active Visas, or those with performance concerns. All resident files will need to have the necessary documents present. Examples include medical school graduation certificates, medical licenses, and resident contracts, as well as a robust collection of evaluations for the site visitor to review. You may additionally be asked to provide them with examples of faculty member evaluations and rotation evaluations to demonstrate that the evaluation process is reciprocal in nature and that the evaluations are being completed as intended. Likewise, documents like PLAs, goals and objectives, or examples of semi-annual review documents are often asked to be reviewed. Knowing where all these documents are in the residency management system or having paper copies readily available in resident files or program binders is important as the site visitor is limited on time. Disorganization or the inability to readily access the requested information will be noted. If there are required rotations outside of the SI's purview, or in another city or state to meet the criteria for a mandatory rotation, the site visitor will also likely focus on these rotations with the documentation and interviews with the residents.

References

1. ACGME Program Requirements for Graduate Medical Education in Pediatrics. ACGME-approved major revision: February 4, 2024; effective July 1, 2025.
2. Kemper KJ, Schwartz A, Pediatric Resident Burnout-Resilience Study Consortium. Bullying, discrimination, sexual harassment, and physical violence: common and associated with burnout in pediatric residents. Acad Pediatr. 2020;20(7):991–7. https://doi.org/10.1016/j.acap.2020.02.023. Epub 2020 Feb 27.
3. Kemper KJ, Schwartz A. Update on mistreatment and burnout in pediatric residents. Acad Pediatr. 2023;23(5):869–71. https://doi.org/10.1016/j.acap.2022.12.004. Epub 2022 Dec 26.

Starting a New Training Track

7

Amanda Stewart, Yael Smiley,
and Olanrewaju Falusi

Determine the Rationale for a New Track

Program directors (PDs) or future track leaders will need to clearly define the reasons a new track is warranted at their program. A new track could address gaps in current training or leverage local expertise and passion to expand training opportunities in a particular area. For example, several internal medicine residency programs created hospital medicine tracks to address gaps in knowledge about quality improvement and value-based care for graduates pursuing careers in hospital medicine [4].

A needs assessment that solicits diverse perspectives can clarify the goals for a new track. The perspectives of residents, PDs, and institutional officials are fundamental to assessing these goals. Their input can be collected through focus groups, one-to-one interviews, and surveys. Leaders should consider residents themselves as potentially the most important group to provide input into track goals. Depending on the size of the existing residency program, not all residents may be able to, or interested in, providing input. Track leaders may identify key members within the residency such as chief residents or specific residents with self-identified interest in the track's domain. In addition to current residents, potential future residents such as medical students, or residency program alumni, may have valuable different perspectives that are useful to integrate. Residency leadership, such as PDs or associate and assistant program directors (APDs), will have a clear picture of the current state of residency training and can provide insight into educational gaps and resources already existing within the program.

Program leadership should also conduct a broad assessment of institutional and specialty-specific resources. This may include reviewing existing institutional and local resources, such as a community health needs assessment or health equity report, to determine the key elements that should be built into a track to address local health needs. For research-focused tracks, this could include reviewing materials such as institutional reports on grant funding and publications to understand the existing academic landscape, strengths, and areas for resident involvement. A literature search can help reveal standards and approaches other institutions have used in similar projects. For example, in establishing a new pediatric advocacy track, an APD referred to a toolkit [5, 6] published by the American Academy of Pediatrics which had compiled advocacy initiatives that were mapped to educational competencies and used this as a blueprint for the new residency program track. It can also be helpful to

A. Stewart · Y. Smiley · O. Falusi (✉)
Children's National Hospital, George Washington University School of Medicine and Health Sciences, Washington, DC, USA
e-mail: OOFALUSI@childrensnational.org

H. McPhillips et al. (eds.), *Graduate Medical Education in Pediatrics*, Excellence in Medical Education 3, https://doi.org/10.1007/978-3-032-12952-9_7

research other residency programs already providing training in the area of interest to see what educational approaches seem relevant and effective. Sources for this beyond the medical literature include residency program websites and colleagues in professional societies and special interest groups.

A needs assessment may also benefit from directly engaging community members who may be involved in research or receive clinical care from the institution to solicit priorities from the community related to the new track. Community members should be compensated for their time in providing feedback on a potential new training track.

Identify Champions for the New Track

A critical aspect of developing a new training track is to identify key decision makers and obtain buy-in, which is necessary to launch any new program. These individuals and groups may contribute ideas to the formation or implementation of the new track, may provide funding or other approvals that are fundamental to building the track, or may consist of the team that will be involved in leading or participating in the track itself.

At the institutional level, there are many key parties to engage in the process of developing a new residency track. Key among them is the hospital or institutional educational leadership team. This may include existing residency and fellowship PDs or APDs, designated institutional officers (DIOs, the institutional liaison that ensures the program complies with Accreditation Council for Graduate Medical Education (ACGME) requirements [7]), vice chairs of education, deans, department chairs, or others with educational and clinical leadership positions. Their engagement and investment in the program development will improve the curricular strength of the track through their educational expertise, as well as improving program implementation through existing relationships. As they oversee the educational mission and activities of the institution, it is likely that their approval may be necessary for program development and implementation to proceed, so it is critical to engage these leaders early in the process. Those developing tracks may also want to involve key administrative staff who are instrumental to the functioning of the residency program early on to ensure their input is incorporated into the planning process. This will also allow them to voice concerns, such as if additional administrative support will be necessary.

Beyond educational leaders, designing a new training track also requires buy-in from other key institutional partners. Those hoping to develop a new residency track should look to other leadership that may be relevant to their track. For example, if starting a primary care track, existing primary care leadership such as a division chief, department chair, or general academic pediatrics fellowship PD should be engaged early on. These subject matter experts may come on as leadership of the new training track or may simply provide guidance in program development. They may also be instrumental in ensuring appropriate resources exist to implement desired program elements, such as how new primary care track residents' clinic sessions can be distributed within the current clinic(s)' infrastructure. If these resources do not exist, track leaders will need to work with institutional leaders to secure additional funding or support to add resources or may need to rework the planned elements of the curriculum. Similarly, for tracks focusing on advocacy, research, global health, or other specialties, track leaders should engage existing leaders in these domains for similar considerations.

Obtaining Institutional Buy-In

Engaging interested parties to design and implement a new track requires both educational and organizational leadership theories to maximize chances of success. A solid grounding in educational theory that builds in an evaluative component a priori is necessary to ensure that the curriculum is sound and to optimize participants' learning and experiences within the track. Educational theory is unlikely to be sufficient, however, in convincing key decision makers about the value of a new track and persuading an institution to place its limited resources behind a novel venture. Kotter's eight-step process for leading change [8] is one, although certainly not the only, methodology for effecting change at the organizational level. Kotter recommends the following steps [8, 9] which can serve as effective change management principles that track leaders may wish to utilize:

1. Creating a sense of urgency: Why is your track needed right now? Data and stories are helpful to developing an understanding of the need for your track, but urgency is also key to gaining momentum for track development and implementation.
2. Build a coalition: As you engage interested parties, who are your early champions that can work together to push your track forward? Ensure your team includes diverse voices from a variety of different roles to be most effective.
3. Form a strategic vision: What would your residency program, graduate medical education office, or institution look like once your track is created? Could your track be used to recruit or retain talented individuals? Could it be used for promoting the hospital's research or community missions?
4. Enlist a group of volunteers: Once you've identified your champions, what would you like them to do to push your track forward? How can you communicate your vision early and often to ensure the team has a shared mental model as they approach decisions and conversations with other decision makers and interested parties?
5. Enable action by removing barriers: Are there grants or other funding opportunities that you can identify to potentially offset the cost of starting a new training track? What are the concerns or resistance you encounter? Are there data you can find from other similar programs that support your vision and may allay these concerns from institutional leadership?
6. Generate short-term wins: Can you find small wins along the way that you can recognize, celebrate, and advertise to keep the team's momentum going? Be strategic in setting small goals to ensure you get early wins to keep your team motivated.
7. Sustain acceleration: Once you've gotten some wins under your belt, how can you continue to push harder? Can you advocate for additional funding for new track experiences or expanding the number of positions in the track after several years of positive evaluations?
8. Institute change: How does your program contribute to the overall culture and success of your institution? Your goal is for your track to become a core part of the institutional identity, to sustain the change you worked for thus far. Can you continue to evaluate your track in new and creative ways, bringing feedback to institutional leadership frequently, and emphasizing the ways that it aligns with the hospital's mission and vision?

Recruit Leaders for the New Track

An important consideration for institutions that are looking to start a new training track is to decide early on who will lead the new track. The leadership team may include one or more track directors along with rotation directors and faculty to lead educational initiatives outside of rotations. The program should determine how existing personnel will participate in track leadership, such as having an administrative staff person and a designated chief resident to co-manage the track along with faculty.

Faculty should be recruited who have an interest and expertise in the track content as well as in education. For example, a residency program that is hoping to design a research track should approach faculty with a proven track record of research excellence, but especially those who also demonstrate excellence in teaching and mentorship. Track leadership should have dedicated protected time for their roles. This will ensure track leaders have the skills, interest, and time needed to design, implement, and evaluate the curricular elements of the track—all necessary components to ensuring that participants have high-quality training experiences.

Within this newly developed leadership structure, another key decision is whether the new track merits an APD position. This decision may be based on the size of the new track, the existing leadership structure of the broader residency program, and the track's curricular elements. At some larger residency programs, specialized tracks may have a similar number of positions as entire small or mid-sized residency programs [10–12]. Additionally, some specialized tracks have numerous rotations that differ from categorical tracks and require careful coordination within the broader residency clinical schedule. These tracks may then benefit from a dedicated APD to coordinate the various track rotations, provide mentorship to residents participating in the track, manage track recruitment, provide guidance to track faculty such as rotation directors, and handle evaluation of the program and of the residents themselves. Regardless of the track leadership structure, protected time through a dedicated funding source should be provided to track APDs or other leaders to allow them time to manage track curricular, administrative, and clinical demands.

The amount of time needed for track APDs and/or faculty leads may be highest at the beginning, to support designing and implementing the track. The track leader may then be able to reduce the necessary protected time once the track is established and the initial start-up period is complete. However, if the track is expanding in terms of size or additional curricular elements, it may continue to require ongoing high levels of administrative funding and support. The amount of protected time necessary for track leaders will also vary based on the size of the track, the number of and experience of other members of the leadership team, and the amount of administrative support provided to the track by the residency program or institution more broadly. It is also important to note that the ACGME sets minimum levels of full-time equivalents (FTEs) required in a residency program leadership team based on the number of residents. As such, if a program already meets the minimum required FTE, leadership approval for a new APD position with protected administrative time may be more challenging to secure without expanding the number of residents in the program.

Determine Educational Content for the New Track

After completing a needs assessment, generating institutional buy-in, and determining faculty leaders, the overall goals and objectives of the track should be determined and mapped to educational strategies. This process may begin concurrently with the previous steps, as an initial educational plan may be needed to secure leadership buy-in. Education within the new track can be delivered in the form of rotations, conference series, special events, longitudinal projects, and scholarly work. Residents will need protected time to complete the curriculum for the new track, optimally in a way that supports longitudinal and cross-class learning along with individual learning experiences.

Both clinical and non-clinical rotations can help meet track goals. Track-specific clinical rotations can bolster training in tracks where additional clinical experiences supplement career training goals, for example, participating in a rural medicine rotation as part of a primary care track [1]. Non-clinical rotations can leverage the structure of rotations to provide residents with protected time for learning opportunities, such as coursework in another university department [1]. Some tracks may consider offering a degree for participants that complete the track, such as a master of science for research tracks, a master in education or a master in medical education for education-focused tracks, or a master in public health for advocacy- or policy-based tracks. To accomplish this, track leaders will need to establish partnerships with their affiliated university, medical school, or with specific graduate schools within the university. Alternatively, tracks may offer a certification or other accreditation upon program completion, which may have less formal requirements and require less coordination with outside educational entities. Some tracks may choose to offer both, such as a certification in public health versus a master in public health degree, depending on participants' level of commitment and accomplishments while in the program. Outside of university coursework, non-clinical rotations can include education with diverse partners invested in healthcare, such as working with leaders of a quality and safety committee or community-based organizations.

Track-specific lectures should be planned in collaboration with the overall residency educational calendar. For example, an hour during each academic half-day could be reserved for track-specific education. Alternatively, programs may wish to offer this education to the entire residency program. For example, a research fundamental lecture series could be a component of the research track but offered at a time when any resident can attend. Tracks may also choose to require a longitudinal project and scholarly work, which could include publications and other deliverables such as curricula, manuals, bedside teaching modules [13], testimony, community engagement projects, blog posts, or podcasts.

When track-specific education is required of all residents in the track, this ensures that the curriculum is standardized and makes sure the goals are being met by all residents in the track. Some goals of the track may already be met through basic residency program training. For example, learning to conduct a root cause analysis may be a goal of a quality improvement track, and this goal may be met through participation in a residency-wide morbidity and mortality conference series. In other instances, track goals can be met if existing program electives become required for track participants. For example, a health policy rotation may be an elective option for residents in the categorical program but a required rotation for residents in an advocacy track. To meet other goals for the track, new track-specific education may be needed. Track leaders must work within the training guidelines set out by the ACGME to find time for new rotations. This may mean residents in the track have fewer weeks of independently chosen elective time, for example, if a primary care track requires residents to complete a dermatology rotation in lieu of elective time. However, residents who self-select into a particular track are likely to have sought elective rotations connected to the goals of the track, so the reduced elective time may not ultimately be undesirable.

Another strategy to incorporate new track-specific education that preserves elective time is to reduce the number of non-ACGME-mandated weeks of certain rotations (e.g., if residents in a program already complete more weeks of night float or emergency medicine than the ACGME requires). This strategy is likely to be attractive to residents in the track as their elective time remains intact and they have dedicated educational time to meet the goals of the track. Track leaders will need to advocate for this time and be mindful that outside factors could threaten these rotations as program needs change (e.g., due to ACGME changes or shifting needs for inpatient coverage). It is also important to consider the way differences in schedules will be perceived by residents who are not in the specialized track, and that development of a new track ideally does not lead to increased clinical time for non-track residents. It can be helpful for track residents to have the same amount of inpatient shifts and backup call, even if distributed differently throughout the year, to avoid resentment from residents outside the new track.

Ultimately, participants' schedules will need to be designed in such a way that allows participation in rotations, lectures, projects, or other track requirements. Depending on the time required to complete these additional curricular elements, some tracks could be extended beyond the traditional number of years for categorical residency.

Funding Positions for the New Track

A final key element for a new training track is how track positions will be funded. Initially, programs may be asked to convert positions from a categorical training program into positions for the new track. This requires careful consideration of the planned schedule and additional elements of the new training program and their potential impact on the clinical demands of the institution. Thus, it is key to consider early while planning for the track with institutional leaders. Another route that programs may choose is to apply for additional training positions through the ACGME, which must approve additional positions within each institution "based on an assessment of the program's resources and ability to provide the required elements for education in the specialty or subspecialty." [14] Program funding, used for resident salaries and benefits, as well as other administrative and operating costs [15], will likely come via the Children's Hospital Graduate Medical Education [16, 17] Program (for programs based in free-standing children's hospitals) or Graduate Medical Education [18, 19] Program (for programs that receive funding through Medicare), or through additional funds provided by the institution for resident salary and benefit support as well as additional faculty and staff FTE. Particularly for programs that address a workforce shortage need, such as primary care tracks or those based in rural or underserved areas, funding may be available through state legislatures, federal funding through the Health Resources and Services Administration, or other private grant sources [15]. So, the process of applying for additional program positions may require special buy-in from the DIO as well as legal and policy experts, such as the institutional government affairs team. Once the value of a new training track has been established, especially if grant funding lapses, hospitals may choose to fund additional training program positions out of institutional resources [20]. This would be expected to require buy-in at the highest levels of hospital leadership (e.g., executive level or "C-suite" officials) and is more likely if there is a determination of the importance and value of the track for the broader institution (such as through advertising, recruitment and retention of faculty, or community benefit).

Recruit for a New Track

There are several considerations regarding recruitment for a new track. Program leaders must decide if the track will be a separate match through the National Resident Matching Program (NRMP), or an educational experience resident can opt into once in the program. The advantages of offering a match through the NRMP are that it clearly defines the number of residents who can be in the track and formalizes the application and selection processes. Programs should advertise the new track to potential applicants (e.g., through the institutional website, at residency fairs, and educational conferences) and make clear if applicants can apply to, and rank, multiple tracks at one residency program. Track leaders must also lay out selection criteria for applicants to the track. These criteria may be distinct from those used by other tracks at the same residency program. For example, a research track may prioritize candidates with advanced degrees (e.g., PhD, MSc) or prior publications more heavily than the categorical program. Despite this, it may be worthwhile to have all track applicants interview for the categorical program as well as the specialty track to make sure the applicants meet all the selection criteria for the categorical program in terms of medical knowledge, clinical skills, and desired personality/character traits, along with the track-specific selection criteria. When creating a new track through the NRMP, there are risks related to the match process. The program should determine what occurs if there are unmatched positions in the track, for example, reverting to categorical positions. The new track may be more competitive or less competitive than the categorical track, but this will not become clear until match data are available. Offering tracks can change the number and quality of applicants to the entire residency program. One family medicine residency program found that in the years following the creation of a scholarly track, their program received significantly more applications for residency, and the applicants had higher scores on standardized tests and medical school evaluations [21].

If a track is not part of an NRMP match, programs have multiple options regarding recruitment and selection. Some tracks may offer participation to a limited number of residents, whereas some may be available to any resident who wants to participate. Programs could require track selection at a particular point in residency. For example, residents may be asked to apply to the track at the start of their intern year to participate in a longitudinal experience across their entire residency. Alternatively, programs may choose to let new interns explore various tracks and solicit applications after a designated period of time, such as 6 or 12 months. Another option that offers the most flexibility is to allow residents to opt into the track at any time; however, with this model, residents may not complete all curricular elements of the track. When residents do not have to rank a preferred track via NRMP, programs may also have the flexibility to allow residents to pursue multiple tracks during residency.

Postgraduate or Other Non-Residency Tracks

Although many new training tracks are residency tracks, there may be opportunities for designated training tracks for fellowship trainees, other postgraduate trainees, or faculty. These tracks would be expected to have unique funding structures and requirements, as they are unlikely to fall under the purview of the ACGME (in contrast to ACGME-accredited fellowship training programs). They may be multidisciplinary and thus have multiple accreditation or governing bodies' regulations to consider or may be less strictly regulated if there are no formal degrees or certifications conferred on participants upon completion. Postgraduate tracks may also be smaller than residency tracks; thus, attention should be paid to program sustainability while designing, implementing, and evaluating these new training tracks. These tracks may increase awareness of various training opportunities within and beyond the institution that are also of interest to residents in specialized tracks. They may also increase the institution's available residency track faculty and mentors through advanced training of postgraduate and multidisciplinary faculty and staff.

Postgraduate training tracks may aim to bring together specific groups, such as women [22] or those who come from groups that are underrepresented in medicine [23, 24], to provide a forum for community and skills-building. They may also be aimed at participants with a shared interest or academic focus. These programs can exist at the institutional level or outside of the institution, such as through professional societies. Programs aimed at providing participants with leadership [25], educational [26, 27], or research [28] skills exist at multiple institutions. Many professional societies have programs with similar goals, which bring together participants from a variety of institutions. The Academic Pediatric Association, for example, has multiple training programs to enhance participants' policy or medical education skills (Health Policy Scholars Program [29], Educational Scholars Program [30]), and the Robert Wood Johnson Foundation provides research training through its National Clinician Scholars Program [31]. Institutional tracks typically require leadership approval for participation, such as agreement by a participant's fellowship PD, division chief, or department chair. Those outside of a clinician's institution likely still require leadership buy-in, which can be monetary, such as contributing funding or protected time for their staff's participation, or less formal, such as approval to participate in a program without financial support.

Postgraduate or faculty tracks may take advantage of the fact that many fellowship programs or faculty positions have some academic protected time built into existing schedules. This means that programs, at least initially, could potentially be designed to enhance participants' skills or provide key training or faculty development experiences without additional dedicated funding [32]. This can allow track leaders to evaluate the program and use data and evaluation metrics to apply for funding to expand or otherwise improve support for pilot programs.

As leaders are looking to start a new postgraduate training track, the application process will need to be designed to fit the needs of the particular track from the start. These tracks are unlikely to use the NRMP application process that is used for residency and fellowship training programs (at least initially). In the early stages of a new postgraduate track, the application process may be less formal, potentially utilizing "word of mouth" or leaders' existing networks to recruit participants. This process may become increasingly formal as awareness and interest in the track improve, leading to a higher number of applicants.

As with any new training track, the curricular elements of a postgraduate training track should be thoughtfully designed with educational theory at the forefront and leaders should use any existing literature or internal data to inform the design of their track. Additionally, compared to residency training tracks, leaders of postgraduate training tracks may benefit from building flexibility around scheduling and into curricular elements of the program early on. As postgraduate and faculty development tracks are likely to include participants from a broader range of clinical specialties, participants' interests and clinical schedules may vary widely. For example, a postgraduate multidisciplinary advanced advocacy training program found that flexibility around scheduling was key to its success, as participants were from disciplines with a mix of shift schedules, clinic-based schedules, research blocks, and service weeks or months [32]. Similarly, as postgraduate track members are further along in their careers, they may have defined academic interests. Therefore, tracks should balance ensuring there are core competencies that all participants achieve while tailoring curricula to individuals' specific interests to optimize the program's effectiveness.

Evaluate the New Track

After implementation, program leaders must determine how to evaluate the new track. The Kirkpatrick Model for evaluation [33], typically cited in curriculum development, provides a framework that is also useful in planning the evaluation of a track.

Kirkpatrick Level 1 (participants' reaction, satisfaction, and engagement) and Level 2 (knowledge, attitudes, or self-assessed skills) may be measured by surveys related to specific learning experiences or as track-wide evaluations. Individual rotations from the track can be evaluated using residency-wide processes. It may be more challenging to create an evaluation that captures non-rotation experiences in the track, such as longitudinal projects and lecture series. Sending surveys to residents who are in the track can yield useful information, although this may have limitations due to the number of residents eligible to take the survey and the response rate. Track-specific questions added to residency-wide annual program evaluations may be a strategy that yields a better response rate but may offer less detail about the track. It is also important to note that resident evaluations of a track are subject to program-wide factors. For example, residents in a primary care track may express that frequent backup calls to cover inpatient services affected patient continuity in the outpatient setting. Track leaders can advocate for program-wide needs (like backup coverage) to minimally interfere with track experiences, but the degree to which this is possible may be outside the control of the track leaders, even though it may significantly affect the resident experience.

Level 3 (change in behavior with application of learning) may require strategies that are more time- and resource-intensive but provide richer and more actionable data than lower-level evaluation methods. The methods used must align with the learning objectives, such as observation by faculty to assess teaching skills of a resident in a medical education track or review of EHR documentation for a primary care track resident. The depth of evaluation desired, and needed faculty time, may help support the need for protected FTE for track leadership. Level 4 (patient/community/societal level results or return on organizational investment) may be challenging to attribute to educational interventions, but surveying alumni can show if the goals of the track are being met by individuals who completed the curriculum and are now in practice. If alumni continue to use the skills they developed during the track, this underscores the relevance of the track goals and the impact of the curriculum. Feedback from evaluations can be used for continued justification of the track and program improvements. Track funders may have specific priority outcomes such as post-residency career paths, changes to the practice environment, residency recruitment statistics, or other outcomes. Track leaders should work to evaluate these metrics rigorously, as existing or future funding may be contingent upon success in these domains.

Conclusion

Creating a new residency track is a complex but potentially rewarding endeavor that requires careful planning, strong institutional support, and ongoing evaluation. The process begins with identifying the rationale and conducting a thorough needs assessment to determine the goals and structure of the track. Securing buy-in from key individuals, recruiting passionate and qualified leaders, and designing an innovative curriculum tailored to the track's objectives are all critical steps. Funding considerations, recruitment strategies, and integration with existing residency program structures and culture must also be thoughtfully addressed.

Once implemented, rigorous evaluation of the new track is essential to demonstrate its value, identify areas for improvement, and justify its continuation or expansion. This evaluation should encompass multiple levels, from participant satisfaction to changes in behavior and, ideally, long-term career outcomes. By following a structured approach to development, and maintaining a commitment to continuous improvement, residency programs can successfully establish new tracks that enhance educational opportunities, address evolving healthcare and societal needs, and prepare residents for diverse career paths in pediatrics.

References

1. Paradise Black NM, Black EW, Rivkees SA. Implementation of a novel track-based pediatric residency training program. J Pediatr. 2014;165(6):1076–7. https://doi.org/10.1016/j.jpeds.2014.08.053.
2. Lichtenstein C, Hoffman BD, Moon RY. How do US pediatric residency programs teach and evaluate community pediatrics and advocacy training? Acad Pediatr. 2017;17(5):544–9. https://doi.org/10.1016/J.ACAP.2017.02.011.
3. Thomas PA, Kern DE, Hughes MT, Chen BY. Curriculum development for medical education: a six-step approach. Johns Hopkins University Press; 2015.
4. Sweigart JR, Tad-Y D, Kneeland P, Williams MV, Glasheen JJ. Hospital medicine resident training tracks: developing the hospital medicine pipeline. J Hosp Med. 2017;12(3):173–6. https://doi.org/10.12788/JHM.2703.
5. Community Pediatrics Training Initiative. Accessed 30 July 2024. https://www.aap.org/en/advocacy/community-health-and-advocacy/community-pediatrics-training-initiatives/.
6. Hoffman BD, Barnes M, Ferrell C, et al. The community health and advocacy milestones profile: a novel tool linking community pediatrics and advocacy training to assessment of milestones-based competence in pediatric residency training. Acad Pediatr. 2016;16(4):309–13. https://doi.org/10.1016/J.ACAP.2016.03.006.
7. D'souza RS, Langford B, D'Souza S, Rose S, Long T. Characteristics of designated institutional officials and sponsoring institutions of ACGME-accredited training programs. J Grad Med Educ. 2021;13(1):70. https://doi.org/10.4300/JGME-D-20-00313.1.
8. The 8-Step Process for Leading Change | Dr. John Kotter. Accessed 29 July 2024. https://www.kotterinc.com/methodology/8-steps/.
9. Kitson C. Leading change. Ment Health Today. 2007;(January):16–8.
10. PLUS: Pediatric Leaders Advancing Health Equity Program | Department of Pediatrics. Accessed 11 Aug 2024. https://pediatrics.ucsf.edu/graduate-medical-education-programs/san-francisco-residency/programs-tracks-and-pathways/plus.
11. Leadership in Advocacy, Under-resourced Communities and Health Equity (LAUnCH) Track | Children's National Hospital. Accessed 11 Aug 2024. https://www.childrensnational.org/for-healthcare-professionals/healthcare-education/graduate-medical-education/residencies-and-fellowships/pediatric-residency-program/curriculum-overview/residency-training-tracks/launch-track.
12. Tracks - BCRP. Accessed 11 Aug 2024. https://bcrp.childrenshospital.org/program/tracks/.

13. Regan L, Stahmer S, Nyce A, et al. Scholarly tracks in emergency medicine. Acad Emerg Med. 2010;17(Suppl 2). https://doi.org/10.1111/J.1553-2712.2010.00890.X.
14. ACGME Answers: Explaining GME Position Allotment. Accessed 29 July 2024. https://www.acgme.org/newsroom/blog/2022/acgme-answers-explaining-gme-position-allotment/.
15. Barajaz M, Turner T. Starting a new residency program: a step-by-step guide for institutions, hospitals, and program directors. Med Educ Online. 2016;21(1). https://doi.org/10.3402/MEO.V21.32271.
16. Everything you need to know about CHGME. Accessed 29 July 2024. https://www.childrenshospitals.org/content/public-policy/fact-sheet/everything-you-need-to-know-about-chgme.
17. Coughlin CG, Michelson KA, DeLong AJ, Stewart AM. Federal funding for children's hospitals: challenges and critical shortages for pediatric care. Pediatrics. 2023;152(4). https://doi.org/10.1542/PEDS.2023-061714/193944.
18. Eden J, Berwick D, Wilensky G, Medical Education C on the G and F of G, Services B on HC, Medicine I of. GME Financing. In: Graduate medical education that meets the nation's health needs. National Academies Press (US); 2014. Accessed 29 July 2024. https://www.ncbi.nlm.nih.gov/books/NBK248024/.
19. Graduate Medical Education Funding. Accessed 29 July 2024. https://www.ncsl.org/health/graduate-medical-education-funding
20. Lichtenstein C, Cora-Bramble D, Ottolini M, Agrawal D. Is there a return on a children's hospital's investment in a Pediatric residency's community health track? A cost analysis. J Community Health. 2018;43(2):372–7. https://doi.org/10.1007/S10900-017-0433-5.
21. Celebi JM, Nguyen CT, Sattler AL, Stevens MB, Lin SY. Education for Primary Care Impact of a scholarly track on quality of residency program applicants Impact of a scholarly track on quality of residency program applicants. 2016;27(6):478–81. https://doi.org/10.1080/14739879.2016.1197049.
22. Women at Children's Hospital (W@TCH) | Children's National Hospital | Children's National Hospital. Accessed 24 July 2024. https://www.childrensnational.org/about-us/dei/women-at-childrens-hospital
23. Guevara JP, Adanga E, Avakame E, Carthon MB. Minority faculty development programs and underrepresented minority faculty representation at US Medical schools. JAMA. 2013;310(21):2297–304. https://doi.org/10.1001/JAMA.2013.282116.
24. Childs E, Yoloye K, Bhasin RM, Benjamin EJ, Assoumou SA. Retaining faculty from underrepresented groups in academic medicine: results from a needs assessment. South Med J. 2023;116(2):157. https://doi.org/10.14423/SMJ.0000000000001510.
25. Fundamentals of Leadership Program | The Center for Faculty Excellence at the GW School of Medicine and Health Sciences. Accessed 28 July 2024. https://cfe.smhs.gwu.edu/fundamentals-leadership-program.
26. The SMHS Academy of Education Scholars | The Center for Faculty Excellence at the GW School of Medicine and Health Sciences. Accessed 28 July 2024. https://cfe.smhs.gwu.edu/smhs-academy-education-scholars.
27. Boston Children's Hospital Academy for Teaching and Educational Innovation and Scholarship | Office of Faculty Development | Research | Boston Children's Hospital. Accessed 28 July 2024. https://www.childrenshospital.org/research/office-faculty-development/boston-childrens-hospital-academy-teaching-and-educational-innovation-and-scholarship.
28. Pediatric Health Services Research Fellowship | Department of Population Medicine. Accessed 28 July 2024. https://www.populationmedicine.org/teaching/fellowships/pediatric-health-services-research-fellowship.
29. Health Policy Scholars Program (HPSP) - Academic Pediatric Association. Accessed 24 July 2024. https://www.academicpeds.org/program/health-policy-scholars-program/.
30. Educational Scholars Program (ESP) - Academic Pediatric Association. Accessed 24 July 2024. https://www.academicpeds.org/program/educational-scholars-program/.
31. About Us | NCSP National Clinician Scholars Program. Accessed 24 July 2024. https://nationalcsp.org/about-us.
32. Stewart AM, Greenberg J, Barnes KW, Winn A. Innovation in advanced advocacy training through clinician partnerships with institutional government relations. Acad Pediatr. 2024; https://doi.org/10.1016/J.ACAP.2024.06.010.
33. Kirkpatrick JD, Kirkpatrick WK. Kirkpatrick's four levels of training evaluation. Association for Talent Development; 2016.

8 Developing One's Residency Leadership Team

Margaret (Meg) McNamara
and Michelle Thompson

Building Your Residency Leadership Team

Building your team is one of the most exciting and important responsibilities that you undertake early in your term as program director (PD). The thoughtful selection of your teammates is critical for success in your own role as well as for how your program develops and supports your residents. It is also central to the enjoyment of your work together. You have several teams to think about: your core faculty team, your administrative staff team, the chief residents, and your informal "back-up" team when you need mentorship, advice, or assistance in getting things done.

There are a variety of factors to consider in building your team, including compliance with Accreditation Council for Graduate Medical Education (ACGME) requirements, program needs, work styles and personalities, and balancing perspectives and skill sets. The first thing to know is the full-time equivalent (FTE) allocated for your team. For both faculty and administrative team members, FTE for program leadership is based, at a minimum, on ACGME program requirements related to the number of trainees in your program [1]. This provision ensures that even institutions without significant resources have the essential complement of people needed to run the program. You may be able to negotiate additional FTE with your Department Chair, Vice Chair of Education, or Designated Institutional Officer (DIO) if you can make a compelling case to demonstrate the need, and resources are available. Depending on reporting and revenue streams within your institution, you may have significant influence or very little input about the administrative staff who support the program, which we will discuss in detail later.

Your core faculty team needs to be comprised of the key people who regularly work with you to execute your vision, give you honest feedback, help you to avoid pitfalls, and share the load in tackling challenges, as well as the rewards and satisfaction when things go well. If the FTE that your institution provides for the PD position exceeds what is required by the ACGME based on program size, consider your overall responsibilities to determine if it will be more advantageous to keep that time for your own work versus redistributing it to an associate program director (APD). It is helpful to continue enough of your own clinical work to ensure that you have some interactions with residents outside of your administrative leadership role and that you stay in touch with issues and workflows in the clinical learning environment, since this may influence some of

M. (Meg) McNamara (✉)
University of California San Francisco,
San Francisco, CA, USA
e-mail: Margaret.McNamara@ucsf.edu

M. Thompson
CHLA, Los Angeles, CA, USA

H. McPhillips et al. (eds.), *Graduate Medical Education in Pediatrics*, Excellence in Medical Education 3, https://doi.org/10.1007/978-3-032-12952-9_8

your priorities as PD. The ACGME requires the program director to participate in clinical activity consistent with their specialty.

Beyond FTE allocation, there are no hard rules from the ACGME or the Association of Pediatric Program Directors (APPD) about how to structure the core faculty team. It is advisable to consult your Chair and/or your institution's GME office to understand if there are any restrictions on how you approach this process. Early decisions include whether to allocate the same amount of FTE to each APD and whether you will have different "levels" within the team (i.e., Associate and Assistant PDs who may be more junior versus all Associate PDs). How you determine this depends on how you decide to structure their responsibilities to complement your skills and meet the needs of your program. Some PDs assign APD duties based on content or a focus area (e.g., recruitment, assessment, curriculum, and mentoring) while others do so related to clinical sites or services (e.g., inpatient, outpatient, continuity clinic, and individualized curriculum), or some other combinations. Some programs have the same FTE allocated for each APD with an expectation of equal contribution, with some shared common tasks, such as advising, rotation oversight, and the clinical competency committee, and with more fluid assignments of projects or activities based on what is needed. There is not one "right way" to do this; think about what seems most useful and beneficial to support you in your role as PD and to serve the program. Consider reaching out to other programs that are similar in size and/or mission, both inside and outside your institution, to discuss the pros and cons of the different ways to structure the team.

How do you know who you want on your team? It may take you some time to figure out who you want or need to have on your leadership team. This is highly variable depending on whether you are new to an institution or you were already a core member of the residency leadership team before starting as PD. Who are the current members of your team, how do they work together, and how will they work with you in your new position? What are the pressing needs of the program, and is this the right group to address them? Who are the teammates you need to implement your vision? [2]. You may be stepping into a position where there is a well-functioning team that needs little or no adjustment, or perhaps it is time for a substantial change to optimize the team's effectiveness. The pace of building your team will depend on several factors, including timing in the academic year as this relates to appointments and FTE allocation, prior commitments that may need to be honored, and how much time you need to assess areas in the program that require development or change.

If there is already an established leadership team, meet with each of them individually to hear their opinions about what is going well and what are the areas of challenge, as well as to assess their level of interest and commitment in continuing to serve in their role. Be sure to include other perspectives as you solicit this information about what is going well and what needs attention so that you have a fuller understanding of your tasks. Make sure to include perspectives from staff, residents of all levels, and other stakeholders. If you plan to make changes to your team, it is advisable to talk in advance with your Chair/Vice Chair of Education to be sure that you have their support and understand any limitations or unseen implications (local politics, etc.) before you act.

When you decide to add or change positions, a formal process with an open call to the faculty, even for part-time roles, is considered best practice. We do not always know who is interested in getting more involved in GME leadership, and there may be fresh perspectives from people who bring new ideas and skills to your team. An open call has the advantage of encouraging a diverse applicant pool, including those who have been historically excluded from leadership roles. Diversity encompasses a variety of factors, including race, ethnicity, age, gender and gender identity, people with disability, and life/work experience. There is ample, longstanding evidence in the literature about the benefits of diverse teams in improving effectiveness and increasing innovation. Everyone on the leadership team needs to be committed to supporting diversity and creating a culture of belonging in your program and the workplace. Your trainees, colleagues, and applicants will take note of who is on your team and who has a seat at the table. Representation matters and a diverse leadership group may help promote a sense of belonging for those residents from backgrounds who are historically under-represented in medicine. Diversity in your leadership team also aligns with the ultimate goal of the field of Pediatrics to develop a more representative workforce to serve our children and families and to advance health equity [3]. The AAMC's GWIMS Equity Recruitment Toolkit is a helpful resource with strategies for best practices, including implicit bias training, holistic applicant review, and standardization in interviewing processes [4].

Another critical area to reflect on is who will help round out your team to complement your leadership style and fill in any gap areas. For example, if you are someone who tends to be "big picture," make sure you have teammates who are detail-oriented and will focus on the nuances. If you are very focused on relationships, look for someone who brings a more data-driven perspective. If you are highly risk averse or conflict avoidant, bring others on board who will help push you beyond your comfort zone. If you are an inpatient subspecialist, consider including outpatient General Pediatrics colleagues to inform decisions in that arena. In addition to your APDs, Site Directors are required at each clinical site. These roles may involve a small stipend from the clinical site or division or may be filled by an APD.

When the core faculty team is established, it is important to clearly outline roles and responsibilities in writing. At the outset, plan at least twice-yearly performance review meetings for bi-directional feedback in addition to a formal written performance assessment in the spring of each academic year. These touch points set the stage for open and direct discussion about each party's level of satisfaction with the role and can help (re)set expectations. Consider how often your direct reports will meet with you; initially, this may be as often as weekly while you develop your working relationship and establish what needs to be done and how best to do it. There is a lot of work involved in running a program; so, make the most of meeting times and do not meet for the sake of just meeting. Consider asking your APDs to send you a written agenda at least a day before you meet so that you can add to it and/or determine if it is more productive for you to cancel.

As you start your work together, it is key to set expectations about when and how the team will meet to create shared mental models for what needs to be done and how to do it. You may want to employ a standardized tool to illuminate individuals' approaches to work and leadership (e.g., Meyers–Briggs, DISC Assessment). This information can be very helpful to you so that you can intentionally assign projects or working groups based on complementary work styles and skills within your leadership team. Holding periodic (e.g., annual or biannual) retreats for your leadership group can aid in strategic planning for your program and help create an aligned vision as well as strengthen relationships and promote camaraderie among members of the leadership team.

In addition to developing collaboration, effectiveness, and *esprit de corps* with your leadership team, you also want to invest in developing individuals on the team. You can demonstrate your commitment to their growth and development by regularly assessing whether their professional development goals are identified and being met. If they are interested in expanding their networks or advancing skill sets or leadership development, you can assist by sponsoring or referring them for opportunities within your department or institution, or extramural professional organizations. For team members who consistently perform at a high level, look for opportunities to nominate them for awards or for them to participate in courses or programs that could elevate their profiles. You can sponsor their attendance at relevant conferences (e.g., APPD, ACGME, AAMC) and offer to connect them with their counterparts in other programs to develop their portfolios as medical educators. The APPD Fall Meeting traditionally focuses largely on support and key knowledge content for leaders who are new to their roles in GME pediatrics; the annual ACGME meeting may also be helpful for leaders who would benefit from an overview of GME requirements. The APPD Spring Meeting offers a broader platform with topics that are relevant for educators and leaders across the spectrum of pediatrics GME.

Even as you think about building your team now, it will not be long until you may also begin to consider succession planning. Programs and institutions vary in how PDs are selected. Some programs routinely identify an APD who is the "heir apparent" when the PD steps down. Some institutions require a formal search, whether that be local, regional, or national. In any case, it is a good idea to begin "legacy planning" even a couple of years into your role as PD. For places that require an open search, this can help assure that those on your team with an interest have the skills and knowledge to apply for the PD job when you are ready to step away from the role.

Running a residency program is a complex and demanding operation that requires an excellent administrative team. Just as for the core faculty team, FTE for program administration is based, at a minimum, on ACGME program requirements related to the number of trainees. At the outset, determine how the staff administrative team is hired and supervised. Many academic programs have parallel structures with separate budgetary and reporting lines (i.e., academic/faculty and administrative), whereas, in some other programs, the PD may have more direct responsibility for the administrative staff. If the PD is not the direct supervisor for the administrative team, ensure that there is an effective mechanism in place for you to provide feedback and oversee their performance. It is essential for coordinators to understand the many facets of GME and be adequately detail-oriented because there are so many requirements and deadlines to manage. You need a residency coordinator who is trustworthy and on whom you can depend to accomplish many high-stakes administrative tasks that need to be done accurately and punctually to comply with requirements of institutional, funding, licensing, and accreditation bodies. Larger programs may have multiple administrative staff and can consider having an overall program manager who oversees coordinators who are assigned various projects and/or tasks. With multiple staff, some degree of cross-training is highly desirable to prevent a crisis in program management when someone inevitably needs to emergently take time off or unexpectedly leaves the position.

The administrative team works hard and often under pressure, managing many competing priorities and deadlines. Soliciting and valuing their ideas about optimizing the workflow goes a long way in creating a strong team dynamic, high morale, and more job satisfaction. Your administrative staff also possess valuable information regarding interpersonal communication skills and professional behaviors of applicants and residents; it is wise to seek their feedback before ranking intern candidates or selecting chief residents. As you work with the administrative team, ensure that you provide them with context for their work and responsibilities so that they develop a greater understanding of their role in supporting developing pediatricians and the importance of their contributions to GME. Just as with your core faculty team, look for ways to recognize the important contributions of these administrative professionals. This may include sponsoring attendance at professional conferences, nominating them for awards, engaging them in academic projects, and advocating for their compensation or advancement. Supporting your program coordinators in pursuit of Training Administrators for Graduate Medical Education (TAGME) certification can boost their professional development and leadership potential. In addition, APPD's Leadership Empowerment for Advancing Pediatric Education Specialists (LEAPES) is a yearlong leadership program for coordinators, managers, and educational specialists who want to enhance knowledge, skills, and networking to advance their GME careers.

The next team to consider is your chief residents. It is not an exaggeration to say that having the right chief residents can make or break a year. They need to be strong clinicians and teachers. In addition, they must have a high level of professionalism, demonstrate excellent communication and conflict management skills, be capable of performing administrative duties, and be willing to serve as leaders. These roles and responsibilities can be especially challenging given their proximity to the residents as near-peers. It is an extremely difficult job! It is also a role that almost inevitably results in tremendous growth and development, which most former chiefs are glad to have experienced, even if they are ready to be done when the year is over. There are many variations on chief resident selection, so you have a lot of latitude in how you do this. Across the country, some programs are having increasing difficulty in recruiting chiefs due to the demands of the job, along with the potential of relatively lower earnings compared to alternative positions. In cases where graduating senior residents are not identified to fill these important positions, there are various potential solutions. Some programs hire graduates from other programs to serve in this role, some have current senior residents assume "chief duties" for several months of the year, and others offload traditional chief responsibilities to faculty and administrative team members.

Typically, chief resident selection is geared toward the second-year class since commitment to a chief year will affect their timeline for job/fellowship applications, but this also depends on the factors noted earlier. With the recognition that selection methods may involve bias, programs can employ strategies to mitigate bias by using holistic review, engaging multiple diverse representatives in the selection process, and assessing for evidence of bias in past or current selection [6]. There are many ways to select chiefs, with one major decision being whether you will ask a resident to serve in this capacity or whether you invite residents to apply. In either case, the PD and APDs can identify candidates they would like to encourage in this role. To expand the pool, you might also ask residents, fellows, and faculty for nominations. You may want to review CVs as well as their performance in residency. This may help inform a decision about whether candidates have the requisite skills to succeed. It is advisable to ensure that potential chiefs understand the position so that they are prepared to support the program and can thrive in the job; be sure that their perception is generally in line with your expectations for the role. This could be accomplished through a brief written candidate statement outlining why they want to be chief or through interviews with the PD, APDs, site directors, or other key stakeholders. A formal application process can be very informative but may also come with some potential complications. For instance, when there are more people interested than positions available, not being selected may adversely impact morale. In general, if you choose to conduct interviews, it is good practice to have a confidential process to honor some residents' preferences for peers not to know they are applying, and to use standardized questions so you can compare answers among candidates to help mitigate bias in the selection process. Interviews can provide valuable information when you notice what questions candidates have about the job and can assess their level of commitment and enthusiasm for the various aspects of the position. Consider what candidates stand to gain from the year in addition to what you need from them and what they will bring to the program. It is critical to think about the entire chief team in addition to the individual candidate's skills and qualities. You want to balance strengths, skills, and personalities. Be thoughtful about how you will create the team of chiefs, since they need to work closely together and with the whole leadership team.

Another team you will want to focus on building is your "back-up" team. Moving into the role of PD may shift the dynamics of many of your professional relationships. If you continue to work in the same institution, some people may perceive you in your new role as PD to have new "positional power" that could change interactions with some of the key people with whom you previously consulted. If you move to a different program, you may be starting from scratch, and it is then even more important to identify some trusted colleagues who can provide counsel in tough situations or just provide a listening ear. Your longstanding mentors will continue to be crucial to support you in your new role, especially since they likely already know your strengths and weaknesses and, hopefully, can be confided in without fear of judgment when you need feedback or advice. The Chair and/or Vice Chair of Education for your Department are important allies in moving forward with some strategic initiatives or backing you up in cases of significant conflicts or challenges. The GME office (e.g., Associate Dean of GME and/or DIO) will often have useful experience, precedents, or guidance to share on a wide variety of issues or decisions. Peer PDs within your institution can be very helpful consultants who may be willing to band together to tackle local challenges or share best practices and resources. In addition, peer PDs from other pediatric programs can offer invaluable consultation, provide moral support, or serve as thought-partners to brainstorm and collaborate. Find individuals in health system leadership (e.g., the C-suite and Nursing leadership) who can be partners when issues arise in the clinical learning environment, where you may have some influence but insufficient leverage to effect change. Other key informants to identify are colleagues from the disability services management, human resources, labor & employee relations, and legal department. These professionals can provide critical assistance with questions related to accommodations requested by residents, parental or family medical leave, professionalism issues, union contracts, and much more. Liaisons within the ACGME, state licensing board, and American Board of Pediatrics (ABP) are extremely helpful with navigating issues around program requirements, accreditation, and trainee credentialing and certifications.

Finally, a quick note to highlight the importance of developing self-awareness in effectively leading others on your team. Routine engagement in self-reflection and developing self-awareness promotes personal growth and strengthens relational skills. Managing your own well-being and modeling self-care positively impacts the well-being and effectiveness of the entire team [5]. Seek out resources for further developing your leadership skills, such as institutional and professional society-sponsored courses and peer coaching programs. Explore with your Chair or GME office whether there is funding available to support executive coaching or leadership development courses. The APPD LEAD Program is an example of an outstanding 10-month leadership development program for both residency and fellowship program directors. The American Association of Medical Colleges (AAMC) Group on Resident Affairs GME Leadership Competencies published online in 2023 and the ACGME also have some important leadership development resources [6, 7]. As previously mentioned, lean on your network of trusted mentors and peer PDs.

Building a great leadership team is highly impactful and a major opportunity to positively influence your program for years to come. Finding energetic, motivated, committed colleagues who want to invest in your residents' education and training alongside you has the capacity to significantly improve your program and add immeasurably to the enjoyment and satisfaction that you derive as PD. Choose wisely. Go team!

References

1. Accreditation Council for Graduate Medical Education (ACGME). Program Requirements for Graduate Medical Education in Pediatrics. 2024. https://www.acgme.org/globalassets/pfassets/programrequirements/2025-prs/320_pediatrics_2025.pdf.
2. Watkins MD. Build your team. In: The first 90 days. Harvard Business Review Press; 2013. p. 165–98.
3. Elliott TC. How do we move the needle?: building a framework for diversity, equity, and inclusion within graduate medical education. Fam Med. 2021;53(7):556–8. https://doi.org/10.22454/FamMed.2021.199007.
4. American Association of Medical Colleges (AAMC) GWIMS Equity Recruitment Toolkit 2023. https://www.aamc.org/media/23651/download.
5. Shanafelt T, Trockel M, Rodriguez A, Logan D. Wellness-centered leadership: equipping health

care leaders to cultivate physician well-being and professional fulfillment. Acad Med. 2021;96(5):641–51. https://doi.org/10.1097/ACM.0000000000003907.
6. Gustafson S, Poitevien P, Acholonu R, Blankenburg R, Fromme HB. Opportunities for mitigating bias in the process and priorities for pediatric chief resident selection. Acad Pediatr. 2022. PubMedID 34902563.
7. American Association of Medical Colleges (AAMC) Group on Resident Affairs GME Leadership Competencies: Monograph and Self-Assessment Tool. Fall 2023. https://www.aamc.org/career-development/affinity-groups/group-resident-affairs/aamc-gra-gme-leadership-competencies.

9 Program Director Career Advancement and Leadership

Rebecca R. Swan and Brian Lurie

Mentorship

Guidance provided by those more experienced is important for all professionals, and this is true for program directors. Mentorship is critical for support, goal setting, networking opportunities, and accountability, as well as perspective and feedback.

Mentors and/or sponsors should be sought at multiple levels for different potential purposes. A program director requires knowledge of important departmental and institutional politics that impact the clinical and education environments. Mentorship is also important for guidance on career planning, including staying on track for promotion within your institution, next steps in obtaining leadership skills, and identifying opportunities for advancement, including local, regional, and national roles.

Department

Program directors should seek mentorship specifically around leadership and administrative skills. Within the department, the mentor may be a division chief, a more seasoned program director, or the Vice Chair of Education. It is important to establish a relationship with the mentor, including regularly scheduled meetings. One needs to set goals as well as have bi-directional expectations for the next 1, 5, and 10 years. As goals are set, the program director can discuss the necessary skills to achieve them with mentors, including self-assessment of current abilities and opportunities. Additionally, program directors should recognize the importance of establishing a relationship with the Chair. Education is only *part* of the mission of most departments but must remain a focus. Educational leaders help chairs maintain that focus and, in turn, chairs can offer mentorship and career guidance to the other members of their leadership team.

Institutional

Institutional mentors are also important for program directors, as they represent knowledge and experience within the broader graduate medical education environment locally. Mentorship at this level may be more senior program directors in other departments or leadership within the

R. R. Swan (✉)
Vanderbilt University Medical Center,
Nashville, TN, USA
e-mail: rebecca.swan@vumc.org

B. Lurie
Brown University Health - Hasbro Children's,
Providence, RI, USA

H. McPhillips et al. (eds.), *Graduate Medical Education in Pediatrics*, Excellence in Medical Education 3, https://doi.org/10.1007/978-3-032-12952-9_9

Graduate Medical Education (GME) Office, for example, the Designated Institutional Officer (DIO). These mentors can be excellent resources to help orient new program directors, both in structured programs through the GME office and through sharing lessons learned. It is important to have trusted resources to ask institutional-specific GME questions, to brainstorm problems (including navigating departmental conflicts), to commiserate challenges, and to receive trusted feedback.

Extra-Mural

Developing extra-mural mentorship may take time. The Association of Pediatric Program Directors (APPD) is an organization that allows program directors to build a community through annual meetings as well as regional connections throughout the year. Establishing a relationship with more senior program directors in pediatrics allows mentorship that is naïve to the internal politics of an institution, which can be helpful when discussing issues involving personnel; they also often have innovative ideas for problems and can assist with career planning based on their experiences and journeys.

Skill Building

Leadership Skills

A program director is selected based on recognition of leadership skills and achievements as an educator, and potential for growth in both areas. This decision can be made by a search committee, a Vice Chair of Education, a Department Chairperson, some combination of these, or another administrator. That said, there are specific skills that a program director needs to be successful.

A program director is primarily the leader of the training program. Much has been written about being a leader, and much has been studied about what it takes to be a good leader. Certain attributes and skills are consistently mentioned. Honesty and credibility are the most common attributes looked for in a leader. A team needs to be able to trust their leader before they are going to follow them. Honesty, ethics, and values are closely inter-related and often noted in descriptions of strong leaders as the characteristics most desired to be emulated. Jim Kouzes and Barry Posner published *The Leadership Challenge* in 1983 on this topic; the seventh edition came out in 2023.

Being able to share a vision for the program in an optimistic manner is another important skill. Program directors must be able to develop a long-term vision for the program and communicate that vision to others. This includes setting goals and objectives as well as creating a strategic plan for achieving them. Maintaining the status quo is management; leading into the future through creativity and innovation with teamwork is the role of a leader. It is about inspiring trainees and faculty, especially in times of change, challenge, or uncertainty. Expanding programs, offering new rotations or new clinical sites, responding to Accreditation Council for Graduate Medical Education (ACGME) citations, or navigating the unexpected, like a pandemic, require a leader who has appropriate leadership skills and styles for each of those situations. A program director may have a certain leadership style that has worked in the past but will need to pursue education on other styles to broaden their toolkit in navigating challenges.

Leadership also requires adaptability, which relies on emotional intelligence to respond to circumstances, situations, and individuals. Daniel Goleman, a psychologist who has written extensively on leadership styles, describes a framework of six leadership styles based on emotional intelligence [1]. Emotional intelligence requires understanding and managing one's own emotions while also understanding and responding to others' emotions. Understanding these styles and developing the skills to utilize different styles as situations dictate is important for leadership success. Utilizing a leadership style inventory or assessment, with appropriate guidance or coaching to build skills, can be helpful; these are often part of structured leadership courses recommended for career advancement. The Leadership Practices Inventory [2] is an example of such a tool that is frequently utilized as both a self-assessment and an assessment by supervisors and direct reports. The inventory provides both quantitative and qualitative feedback on leadership behaviors to identify strengths and areas for improvement.

Program directors should consider the utility of executive coaching. This type of leadership coach works with senior-level leaders to refine skills around strategic thinking, decision making, and communication. This is a resource to be considered as part of negotiations for a new role or position, to provide for the cost and time commitment.

Personnel Management and Team Building

Personnel management and team building is an important task for a program director. A program director is in the unique position of being "middle management," leading trainees and faculty in the education environment, and the skills of leading direct reports are different than directing peers. The first team for a program director to consider is the program leadership team: program coordinators or managers, associate program directors, and chief residents. A program director cannot function alone, and job satisfaction is clearly related to having a supportive team structure. Program directors must be able to build and maintain a cohesive team of faculty members and residents, fostering a collaborative and supportive environment.

Members of the leadership team may have clearly identified roles, for example, the coordinator or manager; both human resources and the ACGME provide guidance for these positions. Coordinators or managers, depending on the tenure of a job, may provide an important historical perspective on both the program and department. Providing feedback and career development opportunities for these important staff members plays a key role for the program director, as being a leader includes supporting and advocating for the careers of team members.

Associate program directors' positions vary between institutions. Some have well-delineated roles, for example, organizing retreats, managing committees, and taking responsibility for specific aspects of curriculum or recruitment. Others have more fluid positions where they work to assist the program director more generally. It is preferable to have job descriptions with expectations and deliverables, recognizing that a transition to a more structured team should be gradual and discussed openly with all involved parties, especially in the situation of a program director coming into a new institution.

Chief residents are in a unique role, serving as junior faculty for a year. Program directors are often responsible for the selection of these leaders and thus have the opportunity to mentor them in their professional development, in addition to collaborating with them to lead the residency program.

There are other skills that program directors will draw upon daily. They must be able to manage their time effectively, balancing administrative tasks with clinical responsibilities and teaching duties. The program director must participate in clinical activity consistent with the specialty (ACGME). This provides credibility as a clinician-educator and role-model for the trainees and faculty, as well as helps the program director maintain clinical skills for future positions. Program directors must be able to make informed decisions quickly and effectively, weighing the pros and cons of different options and considering the impact on the program and its stakeholders. At the same time, there is space for brainstorming and collaboration with others, to build morale and constructive interaction during team retreats and other team-building events.

Program Management

Program directors' primary responsibilities involve maintaining accredited programs to allow graduation of board-eligible trainees. This requires an understanding of the ACGME program for curriculum and program structure, as well as faculty and leadership. In addition, program directors need to be aware of the policies and procedures for board-certification and documentation requirements. This includes an understanding of standards for certification as well as nonstandard training pathways. Program directors wishing to advance in areas of program and/or trainee certification can pursue involvement in national organizations to consider redesign of standards or requirements, as well as participation in pilot studies of such redesigns; involvement in national activities with these organizations leads to networking and collaborations, important for career advancement both within a home institution and beyond.

Communication Skills

Communication skills are central to effective leadership. Program directors must communicate effectively with trainees, faculty, staff, and administration in order to ensure the program runs smoothly. Communication is bi-directional by all parties; it is important for leaders to know when to talk and when to actively listen. Open communication is important with the goal of being appropriately transparent about visions and challenges. Ensure communication is clear, with specific goals and follow-up identified. Practice asking open-ended questions as well as providing feedback. Acknowledge information received, including feedback, act on it if possible, and report back on the outcome.

Leading from the Middle

Managing from the middle is an important challenge to address. Supervising trainees, leading direct reports on the leadership team, and managing faculty as part of the education team are all critical aspects of the role of program director; success with these elements is important for career advancement in higher leadership roles. Additionally, the program director has a unique relationship with the department chair. The chair must balance the needs of the residency program, including ACGME accreditation requirements, with the needs of the overall department, which includes the clinical and research missions in addition to the education mission. This can result in the need to negotiate and compromise, with a goal of maintaining a supportive working relationship with the chair.

Once a program director is settled into the role, it is useful to assess current skills and gaps in skills, both for the current job as well as for future roles in leadership. Self-assessment can be useful, but asking mentors or utilizing tools such as 360 assessments can also be valuable. The skills a program director uses daily provide the portfolio of translatable skills for the next leadership role in the future.

Change Management

One of the essential skills for a leader, especially a program director, is leading change to transform the organization due to internal motivation or external factors. This can be a challenge when a program director is functioning as both a manager and a leader. A manager is charged with implementing processes and maintaining an organization. A leader, on the other hand, focuses on innovation and adapting an organization to changes. Being able to articulate the vision and rationale for change, organize a team to implement the changes, and remain open to feedback in a non-defensive manner are advanced leadership skills. Advanced roles in organizations, either in medical education or operations, rely on leaders who can lead and manage change [3].

Running Meetings

As one assumes higher leadership roles, running a meeting becomes more of a responsibility and less of a participatory activity. Program directors require strong skills in running meetings to ensure that they are productive, efficient, and effective. There is a skill to running effective meetings, to ensure goals are accomplished and the correct participants are involved who feel valued and heard. Setting agendas, determining correct attendees, assigning responsibilities, and ensuring follow-up on tasks and deliverables are all important aspects of effectively running meetings.

Negotiation Skills

Program directors require strong negotiation skills to successfully navigate the complex and multifaceted healthcare education environment. Negotiating is classically described as a skill that physicians are often not well prepared for or comfortable with. Yet, it is a critical skill for leaders, both negotiating personally as well as for their teams and programs. Preparation is an important part of negotiating, and involves understanding goals, potential areas for compromise and how leadership styles factor into the process. Communication plays a role here, both active listening as well as clearly stating one's own interests and needs to prevent misunderstandings.

Conflict Management

Program directors must be able to manage conflicts and disagreements between residents, faculty members, and other stakeholders in a professional and diplomatic manner. Conflict is ubiquitous in work or team environments when people have differing opinions, beliefs, or ideas. If managed well, it can lead to positive change; if not, it can be destructive and undermine progress toward goals and leadership stability. Depending on personality type, conflict management is a skill often self-assessed as deficient or "less confident." A commonly referenced framework to approach conflict is the Thomas–Kilmann Conflict Mode Instrument, which approaches conflict management through two dimensions: assertiveness and cooperativeness [4]. This instrument has been used in leadership courses for healthcare leaders since first described in the 1970s. This framework explains conflict and allows a self-assessment of preferred conflict management styles. Once a leader understands his or her preferred style or styles to manage conflict, he or she can better understand when other styles might be more advantageous and then begin to develop those skills.

GME Finance

Graduate medical education financing is one of the most challenging topics for program directors. It is a complicated issue because of the complexities of funding, both at the institutional and national levels. Program directors are encouraged to have a basic understanding of funding to be able to advocate for their programs. Learning basic financial terms to help manage resource allocation when considering program expansion or development, in addition to other budgetary nuances, is a skill that is important for advancement in educational leadership. Knowing who completes the program or education budget and asking to review it as well as meeting with the department financial administrator is a starting point to understand finances. Establishing regular meetings with the financial leadership to understand pressures as a department and system that impact the program's budget can be useful. Having this knowledge is paramount to being transparent with trainees about funding decisions.

Career Advancement

As a program director, there are several career advancement opportunities to consider. These include higher leadership roles within academic medicine. Many program directors advance within their own institutions or are recruited to other institutions to higher positions, such as Vice Chair of Education, DIO, Associate Dean, and Dean roles. Program Directors can also become leaders in professional organizations, such as the American Academy of Pediatrics (AAP), the American Board of Pediatrics (ABP), the American Osteopathic Board of Pediatrics

(AOBP), the APPD, and the ACGME. Although some are voluntary roles, some are career advancement into paid positions. Program directors can provide consulting services to other residency programs or medical institutions to help them improve their programs, either as visiting professors or consultants. These experiences can help shape the trajectory of career paths for program directors.

The Association of American Medical Colleges (AAMC) Group on Resident Affairs (GRA) published an online reference entitled *2023 AAMC GRA Graduate Medical Education Leadership Competencies (GMLECs)* in 2023 [5, 6]. This publication is a useful resource for program directors seeking career advancement, both within graduate medical education and elsewhere. The leadership competencies were presented in a framework of four domains of leadership competencies necessary for success as an institutional-level GME leader: foundational attributes, leadership capabilities, knowledge and skills, and essential functions.

Foundational attributes encompass those personal qualities that a person brings to the leadership role. These include emotional intelligence, communication, professionalism, commitment to the team, and being values driven. Communication as an effective leader requires active listening and clear communication styles appropriate for the team. An environment built on trust welcomes feedback and learns from it. A leader role models integrity, humility, and personal responsibility, and in doing so, inspires the same in others. One's adaptability with change and ability to learn from mistakes, focus on system-thinking oriented to results, and the courage to accept risk and inspire others to do the same are all part of foundational attributes.

Leadership capabilities encompass the skills needed to be successful in achieving the institutional GME mission. This includes the development and evaluation of educational programs and learning environments, role-modeling inclusive and diverse partnerships, and relationships, developing others on the team to advance the GME mission, and building synergy among the stakeholders to achieve overall goals. Understanding organizational structure and policies to allow quality improvement, innovation, and effective strategic planning is also a critical leadership ability.

As program directors consider career advancement, the skills to build relationships to achieve GME and institutional goals are important to consider. Often, advanced roles include working across groups that have disparate goals but have interdependent working relationships. Fostering diversity of thought, backgrounds, and ideas, pursuing partners appropriate for the mission and vision, and managing conflicts are vital skills.

Successful institutional GME leadership embodies developing the people on the team. Understanding adult learning theory and education methodology, as well as applying interprofessional education principles, is an important starting point. Professional development for program directors as well as program managers, both development and support, will be the responsibility of an institutional GME leader.

The influence of the health care environment on GME is an important concept to understand, as GME impacts clinical operations and other policies. Institutional GME leaders are seen as experts on institutional and program requirements of the ACGME and other accreditation bodies, both in understanding and operationalizing. Financial skills around budgeting and reporting are expected at this level as well. Additionally, a baseline understanding of relevant laws as well as a collaborative relationship with Human Resources and general counsel are critical.

Essential functions of the institutional GME leader center around obtaining and maintaining institutional and program accreditation. This involves working with the Graduate Medical Education Committee (GMEC), program leadership, and the leadership (including safety and quality officers); a multitude of metrics are required to be followed. Supporting and providing professional development for GME leaders, staff, and faculty is another essential function. These functions are all done within a culture of sustained personal professional development, to encourage and role model innovation and continuous improvement.

The described skillset is not exhaustive but certainly covers much of what a program director would need as a successful graduate medical education leader and beyond. The AAMC provides a GME Leadership Competencies Self/Multi-Rater Assessment Tool [5, 6] that a program director can utilize not only to assess current skills but also to identify areas for growth. Those growth areas can be used to identify resources to prepare for an advanced role in the academic medical setting. Although there are limited leadership development programs specifically for these roles [7], there are opportunities available and focused resources to address specific skill deficits and interest areas.

Skill Building

Graduate Degrees

Graduate degrees are viewed as a benefit when transitioning into leadership roles in medical education, in addition to aiding in the ability to maintain and innovate residency programs. If a program director is interested in advancing their leadership career in medical education, there are graduate degrees, certifications, and courses to help with professional development and enable the cultivation of necessary skills. When considering a graduate degree, multiple options exist, many with different methods and modalities of learning to fit into busy schedules and concurrent job responsibilities. Some of these programs offer part-time options and may include combinations of in-person and virtual learning activities, coaching, mentorship, and group or individualized projects. A selection of these degrees is discussed below, although by no means is this an exhaustive list.

A Master of Education (MEd), a Master of Science in Health Professions Education (MS-HPE), and a Master of Science in Medical Education Leadership are all programs designed to provide a foundation in adult learning theory, curriculum development, educational design, integration of educational technology, and creating and maintaining assessment tools. By earning these types of degrees, learners develop the skills and foundations to complete both qualitative and quantitative research projects to help advance medical education. Programs often help participants become better teachers and provide different modalities for delivering educational content, including advances in educational technology. By obtaining a Master of Education, one develops the leadership skills to be innovative, motivate others to be educational scholars, and develop competencies to implement and maintain programs.

Master of Health Professions Education (MHPE) is a degree program which is a competency-based educational experience that focuses on the theory, research, and practice of education as it applies to health professions environments. In many MHPE programs, the core content can be categorized into five domains: (1) teaching and learning; (2) curriculum development; (3) program evaluation and learner assessment; (4) educational research methods; and (5) leadership and management. Moreover, many MHPE programs can be tailored to the learner's needs and interests, and specific tracks can be crafted to further enhance the relevance of the MHPE degree to GME leadership activities [8].

Another degree one can consider is a Master of Business Administration (MBA). There are programs that are specifically designed for physicians or those in the healthcare industry. These programs focus on developing business acumen, learning economics and finance, especially as it may pertain to the healthcare industry. They promote innovation to improve clinical outcomes, provide education around healthcare policy, and encourage thinking about value-based care. Many programs contain curricular aspects focusing on change management both locally within an institution and as regionally and nationally in addition to teaching ways to think through marketing strategy.

Some program directors have opted to enroll in MBA programs not specifically designed for physicians. These programs offer a similar curriculum, but the student cohort provides additional exposure to leaders in a variety of industries. Working on team projects with leaders from different fields, with different perspectives, experiences, and ideas, can be particularly challenging and enriching.

Many in program leadership have chosen to obtain their Master of Public Health (MPH). These programs typically focus on population and community health and provide skills to promote wellness for patients and populations; these skills can be applied to individual learners, programs, and departments. Many executive MPH programs are targeted towards those in healthcare and include similar education as an MBA, including organizational leadership and management, health policy, advocacy, and health systems. One will develop skills in program design, evaluation, change management, and research techniques. These programs are usually 2 years in length and are designed to be completed while working full time.

Finally, degrees such as Master of Healthcare Administration (MHA) and Master of Health Management (MHM) are designed to provide competencies in managing a healthcare system, focusing on finance, human resources, and leadership. These degrees will provide education around change management, finance, budgeting, healthcare law, ethics, and health policy. These programs will provide skills enabling one to enhance organizational effectiveness [9].

Other Resources

Program directors do not have to pursue another graduate degree for career advancement. Many medical education organizations offer certificate courses, which can help develop leadership skills and provide the needed tools to both effectively run a residency program as well as pursue the career role. The Association of American Medical Colleges (AAMC) offers multiple opportunities for career and leadership development, particularly designed for those who wish to advance in academic medicine. The CORE Leadership Development program is a series of progressive learning experiences addressing the most pressing challenges in healthcare (4). The objectives of this training include the following:

- Helping cultivate one's abilities to lead collaboratively and drive change at their institution.
- Aligning organizational culture to lead change initiatives.
- Developing a systems-thinking approach to decision making and strategy implementation.
- Discovering techniques for influencing others [10].

This program is different from other certificate programs as it aims to expand leadership knowledge as it pertains to medical education, health care, medical research, and community collaborations and helps grow one's ability to lead on their own professional journey, lead teams, lead the department and the mission, and lead the institution.

Another opportunity provided by the AAMC is the GME Leadership Development Certificate Program, which is targeted towards both new and experienced GME leaders. The objectives of this program are as follows:

- Develop and enhance regional and national networks of professional peer groups.
- Understand the differences between management and leadership.
- Develop an educational mission.
- Strengthen the understanding and competency in financial principles around GME.
- Change management techniques and ways to implement in your institution.
- Better understanding of ACGME principles.
- Teach ways to integrate innovation into culture.
- Develop ways to lead the GME enterprise in the role of advocacy for trainees and faculty [10].

Depending on a program director's interests, areas for development, or needs of their program, the AAMC also offers the Healthcare Executive Diversity and Inclusion Certificate Program, designed to develop the competencies leaders need to drive diversity as a core component of excellent healthcare. The Leadership Education and Development Certificate Program (LEAD) is a one-year program which utilizes cohort style learning and self-reflection to enhance one's abilities to develop a strategic vision and set direction, mentor, and coach others, manage effectively, and build within one's organization [10].

The Association of Pediatric Program Directors (APPD) also offers courses in leadership development. Leadership in Educational Academic Development (LEAD), launched in 2012, provides a unique opportunity for pediatric academic leaders in medical education to engage and learn from seasoned program directors, pediatric educators, and other national leaders in pediatrics. Designed for program directors, associate program directors, fellowship directors, associate fellowship directors, and clerkship directors, APPD LEAD is a nine-month educational program that provides outstanding training for educators aspiring to develop the knowledge and skills needed to advance leadership skills in medical education. The LEAD curriculum focuses on organizational leadership, competency-based curriculum development, faculty development, residency and fellowship program administration, scholarship, and career development. The curriculum is paced over three educational conferences, with additional group activities, readings, and project work expected between conferences [11].

Designed for members of the APPD in their first 3 years in a leadership role and who identify as underrepresented in medicine, the Fostering UIM Education Leadership (FUEL) Program aims to increase diversity in pediatric medical education leadership through professional development and mentorship of underrepresented in medicine early career faculty. Participants are exposed to the many careers in pediatric medical education, as well as the professional development opportunities and educational leaders within the APPD community. The program is based on mentorship, sponsorship, and representation with a focus on experiential learning. Program features include an overview of careers in medical education, promotion in education leadership roles, personal career planning, panel discussions and speed mentoring with UIM educational leaders, networking with APPD leadership and members, and membership in the UIM in Pediatrics GME Learning Community [11].

The Academic Pediatric Association also offers multiple faculty development opportunities. One which may be particularly interesting to Program Directors is the Advancing Pediatric Leaders (APL) program. Those who apply need to have at least 5 years at the rank of assistant professor and must be serving in or have accepted a leadership position. Objectives of the program include developing knowledge, skills, and behaviors to apply in leadership, education and coaching, advancing visibility and promotion of scholarship within one's organization and within the APA, and expanding networking opportunities [12]. This program offers personal as well as peer group coaching, a hybrid curriculum using monthly virtual sessions to supplement two in-person meetings during spring Pediatric Academic Society meetings.

Service and Leadership Opportunities

Service and leadership roles are often expected for faculty positions and required for promotion at academic institutions. When planning career goals, meeting with mentors to consider what positions are available and what skills and experiences are needed for them is an important first step. Additionally, it is important to consider how to develop a local, regional, and national presence, which will assist in attaining positions and opportunities as they arise, as well as in building one's portfolio for academic advancement.

Understanding the opportunities that exist in pediatric medical education and logical steps for an individual are important starting points. Within a department, the role of Vice Chair of Education (VCE) is a logical progression in career advancement for a program director. The role of Vice Chair of Education first appeared in the literature in 2010, with the roles and responsibilities of this position varying per institution. The role was created in response to increasing demands for educational leadership in academic departments [13].

The Vice Chair of Education is defined at most places as the educational leadership position responsible for providing oversight to all learners on the continuum from undergraduate medical education (UME) through GME, to promote the educational mission of the department. In a study by McBride et al., published in *The Journal of Pediatrics* in 2020, about a quarter of those surveyed held this position in addition to other leadership positions with education in their department, such as program director or fellowship director, and the majority were mid-career or senior faculty holding the academic rank of associate professor or professor. Most institutions provide allotted FTE time to the role, while some include the position in other educational responsibilities the person currently holds. Only a small percentage receive additional salary. The VCE reports directly to the chair of the department [14].

Unlike residency and fellowship directors whose responsibilities are in part defined by the ACGME or clerkship directors whose responsibilities are defined by the Liaison Committee on Medical Education (LCME) or the Commission on Osteopathic Accreditation (COCA), there are no established guidelines for the Vice Chair of Education. While reviewing the literature, similar themes emerged when comparing the position of Vice Chair of Education in Pediatrics, Internal Medicine, Surgery, and Emergency Medicine, and fell into the categories of administrative, clinical, education, and research. All involved some component of providing oversight of all the educational programs from UME to GME including ensuring the accreditation and quality of these programs, collaborating on curricula development, faculty development, mentorship of faculty, fellows, residents, and students, promotion of medical education scholarship, recruitment, and management of the educational budget [13–16].

Institutionally, another opportunity for increased leadership responsibility includes participating in or becoming the chair of the Graduate Medical Education Committee (GMEC). According to the ACGME, any sponsoring institution with multiple accredited programs must have a GMEC comprised of the Designated Institutional Officer (DIO), representatives from different programs, residents, and a quality improvement or patient safety officer. The responsibilities of the committee include oversight of the quality and educational experiences of their ACGME-accredited programs; oversight of the sponsoring institution's accreditation; development, review, approval, and institution of GME policies and procedures; and many others which can be found on the ACGME website [17].

Many residency program directors advance on to the roles of either the Designated Institutional Official (DIO) or the Dean of Graduate Medical Education. The DIO's responsibilities include ensuring compliance with ACGME institutional, common, and program (residency and fellowship) specific requirements [17]. The DIO has responsibility for and leads or works collaboratively with the GMEC and must do the following tasks:

1. Approve program letters of agreement (PLAs) that govern relationships between each program or participating site, providing a required assignment for residents/fellows in the program.
2. Oversee submissions of the annual update for each program and the sponsoring institution to the ACGME.
3. After GMEC approval, oversee the submission of applications for ACGME accreditation and recognition, for new programs, requests for voluntary withdrawal of programs, and requests for changes in residency and fellowship program complements [17].

Program directors of different GME training programs at that institution will have a reporting relationship with the DIO. The DIO is responsible for the Office of GME and will have oversight over the education and training of interns, residents, and fellows. Furthermore, the DIO maintains the Clinical Learning Environment and will monitor compliance with clinical and educational work hours, ensure wellness, encourage, and support scholarly activities, and monitor and help develop action plans to address citations and areas for improvement identified by the ACGME [17].

The position of Dean of Graduate Medical Education is similar to the DIO, with roles and responsibilities varying based on the institution. As with the DIO, a common responsibility includes collaboration with program directors and hospital leadership to cultivate an inclusive learning environment for GME faculty, staff, residents, and fellows. The Dean of Graduate Medical Education also helps to develop GME programs and ensures continual improvements, monitors quality initiatives, reviews annual program evaluations, and leads the annual institutional review. In addition to providing oversight to GME programs, the Dean of Graduate Medical Education helps develop and implement educational best practices [18].

National Service and Leadership Opportunities

Serving on committees or in leadership roles of national organizations is a way to gain experience in preparation for career advancement. These activities may also count as scholarship and development of a national reputation at many institutions, both of which are necessary for academic promotion. Below is a description of some organizations program directors can join, which provide multiple opportunities for both participation and leadership.

The Association of Pediatric Program Directors' (APPD) mission is to ensure the health and well-being of all children, serving pediatric programs by leading the advancement of medical education, the development of a diverse workforce, the cultivation of an inclusive clinical learning environment, and the promotion of educational innovation and research [11]. There are many opportunities for service and leadership within the APPD. Sharing scholarship through leading enhanced learning sessions and presentations at the Annual Fall and Spring meetings, Pediatric Medical Education Conference, and APPD Forum for Fellowship Directors are accessible introductions to involvement in the APPD. Volunteering to review submissions for or serve on the planning committee for one of these meetings is another opportunity to develop leadership and managerial skills.

APPD leadership hosts virtual cafes as an opportunity for members to come together and learn from one another [11]. Volunteering to co-host on a topic of interest and knowledge is an excellent way to share expertise and begin to build a reputation. Topics have ranged from best practices around faculty development to lessons learned in the post-match scramble.

APPD's regional structure allows additional leadership opportunities. The organization is divided into eight regions, each led by elected regional chairs whose responsibilities include communicating with their regions, leading regional meetings (both at the annual APPD meeting and in between), promoting scholarship within their regions, participating on the Council of Regional Chairs, and reporting region activities to the Board of the APPD. One can also serve as the Chair for the Council of Regional Chairs, which is a two-year term with the option for a second term [11].

Learning Communities (LC) are a group of APPD members who share learning interests and goals, with the LC providing a platform for deeper learning and innovation. Currently, 12 learning communities allow for collaboration on learning and projects, as well as the development of quality improvement and research initiatives. There are leadership opportunities available within the LC structure, including serving as the chair or vice chair of a community. A new LC can also be formed if there is an area of interest not being met by a current LC. The leaders of all the LCs serve on the Council of Learning Communities, which has additional responsibilities to the Board of the APPD. The position of chair of the Council of Learning Communities is another leadership role to consider in this area [11].

Elected leadership positions also exist within the APPD. The Board consists of the President, President-elect, Secretary-Treasurer, Immediate Past President, and three Members At-Large. The

Nominations Committee, led by the immediate Past President of the APPD, consists of two positions elected by members of the APPD. Section-specific Executive Committees for Program Directors, Associate Program Directors, Fellowship Directors, and Vice Chairs of Education exist, providing additional opportunities for elected leadership positions [11]. These leaders are responsible for sub-sessions at the Spring and Fall APPD meetings. Throughout the year, opportunities to participate in special projects or apply for grants with the APPD are advertised through email communication. Both the Annual Fall and Spring APPD meetings often offer opportunities to become involved in planning activities. Participating in these activities builds a network of collaborators, establishes a national reputation, and creates a foundation for success with elected positions later.

More information on these opportunities is available on the Association of Pediatric Program Directors website.

The Academic Pediatric Association's (APA) mission is to nurture the academic success and career development of child health professionals engaged in research, advocacy, improvement science, and educational scholarship to enhance the health and well-being of all children [12]. Within this organization, multiple faculty development programs and leadership opportunities are available. As with APPD, the APA is divided into regions, each led by three regional chairs. The regions are geographically based and work towards goals that will benefit the membership of the Academic Pediatric Association at large. Participating in regional activities is a terrific way to network, develop innovative collaborative projects, and help select trainees and young investigators to receive grant funding [12].

Special Interest Groups within the APA are opportunities to network with colleagues who share a similar interest. They allow for the ability to discuss issues concerning relevant topics to the SIGS, and work towards goals that will benefit the APA membership. SIGS of interest for the program director include faculty development, mid-career faculty, quality improvement, global health, advocacy training, e-learning in medical education, simulation-based medical education, etc. There are multiple opportunities for leadership, including chairing individual SIGs [12].

Members can be elected to serve on the Board of Directors in the following positions: President, Secretary/Treasurer, Chair of Membership, Diversity and Inclusion Committee, Chair of Education Committee, Chair of Research Committee, Chair of Public Policy and Advocacy Committee, Chair of Health Care Delivery Committee. Members can also volunteer to be on any of the above-mentioned committees to gain national leadership experience [12].

The Academic Pediatric Association also offers faculty development programs, which provide leadership skills and opportunities to apply learned skills. If skills already exist, members can serve on the council and as leadership. These programs include the Health Policy Scholars Program, Research Scholars Program, Quality and Safety Improvement Scholars Program, Educational Scholars Program, Advancing Pediatric Educator eXcellence (for hospitalists), and Research in Academic Pediatrics Initiative on Diversity. Of particular interest to program directors may be the Advancing Pediatric Leaders program mentioned earlier in the chapter [12].

To learn more about the Academic Pediatric Association and its regions, special interest groups, and opportunities to join committees and leadership roles, please visit the Academic Pediatric Association website.

An aspirational goal for program directors is the National Academy of Distinguished Educators in Pediatrics (NADEP), an APA academy of medical educators that advances pediatric educators, educational scholarship, and pediatric educational programs for learners across the continuum of medical education. An honorary service academy, NADEP envisions an expansive, diverse, and inclusive community of pediatric educators who collaborate to enhance pediatric education's role in improving health. Members who have demonstrated their dedication to promote equity, diversity, and inclusion, innovation, collaboration, high-value education, and resilience of pediatric educators may apply to be accepted to this prestigious group [12].

The American Board of Pediatrics (ABP) is another national organization with opportunities for professional involvement. With the mission to certify pediatricians who meet standards of excellence and are committed to continuous learning and improvement, the ABP offers program directors committees and boards to serve on, as well as panels for feedback on topics such as education in pediatrics to continuing certification program development [19]. The ABP also offers opportunities to write and edit certifying exam materials. As Entrustable Professional Activities (EPAs) become incorporated into evaluations, program directors can become local, regional, and national CBME champions. Many other ABP committees are open for national involvement. If interested, please visit the American Board of Pediatrics website for more information [19].

The American Osteopathic Board of Pediatrics serves as the primary certifying body for graduates of osteopathic medical schools who have completed pediatric residency training. Opportunities for service and leadership as an AOA-certified osteopathic pediatrician include joining their board of directors, being a subject matter expert, and participating as an examiner. Board members help establish and maintain standards for certification of osteopathic physicians in the practice of pediatrics. Subject matter experts participate in exam writing, and examiners assist in the administration of written, oral, and clinical examinations [20].

Another organization with opportunities for leadership and scholarship is the American Academy of Pediatrics (AAP), where one can join or lead different sections, councils, and committees. Sections are groups for members who share a specialty, area of interest, or stage of life; councils are designed around subspecialties or multidisciplinary fields with the goal of serving as a source of expertise for the AAP. Committees are appointed by the AAP Board of Directors to address current issues and develop policies. One of particular interest to program directors is the Committee on Pediatric Education, whose goal is to advance pediatric education across the continuum and discuss emerging innovations within the field related to research, curricula development, faculty development, practice issues, and legislative proposals impacting pediatric education [21]. Members of the AAP can also join their local chapters, allowing for regional and state-level collaboration, advocacy, and education. Elected leadership opportunities are available in many of these experiences.

Program Directors may choose to take an active role with the Pediatric Academic Societies (PAS) as a way to gain national leadership experience. PAS connects the academic pediatric community to advance scientific discovery and promote innovation in child and adolescent health. There are opportunities to serve on a variety of committees, either as a member or a leader, throughout the year, in addition to helping plan the annual meeting. The meeting is produced through a partnership of the American Academy of Pediatrics, the Academic Pediatric Association, the American Pediatric Society, and the Society of Pediatric Research [22]. For the meeting, one can serve as a workshop reviewer, abstract reviewer, or session moderator. Additionally, there are many opportunities to present one's own scholarly works, whether in workshops, scholarly sessions, or poster and abstract presentations.

Finally, the Accreditation Council for Graduate Medical Education (ACGME) is an organization that accredits residency and fellowship programs. Program directors can be nominated to serve on the review committee (RC) to help set standards and ensure compliance of programs with these standards [17]. This is a selective opportunity that provides excellent leadership and networking opportunities.

Regardless of the pathway chosen, both in terms of additional training or positions attained, program directors can use each committee role and leadership opportunity as a chance to build tools and develop networks. This includes institutional committees that may not be education related but can still offer insights into organizational operations and project development. Look for chances to gain skills, meet leaders to emulate, and give advice to advance your career with every opportunity.

Conclusion

Program directors are selected based on a record of leadership as clinician educators and potential for success as program administrators. This role requires enhancement of current skills as well as active attainment of new skills, relying on the establishment of mentors for support and encouragement. Resources can be found intramurally and extramurally, with much offered through professional organizations. This expanded skillset will allow not only success as a program director but also consideration of career advancement in medical education leadership and beyond. There are many opportunities for career advancement for Pediatric residency program directors, both within their academic institutions and in the broader medical community. By continuing to develop their skills and knowledge, program directors can advance their careers and make significant contributions to the field of medical education.

References

1. Goleman D. Leadership that gets results. Brighton: Harvard Business Review Press; 2017.
2. Kouzes JM, Posner BZ. The leadership challenge. 6th ed. New York: Jossey Bass; 2023.
3. Hiatt J. ADKAR: a model for change in business, government, and our community. Colorado: Prosci Research; 2006.
4. Mossanen M, Johnston SS, Green J, Joyner BD. A practical approach to conflict management for program directors. J Grad Med Educ. 2014;6:345–6. https://doi.org/10.4300/JGME-D-14-00175.1.
5. Group on Resident Affairs, Association of American Medical Colleges. 2023 AAMC GRA Graduate Medical Education Leadership Competencies (GMLECs); 2023a. 2023 AAMC GRA GME Leadership Competencies. Accessed 1 Aug 2024.
6. Group on Resident Affairs, Association of American Medical Colleges. 2023 AAMC GRA GME Leadership Competencies Self/Multi-Rater Assessment Tool; 2023b. https://www.aamc.org/media/75326/download?attachment. Accessed 5 Jan 2024.
7. Servey JT, Hartzell JD, McFate T. A faculty development model for academic leadership education across a health care organization. J Med Educ Curric Dev. 2020;7:2382120520948878. https://doi.org/10.1177/2382120520948878.
8. Artino AR Jr, Cervero RM, DeZee KJ, Holmboe E, Durning SJ. Graduate programs in health professions education: preparing academic leaders for future challenges. J Grad Med Educ. 2018; https://doi.org/10.4300/JGME-D-18-00082.1. PMID: 29686748; PMCID: PMC5901787.
9. Grey S. Earning a master's in healthcare administration: here's what you should know. Forbes Advisor. 2024; https://www.forbes.com/advisor/education/healthcare/healthcare-administration-masters-degree/
10. Association of American Medical Colleges. https://www.AAMC.org. Accessed 9 Aug 2024.
11. Association of Pediatric Program Directors. https://www.APPD.org. Accessed 9 Aug 2024.
12. Academic Pediatric Association. https://www.academicpeds.org. Accessed 9 Aug 2024.
13. Papanagnou D, Messman AM, Branzetti J, Diemer G, Hobgood C, Hopson LR, Regan L, Zhang XC, Gisondi MA. The vice chair of education in emergency medicine: a workforce study to establish the role, clarify responsibilities, and plan for success. AEM Educ Train. 2019; https://doi.org/10.1002/aet2.10407. PMID: 32072103; PMCID: PMC7011427.
14. McBride A, Li S, Turner T, Vinci R. Roles, responsibilities, and value of a vice chair of education in academic pediatric departments. J Pediatr. 2020; https://doi.org/10.1016/j.jpeds.2019.10.072.
15. Brownfield E, Clyburn B, Santen S, Heudebert G, Hemmer PA. The activities and responsibilities of the vice chair for education in U.S. and Canadian departments of medicine. Acad Med. 2012;87(8):1041–5. https://doi.org/10.1097/ACM.0b013e31825cf71a.
16. Whaley Z, Palenzuela D, Dzara K, Berkowitz LR, Moses J, Petrusa E, Phitayakorn R. Characterizing the role of surgical vice chair of education: stakeholder needs and current practices. J Surg Res. 2024;293:497–502. https://doi.org/10.1016/j.jss.2023.09.038. Epub 2023 Oct 10. PMID: 37827027.
17. Accreditation Council for Graduate Medical Education. https://www.ACGME.org. Accessed 9 Aug 2024.
18. Yanoff J. Leadership in graduate medical education. In: Contemporary topics in graduate medical education. IntechOpen; 2019. https://doi.org/10.5772/intechopen.85736.
19. American Board of Pediatrics. https://www.abp.org. Accessed 9 Aug 2024.
20. American Osteopathic Association. https://www.certification.osteopathic.org. Accessed 9 Aug 2024.
21. American Academy of Pediatrics. https://www.aap.org/en/community/aap-committees/committee-on-pediatric-education/. Accessed 9 Aug 2024.
22. Pediatric Academic Society (PAS). https://www.pas-meeting.org. Accessed 9 Aug 2024.

Part III

Recruitment and Transition to Residency

Recruitment

10

Uchenna Anani and Lahia Yemane

Reflections to consider

- What are the program's mission, vision, and values? Do they need to be updated? Do they align with the department, hospital, graduate medical education (GME) office, institution, and local community needs?
- What are the strengths and unique aspects of the program?
- What are the challenges or areas for opportunity in the program?
- What is the program doing to support diversity, equity, and inclusion (DEI)?
- What attributes (e.g., experiences, skills) make for a successful resident in your program?
- How would you define a successful match for your program?
- Looking at prior recruitment outcomes, have the program's mission, vision, and values been reflected in the match results? If not, why?

U. Anani
Vanderbilt University Medical Center,
Nashville, TN, USA

L. Yemane (✉)
Stanford University School of Medicine,
Palo Alto, CA, USA
e-mail: lyemane@stanford.edu

Nuts and Bolts

Establishing Your Team

Recruitment has many phases, and each requires its own plan and clarity in role assignments. Generally, the Program Director and a Program Coordinator oversee the process, but how you build your broader recruitment team will depend on many factors.

Reflections to consider

- What is the size and complexity of the program(s) you are recruiting for? Is it categorical only, or are there additional tracks and/or combined programs?
- Are there key stakeholders in the residency program, department, or hospital to engage on the team? If so, what roles make the most sense for them?
- What role do residents play in the recruitment process (e.g., do they serve as interviewers, lead social events, etc.)?
- Is your program within an institution with a centralized GME office? If so, what is their degree of involvement, resources, and expectations for your program's recruitment processes?

H. McPhillips et al. (eds.), *Graduate Medical Education in Pediatrics*, Excellence in Medical Education 3, https://doi.org/10.1007/978-3-032-12952-9_10

There is significant variability in the involvement of GME offices in recruitment across institutions, so it will be important to clarify this early on to determine what they will provide versus what the residency program needs to do on its own. If you have a larger residency program and/or multiple tracks or combined programs, it is likely you will have a larger applicant pool and need more people on your team for reviewing application files and conducting interviews. Some larger programs also have a faculty member who has a dedicated role to lead recruitment in partnership with the Program Director and Program Coordinator. There are also times when there are strategic goals in recruitment that require you to involve specific stakeholder groups. For example, some Department Chairs may request to be actively involved in the interview process to ensure alignment with departmental priorities. Likewise, programs with a physician-scientist track may involve departmental research and fellowship leaders, who can help evaluate applicants' research potential and articulate available scholarly opportunities.

The importance of having a program coordinator to oversee recruitment cannot be overstated; the coordinator is the member of the residency team who engages the most with applicants throughout the entire cycle and must work closely with the recruitment team on all associated processes. As mentioned above, with program size and complexity, you may need multiple program coordinators involved in supporting recruitment. There is variability in program coordinator roles across programs, so it is important to set expectations. When determining roles, important areas to consider are: recruitment website updates, social media, application review, sending out interview invitations, interview day logistics, and compiling file and interview information for rank order list (ROL) creation. For example, some programs have the program coordinator involved in screening applications and/or doing full file reviews before interviews. If you plan to do this, you must ensure that you have a clear rubric for them to follow and a process to flag files that need additional review.

Electronic Residency Application Service (ERAS), Thalamus, and the National Resident Matching Program (NRMP)

There are distinct services that are needed for different components of the recruitment process, and each requires separate, yearly registrations and careful review of updates in timelines, rules, and processes. Your residency program and any associated tracks that have separate matches, will each need individual registrations for each service. The Electronic Residency Application Service (ERAS) is where applications are submitted to programs for review, and the National Resident Matching Program (NRMP) is where applicants and programs submit their Rank Order List (ROL) and "The Match" takes place.

ERAS, a service of the Association of American Medical Colleges (AAMC), is a platform to centralize application materials for applicants (i.e., Medical Student Performance Evaluation, Personal Statement, Letters of Recommendations) and deliver them to an applicant's desired programs for review. ERAS has many functionalities to allow programs to screen, filter, and select applications, but what specific features are utilized is up to the residency program to decide in their recruitment plan. In 2023, the AAMC announced a new collaboration with Thalamus to streamline GME recruitment. Thalamus is a private company that started in 2013 with the goal to provide a centralized platform for interview management between GME programs and applicants (Thalamus Core) and has expanded to provide additional services in creating interview day schedules (Itinerary Wizard), data & analytics dashboard (Cerebellum), and more. With this collaboration, the previous ERAS Interview Scheduler tool has now been replaced by Thalamus Core. To learn more about Thalamus and the services offered, visit the following website: https://thalamusgme.com/.

After interviews and the ROL are completed, the finalized ROL is inputted into NRMP. Created in 1952, the NRMP is a private, non-profit organization that uses a mathematical algorithm to match applicants into GME training programs based on ROL preferences. A vast majority of specialties use NRMP, including Pediatrics. Per a certain timeline provided each year, both applicants and programs confidentially submit their ROL. Of note, the program ROL can be uploaded into NRMP manually or downloaded from ERAS/Thalamus by anyone on the recruitment team, but it can only be officially certified by the Program Director. With the yearly registration for NRMP, programs must also attest to follow the "All in Policy" for PGY-1 positions, which states that by virtue of registering for the Match, programs will attempt to fill all positions through it or another national matching plan [1]. Related, programs need to decide each year if they will opt-in to participate in the Supplemental Offer and Acceptance Program (SOAP) that takes place during match week to fill any unfilled positions after the main Match. Also, programs with multiple tracks or combined programs may decide to revert unfilled positions into another track, which is most commonly into categorical positions. Although not common, if a program decides not to participate in SOAP or revert positions from one track to another, they are not allowed to make offers for unfilled positions until after the SOAP process finishes. See upcoming sections on "Match Week" and "Special Considerations" for additional information.

Recruitment Cycle

The COVID-19 pandemic has forever changed the landscape of medical education, including recruitment. With the transition to virtual recruitment in 2020, there was swift collaboration across the pediatric community; the recruitment action teams were formed with representation from the Association of Pediatric Program Directors (APPD), Council on Medical Student Education in Pediatrics (COMSEP), Council of Pediatric Specialties (CoPS), Association of Medical School Pediatric Department Chairs (AMSPDC) and learner groups: NextGen Pediatricians, and FuturePedsRes [2]. The recruitment action teams put forth recommendations to support both applicants and residency programs during this transition; since then, they have continued to provide yearly recommendations and resources [3].

In the following sections, we will expand in more detail about each of the phases of the cycle, but briefly:

- Seeking out applicants: What are your outreach strategies to get applicants to apply to your program (website, social media, conferences)?
- Application review: How are you using holistic review principles to align your file review process with your program's mission? Do you have a standardized rubric?
- Interview day: Who conducts interviews? Do you have structured or unstructured interview questions?
- Creation of rank order list: What weight do you give to different elements of the application (file review, interview)? Who is involved in the final rank list decision?
- Match week: Do you have a plan in case you don't fill all your positions and need to participate in the Supplemental Offer and Acceptance Program (SOAP)?
- Post-match review: Did your match results align with the mission, vision, and values of our program? How are you using match outcomes and any post-interview surveys to assess areas for growth with the next recruitment cycle?

Seeking Out Applicants

Pre-application outreach is very important to increase visibility of the mission, vision, and values of your residency program. Again, you want to think about your ideal residency applicant and the potential best avenues to reach them. Regardless of the outreach formats you decide to take, you want to have an overarching strategy of what message you are trying to convey about the program, including unique aspects, strengths, and if there are common misconceptions. Traditionally, applicants use various websites to learn about potential programs, such as the American Medical Association Fellowship and Residency Electronic Interactive Database (FREIDA), the AAMC Residency Explorer, Residency Navigator, and more. It is also important for programs to be aware of open dialogue sites like Reddit and Student Doctor Network, which are widely viewed by applicants but may have outdated or inaccurate information shared anonymously; there may be misconceptions stated there that you want to address proactively as part of your recruitment strategy. The cornerstone of where to access comprehensive information about a program's mission, strengths, and structure is the residency website. So, it is important that the website is regularly maintained and has accurate and up-to-date information. Related, also make sure that pictures are authentic (i.e., current residents vs outdated or stock images) and are truly reflective of your program. There have also been increased calls for more transparency on websites about what programs are looking for in applications (e.g., number and types of letters of recommendation, specific types of clinical rotations, additional requirements for international medical graduates).

With the transition to virtual recruitment, there was increased emphasis on residency programs and program directors to have a larger social media presence [4, 5]. Although studies show that virtual recruitment is generally viewed favorably by both programs and applicants, challenges remain in assessing program culture, engaging directly with residents, and getting a sense of the city [2, 6, 7]. Programs consider addressing these gaps through the use of photos, videos, and social media content on their program website and/or platforms such as X (formerly Twitter) and Instagram, which applicants increasingly use [8]. Examples include hospital tours, a day in the life of a resident at various clinical sites and teams, things to do on the weekends, features highlighting key strengths or initiatives of the program (e.g., DEI efforts), and resident takeovers. These platforms can be effective in reaching broader audiences, helping programs craft and tailor the messages they want to convey in real-time, and more actively engage current residents in recruitment since they are more social media savvy and understand what an applicant would want to see. On the other hand, it is essential to have a clear plan for who will manage and maintain the platforms, how resident-generated content will be reviewed and approved, and how all materials will remain aligned with institutional communication and social media policies. Without having a clear plan in place, challenges can occur; there have been numerous examples of controversy in the past few years regarding if a post from a residency social media platform was reflective of institutional views.

Webinars are another way to engage broadly with prospective applicants. In response to virtual recruitment in 2020, FuturePedsRes, APPD, and COMSEP collaborated to create a centralized webinar series as a more streamlined way for applicants to learn about programs [9], which has evolved over time in structure and format. Many residency programs or GME offices also host their own virtual open houses (or "first looks") as another opportunity to engage more in-depth with program leadership and current residents.

As more medical students are attending conferences to present research and network, this creates another opportunity for recruitment. For example, many students attend the American Academy of Pediatrics National Conference and the Pediatric Academic Societies Conference, which have the opportunity for hospital and institutional exhibitor booths. Your residency program should check with the hospital and institutional marketing teams to see if they have a booth and opportunities to collaborate, which could also strengthen your strategic alignment with those groups. If you are a program that is focused on supporting physician scientists, you can consider attending the American Physician Scientists Association meetings. To engage with underrepresented in medicine (UIM) medical students, there are yearly conferences that have residency fairs: Student National Medical Association (SNMA), Latino Medical Student Association (LMSA), Asian Pacific American Medical Student Association (APASMA), and Association of Native American Medical

Students (ANAMS). These organizations each have national conferences; however, for programs focused on recruiting from the local community, it may be beneficial to prioritize their regional conferences as well. At the residency fairs, you can have your own booth as a residency program or collaborate if your institution has other GME programs or a DEI office.

Historically, doing visiting rotations (i.e., clinical rotation outside of your medical school) in pediatrics was not as common as in other specialties. However, with the transition to virtual recruitment and shift from metrics to pass-fail (e.g., USMLE Step 1 score and clinical rotation grades), visiting rotations have gained increased significance for programs [10, 11]. Prior to virtual recruitment, visiting rotations were a way for students to show interest in a residency program and strengthen their application; now, it also provides them an in-person experience they wouldn't have on a virtual interview to see first-hand the culture of the program and interact with residents. Since 2020, funded visiting rotations in Pediatrics geared towards recruiting UIM medical students and other students with an interest in serving under-resourced populations have also gained popularity. APPD, in collaboration with COMSEP, maintains a repository of many of these visiting rotation offerings and is a good source for more information: https://www.appd.org/careers-opportunities/urim-opportunities/. See the upcoming section on "Underrepresented in Medicine (UIM)".

Importantly, your recruitment outreach should also have long-term strategies to build pathways before medical school, which is included in the framework by Gonzaga et al. [12]. Check with your department, hospital community engagement offices, and affiliated or surrounding medical schools to see if there are local pre-collegiate pathway programs that your residents and faculty can engage with. There are also national pathway programs, such as the Summer Health Professions Education Program (SHPEP) and Health Careers Opportunity Program (HCOP), that focus on preparing college students from disadvantaged backgrounds to enter health professions schools. If you are near a college or university, find ways to interact with the pre-medical organizations to start building connections; once in a medical school, partner with the local pediatrics interest groups, SNMA, LMSA, APAMSA, and ANAMS, to help encourage more medical students to enter the field of pediatrics.

In summary, there are many methods (websites, social media, webinars, conferences, pathway programs) to conduct applicant outreach, so it is important to work with your team to identify which avenues will work best for your program and goals.

Application Review

Application Materials and Components

There are several components to a residency application that may be considered in your review for applicant selection. Those materials currently include the following:

1. MyERAS application/CV: This contains an applicant's general information, contact information, AAMC ID, most recent medical school, current work authorization status, as well as self-identified demographic information, program signals#, geographic* and setting** preferences, medical licensure, state medical license, undergraduate/medical/postgraduate education and training, honors/awards, memberships in honorary/professional societies, publications, and selected experiences^.
   - #Program signals refer to an applicant identifying interest in obtaining an interview at a specific residency program. The number of program signals allowed depends on the specialty and is determined annually by each specialty in conjunction with ERAS. Programs can see which applicants identified their program via a program signal as of particular interest.
   - *Geographic preference refers to U.S. Census divisions in which appli-

cants prefer to reside/practice. There are nine divisions/regions, and applicants are allowed to list up to three geographical preferences in their ERAS application. Applicants are also allowed to designate "no preference" if they are not geographically focused in their search. For each of these options, applicants can provide an explanation (if desired). Geographical preference is in addition to and separate from the program signal (see above).

- **Setting preference refers to the type of city or setting (urban, rural, suburban) that applicants prefer to reside/practice.
- ^Applicants are allowed to identify and describe up to ten experiences/activities that can be categorized into eight types (education/training, military service, professional organization, research, teaching/mentoring, volunteer/service/advocacy, work, and other extracurricular activity, club, hobby). Of these ten experiences, three can be designated as the most meaningful experiences.

2. Medical school transcripts (including core rotations, electives, acting/sub-internships)
3. Medical student performance evaluation (MSPE), which contains a summary of clerkship grades and evaluations
4. USMLE or COMLEX score transcripts (Steps 1–3 for USMLE and Levels 1–3 for COMLEX)
5. Personal statement
6. Letters of recommendations

It is important to note that the residency application process has undergone rapid change in the past 5 years (2020–21) with the COVID-19 pandemic. This is the most current information as of the publication of this book; however, specifics may change.

Establish Your Process

Before diving into your application review, it is important to refer to your program's mission, vision, and values (see section on "Getting Started: Overarching Goals"). Your program's mission will serve as the foundation to help guide and formulate your program's desired outcomes and bring clarity and direction to your recruitment process [13]. Every program has a different mission; therefore, what programs are looking for in applicants may vary. The goal of the application review process and interview is to assess how the applicant has demonstrated the skills, attributes, and experiences that are most valued by your program and align with your program's mission.

As you design your application review process, it is also important to consider if you will utilize an initial limited screening process to determine interviews offered or if you will do full file reviews of all applicants upfront to determine interviews offered. Also, with the utilization of program signals and geographic preferences, you will want to decide how your program will, or will not, weigh those in the review process. In the past, an initial limited screening process with the use of ERAS filters for metrics was commonly used by specialties and/or programs with a very high number of applications to reduce the total number of applications that would be manually reviewed. However, this practice has become less common with the transition of USMLE Step 1 and COMLEX Level 1 to pass-fail and the increasing emphasis on the use and importance of holistic review.

Holistic Review

Recognizing the importance of a diverse workforce to help eliminate health disparities, the LCME in 2009 and ACGME in 2019 created standards that all medical schools and GME programs should engage in recruitment and retention of a diverse and inclusive workforce across the medical education continuum [14, 15]. Holistic review is defined by the AAMC as "a flexible, mission-driven approach to recruit and assess an individual's competencies by considering their experiences, attributes, competencies and metrics (EACM) in order to select applicants who will best contribute to the program's unique goals, learning environment, and the practice of medicine." [16] To help guide the development of a holistic review process and standardized scoring rubrics, your team can utilize the AAMC's Applicant Criteria Identification and Prioritization worksheets and Holistic Application Review Rubric development templates [16]. It is important that your team mutually agree upon the goals of recruitment and what you want to prioritize. These tools can help your team identify, refine, and prioritize which EACMs you want to focus on to ensure consensus and buy-in.

Historically, metrics were heavily used for applicant screening and selection, but literature has shown there are racial and ethnic disparities in USMLE scores, clerkship grades, MSPEs, and induction into medical honor societies [17–19]. Importantly, studies have also demonstrated that many of these metrics do not correlate to future clinical performance, which led to calls for rethinking their importance in residency selection [20, 21]. Utilizing a mission-driven approach that does not rely solely on metrics can serve as an equitable recruitment strategy that will help to broaden and enrich your selection pool of highly qualified applicants and support workforce diversity. Implementing holistic review and decreased emphasis on Step 1 scores were found to be effective in a scoping review on interventions to increase racial and ethnic diversity in GME [22]. For example, if your program's mission prioritizes training of pediatricians who are committed to serving marginalized communities who primarily speak Spanish, implementing a holistic application review that prioritizes an applicant's experiences and attributes that align with these values such as shared lived experiences, dedication to service of marginalized communities, or fluency in Spanish, can help to bring diverse applicants to serve your local community. Personal statements have also become very important for holistic review as an opportunity for applicants to share their unique story and the broader context of their application, which usually involves their lived experiences, challenges, and aspirations.

There are several barriers that have challenged the adoption and utilization of holistic review practices within GME. Some of these barriers include the amount of time and labor required of the recruitment team to review applications, the lack of buy-in and consensus-building on goals within your recruitment team, and the lack of standardized scoring rubrics [13, 23]. The implementation of holistic review can vary quite a bit across programs and institutions. Variables such as the number of applications you are reviewing, the complexity of your application scoring rubric, and the number of members in your team can greatly influence the number of resources and amount of time needed to perform these tasks. Understanding your team's structure and capabilities is a necessary and practical early step as you tailor your holistic review process. In a study of three specialties at a single institution, Swails et al. [24] demonstrated the effectiveness of using mission-aligned experience and attribute filters in ERAS as part of the screening process as opposed to metrics. Results showed improvement in the diversity of their screened applicant pools and demonstrated how you can help address the barriers of time and labor in manual application review. Also, in recognition of the time needed for holistic review, the APPD Residency Recruitment Action Team (APPD RRAT) annually recommends a minimum time period between the time programs have access to ERAS applications and sending initial interview invites.

There are two major types of scoring rubrics that programs can consider: single-criterion and multi-criterion rubrics. Single-criterion rubrics use a detailed descriptor for each level of performance or practice described for an attribute, competency, and/or metric for the reviewer to assess. A very basic example of this might include evaluation of individual criteria, including leadership, commitment to service, distance traveled, and academic achievement, with a rating of each criterion on a scale of 1–5, with 1 being the lowest and 5 the highest. Advantages of single-criterion rubrics include the evaluation of more individual criteria or areas of strength for applicants and the ability to apply higher or lower value to the individual criteria.

Disadvantages primarily include that they can be more time-consuming, tedious, and overall burdensome for reviewers to fill out and complete. In contrast, a multi-criterion rubric brings all the criteria together and pairs them with a single rating scale. An example of a multi-criterion rubric might include the combination of key attributes, such as grit, resilience, cultural humility, and leadership, and assigning an overall score of 1–5. Advantages of this format include assigning one singular value as opposed to assigning scores for several different categories, resulting in less time needed to fill out. The disadvantages are that this format does not allow for more individual evaluation of strengths. Ultimately, it is up to you and your team to decide which format and EACMs are best suited for you to prioritize in your application review, but keep in mind that for whatever rubric style you decide upon, it's important that you have clear scoring anchors that define what each rating means for more consistency.

Artificial Intelligence Use in Recruitment

There has been an increasing use of artificial intelligence (AI) in UME and GME recruitment by both applicants and programs. For residency programs, studies are revealing how AI models can be used to make application review more holistic, consistent, and less time and labor intensive; however, their sole use over human review is being cautioned since AI-based tools have their own limitations and may also perpetuate biases [25, 26]. For applicants, it has been used to varying degrees with writing personal statements, which has been a point of controversy for program directors. Of note, the AAMC does state that "the use of AI tools is acceptable for brainstorming, proofreading, or editing the personal statement, but the final submission [of your personal statement] should represent your own work." [27] Since its use is rapidly evolving, many institutions are developing guidelines for students and programs around effective and ethical uses of AI.

Underrepresented in Medicine (UIM), Considerations for Supreme Court Decision on Race-Conscious Admissions in Higher Education and Employment Laws

The AAMC defines underrepresented in medicine (UIM) as "those racial and ethnic populations that are underrepresented in the medical profession relative to their numbers in the general population" [28] and typically refers to Black or African American, Hispanic/Latino or of Spanish Origin, Native Hawaiian or Pacific Islander, and American Indian or Alaska Native. Prior to 2003, it was more narrowly defined as "underrepresented minority," which included Black, Mexican American, Native American (that is, American Indian, Alaska Native, and Native Hawaiian), and mainland Puerto Rican. This updated definition intends to allow flexibility with changing demographics and consideration of regional or local representation. Page et al. [29] found that many academic health centers were using the term UIM to include sexual orientation, disability, and socioeconomic factors; they note the importance of broadening the definition while also being cognizant of the historically underrepresented racial and ethnic groups.

A critical distinction in determining what legislation applies to your residents in relation to recruitment is how your individual institution defines them (i.e., are residents considered students or employees). If residents are considered employees, which is more common, their selection processes must be in accordance with Equal Employment Opportunity and any applicable state laws; for example, some states have had anti-affirmative action laws in place for many years. If your residents are considered students, then the 2023 Supreme Court decision (*Students for Fair Admissions Inc. v. President and Fellows of Harvard College and Students for Fair Admissions Inc. v. University of North Carolina)* [30] to eliminate the consideration of race in higher education admissions applies to them. Notably, in the updated core principles of the AAMC Holistic Review definition, it states that "...While programs may not make selection decisions based on protected applicant characteristics (e.g., race, sex, disability, etc.) schools can consider an applicant's discussion of any personal experience—even those related to race, sex, or other protected characteristics—to illustrate examples of mission-aligned experiences or qualities sought by the program." [16] Regardless of how residents are defined, it is important that your residency program partners with the Offices of General Counsel and Human Resources at your institution to ensure that you can maintain your goals for a diverse and inclusive workforce while preserving compliance with federal, state, and institutional laws. Also, this discussion relates specifically to selection and does not apply to UIM outreach; see section on "Seeking Out Applicants" for more information.

Interview Days: Planning, Preparing the Team, Invitations

As you set up your recruitment processes, you will want to determine how many interview days you will have and over what time period. Many factors go into this including the size of your program(s), historical data (e.g., match results and total number of applicants on your ROL needed to match), number of applicants you can accommodate per day, and schedule of key recruitment team members, including residency leaders and interviewers. In terms of interviewers, ideally, you want to have a broad representation across faculty, trainees, roles, specialties, and identities. Virtual recruitment has allowed for increased capacity and accessibility of interviews, and some programs have even been able to engage residency alumni.

Before the interview preparation begins, it is recommended that you have a meeting with everyone involved and outline your program's mission, vision, values and goals of recruitment, including virtual platform and interview day logistics. It is ideal to share a broad overview of the program so interviewers can answer questions from applicants, highlight the key strengths, and review NRMP rules of conduct during interviews. Applicants highly value speaking to faculty and residents during interviews, so it is important to actively engage them in the process. Many institutions also require unconscious bias training for everyone involved in recruitment. If you have a scoring rubric for the interview, like your file review, you will want to have clearly defined scoring anchors.

The APPD RRAT, in alignment with the NRMP policies, puts forth yearly recommendations for applicants and residency programs around sending and accepting interview invitations. As mentioned previously, to encourage holistic review, the APPD RRAT recommends programs wait a minimum amount of time before sending interview invites. Per APPD RRAT, programs should not send more invites than there are interview spots available, and interview offers should be sent late in the afternoon when applicants are typically less clinically busy. Also, applicants should have at least 48–72 hours to respond to invitations offered and should notify programs if they will not be interviewing as early as possible and cancel previously scheduled interviews no later than 2 weeks from the scheduled date. Lastly, programs should inform applicants if they will be offered an interview, waitlisted, or not offered an interview by early December.

Your program coordinator is typically in charge of scheduling and coordinating interviews. When sending invitations, it is important to inquire if any accommodations during their interview day are needed (e.g., allotted time to breastfeed or pump, closed captioning for applicants with hearing impairment). Once invitations have been accepted, it is ideal to have clear and simple communication with applicants about their interview day; many programs have created customized websites or landing pages with associated materials and virtual platforms linked. Information to share with candidates ahead of time may include the following: [3, 31],

- The virtual platform to be used (e.g., Thalamus, Zoom, Teams, Webex).
- Standardized recommendations to applicants on navigating the virtual platform and preferred virtual backgrounds.
- Specific information on back-up procedures if or when technical issues arise (e.g., exchange of phone numbers).
- The schedule for the interview day, planned format for the interview(s).

It is also helpful to perform an interview day run-through with key team members before your interview days begin to address any potential technical challenges or unanticipated issues with the flow of the day that can be addressed beforehand.

Navigating the Interview Day

The general structure of interview days is similar across programs and has not changed significantly with the move to virtual recruitment, except for not having walking tours of clinical sites. The day usually begins with a welcome from the PD, then a presentation by the PD or chiefs, followed by interviews. Some programs have virtual tours, have applicants attend their teaching conferences (morning report, noon conference, portion of academic half-day) and, depending on how they structure their socials, schedule some informal time during the interview day to speak with residents. It is ideal to have interviews on a single day and not spread across multiple days to make scheduling easier for applicants, although this may not be feasible with combined residency programs.

Lastly, applicants find it very valuable to have optional virtual socials as an informal opportunity to engage with residents; these typically happen in the evening and do not have to be specifically tied to their interview day as opposed to in-person interviews. These socials are usually run by chiefs and/or residents with coordinator support on logistics. It is great to get engagement across all PGY levels and especially from PGY1s since they most recently went through the process and can highlight what was most important for them when considering programs. These sessions can also offer opportunities for UIM, LGBTQ+, and other groups to have an informal chance to meet members of their community at the program in a safe and comfortable environment. It is important that beforehand, programs inform applicants that attendance at these sessions is optional and will not weigh into their evaluation or impact their rank order by the program.

Interview Techniques and Assessment

Before interviews begin, you want to decide what the goal of the interview is within the larger recruitment process and what format and people would be needed to best accomplish it.

Considerations include the following:

- Number of interviews per applicant
- Time length for each interview
- Interviewer pool (Who can interview? Faculty, residents, and/or fellows?)
- Interview format (1:1, panel)
- Interviewer assignment—aligning the interviewer with an applicant of shared interests or affinity groups, when applicable
- Use of structured vs. unstructured interview questions
- Use of blinded interviews or screening of certain aspects of the applicant's file from the interview

For example, if your goal is to convince applicants that your program is the best fit, then you may have a more non-structured, conversational interview approach and include residents. However, if you are trying to explore specific areas of their application or mission-aligned attributes or competencies, you may consider standardized behavior-based interview questions, which have also been shown to reduce bias in applicant assessment [32]. In most cases, programs try to do a blend of unstructured and structured questions. There is also the Multiple Mini Interview (MMI) format, used more commonly in UME recruitment, that uses anywhere from 6 to 12 brief sessions or stations, in which each interviewer evaluates a non-medical question asked to the applicant that is designed to assess their non-academic qualities and attributes. Evidence has shown that the MMI format provides a better prediction of an applicant's overall success and strengths and effectively minimizes interviewer bias [33].

Based on your decided goal of the interview and our earlier discussion of holistic review and decreasing over-reliance on metrics, many programs have moved away from interviewers having full access to an applicant's file. Evidence has shown that blinding interviewers to information like USMLE scores, photos, and certain demographic information can minimize bias and increase UIM recruitment [22, 33]. Options include only providing the personal statement, CV, LORs, or no information at all. Programs that have residents as interviewers typically allow them even more limited access to applicant files than faculty. Regardless of what you choose, it is helpful to tell applicants upfront what to expect in terms of interview structure to reduce anxiety.

Importantly, whether in-person or virtual interviews, bias exists. Virtual interviews have had many benefits to applicants and programs but also brought forth new considerations. During the early transition, Marbin et al. [31] wrote a practical perspective to highlight common biases in interviews and their potential exacerbation with virtual format and strategies programs can implement to mitigate them. Ruedinger et al. [34] shared five evidence-informed strategies that can be used in real-time for interviewers to mitigate bias: individuation, perspective taking, mindfulness, stereotype replacement, and counter-stereotypic imaging.

Consistent with the file review process, you will want the interview scoring rubric to have clearly defined anchors. Keep in mind, faculty and residents are busy, so you want to balance comprehensiveness of the scoring rubric with what will be easy for them to complete in a timely manner with the most useful information. With the transition to virtual interviews, many programs have moved to electronic surveys and tools to enter scores, which makes compiling data much easier for the program coordinator.

Post-Interview Communication and Second Looks

The NRMP Match Code of Conduct has clear guidelines that programs must limit post-interview communication with applicants to only sharing clarifying information about the program and cannot ask applicants their ranking intentions. The goal is to prevent undue pressure on applicants but can also be tricky because communication from both sides can be perceived differently. Therefore, it is also important that you educate everyone on your recruitment team about how to handle the correspondence they receive. Although it is discouraged, letters of intent are commonly sent by applicants who may share with programs that they are their first choice, top choice, or very highly ranked, and there is variability in how programs approach responding and if it influences the program rank list. Post-interview communication has been shown to influence applicants and contribute to disparities in ranking. In one national study of academic orthopedic surgery residency programs, it was found that 17% of applicants altered their rank list when contacted by a program, 20% felt pressured to reveal their rank position to a contacting program, and 8% were asked to rank a program #1 in exchange for the program to also rank them to match [35].

Therefore, in alignment with the NRMP Match® Code of Conduct, the APPD RRAT has recommended that applicants not engage in post-interview communication unless for the following reasons:

1. A thank you note (which is optional)
2. Specific follow-up questions from the interview day
3. Updates to provide to an application (e.g., new publication or award)

Additionally, programs should not engage in post-interview communication unless it is for the following reasons:

1. To provide a follow-up email/message with contact information of leadership/interviewers (maximum of 1 follow-up notification)
2. Provide a program update that goes out to all applicants after interviews have concluded (maximum of 1)
3. To reply to an applicant's questions (Note: Post-interview communication is permitted for responding to specific questions or for linking with mentors and/or research colleagues.)

The use of second look visits had been in practice before the transition to virtual recruitment but has gained increased attention. On the one hand, the biggest challenge with virtual recruitment is applicants getting to know the culture of a program and interacting directly with residents, so the opportunity to go visit a select number of their top programs is appealing. On the other hand, offering in-person visits can put an undue financial burden and extend the interview season for both applicants and programs. However, the biggest concern in offering these is putting undue pressure on applicants. Although these second looks are said to be optional, studies have shown that applicants may feel they must go to improve their ranking in the program [36, 37]. To eliminate this concern, for the 2025–26 recruitment season, pediatrics is officially joining the NRMP Voluntary Rank Lock Pilot, which means that programs will have to formally lock their rank order list with the NRMP before conducting second looks.

Rank Order List

The rank order list (ROL) is the final numerical listing of interviewed applicants, from first to last choice, that a program will place in NRMP for The Match. As the program develops its scoring rubrics for file reviews and interviews to align with the mission, vision, and values of the program, it is ideal that you decide at the beginning how much weight you want to give to all your application components, which will be unique for every program. For example, some programs may give more weight to certain elements in the initial screening process, but less at the time of the final rank list. As you make your ROL, you must also decide if you want to rank all interviewed applicants or if there are some that you would not rank at all. Depending on the size of your program, the number of applicants you are ranking, and prior match outcomes, you should consider whether your program is willing to leave a position unfilled rather than rank an applicant who may not be a suitable candidate.

There is variability in how programs integrate discussion of the ROL throughout the recruitment cycle. Some programs will generate a ROL in real-time during periodic post-interview meetings, while others wait until the end of the season when all interviews are completed. Since the final ROL is seen as the most sensitive process of the recruitment cycle, one thing to consider for real-time ROL generation is who is part of the post-interview meetings and what information they have access to. For example, some programs have current residents serve as interviewers, but given that applicants may become their co-residents, they do not give residents access to certain elements in the applicant's file or see the final ROL. It is also important to remind everyone involved in recruitment that the process is confidential; there should also be no discussion between programs or applicants about their ROL position, which would be considered an NRMP violation.

Once you have finalized your ROL, it must be entered into the NRMP R3 system. This can be done by the program coordinator, recruitment lead, or PD; however, it is required that the ROL be officially certified only by the PD. The PD can make edits and recertify unlimited times prior to the NRMP ROL deadline, but if it is not certified, then the program will not match applicants, which unfortunately has happened before, so be very diligent in double-checking. As a note, ROL certification is different from a ROL lock. As pediatrics moves into the NRMP Voluntary Lock Pilot, this distinction will be very important; once a list is LOCKED, no changes can be made.

Match Week

Match week is the culmination of lots of hard work during the recruitment cycle and also a time of excitement and stress for applicants and programs. Each year, there is a specific calendar that is provided by NRMP to outline the week's events. On Monday of match week, the PD and PC will receive an email from NRMP notifying them if they have filled all their main match spots; applicants are also notified at the same time if they have matched. If all spots are filled, there is nothing for the program to do until Thursday when they receive the list of matched applicants, but this must be kept confidential until applicants are notified on Friday at noon Eastern time.

For programs that are notified on Monday, they did not fill all residency spots. If they opted in at the time of yearly NRMP registration, they would participate in SOAP (Supplemental Offer and Acceptance Program). Understandably, this news can be disappointing and sometimes shocking, so it is okay to acknowledge those feelings, but the program must also be prepared to quickly switch gears and start the SOAP process on that same day. If going into the ROL process you had concerns about not filling your spots and/or have needed to SOAP in the past, it is ideal to have a plan set up ahead of time in terms of who will be part of the team and your file and interview processes. Since SOAP is a time-intensive process over just a few days, it is recommended that the PD, PC, and other key members block off time on their calendar for application review and interviews. Big picture, SOAP is a process to help connect unmatched programs with eligible unmatched applicants; it is not another match, but rather a sequence of offers made by programs based on a generated preference list. Over a few days, programs will receive new applications to their program in ERAS, review files, conduct interviews of chosen applicants, and then develop a preference list. During the four SOAP offer rounds, which take place on Thursday of match week, programs will make offers based on the preference list, and then applicants can decide to accept or decline the offer. Of note, the preference list can be modified before each round and must be certified before the next round. As a reminder, by opting into SOAP, programs cannot make offers to any applicants outside of that process until SOAP concludes, which is typically Thursday evening. Ideally, by the end of SOAP, you will have filled the unmatched spots and have a full complement for Friday's match day. If you still have unfilled spots after SOAP concludes, you are no longer bound by NRMP match rules and the process of filling spots is determined by the program, which is also the case for most non-PGY1 spots or off-cycle recruitment. Even after applicants are matched into your program, regardless of if you needed to SOAP or not, there should not be any discussion of their rank position as that can create bias and interpersonal challenges even before joining the program. Please refer to the NRMP website for additional information about Match Week and SOAP: https://www.nrmp.org/.

Post-Match Review

Shortly after match week, it is helpful to debrief the recruitment season with your team while it is fresh on your minds. You can consider doing a strengths, weaknesses, opportunities, and threats (SWOT) analysis or other quality improvement framework to help plan new improvements for the next cycle. Information that can aid this process include detailed match results (and comparison to prior years), if you have post-interview surveys from applicants, feedback from interviewers and the residency leadership, and national specialty data. Recruitment involves a lot of data; therefore, there is an opportunity to look granularly at each stage (applied, invited to interview, interviewed, matchable range, match) and across different factors (e.g., UIM, geography, medical school type) and make targeted interventions. For example, if you have a high percentage of UIM applicants, but very few are invited to interview, you may want to evaluate your holistic file review process; or, if you are getting very few applicants from a specific geographic region, you may want to evaluate your outreach practices.

Special Considerations

Categorical Tracks and Combined Programs

If your categorical program has specialized tracks (e.g., physician scientist, health equity, primary care) or combined programs, they each require their own ERAS and NRMP accounts since they have their own application and match. ERAS also has features that allow residency programs to see if applicants are applying to more than one of their programs. As such, for each track or combined program, you will need to decide whether any unfilled positions should participate in SOAP or be converted back to categorical positions. The standard combined programs in Pediatrics include: Pediatrics-Anesthesia, Pediatrics-Emergency Medicine, Pediatrics-Medical Genetics, Pediatrics-Physical Medicine and Rehabilitation, Triple Board (Pediatrics-Psychiatry-Child & Adolescent Psychiatry), and Medicine-Pediatrics. There are also non-standard programs, with the most common being Child Neurology. Since combined programs typically live within two clinical departments, it is crucial to have clear communication and collaborative plans between the combined and two associated categorical programs about the recruitment cycle, especially because many applicants will dual apply. The programs will need to decide how they want to do the combined program application reviews, which may look different than the two categorical programs, and how to structure the interview day(s).

Transfers Between Programs

There are situations where a pediatric resident wants to switch programs or a non-pediatric resident wants to switch specialties. It will be important to speak with your GME office to clarify institutional policies and funding implications (e.g., is this replacing another resident or unfilled spot or increasing the total number of residents in the program? Are there limitations based on how much training a resident has already completed?).

For switching specialties, the resident typically applies for pediatric residency per the usual ERAS and NRMP processes or occasionally outside the Match. Given that they were in a different specialty, it is unlikely that any of their prior years of experience will count towards meeting pediatric requirements. For current pediatric residents who are transferring programs, this is done outside the Match. There are multiple methods for inter-program transfers within pediatrics. Programs can advertise if they have a position that is now available or, more commonly, residents reach out to programs of interest to inquire about open positions as they are seeking a move for personal or professional reasons. Like the typical recruitment processes, programs may request to see the same application materials submitted in ERAS and conduct interviews. It is critical that programs speak directly to their current program director to get feedback on their clinical and professional performance up to that point and elicit any concerns. Prior to finalizing a transfer, the new program and applicant must be in agreement about key issues: (1) credit for completed rotations at prior program: there should be a careful review of their rotations to determine what meets criteria for completion at the new program and (2) anticipated start dates and graduation, which may be impacted by the first issue and if they need to relocate.

Summary

Recruitment is a key component of having a successful residency program and requires a lot of strategy, planning, resources, and time. Central to the process is evaluating your program's mission, vision, and values and then translating those into a mission-aligned holistic review process of experiences, competencies, attributes, and metrics that you will look for in applicants' files and during interviews. The current landscape of recruitment is dynamic as specialties decide on if they want to remain with virtual interviews or go back to in-person and second look considerations. Pediatrics will participate in the NRMP Voluntary Lock Pilot for the 2025–26 recruitment season. Therefore, it is important to stay up to date with national recommendations from the APPD RRAT, ERAS, and NRMP. Also, make sure to dedicate time to reflect on your match outcomes. Review your outcomes to see if they align with your recruitment goals and if there are opportunities for improvement and revisions in your recruitment processes. As one recruitment season ends, another one quickly begins!

References

1. Main Residency Match All in Policy. NRMP. 12 Nov 2021. Accessed 31 July 2024. https://www.nrmp.org/policy/main-residency-match-all-in-policy/.
2. Frohna JG, Waggoner-Fountain LA, Edwards J, et al. National pediatric experience with virtual interviews: lessons learned and future recommendations. Pediatrics. 2021;148(4):e2021052904. https://doi.org/10.1542/peds.2021-052904.
3. Residency and Fellowship Recruitment Action Teams Resources. Association of Pediatric Program Directors. Accessed 7 Aug 2024. https://www.appd.org/resources-programs/recruitment/.
4. Heitkamp NM, Morgan LE, Carmody JB, Heitkamp DE. Pediatric program directors should have an active presence on twitter. Acad Pediatr. 2021;21(2):201–4. https://doi.org/10.1016/j.acap.2020.11.016.
5. Lee DC, Kofskey AM, Singh NP, King TW, Piennette PD. Adaptations in anesthesiology residency programs amid the COVID-19 pandemic: virtual approaches to applicant recruitment. BMC Med Educ. 2021;21(1):464. https://doi.org/10.1186/s12909-021-02895-2.
6. Wang S, Denham Z, Ungerman EA, et al. Do lower costs for applicants come at the expense of program perception? A cross-sectional survey study of virtual residency interviews. J Grad Med Educ. 2022;14(6):666–73. https://doi.org/10.4300/JGME-D-22-00332.1.
7. Huppert LA, Hsiao EC, Cho KC, Marquez C, Chaudhry RI, Frank J. Virtual interviews at graduate medical education training programs: determining evidence-based best practices. Acad Med. 2021;96(8):1137–45. https://doi.org/10.1097/ACM.0000000000003868.
8. Fuller CC, Deckey DG, Brinkman JC, et al. General surgery residency applicants' perspective on social media as a recruiting tool. J Surg Educ. 2022;79(6):1334–41. https://doi.org/10.1016/j.jsurg.2022.06.003.
9. Neelakantan M, Heitkamp NM, Blankenburg R, Frohna JG. The #PedsMatch21 webinar series: coordinated specialty-level communication during the virtual residency application cycle. Acad Med. 2022;97(7):1012. https://doi.org/10.1097/ACM.0000000000004623.
10. Kindler R, Kahn J, Uddin A, Petersen KH. Underrepresented applicants post-USMLE pass/fail: a national survey of competitive residency directors. J Med Educat Curri Develop. 2024;11:23821205241254161. https://doi.org/10.1177/23821205241254161.
11. Kremer TR, Kremer MJ, Kremer KP, Mihalic A. Predictors of getting a residency interview: differences by medical specialty. Med Educ. 2021;55(2):198–212. https://doi.org/10.1111/medu.14303.
12. Gonzaga AMR, Appiah-Pippim J, Onumah CM, Yialamas MA. A framework for inclusive graduate medical education recruitment strategies: meeting the ACGME standard for a diverse and inclusive workforce. Acad Med. 2020;95(5):710–6. https://doi.org/10.1097/ACM.0000000000003073.
13. Williams C, Kwan B, Pereira A, Moody E, Angus S, El-Bayoumi J. A call to improve conditions for conducting holistic review in graduate medical education recruitment. MedEdPublish. 2019;8:76.
14. Standards, Publications, & Notification Forms | LCME. Accessed 8 June 2020. https://lcme.org/publications/#Standards.
15. Common Program Requirements (Residency). Accreditation Council for Graduate Medical Education (ACGME). Accessed 1 July 2023. https://www.acgme.org/programs-and-institutions/programs/common-program-requirements/.
16. AAMC Holistic review. AAMC. Accessed 12 Aug 2024. https://www.aamc.org/services/member-capacity-building/holistic-review.
17. Lucey CR, Hauer KE, Boatright D, Fernandez A. Medical education's wicked problem: achieving equity in assessment for medical learners. Acad Med. 2020;95(12S):S98–S108. https://doi.org/10.1097/ACM.0000000000003717.
18. Low D, Pollack SW, Liao ZC, et al. Racial/ethnic disparities in clinical grading in medical school. Teach Learn Med. 2019;31(5):487–96.
19. Yemane L, Omoruyi E. Underrepresented in medicine in graduate medical education: historical trends, bias, and recruitment practices. Curr Probl Pediatr Adolesc Health Care. 2021;51:101088. https://doi.org/10.1016/j.cppeds.2021.101088.
20. McGaghie WC, Cohen ER, Wayne DB. Are United States medical licensing exam step 1 and 2 scores valid measures for postgraduate medical residency selection decisions? Acad Med. 2011;86(1):48–52. https://doi.org/10.1097/ACM.0b013e3181ffacdb.
21. Prober CG, Kolars JC, First LR, Melnick DE. A plea to reassess the role of United States medical licensing examination step 1 scores in residency selection. Acad Med. 2016;91(1):12–5. https://doi.org/10.1097/ACM.0000000000000855.
22. Mabeza RM, Christophers B, Ederaine SA, Glenn EJ, Benton-Slocum ZP, Marcelin JR. Interventions associated with racial and ethnic diversity in US graduate medical education: a scoping review. JAMA Netw Open. 2023;6(1):e2249335. https://doi.org/10.1001/jamanetworkopen.2022.49335.
23. Zastrow RK, Burk-Rafel J, London DA. Systems-level reforms to the US resident selection process: a scoping review. J Grad Med Educ. 2021;13(3):355–70. https://doi.org/10.4300/JGME-D-20-01381.1.

24. Swails JL, Adams S, Hormann M, Omoruyi EA, Aibana O. Mission-based filters in the electronic residency application service: saving time and promoting diversity. J Grad Med Educ. 2021;13(6):785–94.
25. Burk-Rafel J, Reinstein I, Feng J, et al. Development and validation of a machine learning-based decision support tool for residency applicant screening and review. Acad Med. 2021;96(11S):S54. https://doi.org/10.1097/ACM.0000000000004317.
26. Mahtani AU, Reinstein I, Marin M, Burk-Rafel J. A new tool for holistic residency application review: using natural language processing of applicant experiences to predict interview invitation. Acad Med. 2023;98(9):1018–21. https://doi.org/10.1097/ACM.0000000000005210.
27. Personal Statement. Students & Residents. AAMC. Accessed 9 Jan 2025. https://students--residents.aamc.org/applying-residencies-eras/publication-chapters/personal-statement.
28. Underrepresented in Medicine Definition. AAMC. Accessed 1 Dec 2021. https://www.aamc.org/what-we-do/equity-diversity-inclusion/underrepresented-in-medicine.
29. Page KR, Castillo-Page L, Poll-Hunter N, Garrison G, Wright SM. Assessing the evolving definition of underrepresented minority and its application in academic medicine. Acad Med. 2013;88(1):67–72. https://doi.org/10.1097/ACM.0b013e318276466c.
30. Supreme Court of the United States. Students for Fair Admissions, Inc. v. President and Fellows of Harvard College (06/29/2023). Published online 2023.
31. Marbin J, Hutchinson YV, Schaeffer S. Avoiding the virtual pitfall: identifying and mitigating biases in graduate medical education videoconference interviews. Acad Med. 2021;96(8):1120–4. https://doi.org/10.1097/ACM.0000000000003914.
32. Langhan ML, Goldman MP, Tiyyagura G. Can behavior-based interviews reduce bias in fellowship applicant assessment? Acad Pediatr. 2022;22(3):478–85. https://doi.org/10.1016/j.acap.2021.12.017.
33. Bergelson I, Tracy C, Takacs E. Best practices for reducing bias in the interview process. Curr Urol Rep. 2022;23:319–25. https://doi.org/10.1007/s11934-022-01116-7.
34. Ruedinger E, Evans YN, Pham DQ, Hooper L. Just-in-time strategies to reduce the effect of interviewer bias during trainee recruitment. Acad Pediatr. 2024;24(5):709–13. https://doi.org/10.1016/j.acap.2024.01.020.
35. Brooks JT, Reidler JS, Jain A, LaPorte DM, Sterling RS. Post-interview communication during application to orthopaedic surgery residency programs. J Bone Joint Surg. 2016;98(19):e84. https://doi.org/10.2106/JBJS.15.01364.
36. Garner HW, Christiansen JD, Blumenfeld SG, et al. Perspectives of US medical residency and fellowship applicants on no-stakes campus visits. J Grad Med Educ. 2024;16(4):475–8. https://doi.org/10.4300/JGME-D-23-00842.1.
37. O'Connor AB, Blatt AE, Fletcher KE, et al. Multicenter study of optional in-person visits to residency programs after virtual interviews. J Grad Med Educ. 2023;15(6):692–701. https://doi.org/10.4300/JGME-D-23-00370.1.

11 Transition from Medical School, Orientation, and Onboarding

Emma Omoruyi and Veronica M. Gonzalez

Introduction

The transition from undergraduate medical education (UME) to graduate medical education (GME) is a significant milestone in the journey of medical professionals. The evolving identity from medical student to resident physician can invoke a myriad of emotions for the trainees. It can be exhilarating, offering the promise of new responsibilities and the opportunity to put years of academic learning into clinical practice. However, it can also be stressful and anxiety-provoking as new residents grapple with their new roles and responsibilities. For many incoming residents, this transition involves significant life changes, such as relocating to a different city, state, or country, which adds another layer of complexity to an already challenging time.

Institutional and individual program onboarding and orientations before the start of residency training play a crucial role in easing this transition. These orientations allow interns to learn and understand the various aspects of their new institution and clinical learning environment. Orientation sessions are designed not only to impart critical information but also to reinforce and highlight particularly challenging areas for interns during this transition process. DiMarino et al. [1] pointed out that although many skills and topics addressed in medical school are broadly applicable across specialties, several institution- and specialty-specific areas are essential to cover during orientation. These include understanding the institutional culture, health disparities prevalent in the surrounding community, and the nuances of the institution's electronic health record (EHR) system.

In August 2021, the Undergraduate Medical Education to Graduate Medical Education Review Committee (UGRC), tasked by the Coalition for Physician Accountability (CoPA), presented a series of recommendations [2] aimed at comprehensive improvements in the UME to GME transition. One of the key recommendations from the UGRC is that residency training programs should include robust orientation and ramp-up sessions at the start of the internship. These sessions should go beyond an introduction of institutional and programmatic logistics, policies, and system utilization and include information regarding patient demographics, an overview of health disparities, and opportunities to engage and connect with the community. This is also a time to introduce and promote the institutional culture by inviting various key leaders, faculty members, and peers. This holistic approach to orientation is intended to provide new residents with a well-rounded understanding of their new

E. Omoruyi (✉) · V. M. Gonzalez
McGovern Medical School at UTHealth Houston, Houston, TX, USA
e-mail: Emma.A.Omoruyi@uth.tmc.edu

H. McPhillips et al. (eds.), *Graduate Medical Education in Pediatrics*, Excellence in Medical Education 3, https://doi.org/10.1007/978-3-032-12952-9_11

professional environment, fostering a sense of belonging and preparedness.

The onboarding process begins almost immediately after the Main Residency Match hosted by the National Resident Matching Program (NRMP). There will be multiple competing deadlines for required documentation before their start date to ensure they are cleared to commence clinical duties as resident physicians. Depending on the program's size, some will solely rely on their program coordinators to initiate onboarding. In contrast, others will coordinate their transition activities with their respective GME offices and other departments to ensure a cohesive and comprehensive onboarding process.

The importance of a well-structured orientation cannot be overstated. Streamlined orientation processes support trainee well-being and improve patient safety. For many entering residents, this is their first "real" job. Effective onboarding and orientation programs ensure that residents are familiar with employment policies and receive education that optimizes their success in their specific clinical environment, even before their first official day. Moreover, like other employees, the UGRC advises that residents should be compensated for attending these orientation sessions [2], recognizing the importance of this time as an investment in their future success and well-being.

Under the guidance of the program director, program leadership should meet with all incoming residents to create individualized learning plans (ILPs) to foster learning and growth from day one. This assessment helps identify any gaps or specific needs of the individuals, ensuring that the orientation is tailored to address these needs effectively. For example, during orientation, a new intern may perceive gaps in their clinical knowledge relative to their peers, leading to anxiety about patient care. Through an individualized learning plan, program leadership provides targeted support, pairing the intern with a faculty and/or senior resident mentor and incorporating structured board review, case-based learning, and targeted readings. Regular formative feedback helps track progress and refine learning strategies. This personalized approach builds confidence, reinforces knowledge, and ensures the intern grows at their own pace while effectively caring for their patients.

Additionally, orientation is not merely a time to disseminate information but also an opportunity to establish shared values, program expectations, and institutional policies. It is a critical period for new interns to bond and spend meaningful time together, building the camaraderie and support networks that will sustain them through the challenges of residency.

Effective orientation and onboarding programs are essential in preparing new residents for the complexities of their roles. By addressing the multifaceted needs of incoming residents, programs can ensure they are well-equipped to manage their responsibilities. This not only enhances the residents' experience but also has a positive impact on patient care and safety. The transition from UME to GME is a crucial period that requires thoughtful and comprehensive planning. By implementing robust orientation programs, institutions can support new residents in navigating this challenging phase, setting the stage for their future success as healthcare professionals.

In this chapter, we present strategies to effectively orient and onboard new residents, discussing the nuances, challenges, and ethical considerations involved in the process. We aim to provide readers with actionable insights and practical guidance to create onboarding and orientation programs that meet new residents' immediate needs and lay the foundation for their long-term success and well-being in their medical careers. Through careful planning and execution of onboarding and orientation processes, program directors can significantly influence the quality of the residency experience, ultimately contributing to better outcomes for residents, their patients, and the program.

Preparing for Resident Onboarding

Setting Onboarding Expectations

Currently, there are no published guidelines that specify when the onboarding process for medical residents should begin or outline the structure of orientation programs. Pediatric residency programs are heterogeneous, varying in size and affiliations. They can range from small to large and be university-affiliated or community hospitals. Programs may be linked to freestanding children's hospitals or be a part of a hospital within a hospital (i.e., a children's hospital attached to an adult hospital). Additionally, they may or may not include fellowship programs. Regardless of the program type, it is essential to have a clear onboarding and orientation plan tailored to meet the specific needs of each program.

As we discuss how to prepare for the new influx of interns, it is important to understand what onboarding entails. In an article published in *Forbes Advisor*, Crail and Haskins [3] describe employee onboarding as a comprehensive process that involves paperwork, workstation setup, defining role expectations, and facilitating social introductions. It aims to efficiently integrate new employees into the company, covering legal requirements and easing their transition into the workplace community. Some of the best practices for onboarding published by the Society for Human Resource Management Foundation (SHRM) [4] are to have a written onboarding plan and be explicit with new employees regarding objectives, timelines, roles, and responsibilities. Although jobs in the corporate world are not directly comparable to resident onboarding, the intended purposes and outcomes are very much applicable.

Establish Communication Channels

Once the Match has occurred, it is important to establish contact with the incoming interns through a welcome email as soon as possible. Most programs communicate primarily by email. Some also use dedicated websites that incoming residents are directed to for further details. The welcome email should highlight the specific points of contact for the training program, including telephone numbers and email addresses. Program coordinators, the chief residents, and/or individuals within the institution's GME office will often be the direct points of contact. Additionally, the email should provide an overview of communication channels, important dates, and deadlines that they need to be aware of in the coming weeks and months leading up to their start date.

Practical Considerations

The welcome email is the first step to helping the incoming interns establish a sense of connection and belonging within the program. As they wrap up their last year of medical school and navigate the onboarding process, some will face an added layer of stress due to relocating. To alleviate this stress and aid the transition, programs should include practical considerations regarding nearby housing options and any available relocation assistance. It is helpful to highlight areas in and around the campus where most residents live. Some may have children and want to know about neighborhoods with good daycares and schools. It is also beneficial to include transportation options and parking specific to the area. Keep in mind that some are moving to an unfamiliar place, and anything the program can do to ease the transition will increase their level of preparedness and sense of community on their first day.

Onboarding residents involves coordinating several critical tasks simultaneously. In addition to completing the previously mentioned requirements, new residents must also gain access to hospital and clinic systems. This includes acquiring hospital badges, computer passwords, and login information. For institutions accredited by The Joint Commission 2024 [5], residents do not need to be credentialed and privileged by the hospital's medical staff organization. Instead, they practice under the supervision of a licensed physician who holds hospital privileges. However, if residents engage in activities outside the residency program, such as moonlighting, they will need to obtain their own individual hospital privileges. While the Accreditation Council for Graduate Medical Education (ACGME) 2021 institutional requirements [6] do not necessitate Joint Commission accreditation, it is important to verify the process for residents to provide direct patient care while in training.

During onboarding, the program may also work on acquiring lab coats, identification (ID) badges, telecommunication devices (i.e., pagers, cell phones), parking permits, and headshots for display on the program's website or distribution within the department. Follow-up emails with the incoming residents can be used to solicit their schedule requests as well as specialty interests, allowing program leadership to pair them with faculty mentors.

Licensure and Credentialing

Incoming interns will need to be credentialed by the institution for appointment to the program. It is the program's responsibility to ensure the incoming residents' credentials are reviewed and approved. The onboarding process often begins with the distribution of various documents for their review, such as GME policies (e.g., duty hours) and institution-specific policies and procedures. Trainees will need to submit various educational training documents, such as the medical school performance evaluation (MSPE), diplomas or certifications of completion, medical school transcripts, and curriculum vitae (CV). Since they are considered new hires at their institution, they will need to undergo identity verifications (e.g., passports, birth certificates), background checks, and health clearance. Health clearance often comprises proof of immunizations and/or antibody titers, tuberculosis testing, and drug screening.

Depending on the state, residents will either need to be licensed or acquire physician-in-training permits to be able to practice medicine. These licensing applications or permits are filed with the respective state licensing board. It is necessary to obtain identity verification documents and diplomas or certificates, including background checks, to submit for licensure. Some state boards have lengthy turnaround times, and therefore, receipt of these documents promptly is imperative to avoid delays in start dates.

Special Considerations

For international medical graduates (IMGs), there are a few extra steps in the onboarding process. Additional points of contact should be provided to them as some institutions have dedicated specialists or a separate office to manage international affairs. IMGs are required to have an Educational Commission for Foreign Medical Graduates (ECFMG) Certificate and a valid visa to participate in an accredited GME institution in the United States. The most commonly sponsored visa for IMGs is the J-1 visa, although some institutions sponsor IMGs with H-1B visas. It is important to know which visas are sponsored by the institution and ensure that IMGs have the necessary support to navigate these additional requirements.

Coordination with Other Departments

Larger residency programs typically coordinate with various other departments such as human resources, payroll, benefits, and GME office. It will be important that program coordinators and, if applicable, administrators within the GME office monitor the completion of these checklists to ensure incoming residents will be cleared to perform clinical duties on their first day. Delinquent submissions can lead to delays in start dates for the interns. On those occasions when a trainee is not as responsive to communications or timely in their submissions, consider utilizing the chief residents to communicate directly with the incoming resident.

Finally, programs should seek feedback from new residents on the onboarding process. This feedback can provide valuable insights into what aspects of the process are working well and where improvements are needed. By continuously evaluating and refining the onboarding process, programs can ensure that they are meeting the needs of new residents and providing the best possible start to their medical careers.

In summary, the onboarding process for pediatric residency programs is a multifaceted endeavor that requires careful planning and coordination. While there are no published guidelines on when onboarding should begin or how it should be structured, each program must develop a clear and tailored plan that meets its specific needs. Effective onboarding and orientation are crucial for integrating new residents into the program and ensuring their preparedness and well-being as they embark on their medical careers. By addressing the logistical, educational, and social aspects of onboarding, programs can create a supportive environment that fosters success and a sense of community among new residents.

Orientation Planning and Execution

Purpose and Objectives of Orientation

Onboarding and orientation are often used interchangeably. PeopleAdmin [7] describes onboarding as a *process* and orientation as an *event*. Similar to onboarding, there are no published standards of what orientation should comprise for new residents, and yet it is ubiquitous. The duration varies according to the program's size and needs. Ben-Zion et al. [8] found that orientation time ranged from 30 to 120 hours for pediatric residency programs. New resident orientation often contains dense material; hence, it is important to provide it in an engaging and robust manner to maximize the retention of the wealth of information provided to them.

In alignment with the UGRC 2021 recommendations [2], the overarching goal of orientation is to ease the UME to GME transition of new residents from various backgrounds to promote readiness to assume increased patient care responsibilities. While the inclusion of administrative policies and procedures is necessary, a well-structured orientation will take a holistic and comprehensive approach to help new residents understand their new professional environment and introduce them to the culture and values of the institution. This cultural integration is vital as it helps residents align with the institution's mission and vision, thereby enhancing their overall experience and performance. Incorporation of community engagement and socialization opportunities will also foster a sense of preparedness, connection, and well-being.

Typical Orientation Program

Introduction to the Healthcare Facility and Training Institutions

The content and structure of orientation will vary across institutions, given the array of programs; however, many orientation programs will encompass similar components. In a study of emergency medicine residency programs, McGrath et al. [9] found that most orientation presentations were sponsored by the department, while others coordinated with their affiliated hospitals, medical schools, academic health centers, and/or the GME office. Most programs will include an introduction to the training institution and healthcare facility. The goals and objectives of the overall program curriculum are also reviewed. The institution's mission and values are reinforced, and residents are provided with an overview of the ins and outs of each clinical site. During this time, residents are often given tours to familiarize themselves with the layout, key locations, and overall environment of the facility, helping them understand what to expect and where to find essential resources.

Orientation to Specific Patient Populations

In pediatric resident orientation, it is essential to acquaint residents with specific patient populations and specialty areas to ensure they are well-prepared to provide high-quality, specialized care. This component of orientation goes beyond general hospital tours and administrative details to delve into the unique aspects of pediatric care. Caldarelli et al. [10] described the importance of providing residents with an immersive and experiential learning experience by exposing them to the various health disparities that exist within the local community, with an emphasis on understanding the social determinants of health. Incorporating these elements into the orientation program helps pediatric residents build a strong foundation, enabling them to confidently address the complex needs of their patients by recognizing and addressing inequities related to race, socioeconomic status, and other demographic factors. It ensures that they are not only clinically competent but also empathetic and responsive to the unique challenges faced by children and their families in healthcare settings.

Beyond addressing social determinants of health, pediatric resident orientation should also introduce trainees to special populations, including medically complex children and those who require highly specialized care. These patients often have multiple, chronic conditions, neurodevelopmental disabilities, and/or technology dependencies, necessitating a multidisciplinary approach to management. Early introduction of available services to the program's affiliated healthcare system(s), such as complex care and specialty clinics and palliative services, can ensure trainees are equipped to provide comprehensive, compassionate care to children with chronic, complex, and special healthcare needs.

Electronic Health Record and Technology Training

Another important aspect of orientation is providing training on the use of technology and the EHR. As healthcare continues to evolve, the use of technology in clinical practice has become increasingly important. Programs should ensure that new residents are proficient in using the institution's EHR system and other relevant technologies. This training should include not only the technical aspects of using these systems but also best practices for maintaining patient confidentiality and data security. This will ensure residents are prepared for patient care on their first day.

Overview of Policies, Procedures, and Protocols

Often, the densest part of orientation involves covering various institutional and programmatic policies, procedures, and protocols. The GME office and other departments frequently assist with this segment for larger programs. During the onboarding process, residents should have received documentation regarding payroll and benefits (e.g., health insurance, dental, vision, life insurance, short-term and long-term disability, retirement plans, and professional liability insurance). Additionally, a review of family and medical leave policies and information on leaves of absence is included. Orientation is an opportunity to revisit this information, allowing residents to seek clarification and elect their benefits.

An introduction to patient safety and quality improvement (QI) and care transitions during orientation ensures that trainees understand their role in maintaining safe, high-quality patient care. In alignment with the ACGME milestones, interns should receive an overview of variance reporting systems and how to identify and participate in the analysis of patient safety events. In addition, they should also have an opportunity to learn how to participate in QI initiatives. By doing so, interns will be empowered to recognize safety issues and contribute to ongoing improvement efforts. Additionally, structured education on effective handoffs and care transitions, such as using the I-PASS tool, improves efficiency with standardized communication and prevents medical errors. By integrating these foundational principles into orientation, residency programs instill a culture of safety, accountability, and continuous improvement from the very start of training.

Furthermore, orientation generally covers a range of additional topics, including information on the Health Insurance Portability and Accountability Act (HIPAA) and billing compliance, clinical documentation integrity, professionalism, the learning environment, and how to report mistreatment. Other important areas addressed are sleep deprivation/fatigue mitigation, duty hours, wellness, radiation safety, injury protocols, employee assistance programs, mental health support services and referrals, and nearby recreational activities.

Wellness and Self-Care

Programs should offer resources and support for wellness and work–life integration. Residency can be a stressful and demanding period, and it is important to promote a healthy work–life balance to prevent burnout. The ACGME 2024 common program requirements [11] recognize that physician burnout is a serious and prevalent issue that impacts the learning environment, physical and mental health, and patient safety. Residency programs are required by the ACGME to address and support resident self-care and well-being. Programs should provide information during orientation on wellness resources, mental health services, and strategies for managing stress. Providing an overview of this topic during orientation will encourage residents to prioritize all aspects of their health, fostering improved overall well-being and performance throughout their training.

Additional Training

Special Certifications

Before residents are immersed in their clinical settings, they are required to attend skills training for additional certifications. Most pediatric residency programs require attendance in Pediatric Advanced Life Support (PALS) and Neonatal Resuscitation Program (NRP) courses during orientation. Certification in these two sessions ensures that residents are well-versed in managing infants and children in life-threatening emergencies.

Residents as Educators

Residents not only step into a clinical role but also supervise and teach medical students as part of their training. During orientation, it is the program's responsibility to prepare residents for their role as educators by familiarizing them with the learning objectives and expectations of any medical student courses and the pediatric clerkship. This preparation includes workshops and seminars on various teaching methodologies, such as interactive learning, bedside teaching, and small group discussions, ensuring residents understand the curriculum and the specific goals students must achieve during their rotations.

Additionally, orientation should facilitate training on effective teaching practices, providing feedback, and assessing learners. Residents are taught how to create a supportive learning environment that encourages student engagement and critical thinking. They also learn techniques for delivering constructive feedback that helps students improve their clinical skills and knowledge, recognizing their strengths and identifying areas for improvement. Training on evaluating student performance objectively, using standardized assessment tools, and properly documenting and communicating assessment results is also covered. By thoroughly preparing residents for their dual roles as clinicians and educators, the program ensures they are equipped to provide high-quality education and mentorship to medical students, ultimately enhancing the overall learning experience within the clinical environment.

Introduction of Key Personnel

Introducing key members of support people from program leadership, faculty, staff, and various departments during pediatric residency program orientation is crucial for several reasons. Firstly, it fosters a sense of community and teamwork, helping residents understand the network of professionals available to support their clinical, educational, and personal needs. By meeting key personnel from departments such as nursing, administration, social work, and various medical specialties, residents can more easily navigate the healthcare system and know whom to approach for specific questions or concerns. This introduction also highlights the collaborative nature of pediatric care, emphasizing the importance of interdisciplinary communication and cooperation. Lastly, these introductions are vital for creating an integrated and supportive environment that contributes to the residents' success and the quality of patient care.

Socialization

In the McGrath et al. [9] study, the most commonly stated goal of orientation was to provide an opportunity for interns to become acquainted with one another. Beyond familiarization with their training environment and policies, this enculturation typically involves various activities designed to help new residents establish connections and friendships. Many programs incorporate team-building activities and social events such as scavenger hunts, happy hours, and local gatherings where residents and their families are invited. These events foster social ties that support and encourage the residents during their training, as this can be a stressful time in their lives.

Incorporating Mentors into Orientation

Programs should consider implementing a formal mentorship system where faculty members or experienced residents are assigned to new interns. Rather than random pairing, Joe et al. [12] cited that the most common strategies for assigning mentors were based on the mentee's personal interests, gender identity, and career goals. The role of mentors and preceptors during orientation is pivotal. Mentors can provide guidance, support, and advice on both professional and personal matters. This relationship can be invaluable, particularly during the initial months of residency when new interns are adjusting to the demands of their roles. Mentorship programs can also facilitate the development of long-term professional relationships and networks, which are beneficial for career growth and development.

Early introduction and development of individualized learning plans (ILPs) during orientation help tailor the learning experience to each resident's unique needs. Faculty mentors can use this information to provide personalized guidance, fostering a structured and supportive relationship. This approach aims to equip new pediatric residents with the knowledge, skills, and support necessary to succeed in their training. By focusing on both personal and professional growth, mentors help residents build confidence and competence, preparing them for the independent practice of medicine and ensuring their holistic development as future pediatricians or pediatric subspecialists.

The institution and program are instrumental in providing resources for faculty participation in professional development activities, thereby promoting a culture of continuous learning and growth. Introducing mentors early during orientation provides residents with immediate support and guidance. The importance of faculty development initiatives for clinician-educators is increasingly recognized. Wiese and Bennett [13] describe a growing range of key faculty development programs that target core areas, such as teaching skills, assessment, instructional design, leadership, and educational scholarship. These initiatives aim to improve teaching effectiveness and should also encompass strategies for workplace learning, ensuring mentors can provide comprehensive guidance and meaningful support throughout the resident's training.

In summary, the orientation program includes an introduction to the healthcare facility and training sites, familiarizing residents with specific patient populations and specialty areas. It provides an overview of essential policies, procedures, and protocols, and includes training on technology, electronic health records, and compliance. Additionally, new residents are introduced to the support staff and various departments they will interact with. Programs should highlight the importance of teamwork, communication, and professional conduct during orientation. Emphasis is also placed on wellness and self-care, recognizing the importance of maintaining personal health and well-being. These elements are essential for building a cohesive and supportive learning environment.

Introduction to Clinical Environment

Transitioning into clinical responsibilities is a pivotal moment for new residents. They can expect to navigate a complex environment with high patient volumes, diverse medical conditions, and a multidisciplinary team. Understanding their roles, expectations, and team dynamics is crucial. Residents must quickly adapt to the fast-paced nature of clinical settings, learning to balance patient care with administrative duties.

The structure of orientation or onboarding programs to ease this clinical transition should cover a range of topics, including hospital protocols, patient interaction techniques, and initial clinical tasks. Through the GME office, many new trainees will receive comprehensive introductions to electronic health record systems, departmental workflows, and emergency procedures. By gaining a thorough understanding of institutional policies and practical skills, residents build confidence and competence in their new roles and identity as physicians. However, trainees who also need to identify as pediatricians will benefit from more specific elements such as the role of child life, pediatric acute lifesaving skills, neonatal resuscitation skills, and family-centered communication. Utilizing interactive workshops and simulations can help reinforce learning.

Support Networks

In addition to support provided by mentors and advisors, peer support from other pediatric trainees can play a crucial role in guiding new residents through their initial clinical experiences [14]. Having recently experienced this transition to the clinical environment, peer mentors can provide personalized advice, share their experiences, and provide emotional support, helping residents navigate the complexities of clinical practice. Senior peers can offer emotional support, share coping strategies, and foster a sense of camaraderie. These peer networks facilitate the integration of new residents into the clinical setting, helping them overcome challenges and build professional relationships. Peer support groups also create a sense of community, enabling residents to share their experiences and learn collaboratively. Being introduced to the co-residents during orientation could be an invaluable opportunity to develop these critical relationships.

Effective supervision and robust support mechanisms are crucial in the transition from medical student to pediatric resident. These mechanisms ensure that new residents receive the guidance, feedback, and mentorship necessary to develop their clinical skills and professional identity. The roles of senior peers and faculty members are pivotal in this process, providing both oversight and support to new residents. Supervision and support mechanisms are integral to the successful transition of new residents. Senior peers and faculty members each play distinct yet complementary roles in this process. Together, these layers of supervision and support create a comprehensive framework that helps new residents develop their clinical skills, professional identity, and personal well-being, ultimately leading to improved patient care and professional satisfaction.

Orientation should include defining an understanding of these roles and their importance:

Senior Peers

- Clinical Supervision: Senior peers provide day-to-day supervision in the clinical setting. They assist with patient management, help new residents interpret clinical data, and oversee procedures. This hands-on supervision ensures patient safety and allows new residents to learn through direct experience under guided conditions. New trainees' understanding of this form of supervision could remind them that someone is always available to assist them.
- Feedback and Evaluation: Senior peers and faculty should provide immediate, formative feedback. This includes constructive criticism and positive reinforcement after clinical encounters or procedures. Regular, informal feedback helps new residents adjust their practices in real-time and enhances their learning process [15].
- Role Modeling: Senior peers serve as role models, demonstrating professionalism, effective communication, and clinical competence. New residents can observe and emulate

the behaviors and attitudes of their senior peers, which is crucial for their professional development.

- Emotional and Social Support: Transitioning to residency can be stressful and isolating. Peer support groups, often led by senior residents, provide a platform for discussing challenges and successes, further promoting a supportive environment.

Role of Faculty

Faculty members, including attending physicians and program directors, provide higher-level supervision and support. Their roles encompass:

- Formal Supervision: Faculty members are responsible for the overall supervision of resident activities. They oversee clinical decisions, ensure adherence to best practices, and intervene in complex or critical cases. This layer of supervision guarantees that patient care meets high standards and that new residents are supported in their clinical duties.
- Structured Feedback and Evaluation: Faculty conduct regular evaluations through formal mechanisms, such as performance reviews, 360-degree evaluations, and competency assessments. These evaluations are based on direct observation, feedback from peers and patients, and clinical outcomes. Structured feedback sessions, often held quarterly, allow for comprehensive discussions about strengths, areas for improvement, and career development.
- Mentorship and Career Guidance: Faculty members often serve as long-term mentors, guiding new residents through their residency and beyond. They provide career advice, assist with research and academic endeavors, and help residents navigate the complexities of medical practice. This mentorship is crucial for professional growth and career planning.
- Educational Support: Faculty support the educational curriculum of residency programs. They deliver lectures, lead case discussions, and organize workshops and simulation exercises tailored to the residents' learning needs and ensure that they acquire the necessary knowledge and skills.
- Emotional and Professional Support: Recognizing the stress and potential burnout associated with residency, faculty members also play a role in supporting residents' well-being. They promote a culture of openness, where residents feel comfortable discussing their challenges. Faculty can direct residents to wellness resources and provide support for maintaining a work–life balance.

In summary, senior peers offer immediate, relatable guidance and support, while faculty provide structured oversight, formal feedback, and long-term mentorship.

Opportunities for Skill Assessment and Development During Onboarding

The onboarding period offers numerous opportunities for skill assessment and development, utilizing various educational modalities, such as role-play, simulation, and observed structured clinical encounters (OSCEs). These methods not only enhance clinical competence but also foster confidence, communication, and decision-making skills. It's also an opportunity to identify common gaps that may occur during the transition from medical school to pediatric residency [16].

Role-Play

Role-play is a dynamic and interactive technique employed during pediatric intern orientation to simulate real-life clinical scenarios. Interns can engage in role-play to practice patient interactions, including taking pediatric medical histories, conducting physical examinations, and delivering difficult news to patients and families. When done in a psychologically safe manner, this method allows interns to receive immediate feedback from peers and instructors, to refine their communication skills and bedside manner.

Psychological safety in role-play allows interns to work on their communication skills without fear of judgment by fostering clear expectations, supportive facilitation, respectful feedback, and a growth-oriented debriefing process. Role-play also provides a safe environment to make mistakes and learn from them, thereby building confidence in handling similar situations in actual clinical practice [17].

Simulation

Simulation-based training is a cornerstone of skill development during onboarding. Simulations provide a safe, controlled environment for residents to practice and hone their clinical skills. High-fidelity simulations use advanced manikins that mimic pediatric patients, enabling interns to practice and hone their procedural skills in managing common pediatric conditions, emergencies, and procedures. These simulations replicate the high-pressure environment of pediatric emergencies, helping interns develop critical thinking and rapid decision-making skills. Furthermore, simulation allows for the assessment of interns' technical skills, such as intubation and interosseous placement [18]. Simulations often involve interdisciplinary teams, promoting collaboration and communication skills. Residents learn to work effectively with nurses, pharmacists, and other healthcare professionals, which is essential for providing comprehensive patient care and developing their ability to work effectively as part of a healthcare team. Debriefing sessions following simulations are crucial for reflecting on performance, discussing errors, and identifying areas for improvement. These sessions are crucial for the development of reflective learning skills needed for a lifelong learning mindset.

Observed Structured Clinical Encounters (OSCEs)

OSCEs are structured and standardized methods for assessing clinical competence. During orientation, pediatric interns may participate in OSCEs designed to test different aspects of pediatric care. These clinical stations might include scenarios, such as managing a child with asthma, counseling parents on vaccination, or recognizing signs of child abuse. OSCEs provide a comprehensive evaluation of an intern's knowledge, clinical reasoning, and interpersonal skills. The feedback obtained from OSCEs helps interns identify specific areas needing further development and tailor their learning objectives accordingly. A smaller residency program could partner with a medical school by integrating OSCEs into existing medical student assessments, allowing residents to participate as standardized patients, assessors, or peer educators. This collaboration could provide shared resources, faculty support, and standardized patient pools while giving residents valuable teaching experience and ensuring cost-effective, high-quality assessments.

Other Modalities

E-learning modules (training offered online through a digital device) offer asynchronous, flexible, and accessible ways to acquire knowledge on pediatric-specific topics. These types of modules can be spaced throughout the year to help reinforce concepts introduced early.

By integrating role-play, simulation, OSCEs, and other educational modalities, pediatric programs can ensure that interns are well-prepared to meet the challenges of clinical practice, ultimately enhancing the quality of care provided to pediatric patients.

Introducing Pediatric Interns to Assessment and Feedback in Training

Introducing pediatric interns to effective assessment and feedback mechanisms is crucial for their development, ensuring they acquire the necessary skills and competencies for independent practice. This process involves familiarizing them with robust assessment tools, the importance of timely feedback and guidance, and how to address challenges or concerns during training. Preparing interns during orientation for receiving both summative and formative feedback through introducing them to your program's assessment tools and expectations is important.

Assessment tools provide a structured framework to evaluate their clinical skills, knowledge, and professional behaviors. ACGME requires that programs provide trainees with both formative and summative feedback. The ACGME Milestones provide a framework for the growth and progression of the residents during their training. The milestones are not to be used for high-stakes decisions such as graduation requirements and cover a wide range of skills from patient care and medical knowledge to interpersonal and communication skills.

Interns should also be introduced to the concept of direct observation, where faculty members and senior residents observe them in clinical settings to provide real-time evaluations of their performance. This method allows for the assessment of both technical skills, such as performing procedures, and non-technical skills, such as teamwork and communication. Structured clinical observation tools, like the Mini-CEX (Clinical Evaluation Exercise), should be explained and demonstrated to ensure consistency in evaluations.

Providing Timely Feedback and Guidance

Pediatric interns need to understand the importance of receiving timely feedback and guidance to support their development and ensure continuous improvement. Effective feedback should be specific, objective, and focused on behaviors that can be changed. It should be delivered constructively, highlighting strengths while addressing areas for improvement.

For example, interns should be introduced to the "SBI" model (situation-behavior-impact) for providing feedback (CITE). This model encourages faculty to describe the specific situation, the observed behavior, and the impact of that behavior. For example, instead of saying, "You need to improve your communication skills," a faculty member might say, "During the patient encounter yesterday (Situation), you did not explain the diagnosis clearly to the patient (Behavior), which caused confusion and anxiety (Impact)." This specific feedback helps interns understand what they need to work on and why it is important.

The importance of immediate feedback, given during or shortly after clinical encounters, should also be emphasized. This "in-the-moment" feedback allows interns to make adjustments and apply new strategies right away. Program expectations for regular feedback sessions, such as monthly or quarterly evaluations, should be explained to interns. They need to understand where and when they can obtain summative assessments and their role in advocating for formative assessment. These sessions provide opportunities for them to receive comprehensive feedback on their performance. Interns should be encouraged to engage in self-assessment, reflecting on their strengths and weaknesses, and discussing these with a faculty advisor or mentor. This collaborative approach fosters a culture of continuous learning and improvement.

Longitudinal mentorship relationships should be introduced as another important aspect of providing guidance. Mentors and advisors can help interns set goals, develop action plans, and navigate challenges. Explaining the role of mentorship provides interns with a trusted source of feedback and guidance throughout their training.

Addressing Challenges and Concerns During Training

Pediatric interns should be made aware of how to address challenges and concerns that may arise during training, which is critical to ensuring their well-being and success. Residency training is demanding, and interns may face various challenges, including burnout, work–life balance issues, and difficulties in meeting personal and professional expectations.

Creating a supportive and open environment is crucial for interns to feel comfortable discussing their concerns. Orientation is a chance to share how the program directors and faculty create and foster dialogue and anonymous reporting systems. Peer support groups and wellness programs should be normalized during the onboarding period and encouraged as a tool for trainees to cope with stress and maintain their well-being. Formal grievance and support mechanisms should be explained to address serious concerns, such as harassment, discrimination, or significant professional misconduct. These mechanisms should ensure confidentiality, impartiality, and prompt resolution of issues.

Regular assessments and feedback can help in early identification of residents who may be having difficulties. During the orientation and onboarding period, residents should be encouraged to identify areas of strength and challenge and work with advisors and mentors to develop learning goals. This plan may include additional supervision, targeted educational activities, and regular check-ins with faculty advisors.

Challenges and Strategies

One of the most prominent challenges of residency is managing the substantial increase in workload. Interns must quickly learn to balance patient care responsibilities with administrative tasks, all while continuing their education and professional development. Another common challenge is the feeling of imposter syndrome and self-doubt. Despite their rigorous training, many new residents question their abilities and fear making mistakes. This can hinder their confidence and negatively impact their performance. Additionally, navigating the complexities of patient interactions, including communicating with families and working within a multidisciplinary team, can be daunting. These interactions require refined interpersonal skills and emotional intelligence, which are not always fully developed at the end of medical school training. Orientation provides an opportunity to introduce these concepts that should also be reinforced throughout training. To introduce these concepts effectively, program directors might use various tools and resources:

Strategies for Overcoming Challenges

Time Management and Workload Prioritization

Effective time management and workload prioritization are essential skills for pediatric residents. Program directors can play a crucial role by providing structured guidance on these topics. This can include workshops or seminars focused on time management techniques, such as the Eisenhower Matrix, which helps residents categorize tasks by urgency and importance. Encouraging the use of digital tools and apps designed for task management can also be beneficial [19].

Mentorship programs can provide practical advice on setting realistic goals and creating efficient workflows. Experienced mentors can share their strategies for prioritizing patient care while balancing administrative duties and personal time. Furthermore, emphasizing the importance of self-care and work–life balance from the outset can help residents avoid burnout. Ensuring residents understand the necessity of taking breaks, exercising, and maintaining a healthy lifestyle is crucial for long-term success.

Addressing Imposter Syndrome and Self-Doubt

Imposter syndrome and self-doubt are common among new residents and can significantly impact their confidence and performance [20]. Program directors should create a supportive environment where residents feel comfortable discussing these feelings and identify the structural and institutional-level factors that drive these feelings of self-doubt. It is important to normalize these feelings in orientation so that residents who may be impacted by these feelings know how to name the experience and where to reach out for support. One study analyzing data from 2000 to 2014 on residents in ACGME-accredited programs found that the leading cause of death was neoplastic disease, followed by suicide. The study also highlighted that one of the highest-risk periods for resident suicide is during the summer of the intern year, making discussions about mental health an important part of orientation [21].

Implementing peer support groups can also be effective. These groups provide a safe space for residents to share their experiences and offer mutual support. Facilitated by trained moderators, these sessions can help normalize feelings of self-doubt and provide strategies for overcoming them. Workshops focused on building resilience and coping strategies can further assist residents in managing imposter syndrome. Techniques such as cognitive-behavioral strategies, mindfulness, and reflective practice can empower residents to recognize and challenge negative thoughts, fostering a more positive self-image and greater self-confidence.

Highlighting the achievements and progress of residents regularly can also boost morale and reinforce their sense of competence [22].

Seeking Support and Guidance from Peers and Mentors

The importance of seeking support and guidance from peers and mentors cannot be overstated. Program directors should facilitate the development of strong mentorship relationships from the beginning of residency. Pairing new residents with experienced mentors who can provide ongoing support, career advice, and professional development guidance is essential. Encouraging residents to engage in regular, informal meetings with their mentors provides opportunities for residents to discuss their challenges, seek advice, and receive constructive feedback.

Creating a culture of collaboration and teamwork within the residency program can further enhance peer support. Encouraging residents to work together on projects, participate in study groups, and engage in social activities can strengthen bonds and foster a sense of community. This collaborative environment helps residents feel less isolated and more supported as they navigate the challenges of their training. Orientation provides a nice opportunity to establish these bonds through welcome events.

Utilizing Available Resources for Continued Learning and Growth

Program directors should ensure that residents are familiar with the educational tools and opportunities available to them, such as online learning platforms, simulation centers, and library resources.

Structured educational sessions, such as grand rounds, journal clubs, and case conferences, provide valuable opportunities for residents to enhance their knowledge and clinical skills. Encouraging active participation in these sessions can help residents stay current with the latest advancements in pediatric medicine and improve their critical thinking and clinical reasoning abilities.

Finally, promoting a culture of lifelong learning is crucial. Encouraging residents to pursue additional certifications, attend workshops and conferences, and engage in research activities can foster continuous professional development. Providing information on available scholarships, grants, and professional organizations during orientation can support residents in these endeavors.

Ethical and Professional Considerations

By providing guidance on ethical decision-making, addressing professionalism issues promptly, creating a supportive environment, and promoting a balance between patient care and self-care, program directors can equip residents with the skills and mindset needed for a successful and fulfilling residency. It is also an important introduction to the challenges they will face in clinical practice.

Providing Guidance on Ethical Decision Making

Ethical decision-making is a cornerstone of medical practice, particularly in pediatrics, where the vulnerable nature of patients necessitates heightened sensitivity and responsibility. During the onboarding process, program directors can introduce ethical frameworks and principles, such as autonomy, beneficence, non-maleficence, and justice. Case-based learning is an effective method to teach these principles. By presenting real-life scenarios and facilitating group discussions, residents can explore the complexities of ethical dilemmas and learn to navigate them thoughtfully.

Incorporating formal ethics training sessions led by experienced clinicians and ethicists can further enhance residents' understanding. These sessions can cover topics such as informed consent, confidentiality, end-of-life care, and decision-making involving minors and their families. If unable to cover these topics during orientation, programs should ensure ethics training is provided early in the academic year to establish a strong foundation for ethical decision-making. Additionally, encouraging residents to reflect on their values and biases and how these influence their clinical decisions can foster a deeper commitment to ethical practice (Spencer et al. 2022) [23].

Addressing Professionalism Issues as They Arise

During orientation, program directors should clearly articulate the expectations for professional behavior. This includes punctuality, accountability, respectful communication, and adherence to institutional policies. Providing examples of unprofessional conduct and discussing the potential consequences can help underscore the importance of professionalism. Additionally, programs should address professionalism in social media use, including guidelines on patient confidentiality, appropriate online conduct, and adherence to institutional policies regarding digital communication.

Regular feedback mechanisms are essential for addressing professionalism issues promptly. Establishing a culture of open and constructive feedback allows for immediate correction of unprofessional behaviors. Residents should be encouraged to seek feedback actively and view it as an opportunity for growth. Mentorship programs can also play a significant role in fostering professionalism as guides, models, and support for residents in navigating complex interpersonal dynamics.

Promoting a Supportive Environment for Residents to Seek Assistance

Juggling patient care responsibilities with self-care and well-being is essential for preventing burnout and ensuring sustainable practice. During orientation, program directors should highlight the importance of self-care and provide strategies for maintaining a healthy work–life balance. Encouraging residents to set boundaries, prioritize tasks, and take regular breaks can help manage stress and prevent burnout.

Providing resources such as wellness programs, fitness facilities, and access to mental health professionals can support residents in maintaining their well-being. Emphasizing the importance of seeking help early when feeling overwhelmed and normalizing discussions about mental health can also contribute to a healthier training environment.

Regular check-ins with faculty mentors can provide a safe space for residents to discuss challenges and receive guidance. Promoting an open-door policy among faculty can make it easier for residents to approach them with concerns, fostering a culture of openness and support. By promoting self-care alongside patient care, program directors and faculty can help residents develop resilience and maintain their passion for pediatrics.

Diversity and Inclusion Initiatives

Fostering an environment of diversity and inclusion not only enhances the learning experience but also improves patient care by equipping residents with the skills needed to understand and address the varied needs of the communities they serve. As pediatric residency program directors, it is crucial to integrate diversity and inclusion initiatives into the orientation process to prepare trainees for the complexities of contemporary medical practice and help establish the program's culture. Individuals from diverse backgrounds and cultures bring varying levels of comfort and proficiency in navigating diverse environments. So, diversity and inclusion initiatives cannot follow a "one-size-fits-all" approach; they must be tailored to account for each resident's lived experience and competency in fostering inclusive spaces. Effectively meeting learners at their individual starting points is essential to fostering meaningful engagement and development in this area, while also ensuring that minoritized and marginalized residents are supported and not placed in a position where they must repeatedly confront or educate others on foundational aspects of historical oppression. This can be achieved by incorporating diversity and cultural sensitivity training, creating an inclusive environment for residents from diverse backgrounds, and addressing healthcare disparities within the program and community. Encouraging residents to engage in self-reflection and discussion about their own cultural backgrounds and biases can further promote cultural awareness and sensitivity.

Creating an inclusive environment where pediatric residents from diverse backgrounds feel welcomed and supported is critical to their success and well-being. Program directors should actively promote a culture of respect and inclusion by setting clear expectations for professional conduct and zero tolerance for discrimination and harassment. This includes providing training on recognizing and addressing microaggressions and fostering allyship among all staff members.

Mentorship programs can play a significant role in supporting residents from diverse backgrounds. Pairing new residents with mentors who share similar cultural or ethnic backgrounds may provide valuable guidance and foster a sense of belonging. Additionally, creating affinity groups or support networks within the residency program can offer residents a platform to share their experiences, seek support, and advocate for their needs.

Addressing healthcare disparities within the residency program and the broader community is a crucial component of diversity and inclusion initiatives. Pediatric residency program directors should emphasize the importance of understanding and addressing these disparities as part of the residents' training. This can include educating residents about the historical and systemic factors that contribute to health inequities, especially those locally, and encouraging them to consider these factors in their clinical practice (Cruz et al. 2022) [23].

Incorporating community engagement and outreach into the pediatric residency program can provide residents with hands-on experience in addressing healthcare disparities. Collaborating with local organizations, clinics, and community groups can help residents understand the unique health challenges faced by different populations and develop strategies to address them. Service-learning projects and volunteer opportunities can further enhance residents' understanding of and commitment to health equity. Some programs have included walking or bus tours in their orientation to help trainees get a better understanding of the communities their patients live and work in [24].

By making diversity, equity, and inclusion training a core component of the onboarding process, residency programs can cultivate a more inclusive and effective healthcare environment for pediatric trainees/patients and their families.

Program Evaluation and Improvement in Pediatric Residency Programs

An ongoing step in the onboarding process should include feedback in both directions. Trainees should be able to self-assess and receive feedback, and the program should regularly welcome evaluation opportunities. Practical program evaluation and improvement are critical components of maintaining and enhancing the quality of pediatric residency programs, especially with ongoing changes in the pediatric educational environment. Evaluating areas like the resident's experiences and perceptions of the program's inclusivity can help identify areas for improvement. Program leadership should be responsive to feedback and committed to making necessary changes.

The program's various evaluation methods to capture specific aspects of the training experience, including the quality of teaching, the adequacy of clinical exposure, and the effectiveness of supervision, should be introduced to the trainees. It is essential to ensure anonymity and confidentiality to encourage honest and constructive feedback. Additionally, residents should understand the importance of regular and timely feedback, not just at the end of rotations or academic years, to facilitate timely interventions. Engaging residents and preceptors in the feedback process helps build a culture of continuous improvement and accountability within the program.

Because the onboarding process is crucial for acclimating new residents to the demands and expectations of the pediatric residency program, assessing the effectiveness of these processes may involve evaluating how well new residents adapt to their responsibilities and how prepared they feel after the initial orientation period. Early performance evaluations may provide objective data on how well residents apply what they learned during onboarding. Feedback from residents about gaps or areas for improvement in the onboarding process is invaluable for refining and enhancing the program to better meet the needs of future cohorts.

Once feedback and data have been collected and analyzed, developing and executing action plans that address identified issues is essential. This process involves prioritizing areas for improvement, setting clear goals, and allocating resources to support the changes. Those who provide feedback should be part of the planning and execution stages to ensure that their concerns are adequately addressed and that they feel invested in the outcomes. Celebrating successes and acknowledging improvements can maintain momentum and encourage a culture of continuous improvement. These efforts contribute to developing a supportive and effective training environment, ultimately enhancing future physicians' quality of pediatric care.

Conclusion

For program directors, facilitating effective resident onboarding is paramount in ensuring a smooth transition from UME to GME. A well-structured orientation program addresses the logistical, educational, and social aspects necessary for new residents to integrate into their roles successfully. Key components of a successful onboarding process include setting clear expectations, establishing communication channels, and providing practical support such as housing information and system access. A comprehensive orientation helps familiarize residents with institutional policies, patient populations, technological tools, and opportunities for socialization.

The importance of ongoing support and development throughout residency cannot be overemphasized. Continuous mentorship and regular feedback mechanisms are vital in helping residents navigate their evolving responsibilities. Program directors should conduct needs assessments to tailor orientation to individual requirements, ensuring that any gaps in knowledge or skills are addressed early. By fostering a culture of open communication and support, programs can mitigate feelings of stress and isolation often experienced by new residents. Regular check-ins with mentors and faculty, along with peer support groups, provide a robust support system that promotes well-being and professional growth.

Future enhancements in onboarding practices should focus on creating more personalized, experiential, and hands-on learning experiences. Incorporating simulation-based training, role-playing, and OSCEs can significantly improve residents' clinical competence and confidence. Additionally, integrating diversity and cultural humility competency training is essential to prepare residents for the diverse patient populations they will serve and the diverse learning environment. Emphasizing wellness and self-care from the outset helps prevent burnout and promotes a healthy work–life balance.

The onboarding process should be continuously evaluated and improved based on feedback from residents and faculty. Implementing regular assessments and collecting feedback from participants and stakeholders on the effectiveness of the orientation can help identify areas for improvement. Action plans should be developed by the program and executed to address any identified issues, ensuring that the orientation and onboarding process evolves to better meet the needs of future cohorts.

In summary, the transition from medical student to resident physician is a critical period that requires careful planning and support. Effective onboarding and orientation programs set the foundation for residents' success, enhancing their ability to provide high-quality patient care. By continuously refining these processes and addressing the multifaceted needs of incoming residents, program directors can significantly impact the overall residency experience, contributing to better outcomes for residents, patients, and the program.

References

1. DiMarino LM, Boppana RC, Pincavage AT, et al. AAIM recommendations for undergraduate medical education to graduate medical education transition curricula in internal medicine. Am J Med. 2023;136:489–95.
2. Coalition for Physician Accountability. The Coalition for Physician Accountability's Undergraduate Medical Education-Graduate Medical Education Review Committee (UGRC): recommendations for comprehensive improvement of the UME-GME transition. https://physicianaccountability.org/wp-content/uploads/2021/08/UGRC-Coalition-Report-FINAL.pdf. Published 2020. Accessed 19 June 2024.
3. Crail C, Haskins J. The onboarding process: a step-by-step guide https://www.forbes.com/advisor/business/onboarding-process/. Accessed 15 Jul 2024.
4. Bauer T. SHRM foundation's effective practice guidelines series. Onboarding new employees: maximizing success. https://www.shrm.org/about/foundation/products/Documents/Onboarding%20EPG-%20FINAL.pdf. Published November, 2010. Updated February, 2011. Accessed 17 July 2024.
5. The Joint Commission E-edition for Hospital, Release July 1, 2024. Oakbrook: Joint Commission Resources; 2024.
6. Accreditation Council for Graduate Medical Education. Institutional requirements. Accreditation Council for Graduate Medical Education; 2021. https://www.acgme.org/globalassets/pfassets/programrequirements/800_institutionalrequirements2022.pdf. Accessed 15 July 2024.
7. PeopleAdmin. What is onboarding exactly? https://peopleadmin.com/blog/what-is-onboarding-exactly/; 2013. Accessed 21 Jul 2024.
8. Ben-Zion S, Unaka N, Price L, Wallihan R. 68. Evaluating the perceived effectiveness of pediatric intern orientation. Acad Pediatr. 2019;19:e31–2. https://doi.org/10.1016/j.acap.2019.05.082.
9. McGrath J, Barrie M, Way DP. Emergency medicine resident orientation: how training programs get their residents started. West J Emerg Med. 2017;18:97–104. https://doi.org/10.5811/westjem.2016.10.31275.
10. Caldarelli E, Hess JJ, Weaver E, et al. A graduate medical orientation intervention focused on local health inequities. J Grad Med Educ. 2023;15:442–6. https://doi.org/10.4300/JGME-D-23-00016.1.
11. Accreditation Council for Graduate Medical Education. The Program Directors' Guide to the Common Program Requirements (Residency). Accreditation Council for Graduate Medical Education; 2024. https://www.acgme.org/globalassets/pdfs/guide-to-the-common-program-requirements-residency.pdf. Accessed 25 July 2024.
12. Joe MB, Cusano A, Leckie J, et al. Mentorship programs in residency: a scoping review. J Grad Med Educ. 2023;15:190–200. https://doi.org/10.4300/JGME-D-22-00415.1.
13. Wiese A, Bennett D. Orientation of medical trainees to a new clinical environment (the ready-steady-go model): a constructivist grounded theory study. BMC Med Educ. 2022;22 https://doi.org/10.1186/s12909-022-03105-3.
14. Pethrick H, Nowell L, Paolucci EO, Lorenzetti L, Jacobsen M, Clancy T, Lorenzetti DL. Peer mentoring in medical residency education: a systematic review. Can Med Educ J. 2020;11(6):e128.

15. Sargeant J, Lockyer JM, Mann K, Armson H, Warren A, Zetkulic M, Soklaridis S, Könings KD, Ross K, Silver I, Holmboe E. The R2C2 model in residency education: how does it foster coaching and promote feedback use? Acad Med. 2018;93(7):1055–63.
16. Lyss-Lerman P, Teherani A, Aagaard E, Loeser H, Cooke M, Harper GM. What training is needed in the fourth year of medical school? Views of residency program directors. Acad Med. 2009;84(7):823–9. https://doi.org/10.1097/ACM.0b013e3181a82426.
17. Rao P, Hill E, Palka C, Rea K, Jones K, Balzer K, Cornell T, Rooney D, Cousino M. Improving pediatric resident communication during family-centered rounds using a novel simulation-based curriculum. MedEdPORTAL. 2018;14:10733.
18. Mills DM, Wu CL, Williams DC, King L, Dobson JV. High-fidelity simulation enhances pediatric residents' retention, knowledge, procedural proficiency, group resuscitation performance, and experience in pediatric resuscitation. Hosp Pediatr. 2013;3(3):266–75.
19. Todd BR, Traylor S, Heron L, Turner-Lawrence D. Sprint through tasks: a novel curriculum for improving resident task management in the emergency department. MedEdPORTAL. 2020;16:10956.
20. Liu RQ, Davidson J, Van Hooren TA, Julie AM, Koughnett V, Jones S, Ott MC. Impostorism and anxiety contribute to burnout among resident physicians. Med Teach. 2022;44(7):758–64.
21. Yaghmour NA, Brigham TP, Richter T, Miller RS, Philibert I, Baldwin DC Jr, Nasca TJ. Causes of death of residents in ACGME-accredited programs: a 15-year analysis of national data. Acad Med. 2017;92(7):976–83.
22. Rivera N, Feldman EA, Augustin DA, Caceres W, Gans HA, Blankenburg R. Do I belong here? Confronting imposter syndrome at an individual, peer, and institutional level in health professionals. MedEdPORTAL. 2021;17:11166.
23. Spencer SP, Lauden S, Wilson S, Philip A, Kasick R, Mahan JD, Fernandes AK. Meeting the challenge of teaching bioethics: a successful residency curricula utilizing team-based learning. Ann Med. 2022;54(1):359–68.
24. Cross JJ, Arora A, Howell B, Boatright D, Vijayakumar P, Cruz L, Smart J, Spell V, Greene A, Rosenthal M. Neighbourhood walking tours for physicians-in-training. Postgrad Med J. 2022;98(1156):79–85.

Part IV

Curriculum and Educational Design

Curriculum Development 12

Sarah Gustafson, Christiana M. Zhang, and Belinda Y. Chen

Overview of the Kern and Thomas 6-Steps of Curriculum Development in Medical Education

A curriculum is defined as "a planned educational activity," and pediatric program leaders plan educational activities ranging from small lectures to large residency programs [1]. In the Kern and Thomas model, curriculum development consists of six steps, which are iterative and interdependent. Here, we describe the 6-Steps as they apply to pediatric residency programs more generally, and later in the chapter, we will describe how they can be used locally as a framework for curriculum maintenance, enhancement, and revision. This framework should prove useful as you read the other book chapters and consider specific aspects of the program you lead.

S. Gustafson (✉)
University of California, Los Angeles, Los Angeles, CA, USA
e-mail: SGustafson@mednet.ucla.edu

C. M. Zhang · B. Y. Chen
Johns Hopkins School of Medicine, Baltimore, MD, USA

Step 1: Problem Identification and General Needs Assessment

Identifying the Health Care Problem that you expect your educational program to prepare learners to address and conducting a General Needs Assessment to describe the gap between the ideal and current approaches to that problem.

- Identify a healthcare problem. Even if you are responding to a perceived deficit in the training program, ensure that you can articulate how each problem is connected to a larger healthcare problem.
- Conduct a literature review (e.g., PubMed, AAMC MedEdPortal, Association of Pediatric Program Directors (APPD) LESSON, other societal websites) to provide the justification for the curriculum and an understanding of the existing curricula on the topic.
- When forming the general needs assessment, articulate and document the gap between the current state and the ideal state, considering how educators, patients, communities, and current healthcare professionals address the problem.
- A clear problem identification statement will help cast a clearer vision of how the curriculum can guide your trainees towards impacting this "north star."

H. McPhillips et al. (eds.), *Graduate Medical Education in Pediatrics*, Excellence in Medical Education 3, https://doi.org/10.1007/978-3-032-12952-9_12

Step 2: Targeted Needs Assessment

Gathering information for a Targeted Needs Assessment—examining what you know and what you do not know about your learners and the learning environment.

- Consider necessary information about your local context.
- Identify local collaborators.
- Align the curriculum with institutional missions and local needs.
- Consider what information might already be available in the form of rotation evaluations, ITE exam scores, informal comments from trainees, and forums such as housestaff meetings.
- Use sound survey or focus group methods when gathering new information.

Step 3: Goals and Objectives

Articulating clear Goals and Objectives will guide your educational and evaluation methods.

- Goals can be broad and general, whereas objectives should be specific and measurable.
- Learners and instructors should look at the objectives and understand how to determine when learners have achieved the objective and why it is relevant.
- Not all learner objectives are purely cognitive. Also, consider affective, psychomotor skill, and behavioral objectives and their connection to overall healthcare outcome objectives. Classifying the type of learning objectives will help greatly in identifying congruent educational and evaluation strategies.
- The mantra for high-quality objectives from Kern and Thomas is "who will do how much (or how well) of what by when?" Adding details to answer those questions usually makes the objective clearer.
- An alternative model from the business literature is to write SMART objectives (specific, measurable, achievable, relevant, and time-bound) [2].
- Bloom's taxonomy can help identify verbs that clarify the level of cognitive objectives [3].

Step 4: Educational Methods

Choosing congruent and feasible Educational Strategies to optimize the success of the curriculum and manage resources wisely.

- Educational content and methods should align with learner objectives and knowledge of the anticipated learners and their environment.
- Subject matter experts can help to curate knowledge for quick learning and reference.
- Most GME training is expected to be experiential learning from engaging in activities that require the application of the learner's existing expertise and motivate the acquisition of additional knowledge and skills.
- Consider the patient mix at your program and seek to address anticipated experience gaps.
- Residency programs are expected to include scholarly activity and education of others in addition to direct patient care because pediatric specialists and subspecialists need to have broad skill sets to address health care problems.
- Timely, specific, helpful feedback and access to resources can enhance each resident's ability to be a lifelong learner in the care of pediatric patients.

Step 5: Implementation

Planning curricular Implementation to ensure it is sufficiently organized and resourced to be effective.

- Name all involved collaborators.
- List the resources required in terms of people, time, and materials.

- Gain political capital by using the 6-Steps to effectively communicate about the curriculum.
- Decide whether to phase-in pieces of the curriculum, pilot, or launch fully.

Step 6: Evaluation and Feedback

Designing a system for feedback that allows for effective evaluation of both the learners and the program.

- Use a systematic approach to both assess learners and evaluate the program.
- Consider the formative (information for improvement) and summative (final judgment) assessments within the curriculum.
- Align the evaluation with the objectives and educational methods.

Applying the 6-Step Approach to Pediatric GME Programs: Big and Little Gears

When considering larger GME programs as a whole, think of the curriculum development process like an analog clock face with multiple gears behind it (Fig. 12.1). The overarching GME program is the main wheel or "Big Gear," but smaller curricula or "Little Gears" within this larger program are individual 6-Step wheels (Fig. 12.2). The wisdom of this approach is in making clear the context of any curricular changes so that the gears serve their purpose—making the hands of the clock move steadily forward in an integrated way. Building on this clock analogy, the following is how we might approach coming alongside a new PD, going through the 6-Steps as interlocking Big (Arabic numerals) and Little Gears (Roman numerals).

In a curriculum revision process, the 6-Step approach can be applied in two cycles. The first is to focus on the Big Gear and perform a program review using the 6-Steps to establish how the current program curricula compare to the "ideal" specialty or subspecialty GME program and describe a program-specific problem identification. Then, the (Little Gear) 6-Steps can be used to revise specific parts of the overall program.

Example of Big Gear curriculum development:

As a pediatric PD, you should be able to articulate where your program fits into the overall 6-Steps from the ACGME/APPD perspective.

1. Step 1, Problem Identification and General Needs Assessment: Articulate how your program graduates will be prepared to solve the problem of improving care for infants, children, adolescents, and young adults.
2. Step 2, Targeted Needs Assessment: List what is unique about your selection process and your training environment and the local institution where your program resides.

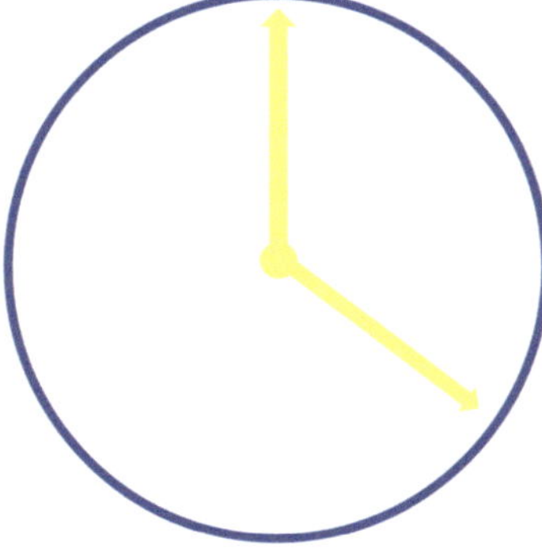

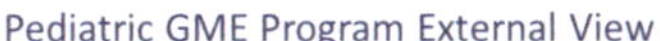

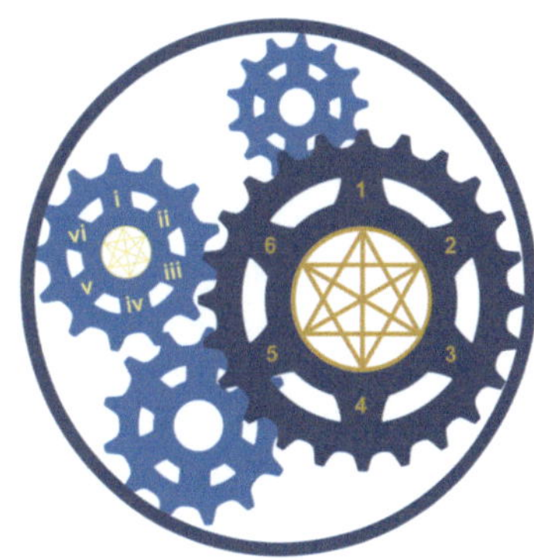

Fig. 12.1 Analog clock of curriculum development. (Used with permission from Dr. Christiana Zhang and the Johns Hopkins Faculty Development Program in Curriculum Development)

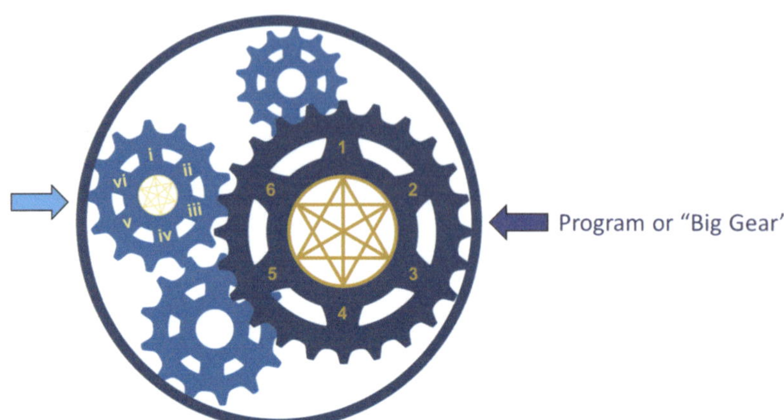

Fig. 12.2 Individual six-step gears within the larger "Big Gear". (Used with permission from Dr. Christiana Zhang and the Johns Hopkins Faculty Development Program in Curriculum Development)

3. Step 3, Goals and Objectives: Look through the goals and objectives set out by the ACGME and APPD and highlight ones that are optional or superficial for most programs but required/emphasized in your program and those that might get overlooked in your program, but are required. There are likely already curricular ideas available to help you fill in gaps quickly, so the core of your program is strong.
4. Step 4, Educational Methods: Map the educational activities in your programs and the clinical/research schedules to ensure all the goals/objectives are covered. Again, there should be plenty of options out there from other programs to inform the core activities that support core goals and objectives.
5. Step 5, Implementation: List the resources and structures in your program that support your trainees and their learning, and the mechanisms needed to keep the key aspects of your program running.
6. Step 6, Evaluation and Feedback: Describe the evaluation plan and design of your program. When do you gather specific data for formative and summative feedback about the learners that can drive program changes to improve performance and outcomes? Start with those that are required by ACGME and accreditation bodies and add or modify to suit local needs and priorities.

Example of Little Gear curriculum development:

Developing a new mental health curriculum within your residency program.

Based on the Big Gear 6-Steps, identify a number of problems that could be addressed and choose a priority problem to focus on next. An example would be: "We are concerned that learners are having to invest too much time learning the logistics of making referrals and we would like to help them increase their learning efficiency so they can devote more time to giving anticipatory guidance before discharge." This becomes the north star for your curriculum revision.

As a program leader, you have the perspective and data to identify who on your core faculty can help shore up parts of the curriculum and provide them with key program information and context to help them develop curricular elements that are likely to succeed.

6-Steps: Zooming-In to the Little Gears

1. Step i, Problem Identification and General Needs Assessment: State your priority problem and how you identified it (e.g., local data on disease prevalence, ITE training scores, self-rated or preceptor-rated abilities, trajec-

tory of milestones progress, or nonparticipation in planned activities). Then query the literature and colleagues to see if others have addressed the same problem. There may be opportunities to learn from and build upon others' successes, or to develop resources to benefit a broader array of learners.

2. Step ii, Targeted Needs Assessment: Based on step i, define and then describe your intended learners. In developing or refining a curriculum for local use, look at data from your program. For a regional or national audience, look at data from national sources such as APPD or other professional organizations. If the desired information is not readily available, consider how much effort it would take to gather that information and how such data might influence your curricular design. As much as possible, reach out to colleagues to adopt or adapt existing resources and help brainstorm ideas to quickly fill gaps and monitor their impact.
3. Step iii, Goals and Objectives: Articulate a clear learning goal that is congruent with the problem identified in Step i and the audience of intended learners in Step ii. Sharing information makes it possible for others (both faculty and learners alike) to focus on writing specific measurable objectives that could drive learning towards that goal. Consider the highest order learning objectives your program can aim for, as well as program or process objectives and their relationship to outcome objectives. Think about Bloom's taxonomy, Kirkpatrick's Reaction levels, and Miller's pyramid. Well-written objectives will help you to more easily match educational and evaluation strategies. So, even though you do not actually collect assessments and evaluations until after curriculum implementation, thinking about "how much/how well" as you are writing your objectives will be helpful.
4. Step iv, Educational Methods: For educational content relative to that objective, encourage your faculty to look to subject matter experts and resources both within and external to your program. Challenge them to identify multiple educational methods that are congruent with their objectives and then choose the one that is feasible with the resources currently available or potentially obtainable.
5. Step v, Implementation: Encourage your faculty to consider how existing administrative structures can accommodate the needs of any proposed educational and evaluation strategies. Keep things simple and use resources effectively to match the needs.
6. Step vi, Evaluation and Feedback: Sometimes you think that your curriculum is working effectively, but a metric was not met or no data were available at all. Data collection takes effort, so look for ways to synergize. What are you measuring that is working? Keep in mind what data access each collaborator needs to avoid reinventing the wheel. Remember how the feedback loop should work: providing reliable information to facilitate mid-course corrections to keep learners on track to their goal.

Diving Deeper into the 6-Steps

Now that we have provided an overview of curriculum development steps, we shall discuss in further detail some curriculum development application examples commonly shared by pediatric GME programs.

Problem Identification and General Needs Assessment

Step 1

Since problem identification involves taking a few steps back and looking at the 30,000-foot view of the problem, pediatric GME programs share a common overall problem identification.

Mission statements of national collaborators are a helpful resource where pediatric program directors can obtain inspiration for program-level problem identification. Use a search engine to browse the mission statements on the websites of the organizations in Table 12.1. For example, the

Table 12.1 Collaborators in pediatrics

Organization	Curriculum content	Assessment data	Examples of collaboration opportunities
ACGME - Accreditation Council for Graduate Medical Education	Requirements for curricular content. Asynchronous material such as Equity Matters.	EPAS/Milestones	Sponsored opportunities for residents and fellows such as *Back to Bedside*
ABP - American Board of Pediatrics	Board content specification outline	Board pass rates Interactive pediatric workforce data	Resources for implementation of EPAs
AAP - American Academy of Pediatrics	Pedialink Equipp	Policy statements and associated references	Sections related to subspecialties and interest groups
APPD - Association of Pediatric Program Directors	APPD LESSON - curriculum content APPD LEARN - scholarship in medical education	National surveys can provide general needs assessment.	Listserve with ability to ask questions
COPS - Council of Pediatric Subspecialties	Webinars and descriptions of different subspecialties	Subspecialty EPAs and milestones	Committees and Action Teams
COMSEP - Council on Medical Student Education in Pediatrics	Curricula transitioning from UME to GME	COMSEP clerkship competencies	Pathway to pediatric residency
FuturePedsRes	Curricular structure and initiatives of peds residency programs	Data on program sizes and highlights by program and region	Pathway to pediatric residency
AMSPDC - Association of Medical School Pediatric Department Chairs	Resources for new chairs	Statements on the pediatric workforce	Committees and Programs

These organizations are excellent sources of national priorities, general needs assessment data, and opportunities for collaboration (through listservs, subcommittees, and meetings)

mission of the American Academy of Pediatrics (AAP) is "to attain optimal physical, mental, and social health and well-being for all infants, children, adolescents and young adults". [4]

The stated mission of the Association of Pediatric Program Directors (APPD) is "to ensure the health and well-being of all children, we lead the advancement of pediatric medical education, the development of a sustainable and diverse workforce, the cultivation of an inclusive learning environment, and promotion of educational innovation" [5]. This mission statement builds on the AAP's mission while including pediatric trainees and will align well with the local pediatric GME problem identification.

Problems common to all pediatric training programs include fewer trainees choosing pediatrics or a pediatric subspecialty, changing health issues, increasing child mental health needs, and shifts in societal demographics. Two of the main conclusions of the National Academies of Sciences, Engineering, and Medicine (NASEM) report on the pediatric workforce landscape highlight the need to adapt curricula to be responsive to changing societal needs: [6]

Conclusion #4.1: The current model of education and training has not evolved substantially in response to the changing context of society and medicine, including the changing health needs of pediatric patients, changing practice patterns, and the changing needs of trainees.

Conclusion #4.2: Pediatric education and training needs to be more responsive to the changing needs of infants, children, and adolescents.

Further defining that problem raises additional questions: What is the core knowledge base and skillset of a pediatrician (as opposed to other health care professionals)? What do parents, society, and healthcare professionals look to pediatricians to do? What gaps do we currently see, and how do we prepare future pediatricians to close those gaps and address future gaps?

Statistics and datasets on pediatric patients may also be helpful. According to the CDC, the leading causes of death in the pediatric population in the USA are accidents, congenital malformations, deformations, chromosomal abnormalities, cancers, and homicides/suicides; thus, every US pediatric residency program should provide education and experiences to equip its graduates to address such health problems. Another approach might be to consider what are the leading causes of pediatric (age 0–17 years old) hospital admissions. According to the healthcare cost and utilization project statistics from 2019 (prior to Covid), 77% of pediatric hospitalizations were for children less than 1 year old. The leading primary diagnosis was respiratory for children under 5 years old, whereas depressive disorders was a leading diagnosis for children older than 10 years [7].

The general needs assessment outlines the gap between what various collaborators (e.g., patients/caregivers, society, healthcare professionals) ARE CURRENTLY DOING related to that health care problem and what they COULD/SHOULD BE DOING based on available knowledge/evidence. Describing this gap provides the foundation for developing creative ways to close those gaps. In medical education, the goal is to determine how education can play a role in closing the gap. Who needs to learn what by when to effect needed change?

Sometimes, current and anticipated shortages in subspecialists can inspire and motivate residents to obtain further training in those subspecialties. But sometimes specific problems within those specialties can best be addressed by training a broader range of clinicians (e.g., primary care) or society (e.g., pediatricians teaching caregivers or educators) to be able to manage more common or treatable conditions on their own.

Awareness of the national needs and priorities in pediatrics are essential in building the case for the local training program. The AAP's Strategic Plan outlines national challenges and opportunities in pediatrics [8]. Current common needs are as follows:

- To address shortages in primary care.
- To address shortages in subspecialty care.
- To address the lack of access to care, especially in rural areas.
- To decrease healthcare disparities and their impact on child health.
- To address the dwindling pediatric workforce pipeline.
- To address emerging areas of importance in pediatrics:
  - Increasing use of value-based payment models.
  - Social and environmental determinants of health.
  - Enhancing the use of technology by patients, families, and providers.
  - Mental health.
- To train advocates and leaders in the field of pediatrics.

Each pediatric GME program exists to contribute to solving the overall problem by training future medical diagnosticians and healers within the context of the community that their clinical program serves and the learning community that the program brings together. For example, one program may have more of a focus on refugee health and another may have a lot of children with inborn errors of metabolism. One may have mostly seasoned clinicians as attendings and another may have a large cohort of researchers in their teaching pool. Having a clear program statement that ties to the part of the overall problem that your residency aims to address can help unite your faculty around purpose and save them time since each person does not need to redo Step 1 for themselves.

Step i

When creating or modifying the problem identification for a specific curriculum within a pediatric training program, problem identification is listed as the first step in connection with the general needs assessment, including the literature review of published articles. Table 12.1 lists some sources of pediatric data and collaborators that may be helpful in this step. In your search, pay particular attention to the introduction or background paragraphs of key literature related to your curriculum. For example, a curriculum on pediatric rheumatology in MedEdPortal [9]:

> Pediatric rheumatologic disease… occurs more frequently than several other chronic pediatric diseases...but is an often under-recognized disease entity owing to the misconception that children are too young to have arthritis.... JIA and other rheumatologic diseases are serious conditions that pose unique challenges and require specialized care to prevent morbidity and mortality.

The authors have used their introductory paragraph to establish a case for their curriculum:

- Establishing that trainees will encounter these conditions.
- Highlighting that there are gaps in understanding or misconceptions among pediatricians.
- Describing the morbidity and mortality associated with the condition.
- Discussing workforce issues with a few subspecialists available.

Other important aspects to consider include costs for society and potential cost savings from interventions. The authors might choose not to include that in the opening paragraph of a publication with a word count limit. However, in a presentation to hospital administration to ask for resources, the costs of delayed diagnosis or misdiagnosis might be more important to highlight.

In addition to pediatrics-focused organizations, consider external partners who have implemented similar curricular changes. For example, learning how family medicine colleagues adapted to their new ACGME requirements can be helpful, particularly if your program's clinical sites co-host learners from that specialty. Consider interprofessional resources and organizations. Learning from other residency programs in other specialties within your institution can provide inspiration and a fresh perspective.

For curriculum-specific general needs assessment, search not only for published curricula, but also for national needs assessment surveys. If the information that you are seeking does not exist, you can consider applying to do a needs assessment. APPD reviews applications for national needs assessment surveys and provides feedback.

Frequently, APPD national surveys are published in *Academic Pediatrics*. Surveys can identify gaps in training. For example, a 2022 survey by Fitzgerald et al. identified that while most program directors rate telemedicine as important, most also did not have a telemedicine curriculum [10]. These data can help provide local justification for resources and show that there is room in the literature for scholarly dissemination.

If a systematic approach is used, each of the 6-Steps may potentially be publishable on its own, depending on the scale of the step work. A national or multi-site survey with an acceptable response rate will be more publishable than a local survey. If there has not been a systematic review performed on the topic, devoting resources to conduct a systematic review may be a welcome contribution to the literature and some help to other educators.

However, program leaders typically have a limited number of resources and time, and spending too much time and resources on one step might delay the implementation of the program, which would be counterproductive to the aim of addressing an important gap. Rigor in the approach to curriculum development is not just for the sake of disseminating educational scholarship—it is also for ensuring that trainees get the highest quality education.

The 6-Steps are traditionally arranged in a circle [1], which reminds us that the CD curriculum development process is iterative, not linear, and also that we must balance our investment in each of the steps. Step 1 is termed the "north star" because it keeps us focused on why we are putting effort into curriculum development and revision. At the completion of this step for this cycle, one should be able to articulate the problem that this curriculum is designed to address and the gap between the current and ideal approaches to that problem from a pediatric educator's perspective.

Targeted Needs Assessment

Step 2

The next step is then focused on knowns and unknowns about your intended learners and their learning environment. Table 12.2 provides a checklist of aspects to consider in the targeted needs assessment.

Each program's response to the national needs may be different, but grounding each in a shared problem can open doors to collaborative relationships and sharing of resources. For example, if an institution is starting something as small as a new subspecialty elective experience or as large as a new pediatric fellowship program, the subspecialty governing bodies' websites or mission statements are a place to search for inspiration and alignment. AAP policy and position statements are also excellent resources for specific topics within pediatric training.

Table 12.2 Targeted needs assessment checklist. This checklist, adapted from Kern and Thomas to be specific to the pediatric GME context, can assist program leaders in systematically considering sources of helpful information about their intended learners and anticipated learning environment

Helpful Knowledge About Your Pediatric GME Learners *(Ideally, much of this can be learned through the application/interview process, assessments built into the GME experience, and only occasionally, further dedicated inquiry)*
Knowledge and skills needed at the end of residency: *Milestones, EPAs, and board exams—but also, do most of your learners plan to go on to subspecialty training or rural primary care practice? Conduct research or teach?*
Medical school training and variable training experiences: *Query those who applied to or matched into your program—what are their known gaps or areas of proficiency? For example, some medical schools have no delivery experiences on their nursery rotation, or maybe you selected learners who all speak the primary language of your clinic population?*
Planned experiences in current curriculum*: Do you have a planned orientation experience or boot camp to ensure a certain baseline body of knowledge/skill/sense of cohesion among the interns?*
Existing proficiencies/practices/perceived & measured learning needs:
Cognitive: *Assess on the first ITE and based on direct observation of clinical performance by preceptors*
Affective: *Set expectations during intern orientation; check-in on wellness and professional identity formation with program leadership and advisors*
Psychomotor: *Assess during trainee orientation or early in rotations through direct observation of trainee performance. OSCEs and formal observed history and physical are examples of assessments.*
Current behaviors/performance/practices: *Ongoing feedback through rotational evaluations/audits, housestaff meetings, informal interviews, or check-ins with chief residents.*
Attitudes and motivations of learners to improve performance: *include each resident in developing an individualized learning plan*
Preferences and experiences regarding different learning strategies:
Synchronous vs asynchronous learning: *Inquire as to whether they prefer to view lectures on their own at double-speed with closed captioning to internalize content more efficiently, or if they appreciate opportunities to interact with a live expert.*
Duration: *Gauge experience with just-in-time nuggets of learning like chalk talks* vs *immersive, focused sessions with simulation or community-based learning.*
Methods: *Consider methods you plan to use that may require more or less orientation depending on prior familiarity. For example, employing visual thinking strategies and art to address tolerance of ambiguity, or VR when some learners struggle with 3D vision.*
Helpful Knowledge aAbout Your Pediatric GME Learning Environment
Related existing curricula: *Speak with local leaders of clinical environments or program directors of different specialties to see if there are areas of overlap or opportunities to collaborate. When gaps are found, search MedEdPortal and APPD for resources already available to your learner/faculty and for connections with other programs for larger programmatic implementation.*

(continued)

Table 12.2 (continued)

Needs of collaborators other than the learners: *Assess staffing of faculty divisions and the capacity to have trainees rotating through the services. Note how your program supports others' goals,* e.g., *completing faculty evaluations needed for promotion.*
Barriers, enabling, and reinforcing factors that affect learning:
Barriers: *Are there attendance records for conferences? Note workforce needs such as nighttime coverage for deliveries that may affect availability for synchronous educational sessions during the daytime.*
Enablers: *Ask the program or GME coordinator if your program already subscribes to nationally available resources such as the AAP model for individualized learning plans? Does your institution provide structures such as a GME-wide learning management system?*
Reinforcing factors: *Review previous end-of-year presentations—are there resident awards to recognize individuals or competitive systems to encourage active learning within teams throughout the year? Query your EMR experts—are there dashboards and reports that can provide information about practice habits and outcomes?*
Resources: *List institution-wide resources* (e.g., *library resources), look at the resource list for individual curricular components.*
Informal and collateral curriculum: *Ask chief residents or fellows in their last year for meaningful insights as near-peers. Directly observe trainee-to-trainee handoff to learn what is being conveyed informally.*

Understanding the context of curricular innovation is key. Other steps of curriculum development, particularly implementation, are strongly tied to the targeted needs assessment. This step includes needs assessment of the intended learners AND their learning environment. The potential sources of information are similar across GME programs. Although the learners by default include future pediatricians, it is important to step back and ask whether pediatric trainees are the ideal targeted learners and whether there are others who should be considered. Similarly, when programs send their residents to different hospitals or clinics, the case mix and culture will affect how and what they learn.

Step ii

Programs can minimize duplication of work by first considering relevant available information, such as rotational evaluations, the program education committee (PEC), ACGME surveys of faculty and residents, and program in-training exam (ITE) scores.

The institutional, departmental, and divisional mission statements may help justify the training program's purpose within the institution. Incongruency between the institution's mission statement and some goals of the training program might highlight a need for diversifying educational experiences through partnerships in the surrounding community or with outside institutions, or by advocating for inclusion of new clinical sites within the institution's network.

Step ii is also where you consider the experiences and perspectives of the other learners and professionals who work alongside pediatric trainees. Incorporating such valuable input can help create a more supportive and collaborative environment as a new curriculum is introduced. If pediatric trainees participate in a quality improvement curriculum related to improving interprofessional communication without including nursing perspectives, then resistance from inpatient bedside nurses or clinic nurses may compromise the impact of the curriculum.

Within the training program, the PEC, consisting of residents and faculty, is a rich source of information from the trainee perspective because PECs review rotational evaluations and note qualitative feedback during meetings. Committee members can also be asked for additional opinions in settings outside of committee meetings.

Programs can also identify gaps in their educational program by using the crosswalk between the ACGME common program requirements and the annual ACGME graduating resident survey [11] and faculty survey [12]. For example, if the resident survey is below national average on residents participating in scholarship, programs can present this information to the faculty, department, and institution, connecting these data with a risk of losing accreditation, and thus motivating educators and potentially mobilizing resources.

Individual learner results, when taken in aggregate, can be helpful in a targeted needs assessment. Aggregate program ITE score reports provide valuable information as to gaps in the trainees' knowledge and an opportunity to refocus the clinical curriculum and board preparation around weaker topics. Aggregate clinical performance evaluations of trainees can also be used to identify areas of relative weakness in the program's curriculum. The program board pass rate can similarly identify a need for increasing board-related content or constructing more robust study plans.

There will always be unanswered questions about learners and the learning environment. Before setting out to try to answer them, ask yourself what you will do with the information if obtained. Will it affect a key decision in the CD process? If not (either because not relevant to this curriculum segment or because decisions about the curriculum have already been made), it may not be worth your time to gather. Also, asking for opinions and then not acting on the trainee's wishes might damage trust.

If the missing knowledge is actionable, then consider the best method to gather reliable information for your targeted needs assessment. Questionnaires are the most commonly used means of collecting information, but informal interviews or focus groups may be better for generating ideas. If others have published on the topic previously or there is a published, validated needs assessment tool, this can save time and help guide a valid interpretation of the data. If you believe the information you gather will yield generalizable information that should be shared with the broader education community, it is wise to seek IRB review.

Goals and Objectives

Step 3

An overall goal of a pediatric GME program is to prepare trainees to be board-certified in pediatrics or a pediatric subspecialty. ACGME-approved competencies and milestones have already been outlined and starting in 2028 the ABP will require reporting on Entrustable Professional Activities (EPAs). Therefore, mapping the GME training experiences to those goals will help learners and faculty alike to remember the purposes of each educational experience. While it is not the PD's responsibility to write every learning objective for every rotation, it is helpful for the program leadership to clarify the program's goals, so faculty can align specific measurable objectives with them. In addition to learner objectives, process or program objectives can promote alignment towards the greater goals of the whole program.

Organizational tools can be used to map and coordinate many parts of a curriculum. These can be spreadsheets and calendar systems or larger integrated learning management systems such as MedHub or New Innovations. At the program level, process objectives can be particularly useful to track the implementation of the curriculum and revisions to the curriculum. Trainees' participation in aggregate can be tracked on a dashboard within the management system. In Step 4, we will expand further on curriculum mapping.

ACGME also requires that trainees receive and review rotational goals and objectives. A system to ensure that they receive the objectives automatically can save time for coordinators and directors while preventing errors. Further efficiency can be introduced through a task management system that sends automated reminders for rotational leaders to review, revise, and upload new objectives to the system on a yearly basis.

As outlined in this chapter's overview, high-quality objectives will reveal all components of "who will do how much (or how well) of what by when." This level of specificity will allow both trainees and educators to see the alignment between the objectives, educational methods, and assessment plans. Rather than the program leadership writing all rotational objectives, educators can develop skills through faculty development on best practices in objective-writing.

In a faculty development session, educators can bring their rotational objectives with them to revise. If they do not have objectives already written, sample objectives from the literature or from another local rotation can be used in an exercise where they critique and refine objectives using the Step 3 "mantra" and identify the objective type.

Step iii

Using an example such as this school health curriculum from MedEdPortal [13], faculty can practice classifying objectives and thinking at the rotation or session level:

By the end of this activity, learners will be able to:

- *Articulate the differences between an individualized educational plan (IEP), individualized health plan (IHP), and a 504 plan, as assessed by a pre- and post-didactic survey.* [cognitive].
- *Explain an IEP, IHP, or 504 plan to a family so that the family feels confident in advocating for its children's needs to optimize their education within schools, as assessed by observed role-plays.* [psychomotor skill].

Faculty can practice creating their own rotational objectives, trade with a partner, and critique each other. Hypothetical examples could look like the following:

- *Affective: Rate as important the school-based interventions for children with chronic illness.*
- *Process objective: Create individual health care plans for at least three patients with chronic illnesses during a school-based rotation.*
- *Healthcare outcome: Patients of the trainees who complete the school health curriculum will have better performance in school.*

While it may be unrealistic to attribute changes in the outcome measure solely to a specific curricular intervention, delineating and tracking a relevant outcome objective can be helpful in ensuring that the significance of attaining a curricular goal remains relevant. Frequently, the information utilized to define the health care problem in Step 1 provides such a relevant health care outcome objective.

Educational Methods

Step 4

Much of residency is experiential learning based on direct patient care. Although based on shared RRC requirements for general pediatrics and specialty experiences, each residency program will have a different patient population and case mix. Residents are not required to log all their patients as medical school students do. But residents and PDs will benefit from tracking the types of patients, diagnoses, and treatments seen in the course of daily patient care. They might note that their patient population does not have all conditions that occur nationally, or that at their flagship quaternary care center subspecialty care is centered around very rare conditions. For example, a resident rotating on an oncology elective at a hospital specializing in bone marrow transplantation might not learn first-hand the initial presentation and treatment of low-risk acute lymphoblastic leukemia. Conversely, a resident based at a community hospital might never treat patients with hemophagocytic lymphohistiocytosis. Comparing ABP Board Content Specifications and data from their institutions, a program director can identify the gaps and ensure there are alternate ways to master all required material.

Step iv

Sharing a list of core conditions and topics for residents to review and "check off" during specific rotations is a common strategy. The APPD LESSON curricula for behavioral mental health and pediatric hospital medicine cover some of the most common conditions with which residents should be familiar by the end of residency.

Programs have incentivized residents to do independent, self-directed learning by creating "houses" and gamifying the process of activities such as completing PREP questions and reading *Pediatrics in Review* articles.

The use of curriculum mapping through a learning management system can track educational methods and their alignment with goals and objectives for each rotation. It is critical to assess for and maintain congruence between educational methods and the institutional and program goals and objectives. Having an annual curriculum review document with changes made and the rationale for the changes can empower program leaders to review and assess proposed future changes in light of lessons learned from the past.

Curriculum Mapping

Curriculum mapping can guide learners and educators alike, improving transparency in the educational process [14]. Watson et al. describe the variations in curriculum mapping and outline categories of curriculum maps in dimensions of (1) the purpose of the map, (2) the content of the map, (3) the map process, and (4) the map display or tool used [15]. By considering the purpose and the intended audiences for your curriculum map before embarking on the project, you can ensure that your efforts are focused and that you will minimize the need to go back to redo your map. Wang provides an alternate viewpoint that curriculum tracing is useful and allows flexibility in a dynamically changing field [16].

High-level curriculum mapping in GME commonly starts with publishing the schedule of clinical rotations, commonly referred to as a "block schedule." During recruitment, programs frequently share the building blocks of the residency curriculum, including a mock schedule to give the applicants an idea of what their years at that program would look like. There are many sources of uncertainty in residency, and a lack of control over one's schedule can contribute to burnout. In this way, curriculum mapping is a critical way to help clarify uncertainties for learners.

Curriculum mapping can help faculty educators to plan experiences that reinforce previous learning and fill specific learner gaps. It allows the curriculum to build over time. Sharing the "curricular arc" with educators is critical for topics that span multiple rotations and specialties. Curricular "tracks" can span years and include not only clinical rotations but also specific experiences such as lectures, workshops, and ongoing research projects.

A curriculum map should include the learning outcomes that are expected by the end of the experience or the end of residency. Clear communication about the expected progression through milestones or criteria for higher levels of entrustment, accompanied by specific opportunities for skill demonstration, can help keep residents from falling too far behind. The curriculum map is also useful for the clinical competency committee's review of the learner's performance. McGill's curriculum map aligning their pediatric residency rotations with EPAs provides an outstanding example of a transparent, well-organized curriculum [17].

Curriculum mapping can clarify for the program leaders where there are gaps and redundancies and where there are opportunities to build additional educational experiences or to cut experiences. Suggested content of the curriculum map include: (1) the expected learning outcomes; (2) curriculum content or areas of expertise covered; (3) student assessment; (4) learning opportunities; (5) learning location; (6) learning resources; (7) timetable; (8) staff; (9) curriculum management; and (10) students.

When communicating to leadership, asking for resources, and enhancing the curriculum, a curriculum map organization of the curriculum clarifies and can prevent misconceptions about the current resources or rotations. A well-organized curriculum can provide a foundation for later dissemination or publication.

Implementation

Step 5

Whether implementing a new residency or fellowship program or a new module within a rotation, consider the resources required in terms of people, time, and materials for the overall curriculum. A systematic approach to implementation is essential to ensure the success of the residency curricula. In the textbook by Thomas et al, Curriculum Development for Medical Education, Table 6.1 outlines a general checklist for implementation [1]. While all curricular work is context dependent, there are many common features of implementation in GME.

Step v In the general needs assessment section, we discussed collaborators who are important national (external) sources of support. Table 12.3 identifies additional internal sources of support. APPD's Program Director Handbook describes the core program leadership team, composed of a PD, Associate Program Directors (APDs),

Table 12.3 Examples of other internal sources of support for the functions of the training program as a whole or for a curricular innovation within the program

People
For the Department Chair, Vice Chair for Education, and the Designated Institutional Official (DIO).
For individual rotations, or for fellowship programs, the Rotation Directors, Division Director, or Medical Director of the relevant specialty.
For individual rotations occurring at sites outside the home institution, Education Site Directors.
If there is interaction of residents with medical students, Clerkship Directors and Assistant and Associate Deans at the medical school.
Committees
At the institutional level, the Graduate Medical Education Committee (GMEC) is a source of support and oversight.
Local committees include the pediatric program-specific committees such as the Program Evaluation Committee (PEC), Clinical Competency Committee (CCC), and committees within the program or department such as Diversity, Equity, and Inclusion or Advocacy Committees.
The PEC can help with the implementation of new initiatives. Passionate residents on the PEC or other departmental committee can be champions for change or improvement of aspects of the curriculum.

Coordinators, and Chief Residents [18]. Ensuring that the team understands and is invested in the mission, vision, and future directions of the program is foundational for the successful implementation of every curricular endeavor from implementing a new residency or fellowship program to improving a component of a rotation. Experts within the APPD community have created resources (e.g., the APD handbook and the newly revised PD handbook) for leaders transitioning into new roles. The APPD Fall Meeting is designed to assist with the transition for new program leaders. The APPD Curriculum Learning Community hosts virtual cafes and provides mentorship to members seeking to learn more about CD in pediatric GME.

Coordinators are key team members who manage communication and operations tasks required for a complex training program. Automation of tasks using an internet-based task manager, with team member assignments, built-in reminders, and scheduled-send emails set up through a learning management system can also streamline communication.

Resident buy-in is key to successful implementation, so clearly communicate the rationale for changes. In addition to formal PEC input, you can incorporate residents' interests and ideas from housestaff meetings and other forums including information from your targeted needs assessments. Current residents and fellows may also become future Chief Residents, core faculty, and program leadership, so having a transparent process and inviting their contributions is also an investment in the future of pediatric GME.

For individual rotations, modules within rotations, or didactics, consider whether to pilot, phase in pieces of the curriculum, or launch fully. Sometimes, a full launch is mandated because of an institutional or ACGME deadline. However, the rotation might technically fit the requirements but still not be in its fully envisioned form. As time goes on, enhancement of the rotation can be planned and implemented (see Ongoing Curriculum Maintenance and Enhancement, below).

Evaluation and Feedback

Step 6

A key aspect of any GME program is providing relevant, accurate feedback to learners, faculty, and program leadership for formative and summative evaluation decisions.

Evaluations occur at the resident, rotation, faculty, and program levels. Sending evaluations electronically, via a learning management system, facilitates compilation of results for both individual-learner and program-level review. Creating a system for reviewing evaluation data and implementing curricular change is necessary, given the volume of evaluations that a residency program manages.

Attendings, other housestaff, other healthcare professionals, and patients directly observe residents in practice and give feedback. Faculty can use standardized checklists to conduct direct observations, such as an observed history and physical, and give formative feedback.

Evaluation formats should also tie-in to milestones, EPAs, and other institution-specific evaluations. Milestones are a required assessment for all residents, determined by the CCC but based on direct observation of patient care, and must be reported to the ACGME. Through the framework of milestones in the six ACGME competency domains of patient care, medical knowledge, systems-based practice, practice-based learning and improvement, professionalism, interpersonal and communication skills, residents are rated based on narrative anchors corresponding to competency levels ranging from novice [1] to expert [4]. Like individual direct observation encounters, milestones are meant primarily for formative feedback to the resident learner.

EPAs or "everyday pediatrician activities" are the essential functions that a general pediatrician should be able to perform. Both milestones and EPAs may be used to identify learners in need of additional support or remediation, and can be used to create an individualized learning plan. The milestones and EPAs should align with program objectives, and EPA curricular components can be particularly useful when developing objectives and determining the best educational methods.

While the CCC is the typical forum for resident evaluation review, the PEC is often a forum for rotation and program evaluation review. The overall program evaluations come from sources such as aggregate rotation evaluations, the annual ACGME survey, GME committee feedback, and aggregate ITE and board pass rates.

Step vi

Aside from required trainee evaluation sources, when implementing a new curriculum or an enhancement, program leaders can consider what sources of data and outcomes will help with course correction or to better assess whether the curriculum is working as intended.

Program leaders can consider whether patient outcomes might be tracked to evaluate the success of the intervention. While it is typically difficult and resource-intensive to measure a patient-level outcome, aim for high-Kirkpatrick level outcomes when possible. Lowest to highest, the four Kirkpatrick levels are reaction (how learners felt about the curriculum), learning (knowledge assessment of the learners), behavior (direct observation of behavior change for the learners), and result (patient outcome change). An evaluation or study can include multiple levels of outcomes.

In the I-PASS study [19], it was found that implementation of a standardized handoff was associated with decreased medical errors. In addition to looking at the rate of medical errors ("result" or level 4 Kirkpatrick), they also observed the percentage of time spent with patients and families ("behavior" or level 3), and trainee report of the quality of handoff ("reaction" or level 1).

Outcomes in a pediatric GME program will not always be clinical. In a 2021 survey of pediatric fellowship directors, the authors found a wide variation in scholarly productivity [20].

Increasing exposure to and mentorship for non-clinical research pursuits, including through dedicated career development sessions, fellow participation in skill-building workshops at regional or national meetings, and identification of departmental, institutional, or even national mentors with training in QI, education, and other disciplines may be helpful.

A lower-level objective related to scholarship could simply be "able to name different types of research studies." However, for programs preparing clinicians to be researchers at the end of training, a more congruent higher-level outcome would be publication or presentation at a national meeting. Aligning educational methods with that aim would involve trainee participation in national workshops and participating in research with a mentor whose research interests and skills closely align.

Ongoing Curriculum Maintenance and Enhancement

Once the key required elements of the residency program are in place, there should be a plan for regular curriculum maintenance and enhancement. The 6-Step approach, with the Big Gear and Little Gears outlined in this chapter, helps here as well.

Through the assessment of the program as discussed in Evaluation and Feedback, areas for improvement, refinement, or innovation can be identified. In addition to the pre-existing sources of data mentioned already in the form of rotation evaluations and ACGME annual surveys, additional questionnaires, focus groups, and formal and informal discussions can assess how a curriculum is functioning. Each of the six steps should be considered as an area for intervention.

Often, curriculum enhancement and modification occur because of new external requirements, whether it is institutional, such as a new policy or the opening of a new clinic, or national, such as the ACGME pediatric program requirements changing. In addition to complying with the new requirements, program leaders must consider how the changes will affect their local learners and learning environment, for example, with the 2025 program updates:

> New rotation requirements include mental health and developmental-behavioral pediatrics. The introduction of these required rotations coupled with a decreased requirement for inpatient time has potential impacts on residents' career trajectories, academic hospitalists' schedules, and preparation for care of hospitalized children [21].

Every program has unique aspects that can help learners to acquire expertise in caring for patients whom their affiliated clinical and research sites serve. Recognizing and explaining their "added value" can help with the recruitment of trainees who will thrive in that environment or benefit from that expertise. Every program cannot be all things to all people, so knowing your program's strengths may help you identify what you can further develop and share with others, just as you may look to other programs for ideas for how to improve what your program can offer.

The community of pediatric educators and program directors, including APPD, is critical in sustaining the local team's motivation and provides a source of expert consultation on the listserv as program leaders enhance their existing curriculum.

Whether faculty have a role in precepting trainees, are called upon to cover additional duties in order to protect educational time for trainees, or are leading curriculum enhancement, consider acknowledgment and invitation for their input and feedback in the process. It is important to set time aside to celebrate and recognize the extended curriculum team, including contributing faculty. Faculty need evaluations for promotion, but the recognition should go beyond electronic evaluation. Particularly for faculty who are invested and innovate in the curriculum, educational awards provide a time to celebrate accomplishments. Likewise, annual resident teaching awards for resident leaders of education can provide a way to celebrate residents.

Dissemination: Making It Count Twice

As you go through the steps iteratively, look for opportunities to make things count twice. By that we mean, look for opportunities to share what you have learned and make things easier for others. To do this best, consider what was hardest for you and what made things easier for you in your process. Then, identify the forum that gathers those who need the benefit of your experience and share it! Many times, though not always, this will translate into something that can be listed in your portfolio as a clinician-educator—a talk, chairing a national group, sharing curriculum segments, writing up significant outcomes and lessons learned, or including the data to help others understand the limitations of your work and how they may apply them to improve their own. Through following the 6-Step approach for curriculum development, you will have already conducted a scholarly approach, fulfilling Glassick's criteria for scholarship: [22, 23] clear goals, adequate preparation, appropriate methods, significant results, effective presentation, and reflective critique.

In addition to helping other programs, dissemination can create opportunities for your program to collaborate with other programs who are interested in similar educational innovations. Presentations at national or regional meetings provide the opportunity for feedback on the innovation through fresh perspectives. Working in curriculum development with educators at other institutions may also make the resulting work more generalizable and easier to implement at other institutions.

In addition to furthering the program and the careers of program leaders, this encourages other faculty educators to participate in educational scholarship. Along with the celebration of pediatric faculty in the form of awards and acknowledgments, curriculum development itself provides opportunities for all faculty to participate in scholarship. For program leadership who contribute to faculty development, make it clear that faculty can create scholarly work for academic advancement, and providing faculty development on the 6-Step framework for curriculum development can enable them to get "credit" for the work that they already do. Later in this book, the program director advancement chapter discusses other aspects of advancement, including scholarly work.

Next Steps in Your Curriculum Development Journey

While initially created to assist medical educators tasked with developing new curricula, this 6-Step framework has also been successfully applied to the revision of existing curricula in response to changing needs. Keeping clear in your mind the problems you are preparing your learners to address and how they merge with clear goals and aims, matched with congruent educational and evaluation strategies, will facilitate successful implementation and future enhancement. As a GME program leader, this model can help you to align elements of your training program to not merely meet the requirements of accreditation bodies, but to prepare your learners for the roles they will serve in society as highly trained board-certified pediatricians and subspecialists better than they could prepare on their own.

Being a program director is being a leader in a complex system that can be challenging, but very rewarding. As you look through the rest of this book, we hope the framework we've presented here is useful for organizing your knowledge about your programs and others like it so that you can contribute to and learn from a community of like-minded clinician-educators. Find the gaps, discuss with others, and discover and share new ways to support, motivate, and equip your faculty and learners to be their best.

References

1. Thomas PA, Kern DE, Hughes MT, Tackett S, Chen BY. Curriculum development for medical education: a six-step approach. 4th ed. Johns Hopkins University Press; 2022. p. 103, Table 6.1.
2. Doran GT. There's a S.M.A.R.T. way to write management's goals and objectives. Manag Rev. 1981;70(11):35–6.
3. Anderson LW, Krathwohl DR, Airasian PW, Cruikshank KA, Mayer RE, Pintrich PR, Raths J, Wittrock MC. A taxonomy for learning, teaching, and assessing: a revision of bloom's taxonomy of educational objectives (Complete Edition). Longman; 2001.
4. About the American Academy of Pediatrics. HealthyChildren.org. Accessed August 9, 2024. https://www.healthychildren.org/English/Pages/about-aap.aspx
5. About the Association of Pediatric Program Directors (APPD). Association of Pediatric Program Directors. Accessed August 9, 2024. https://www.appd.org/about/
6. National Academies of Sciences E, Education D of B and SS and, Division H and M, Board on Children Y, Services B on HC, Well-Being C on the PSW and II on CH and. The pediatric health care workforce landscape. In: The future pediatric subspecialty physician workforce: meeting the needs of infants, children, and adolescents. National Academies Press (US); 2023. Accessed August 10, 2024. https://www.ncbi.nlm.nih.gov/books/NBK599760/.
7. Weiss AJ, Liang L, Martin K. Overview of hospital stays among children and adolescents, 2019. In: Healthcare cost and utilization project (HCUP) statistical briefs. Agency for Healthcare Research and Quality (US); 2006. Accessed August 9, 2024. http://www.ncbi.nlm.nih.gov/books/NBK588376/.

8. American Academy of Pediatrics Strategic Plan. Accessed August 9, 2024. https://www.aap.org/en/about-the-aap/strategic-plan/
9. Gillispie M, Muscal E, Rama J, Falco C, Brown A. Pediatric pheumatology curriculum for the pediatrics resident: a case-based approach to learning. MedEdPORTAL. 14:10767. https://doi.org/10.15766/mep_2374-8265.10767.
10. Fitzgerald M, Bhatt A, Thompson LA, et al. Telemedicine in pediatric training: a national needs assessment of the current state of telemedicine education in pediatric training. Acad Pediatr. 2022;22(5):713–7. https://doi.org/10.1016/j.acap.2021.10.009.
11. ACGME. Resident Survey Crosswalk. Published online July 1, 2023. Accessed August 9, 2024. https://www.acgme.org/globalassets/pfassets/programresources/residentsurvey_cprcrosswalk.pdf
12. ACGME. Faculty Survey/Common Program Requirements Crosswalk. Published online July 1, 2023. Accessed August 9, 2024. https://www.acgme.org/globalassets/pfassets/programresources/faculty-survey_cprcrosswalk.pdf
13. Anderson LR, Yang C, Cotter JM, et al. School health: pediatric primary care curriculum. MedEdPORTAL. 14:10764. https://doi.org/10.15766/mep_2374-8265.10764.
14. Harden RM. AMEE Guide No. 21: Curriculum mapping: a tool for transparent and authentic teaching and learning. Med Teach. 2001; https://doi.org/10.1080/01421590120036547.
15. Watson EGS, Steketee C, Mansfield K, et al. Curriculum mapping for health professions education: a typology. Focus Health Prof Educ. 2020;21(1):91–113. https://doi.org/10.11157/fohpe.v21i1.364.
16. Wang CL. Mapping or tracing? Rethinking curriculum mapping in higher education. Stud High Educ. 2015;40(9):1550–9. https://doi.org/10.1080/03075079.2014.899343.
17. McGill. Curriculum Map in General Pediatrics. Department of Pediatrics. Accessed August 10, 2024. https://www.mcgill.ca/peds/education-training/pgme/programs/generalpediatrics/residencyprogram/cbd/curriculummapping
18. APPD. Program directors' handbook. Published online 2024. Accessed August 10, 2024. https://www.appd.org/program-directors-handbook/
19. Starmer AJ, Spector ND, Srivastava R, et al. Changes in medical errors after implementation of a handoff program. N Engl J Med. 2014;371(19):1803–12. https://doi.org/10.1056/NEJMsa1405556.
20. Abramson EL, Weiss P, Naifeh M, et al. Scholarly activity during pediatric fellowship. Pediatrics. 2021;147(1):e2020013953. https://doi.org/10.1542/peds.2020-013953.
21. New ACGME Peds Program Requirements Present Challenges and Opportunities - The Hospitalist. Accessed August 9, 2024. https://www.the-hospitalist.org/hospitalist/article/37015/pediatrics/new-acgme-peds-program-requirements-present-challenges-and-opportunities/
22. Glassick CE. Boyer's expanded definitions of scholarship, the standards for assessing scholarship, and the elusiveness of the scholarship of teaching. Acad Med. 2000;75(9):877–80. https://doi.org/10.1097/00001888-200009000-00007.
23. Mills DM, Teufel RJ II. Tools for medical education scholarship: from curricular development to educational research. Hosp Pediatr. 2020;10(5):452–7. https://doi.org/10.1542/hpeds.2019-0293.

13 Clinical Curriculum

Stacy Laurent and Ross E. Myers

ACGME Requirements

The practice of general pediatrics has become increasingly complex, notably in outpatient general pediatrics. In addition to providing a medical home for well children, outpatient general pediatricians must also provide a medical home for children with medical complexities. With advancing technology and enhanced medical care, patients with complex medical conditions such as extreme prematurity, spinal muscular atrophy, and cystic fibrosis are living longer and healthier lives. The care for these patients in the general outpatient pediatric office is incredibly important and a cornerstone for their overall health care. With the advent of pediatric hospital medicine fellowship being accredited by the Accreditation Council for Graduate Medical Education (ACGME), all the aspects of pediatric medicine other than general outpatient pediatrics require additional training for board certification. Many pediatric subspecialties are seeing decreased applicants to fellowship leading to a continued under-subscription especially in areas such as nephrology, pulmonology, and infectious disease. This puts even more emphasis on pediatric residency programs to prepare their trainees to practice outpatient general pediatrics in this changing healthcare environment. The ACGME has updated its pediatric residency programs to reflect these changes.

The new program requirements will be covered more in depth elsewhere in this book, but they are central to the clinical curriculum for pediatric residents. Given the changes to the pediatric educational landscape described above and changes within the field of pediatrics, adjustments to the program requirements were made. Additional focus is put on ensuring robust general pediatrics experiences, both outpatient and inpatient, mental health care of children, and subspecialty exposures. A new requirement to expose residents to outpatient subspecialties within the first 2 years of residency may help increase visibility and interest in some of the pediatric subspecialty areas with fewer practicing physicians. With the new requirements, it will be incredibly important for programs and faculty to emphasize what a general pediatrician needs to know from their areas of expertise. Assisting trainees to gain the tools to provide a medical home for patients with any condition will enhance patient care, allow subspecialists to focus on the more severe cases, and help patients lead healthier lives.

S. Laurent (✉)
University of Illinois College of Medicine at Chicago, Chicago, IL, USA
e-mail: sthomps2@UIC.EDU

R. E. Myers
Rainbow Babies and Children's Hospital and Case Western Reserve University School of Medicine, Cleveland, OH, USA

H. McPhillips et al. (eds.), *Graduate Medical Education in Pediatrics*, Excellence in Medical Education 3, https://doi.org/10.1007/978-3-032-12952-9_13

In addition, the requirement for individualized curriculum (IC) remains to ensure the learning and career needs are met for each resident. While the IC is covered separately, it is important to consider it as part of the clinical curriculum, as residents will be selecting various clinical experiences to meet their personal goals.

Clinical Experiences

The ACGME requirements outline the necessary pediatric residency experiences, and the American Board of Pediatrics (ABP) General Pediatrics Content Outline delineates the essential knowledge areas in which the general pediatrician should be proficient. In addition, the ABP Entrustable Professional Activities (EPAs) for General Pediatrics breaks down the activities a general pediatrician is expected to routinely perform both safely and effectively in the care of their patients. Each General Pediatrics EPA includes specific activities and highlights the rationale behind the importance of each area of expertise. Therefore, the clinical curriculum must link both patient-facing, hands-on experiences with additional didactic sessions to ensure mastery of a wide breadth of essential clinical knowledge. Rotation-specific curricula focus on both understanding the clinical environment and supplementing the patient experience with planned educational experiences [1]. As each clinical environment and institution is unique, it is also imperative to adapt the clinical curriculum to enhance the learning experience, utilizing the individual pediatric residency program's mission and aims [1].

Breaking down the 120 weeks of clinical experiences required by ACGME into 40 weeks of inpatient, 40 weeks of ambulatory, and 40 weeks of individualized curriculum leaves 24 weeks of undefined clinical experiences for program needs or innovation [1]. These 120 weeks of clinical experiences are dictated by the ACGME but the curricular content should be targeting not only the program requirements but also program specific mission and aims, as well as addressing standardized test results and graduate surveys [1]. Incorporating social determinants of health and other population and structural needs is integral in providing education for trainees to gain the necessary knowledge to start dismantling health disparities. The ABP general pediatrics content outline is a great way to delineate and strategize where content is being covered and how to supplement the clinical learning environment. Each EPA includes curricular components specific to that activity to support curricular development and is designed to be used across the education continuum.

Building a schedule that comprises all necessary experiences is integral to ensuring requirements are met and clinical experiences are incorporated. By starting with a block diagram, programs can work out how the requirements will be met as a generic schedule and do not need to be specific in terms of order of rotations [2]. The block diagram provides rotation, site identification, rotation frequency and postgraduate year it will occur. Depending on the individual institution's patient volume, pediatric residency programs may need to partner with other institutions to ensure trainees receive all the necessary clinical experiences. Specifics on how to proceed with a program letter of agreement (PLA) are contained within the ACGME common program requirements [3].

Inpatient Curriculum

This requirement is made up of 24 weeks of inpatient medicine (a minimum of 16 weeks of general pediatrics or pediatric hospital medicine (PHM)), 12 weeks of intensive care (ICU) (a minimum of 4 weeks in a neonatal ICU and 4 weeks in a pediatric ICU) and 4 weeks of newborn nursery for a total of 40 weeks of inpatient care experiences [1]. The inpatient experience typically consists of a general pediatric or PHM service where residents care for a well-balanced variety of patients. Some institutions may also have subspecialty pediatric inpatient services where patients are grouped by systems such as neurology or nephrology. These subspecialty inpatient experiences cannot comprise more than

4 weeks of a single subspecialty and cannot exceed 8 weeks total within the 40 required weeks of inpatient [1].

The make-up of the Gen Peds/PHM team is variable by institution but traditionally consists of a PGY-1 and a supervisor, as well as a multidisciplinary team of staff such as bedside nurse/charge nurse, pharmacist, child life, and social worker. In order to provide residents with exposure to the 24-h coverage of a hospital unit, many programs will have resident coverage of patients at night. These teams/coverage care may be variable, made up of different levels of trainees and supervision, depending on the individual institution.

Since daytime team structure and staffing varies by institution, it allows for customization. For example, a teaching senior could be added to a team to not only bolster the educational experience of the residents on the rotation but also as a way for additional inpatient PHM rotation experiences. A teaching senior resident could lead didactic sessions during the day as well as assist the team as needed but may not be responsible for carrying the patient load (especially if average daily census does not allow for additional rounders per ACGME requirement). In a traditional block schedule, this additional senior resident can also allow for fewer transitions when a co-resident needs to leave for their continuity of care clinic. Additional clinical scheduling considerations include adding an admitting resident to start at a later time, which would not take away from the patient load to be carried by the rounding residents.

Multiple of the ABP general pediatrics content domains apply to the Gen Peds/PHM setting and content can be mapped to areas to be covered during a rotation as well as longitudinally over the course of residency. A well-rounded inpatient/PHM curriculum starts with identifying all the ABP general pediatric domains that pertain to that space and determining how the content is covered. Table 13.1 shows an example of mapping ABP content to the clinical curriculum.

For most inpatient units, croup, bronchiolitis, and pneumonia can be expected to be regularly seen and cared for in the clinical setting. Resident education on these topics should be bolstered through journal articles and other educational modalities such as podcasts, webinars, and guidelines (i.e., AAP clinical practice guidelines, pediatrics in review, institutional clinical pathways, Pedialink, etc.). For bronchiolitis, this is also listed as a core competency for Pediatric Hospital Medicine in the *Journal of Hospital Medicine* [4] and is included as a common clinical diagnoses and conditions with specific knowledge, and systems organization and improvement goals outlined by the Society of Hospital Medicine [5]. Utilizing both ABP and PHM core competencies, bronchiolitis could be covered by including the educational resources included in Table 13.1 as part of patient care discussions, as well as rotation-specific didactics.

There are also available online resources, such as Open Pediatrics, which is a free resource and has created a course catalog for pediatric training [6]. This online resource has been studied and shown to prime and augment clinical learning [7]. In addition, the Association of Pediatric Program Directors (APPD) has created a Longitudinal Educational Software Solution and Outcomes Network (LESSON) where education materials that advance the training of future pediatricians are vetted and developed into an online Learning Management System (LMS) [8].

For less common diagnoses or areas of clinical practice that are seen less frequently at an individual institution, didactic or case-based discussions are important to ensure a balanced clinical curriculum. This can be done as "wards cases" where residents present on an interesting case during a morning report, faculty lead lectures on topics not routinely covered during the clinical experiences, webinars, or board review with board-style questions and content discussion. Many pediatric specialty organizations/foundations also offer conferences, online learning opportunities and more specifically for health-care provider use. Using the ABP Domain 12 from above, cystic fibrosis is an important topic but one not commonly seen clinically at all institutions as care is prioritized at cystic fibrosis centers. This would therefore be a topic to ensure was covered through either rotation-specific

Table 13.1 Example of clinical curriculum mapping using ABP content

ABP domain Domain 12: Pulmonology	Subtopic	Example of resource mapping	Example additional resources	
A. Upper airway 1. Infectious (e.g., croup, epiglottitis) 2. Laryngomalacia, tracheomalacia, and vocal cord dysfunction 3. Foreign body **B. Lower airway** 1. Asthma 2. Pneumonia 3. Foreign body 4. Other lower airway (e.g., pulmonary artery sling, bronchitis, bronchiolitis, aspiration pneumonia)	**Bronchiolitis** Regularly seen in inpatient units. Education bolstered through journal articles, podcasts, webinars, and guidelines.	1. Clinical practice guideline: The diagnosis, management, and prevention of bronchiolitis Pediatrics Nov 2014; 134(5): e1474–e1502. 10.1542/peds.2014-2742. 2. Pediatrics in Review article: Bronchiolitis Pediatr Rev. (2019) 40(11): 568–576. 3. Clinical pathway: Children's Hospital of Philadelphia Inpatient Clinical Pathways for bronchiolitis treatment. 4. Online course (video): Bronchiolitis—epidemiology, pathophysiology, diagnosis, and care. 5. Podcast: Treating Bronchiolitis in Children, Children's Hospital of Colorado. 6. Board style question review: pedialink prep questions.	**OpenPediatrics:** Free resource with a pediatric training course catalog	Common pediatric respiratory problems course: Covers upper and lower airways obstruction, pneumothorax
C. Parenchymal, extrapulmonary, pulmonary hypertension, and cor pulmonale			**LESSON (Longitudinal Educational Software Solution and Outcomes Network):** Developed by APPD as a platform to house educational materials that are vetted and developed into an online learning management system (LMS)	Step up to hospital pediatrics (in development), a curriculum for inpatient topics such as admission/discharge criteria, cost-effective care, evaluation and management, at-risk populations, and social determinants of health.
D. Chronic lung disease 1. Prematurity/BPD 2. Congenital lung malformations 3. Cystic fibrosis	**Cystic fibrosis** Important topic not commonly seen at all institutions. Should be covered via didactics or lectures. Can be addressed through case-based discussions, faculty-led lectures, webinars, or board review questions.	1. Pediatric Resident Education in Pulmonary (PREP): A Subspecialty Preparatory Boot Camp Curriculum for Pediatric Residents. *MedEdPORTAL 2021;17:11066.* 2. Cystic Fibrosis Foundation—North American Cystic Fibrosis Conference (NACFC): past conference sessions and plenaries available at the NACFC website.		

didactics or during scheduled conference or lecture time.

Consideration should also be given to opportunities to complete procedures. Both the ACGME requirements and the ABPs EPAs include specific procedures for the general pediatrician as well as highlighting the need to consider career-specific procedures for each resident. Procedural skills education can be done as opportunities arise during clinical rotations but can also be scheduled as sessions with mannequin training, simulation, or didactic sessions. MedEdPortal.org includes many procedural curricula, including options for longitudinal educational models, and the New England Journal of Medicine houses many procedural videos that can be used as part of the educational process.

ICU

As part of the inpatient requirements, residents are expected to complete 12 weeks of intensive care with a minimum of 4 weeks of each neonatal ICU and pediatric ICU [1]. Patient composition and volume is variable by institution, so consideration should be given to the need for supplemental educational experiences for a well-rounded intensive care experience. For PICU, LearnPICU is a trusted source for core pediatric critical care topics as well as references and board study materials [9]. Simulation and videos are critical tools in providing critical care education as preparation before rotations, as well as exposure to scenarios or diagnoses not encountered during the rotation. There is specialized pediatric critical care, such as burn, trauma, cardiac, or neurologic care, which can be experienced via collaboration with nearby institutions or through didactic sessions. Simulation (reviewed in Chap. 19) has been proven to be effective in supplementing critical care education and experience.

Additionally, intensive care training should include procedural skills, many of which are included within the ACGME requirements (i.e., bag-mask ventilation, lumbar puncture, etc.) but also with a focus on procedures applicable to the individual residents career plans (i.e., point of care ultrasound). Procedures can be done via mannequin or simulation to supplement the experiences during rotations.

Ambulatory Curriculum

The ambulatory clinical experience is made up of 40 weeks of primary ambulatory care experiences [1]. This is further distilled to: 8 weeks of general ambulatory pediatrics clinic, 4 weeks of subspecialty outpatient experience (minimum of 2 different subspecialties in the first 24 months of training), 4 weeks of adolescent medicine, 4 weeks of mental health, 4 weeks of developmental behavioral pediatrics and 12 weeks of pediatric emergency medicine and acute illness (minimum of 8 weeks in the emergency department) [1]. This leaves 4 additional weeks of ambulatory experience needed which programs can meet by adding a community/advocacy rotation or additional time in their general pediatrics clinic (would need to be counted separately from the longitudinal continuity clinic experience requirement). A community/advocacy rotation frequently involves select experiences to enhance the residents' understanding of their local community and the complex makeup of the environment their pediatric patients are exposed to. While advocacy education is addressed in an additional Chap. 17, some examples of possible experiences include visiting community resources such as Women Infants and Children (WIC), food banks, or women and children's shelters, getting a library card at a nearby branch and meeting with the children's librarian, public health education, meeting with local legislators or the local American Academy of Pediatrics (AAP).

Designing a curriculum to teach general ambulatory pediatrics clinic outside of a longitudinal continuity clinic can be designed in a number of ways. Programs may place residents in an urgent care or a community private practice. While urgent care could meet the technical ACGME requirement in this area, the emphasis should not only be on acute or sick visits but also incorporate general well care and chronic medical condition management as important facets of general pediatric practice. Chronic medical condition management may be a role of the general pediatrician; at some institutions, this is also done in a team approach in conjunction with a variety of specialists and support staff. Local governments may also have a branch of their department of children and family services dedicated to the care of children with chronic health care conditions or those in foster care.

Developmental behavioral pediatricians often refer patients to a variety of resources, such as speech therapy, physical therapy, occupational therapy, applied behavior analysis, and developmental therapy, all of which are important aspects of care for pediatric residents to understand in the care of their patients. Developmental assessments are done by a variety of community organizations including via early intervention, head start programs and other local programs supporting the development of children and can be a useful resource for exposure to the assessments.

Adolescent medicine often occurs both inside and outside the traditional clinic setting. There are multiple organizations that provide embedded health care as part of their offerings, such as Job Corps, juvenile detention centers, and middle and high schools. Partnering with clinics serving adolescents as part of their care is another way to ensure a broad experience; clinics such as sports medicine, obstetrics/gynecology, and youth centers or clinics serving LGBTQ patients. Inpatient consultation is also a component of adolescent medicine and may include support with eating disorders, sexual health, substance use, behavioral health, or transitions of care. Additionally, there are many unique curricular components within adolescent medicine that should be included in a focused adolescent curriculum. Topics such as confidentiality, media use, eating disorders, sexual and reproductive health, sports medicine, substance use, and transitions of care are a few examples. The AAP has a dedicated Adolescent Health Care Resource for Providers within their patient care resource online, and local AAP chapters may have webinars or other recorded content specific to the care of adolescent patients. The Yale Primary Care Pediatrics Curriculum also includes many adolescent-focused topics, and the Society for Adolescent Health and Medicine has developed a set of educational materials to be used as part of an adolescent medicine curriculum.

Mental health is covered in Chap. 18.

If there is not sufficient volume for developmental behavioral pediatrics, adolescent medicine, and mental health, it can be helpful to partner with nearby institutions or local clinics to ensure adequate exposure to these specialties.

Individualized Curriculum

The individualized curriculum (IC) is covered in Chap. 15 but is an important consideration when developing a clinical curriculum, especially as the IC should be distributed throughout a resident's educational experience. An IC should include subspecialty experiences (exclusive of other inpatient and outpatient requirements) and clinical elective, scholarly experience, and other opportunities.

Program Discretionary Time

The ACGME has designated 24 weeks of pediatric residency to meet individual program needs or innovative experiences [1]. These 24 weeks will be used in a variety of ways depending on the service needs of a hospital system, but more importantly on supporting the program's mission and aims. Examples of clinical experiences fitting this description include:

- Step-down or intermediate care unit.
- Refugee clinic/initial medical exams.
  - Care of the underserved and vulnerable populations is integral to pediatrics, and many institutions have implemented strategies to ensure that refugees are able to seek medical care. Unique to the care of refugee children is the need for medical evaluation of unaccompanied minors for

foster placement and family reunification. Pediatric residencies are well poised to incorporate these experiences into their training programs to fulfill the task of improving and eliminating healthcare disparities and providing compassionate care. There are multiple organizations tasked with fulfilling the federal government's requirements for evaluation and placement. Pediatric residency programs can partner with these organizations to develop clinical and educational opportunities. Many of these visits are time sensitive, which should be taken into consideration when creating the clinical experience. In addition to patient-facing experience, many modules and webinars have been created to educate the pediatric provider in the sensitive care of these patients.

- Residents as teacher.
  - Residents are teachers and it is important to support and educate all residents as everyone enters training with different skills and experiences but are quickly expected to be an expert not only in their clinical field but as educators. Many residents as teacher curriculums have been published including on topics such as giving feedback, leading a team, didactic teaching, and clinical teaching. MedEdPORTAL contains a variety of residents as teacher curriculum and workshops.
- Community pediatrics (if not needed to be counted towards the ambulatory weeks).
- Procedures and simulation.
  - See the corresponding Chap. 19.
- Advocacy.
  - See the corresponding Chap. 17.
- Board preparation.
  - Integral to pediatric residency training is preparation for the initial certifying exam. Utilizing rotation time for studying can allow for protected time to implement study plans, participate in board review courses, or attend dedicated board review didactics. This can be done as a traditional rotation of variable length or longitudinally as a half or full day.
- Research/scholarship.
  - Many programs provide research rotations for residents to learn research/scholarship skills and design, implement, and analyze their scholarly work.
- Wellness/professional development.
  - Resident wellness has appropriately been increasingly prioritized as part of residency training. Some programs have started scheduling wellness rotations where residents prioritize seeing their own healthcare providers, learning about mindfulness and resiliency resources, work on administrative tasks such as meeting with their advisor, completing board prep questions, or a quality improvement project. Additionally, each institution's local resources vary and this serves as an opportunity for residents to learn about what is available as well as utilize services they find helpful. This can be an opportunity to work on both personal and professional goals.
- Parenting elective (see Chap. 27 on trainees who are parents).
  - The transition back to residency training after a new baby is difficult for many reasons, and the wellness of both the resident and their family should be considered.
  - A parenting elective can provide a supportive way of learning from one's own baby.
  - Examples of such an experience has been published including: The Use of Parenting Electives in Pediatrics Residency (Ben-Zion, S et al., Academic Pediatrics, Volume 22, Issue 4, 513–517) and A Structured Neonatal Parenting Elective: An Approach for Parenting Leave During Residency (Cree-Green, M, et al. Academic Pediatrics, Volume 20, Issue 5, 2020, 595–599).
- Supervisory experiences.
  - If not met during the required rotations, these weeks can be used to provide supervisor experience. Rotations such as newborn nursery where a senior resident supervises an intern while not having a patient panel of their own would be an example.
  - Experiences unique to a program.

Block and Longitudinal Curriculum

Tracking how and when educational topics are covered is fundamental to ensuring there is not disproportionate coverage of certain topics while others are missed. The clinical curriculum should be distributed between block and longitudinal curriculum. Rotation-based block curriculum should be outlined within the goals and objectives of the rotation and should include items to fulfill the program's mission and aims. This can be accomplished by utilizing the ABP general pediatric domains (see an example for PHM) and/or the ABP EPAs. Each EPA has expanded curricular components that list specifics that should be mastered. Some of the curricular components are more practice-based (clarifying and focusing the clinical questions to be addressed) while others are clinical knowledge-based (problems generally within the scope of general pediatric practice, based on prevalence and potential morbidity, where the role of the generalist is to recognize, evaluate, and treat) [10].

Figure 13.1 shows an example of utilizing an EPA to track curriculum, which can be found within the commitment to confronting racism on the APPD website: https://www.appd.org/about/curricula-for-anti-racism/. EPA-based tracking can be utilized for both block curriculum (competency in newborn care) and longitudinally (competency in health care payment systems and fiscally sound health care of children).

A longitudinal curriculum is based on the content the trainee will receive over the course of the residency or a portion of the residency. An example of this is the longitudinal continuity of care clinic, as residents will rotate through this experience longitudinally throughout residency. Journals such as Pediatrics in Review include an ABP content spec map matching articles with the ABP board content, allowing for ease with tracking.

Building a curriculum where these topics can be covered twice over the course of a residency assists with competency and reaching residents who may have missed the topic in the first session. This can be done by selecting topics and assigning sessions where they would be covered (i.e., noon conference, academic half day, rotation didactics) or utilizing an existing primary care curriculum in addition to other sessions. The Yale Primary Care Pediatrics Curriculum, for example, is a set of pediatric modules where learners can progress through topics led by a moderator who has access to additional resources [11]. Topics hit on the ABP content domains such as language and literacy development, primer on vaccines, adolescent immunization, formula feeding, childhood nutrition, and many more [11]. These modules can be used in a more formal conference or didactic setting, as well as in the clinical setting between clinic sessions or during a daily or weekly clinic meeting.

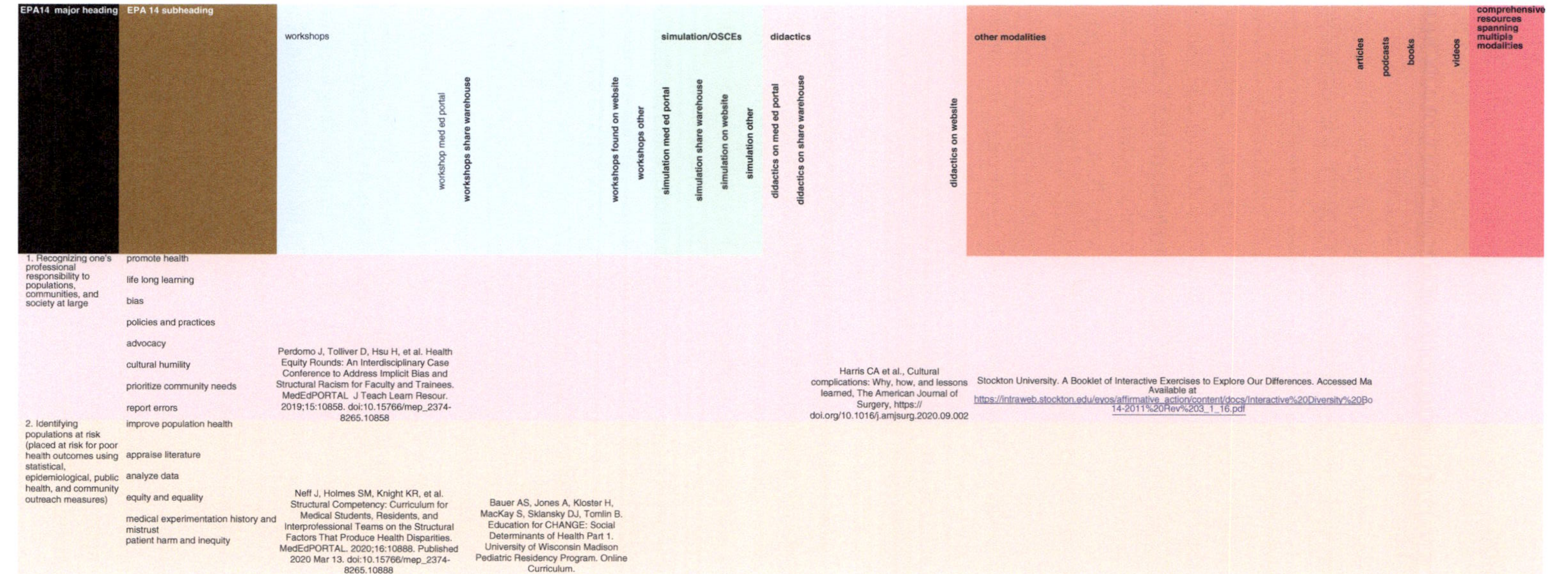

EPA14 major heading	EPA 14 subheading	workshops	simulation/OSCEs	didactics	other modalities	comprehensive resources spanning multiple modalities
		workshop med ed portal; workshops share warehouse; workshops found on website; workshops other	simulation med ed portal; simulation share warehouse; simulation on website; simulation other	didactics on med ed portal; didactics on share warehouse; didactics on website	articles; podcasts; books; videos	
1. Recognizing one's professional responsibility to populations, communities, and society at large	promote health					
	life long learning					
	bias					
	policies and practices					
	advocacy					
	cultural humility					
	prioritize community needs	Perdomo J, Tolliver D, Hsu H, et al. Health Equity Rounds: An Interdisciplinary Case Conference to Address Implicit Bias and Structural Racism for Faculty and Trainees. MedEdPORTAL J Teach Learn Resour. 2019;15:10858. doi:10.15766/mep_2374-8265.10858		Harris CA et al., Cultural complications: Why, how, and lessons learned, The American Journal of Surgery, https://doi.org/10.1016/j.amjsurg.2020.09.002	Stockton University. A Booklet of Interactive Exercises to Explore Our Differences. Accessed Ma Available at https://intraweb.stockton.edu/eyos/affirmative_action/content/docs/Interactive%20Diversity%20Bo 14-2011%20Rev%203_1_16.pdf	
	report errors					
2. Identifying populations at risk (placed at risk for poor health outcomes using statistical, epidemiological, public health, and community outreach measures)	improve population health					
	appraise literature					
	analyze data					
	equity and equality					
	medical experimentation history and mistrust	Neff J, Holmes SM, Knight KR, et al. Structural Competency: Curriculum for Medical Students, Residents, and Interprofessional Teams on the Structural Factors That Produce Health Disparities. MedEdPORTAL. 2020;16:10888. Published 2020 Mar 13. doi:10.15766/mep_2374-8265.10888; Bauer AS, Jones A, Kloster H, MacKay S, Sklansky DJ, Tomlin B. Education for CHANGE: Social Determinants of Health Part 1. University of Wisconsin Madison Pediatric Residency Program. Online Curriculum.				
	patient harm and inequity					

Fig. 13.1 Example of clinical curriculum tracking via entrustable professional activities (EPAs)

Arrangement of Each Clinical Year

Block System Scheduling

The block system has historically been the more common model for scheduling in pediatric residencies. It includes a consistent duration of blocks throughout the year, split into either 26 two-week blocks or 13 four-week blocks. Block assignment is not limited by rotation type and resident continuity clinic would occur one half day per week throughout the year, regardless of the rotation.

X + Y Scheduling

As a way to help pediatric residents have more focus on their rotations and the patients they were caring for in their clinical experiences at the moment, a novel scheduling system to pediatrics was devised in 2018 by five pediatric residency programs. Termed "X + Y" after similar systems were created in internal medicine residency programs, this scheduling system takes outpatient general pediatric continuity clinics away from a traditional model of one half-day session per week to having blocks of time in rotations without any scheduled continuity clinic (X blocks) and other blocks that have continuity clinic (Y blocks). This system was created using the ACGME Advancing Innovation in Resident Education (AIRE) program to enable programs in the pilot to waive one of the ACGME Program Requirements for Pediatrics, where continuity clinics must be scheduled in no fewer than 26 weeks each academic year.

Studies published by the research team for the X + Y AIRE pilot have shown that residents and faculty perceive improvements in both patient care and educational outcomes including improved patient continuity, inpatient workflow and handoff quality, and increased time for teaching in both continuity clinic and inpatient settings (Myers RE, et al. Acad Pediatr. 2021 Sep–Oct;21 (7):1273–1280). These outcomes remained stable or improved at 3 years as well (Myers RE, et al. Acad Pediatr. 2022 Sep–Oct;22 (7):1097–1104.). Given these data, 39 programs joined the AIRE pilot. Different X + Y scheduling systems were utilized from 4 X + 1 Y, 3 X + 1 Y, 6 X + 2 Y, etc. Additionally, within this schedule framework is the X + Y + Z template, which can give programs the flexibility around scheduling. An X + Y + Z schedule typically continues to remove continuity clinic from X rotations (often but not exclusively inpatient experiences), and may have some continuity clinic in both the Y and Z as well as delineate specific subspecialty experiences during Y and Z.

Consider carefully what scheduling system will work best for your program, as it will have an impact on the clinical learning environment for both inpatient and outpatient rotations. Thinking through the pros and cons of X + Y scheduling for each program is one of the most important steps to consider when determining the continuity clinic structure. Identifying key stakeholders of rotations and experiences that will be impacted is a critical first step.

Many possibilities can be created for enhancing clinical curricular offerings by a change to X + Y scheduling. Some of the programs in the pilot have implemented academic half-day educational programs focused on ambulatory pediatrics when groups of residents are on their Y blocks. Others have added experiences with community advocacy organizations and mentoring programs. Utilizing the X + Y structure can help add to the already existing clinical opportunities and experiences for trainees. The updated ACGME requirements removed the 26-week requirement for continuity clinic but continued the 36 half-day requirement and added specificity around time between clinics, stating that there should not be more than 8 weeks between clinic weeks.

Assessment of Clinical Skills

Learner assessment, especially in the realm of clinical skill performance, is a critical piece to ensure that the clinical learning environment is providing the education needed for pediatric trainees to practice pediatric medicine independently. There are several methods one can use to assess the clinical skills of individual learners from direct observation of history taking and physical exam skills to discussions of disease presentation and management among others. Capturing the needed information from various sources, such as faculty, residents, nurses, patients, and families, can be challenging. Evaluation surveys and comments may only paint part of the picture of how a trainee is performing in the clinical arena. The ACGME and the American Board of Pediatrics have developed some tools that may be of use to programs to help with clinical skill assessment.

Clinical Competency Committees (See Chap. 22 on CCCs)

Clinical Competency Committees (CCC) are a requirement from the ACGME to help advise the program director on how the trainees are performing. These can be structured in many ways to help programs gain the information needed to identify how their trainees are progressing and how to better help them gain the necessary skills for promotion to the next training level and for autonomous practice. These groups take the information that has been gathered from evaluations and can provide additional context given their experiences with trainees to better help programs in their overall assessment of individual trainee clinical skills. This committee can also help guide the program director in developing plans to help improve the clinical skills of the trainees to meet the expectations needed.

Milestones

The ACGME Milestones provide a useful framework to help assess trainees on big picture knowledge acquisition and various skills. The anchors used for the various milestones grant faculty and other evaluators the ability to objectively assess learners and show them where they are along a continuum for the individual subcompetencies. The updated Pediatric Milestones 2.0 helps to provide additional clarity in the descriptions for each anchor. Many programs incorporate subcompetency milestones into their learner evaluations, making it easier to know if each trainee is performing and how they are progressing; however, the milestones were not developed with the primary goal of frontline assessment. Proper faculty development in the use of milestones as an evaluation tool is critical in ensuring that program directors and CCC members are receiving accurate information.

EPAs

Entrustable Professional Activities (EPAs) from the American Board of Pediatrics are "observable, routine activities that a general pediatrician should be able to perform safely and effectively to meet the needs of their patients" (https://www.abp.org/content/entrustable-professional-activities-general-pediatrics). These individual activities, unlike the ACGME Milestones, center around the assessment of entrustment levels rather than anchors that describe skills attained. These entrustment levels differ by the individual EPA but usually include "trusted to observe only" to "practice with indirect observation" to "practice independently." This degree of assessment requires faculty, program directors, and CCCs to incorporate various sources of information, including the ACGME Milestones in order to help determine levels of entrustment around the essential activities of a general pediatrician upon graduation. Similar to the ACGME Milestones, faculty development around EPAs, what they are, and what the different entrustment levels mean is critically important to their use in assessment. Having a shared definition of the entrustment levels amongst faculty in a program and around the country will be important, as these are used more in learner assessments.

Summary

Development of a clinical curriculum is a critical puzzle piece of the development and maintenance of a pediatric residency program that meets the needs of future practicing pediatricians. Not only is it important to assess and ensure high quality patient centered teaching during the clinical day but the big picture of mapping and tracking educational domains to ensure a well-rounded education. This can be achieved through the schedule arrangement of each clinical year as well as utilizing both the ABP board content domains and the EPAs through competency-based medical education.

References

1. ACGME. https://www.acgme.org/globalassets/pfassets/programrequirements/2025-prs/320_pediatrics_2025.pdf
2. ACGME block diagram. https://www.acgme.org/globalassets/pfassets/programresources/blockdiagraminstructions_pediatrics.pdf
3. Common program requirements. https://www.acgme.org/globalassets/pfassets/programrequirements/cprresidency_2023.pdf
4. PHM core competencies.
5. PHM section 1 common clinical diagnoses and conditions.
6. Openpediatrics. https://learn.openpediatrics.org/learn/course/internal/view/elearning/2996/common-pediatric-respiratory-problems
7. Online learning and residents acquisition of mechanical ventilation knowledge: sequencing matters. https://pubmed.ncbi.nlm.nih.gov/31688194/
8. APPD LESSON.
9. https://www.learnpicu.com/home
10. ABP.
11. Yale PCPC Talwalkar JS, Smith S, Fenick AM, eds. Yale Primary Care Pediatrics Curriculum, 18th ed.;2024. Available from: http://pcpc.yale.edu

14 Academic/Planned Curriculum

Emily Borman-Shoap, Johannah Scheurer,
and Rachel Poeppelman

The What: Definition and Overview

Broadly, structured education in pediatric graduate medical education (GME) could be used to refer to the entire package of a systematically designed curriculum that integrates didactic learning, clinical experiences, and competency-based assessments to ensure progressive development of pediatric residents' knowledge, skills, and professionalism in accordance with accreditation and institutional standards. In this chapter, we will use the term structured education to refer to planned didactic learning sessions, such as morning report, noon conference, academic half-day, board preparation, boot camps, and simulations.

The residency program leadership team should first begin by taking stock of the entire package of education that a resident will experience from their first days of orientation through to their graduation. Start with the end in mind: What knowledge and skills should a resident acquire during their training? Are there foundational content areas that all residents should experience? If the curriculum varies for residents with different career goals, how might it vary?

As they plan their program-level overall approach to education, residency leaders may find it helpful to consider three main environments for learning: (1) hands-on clinical experiences, (2) rotation-embedded structured education, and (3) structured education planned for all residents. These elements should be considered in how they can be complementary and synergistic to one another in creating an entire curricular package.

Hands-on clinic experiences make a substantial contribution to residents' learning during their training, and the structure and function of experiences will be shaped by many factors. These include ACGME requirements for clinical experiences, available clinical training sites, faculty expertise, and resident future career plans. Some key learning may be so ubiquitous in clinical rotations that it is not necessary to spend substantial additional structured time focusing on a topic. For example, having an explicit noon conference focusing on RSV bronchiolitis diagnosis and management may not be necessary given the prevalence of the diagnosis and numerous opportunities for hands-on learning. However, it is important to continually monitor hands-on clinical learning experiences. Changes to clinical care delivery that are not designed by the residency program can have significant impacts on patient exposure. For example, moving the management of DKA patients to a non-resident team could lead to decreased exposure to an important topic area that was previously learned through hands-on clinical experience.

E. Borman-Shoap (✉) · J. Scheurer · R. Poeppelman
University of Minnesota School of Medicine,
Minneapolis, MN, USA
e-mail: borm0029@umn.edu

H. McPhillips et al. (eds.), *Graduate Medical Education in Pediatrics*, Excellence in Medical Education 3, https://doi.org/10.1007/978-3-032-12952-9_14

Rotation-embedded education includes elements such as adolescent medicine-specific topics covered for all residents who are on the required adolescent medicine rotation, or a case-based teaching session for all residents on their Emergency Medicine rotation. These rotation-embedded structured education sessions often play an important role in providing just-in-time learning opportunities that complement the clinical learning on a rotation. Residency leaders should meet with required rotation leaders on a periodic basis to assess which topics are best covered in smaller didactics embedded within a required rotation versus larger all-program teaching sessions.

Structured education should ensure that all residents receive instruction in the core content areas outlined by the ACGME [1] as well as the ABP [2]. The content and mode of instruction should consider the needs of the learners, available teachers, and the best timing and location. The residency administrative team should have clearly defined roles for all aspects, such as scheduling speakers, supporting just-in-time needs during sessions, and overall quality assurance. Residency programs should also have a robust mechanism for evaluating the effectiveness of their structured curriculum and mechanisms to adapt over time.

In this chapter, we will describe curriculum as didactics or structured educational experiences, including, but not limited to, lectures, simulation-based instruction, flipped classroom, and case-based learning. At the graduate medical education (GME) level, these didactics are often delivered in workshops, noon conferences, academic half-days, and protected teaching time. For GME programs, didactics are the portion of the curriculum and instruction over which educators hold the most direct control. They are a vehicle by which to directly impact our learners' knowledge, skills, and attitudes in a consistent manner, compared to the clinical learning environment in which there exists significant natural variability. Didactics serve an important role in preparing learners for board exams, ensuring delivery of the most vital learning objectives, and can have an added benefit of building community through time spent together learning. Planning didactics for learners also requires an investment of resources both in faculty time, physical space, cost of materials, and learner time. Therefore, educators must ensure that this investment leads to meaningful returns, specifically that the didactics result in the desired in knowledge, skills, and attitudes for the learners.

To provide guidance to curriculum planning teams, program leadership may want to consider various ways of creating a curricular roadmap for their didactic sessions. The type of session will also help to guide the recruitment of the appropriate teachers for various sessions. The following are the possible guiding principles:

- Content-based: working through all ABP content specifications over a prescribed period.
- Thread-based: define threads of topics for the curriculum. For example, each of the 3 years in training covers a different age of patients: newborn-toddler, preschool-school age, adolescent.
- Specialty-specific: each specialty/subspecialty is responsible for "its own" content.
- Session type: different planning team member(s) for different sessions, such as noon conference, morning report, simulations, and academic half-day.
- Competency-based: curriculum aligned with each of the general pediatrics EPAs.
- Domains of competence: medical knowledge (e.g., board review), practice-based learning and improvement, systems-based practice (e.g., root cause analysis, quality improvement education and projects), professionalism (e.g., ethics), interpersonal and communication skills (e.g., communication simulations, leadership training).

The "What": Content Themes in Structure Education

As a residency program plans out the content for its structured curriculum, many resources will be helpful. A mainstay of creating a map for content should include the General Pediatrics Certifying examination content outlines published by the

ABP and the common and specialty-specific training requirements from the ACGME [1, 2]. The general pediatric EPAs also provide a robust roadmap for essential curricular elements [3]. The program should engage in creating a master roadmap of the required content areas from these sources and plan for when and where content will be covered. The following section will explore important content themes that programs should plan to include in their structured education sessions.

Board Preparation

Board preparation (medical knowledge) is a core function of structured curricular time. Programs should consider how frequently they want to cover each topic domain: Will topics be covered over the course of 3 years? Or a program might try to have a set of core topics that repeat every 18 months, or even on an annual basis. If a program elects to have a 3-year roadmap, it is important to make sure that residents have ready access to review materials for sessions that they miss. Programs may wish to create a digital repository of high-yield content from structured sessions that residents can reference as they continue their board preparation. If content is delivered on a repeating cycle, programs may wish to create opportunities for an "advanced session" for residents who have already been exposed to the material in a previous session. The teaching strategies mentioned later in the chapter (team-based learning and game-based learning) are well suited for didactic sessions that are specifically geared toward board review.

Program leaders should ensure that the chief residents and teaching faculty are familiar with the ABP content outline. In addition, sharing your residency program's In-Training Exam results is a great way to help faculty understand the core content that needs to be covered in their sessions.

In order to incorporate ongoing board preparation as a part of a resident's routine, programs may wish to consider small weekly quizzes that all residents are encouraged to complete. A brief review of the quiz answers can be used as the kickoff to an education session. Programs can even consider incentive programs for participation.

Beyond content delivery and practice questions, it may also be helpful to spend some protected time teaching about test preparation and test-taking strategy. Providing guidance about taking practice questions in a mixture of timed and tutor mode, coaching about how to build a study schedule, and support for test-taking anxiety are all topics that could be covered in a structured session on board preparation.

Diagnostic Process: Case-Based Learning and Diagnostic Uncertainty

Case-based learning can be a very effective approach to learning. One aspect that should be explicit in case-based learning is an exploration of the impact of cognitive bias. The opportunity to work through a patient case in a specific and methodical manner creates an excellent opportunity to explore the process of coming to a diagnosis. Residents should be exposed to key concepts in cognitive bias, such as anchoring and diagnostic momentum. The concepts of cognitive bias can be woven into morning report sessions or into more detailed didactic sessions with opportunities to debrief cases [4]. Discussion of working with patients and families during diagnostic uncertainty is another important topic. Simulation sessions related to family communication during diagnostic uncertainty are another potentially effective method [5].

Quality Improvement and Patient Safety

Patient safety and quality improvement is another area where structured education is required to complement the pediatric clinical learning environment. Leaders might consider "system-based" case presentation sessions that focus beyond the medical team to system-based issues and strategies. While trainees should be included in real-time root cause analyses in the hospital system, event frequency and logistic issues may preclude all trainees from engagement. Therefore, leaders must consider alternate structured educational approaches, such as simulated root cause analysis [6]. Quality improvement training may be paired with mentored participation in a quality improvement project, completed by individuals, groups, or the entire residency program, in collaboration with faculty who have relevant expertise. Quality Improvement and Patient Safety teaching is a wonderful opportunity to engage hospital and clinic leadership, and interprofessional team members with expertise.

Procedural Training

Procedural training is yet another area that all residents need to be exposed to and have experience with, yet opportunities in the clinical learning environment may be limited. Therefore, simulated practice during structured learning sessions is prudent. This is an area where program leaders likely need to utilize support from program faculty with content expertise (e.g., general pediatricians for circumcision, pediatric emergency medicine and critical care for positive pressure ventilation, neonatology for emergency umbilical venous line placement). Leaders should also consider non-pediatric faculty whose expertise may be utilized for procedural skill education (e.g., surgery and emergency medicine physicians, advanced practice providers with suturing expertise). While some skills can be learned with low fidelity models (e.g., umbilical line), other procedures and simulation scenarios are best suited to be delivered with high fidelity simulation (e.g., acute patient decompensation).

DEI and Health Equity

Attention to the factors that lead to health inequities, such as structural racism and barriers to care, is a critical element in structured educational programs. Explicitly addressing these issues through a formal conference series, such as Health Equity Rounds, can help to bring issues of social determinants of health and healthcare inequality to the forefront of trainees' minds as they deliver care. In a Health Equity Rounds series, cases are examined for implicit and explicit biases, barriers to care, and the impact on patient outcomes. These series can promote personal self-reflection and intention to change clinical practice [7].

As a program team begins to consider what they will be teaching in their structured education sessions, they should also consider how to best deliver this education. Given the importance of ensuring the effectiveness of didactics, we will begin with a consideration of the best practices for executing effective didactics, rooted in medical education theory and cognitive psychology research. This will not be an exhaustive review but instead will focus on six well-established principles that are particularly relevant to pediatric GME practice. Next, we will give some specific examples of teaching approaches that educators can employ that utilize elements of these best practices.

The "How": Selected Medical Education Best Practice Principles

Principle #1: Maintain Focus on Key Objectives

The exceedingly large volume and complexity of knowledge and skills needed to be a successful pediatrician in the modern world leads to a temptation to squeeze more and more content into a finite amount of didactic time. Yet it is better to successfully achieve a few key learning objectives than to fail to achieve any of a long list of objectives.

This principle is backed up by a cognitive psychology theory—"cognitive load theory" [8, 9]. Essentially, learning happens when information goes through the working memory, of which we all have a finite capacity. Therefore, working memory can act as a bottleneck in the learning process and too much challenging or new content can lead to cognitive overload, which then impairs learning (Fig. 14.1). Overwhelming

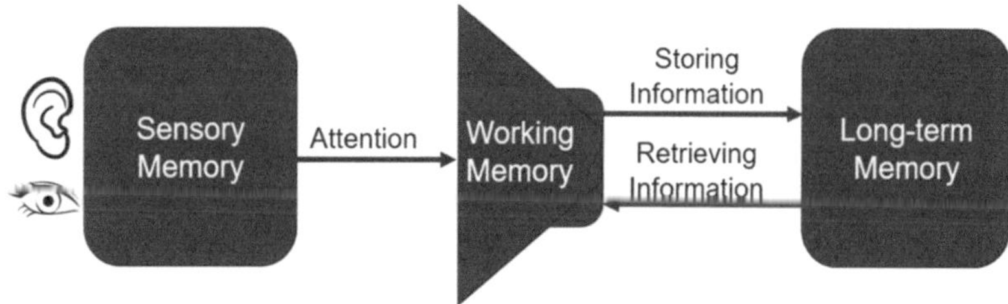

Fig. 14.1 Diagram of the process of moving information from sensory to working to long-term memory. (Adapted with permission Ref. [9])

learners with too many learning objectives and an overfull agenda leads to cognitive overload.

Faculty members should be encouraged to stick to no more than two to four learning objectives per hour of didactic time. This will be HARD. As educators, we always want to teach more and more. Common pitfalls are adding objectives or content that the teacher finds interesting or exciting, or simply wanting to make sure we have "covered" all the material. To ensure that learners achieve the learning objectives, it is imperative to pare down your learning objectives to the most essential ones for your learner population. Be thoughtful about this choice. What are your learners not exposed to elsewhere? What is most difficult for them to learn independently? What is most meaningful for your patient population?

Once the *key* learning objectives for a didactic session have been determined, it is important to constantly refer back to these as a touchstone at all stages of planning and delivery. This is echoed throughout Kern's six-step approach to curriculum design; specifically, every choice made in designing and revising curriculum should trace back to achieving the learning objectives [10]. This is known as "backwards design"—thinking backwards from what you want the learner to be able to do at the end.

One example of backwards design is an approach taken at the University of Minnesota to giving pediatric residents more experience and comfort with initiating high-quality cardiopulmonary resuscitation (CPR). With this key objective in mind, we planned hands-on, low-fidelity simulated mock codes for them during their intensive care rotation. The choice of instructional method (simulation) was made with the key objective in mind. We also chose to have them repeat the first "five minutes" of the code multiple times in the session rather than progressing further down the code algorithm. Certainly, an argument can be made that all aspects of code management are important and should be included. Yet with limited time, we instead chose to focus on successfully achieving one key learning objective rather than simply trying to "cover" several.

The principle of maintaining focus on key objectives extends beyond limiting the number of objectives and the selection of instructional methods. Educators also need to be wary of possible distractions that can lead to cognitive overload [9]. Keep the working memory bottleneck in mind. If your learners are engaged in tasks that don't relate to your key learning objective(s) then they have less of their finite working memory to devote to learning. Common distractors are as simple as overly busy PowerPoint slides, having to search for instructions for a task, or learning how to use a new learning platform. For example, if you want to incorporate polling or audience response in a didactic session, try to be consistent in the technology you use. You want their focus to be on your learning objective(s) rather than the hidden learning objective of learning a new technological tool.

Principle #2: Pacing Is Essential

The way your didactics are paced is crucial. Pacing of content is one of the drivers of learner attention. Too slow a pace can cause learners to lose interest and may fail to challenge them appropriately. Too fast a pace will also risk a loss of attention and doesn't provide the time and space necessary for a learner to adequately process and engage with the material.

Studies suggest a student's attention wanes after approximately 10–15 min of lecturing or any passive learning strategy [11, 12]. This gives us a useful rule of thumb for planning didactic schedules: limit any passive delivery of material to no more than 10–15 min before engaging in a more active learning strategy.

We will delve more into active learning strategies in the next principle, but if your time and resources are limited or your faculty are reticent to redesign a lecture into a more active learning-based activity, there are still some simple and easy strategies you can use to adhere to this rule of thumb. Learner attention can be captured or re-captured with any efforts made at engagement—audience response questions, demonstrations, and embedded discussions [12, 13]. One simple adjustment to an existing lecture is the "pause procedure"—integrating three pauses of 2 min duration into a 1-h talk. During the pause, students are encouraged to discuss with their peers or review their notes. Studies have shown this simple adjustment improves knowledge gains and recall [13, 14].

Principle #3: Employ Active Learning Strategies

Active learning strategies classically seek to drive learning through experience. These experiences can range from clinical encounters to simulation-based learning to gamification. Each type of experience seeks to engage learners in reflection, making connections, and applying knowledge in order to better hold learner attention, promote deeper learning, and improve recall [15].

One popular structure for integrating active learning techniques into didactics is the flipped classroom [16]. In a flipped classroom session, learners are provided with resources to review in advance of didactic sessions. These resources prepare learners with the basic knowledge they will need to engage in meaningful practice and application of concepts in the planned activities of the session. For example, for a didactic session focused on care of technology-dependent patients, learners were sent curated videos to watch in advance explaining core concepts about tracheostomies and the steps needed to perform essential care of a tracheostomy. This allowed for the time spent together in person to be utilized for hands-on, simulated practice with essential care tasks for a tracheostomy patient, such as an emergency tracheostomy change, one of the primary learning objectives.

Gamification is another approach to integrating active learning strategies into didactics. Games can offer open-ended practice, challenging learners to explore principles through problem solving without a fixed goal or specific correct diagnosis. Open-ended practice has been shown to decrease cognitive load, freeing up working memory to devote to learning and building connections with prior knowledge [9]. Further discussion and an example of gamification are included later in this chapter.

Game show mimics, such as Jeopardy and Family Feud, are another way to employ active learning strategies in didactics. "Retrieval practice," or the act of self-testing, is a well-established method of promoting durable learning [17]. A didactic session based around a quiz show such as jeopardy allows your learners to test their own knowledge in a fun and engaging manner. A particularly effective way to use a game show didactic session would be to reinforce topics presented over a longer term, such as either a mid-year or year-end review. Asking your learners targeted questions about objectives covered earlier in the year allows for spaced practice of that material, which has also been shown to promote learning and recall [17].

Principle #4: Harness Peer Expertise

Large group didactic sessions are an excellent opportunity to empower your learners as peer teachers. Within any large group, there is certain to be variation in knowledge and experience levels. Meeting the diverse learning needs of such a group might seem daunting at first, but by highlighting and leveraging the peer "experts" in the group, we can empower our trainees as teachers, help junior trainees to envision themselves meeting objectives, and foster connections. Near peer teachers have also been shown to more effectively target a learner's "zone of proximal development" [18]. Briefly, this is the sweet spot for a learner between concepts that are too difficult or too easy, where the most effective learning happens and where they are challenged but not out of their depth.

Team-based learning, a specific format of a flipped classroom session, is one opportunity to elevate peer "experts." In team-based learning, learners work through a series of tests and application exercises as a team. In a group of learners with mixed levels of knowledge and expertise, this fosters rich peer learning within each small group [19]. This team-based learning exercise will be discussed in more detail below.

Principle #5: Give the Learners Control

The shift to competency-based medical education called for educators to elevate the voice of the learner and leave behind the old "sage on the stage" model to one that centers the learner in all curricular decisions [20]. More recently, medical educators are increasingly recognizing the importance of involving learners not only in the creation and review of curricular materials but also in determining their own individualized path through a curriculum.

By allowing our learners some capacity to shape their own learning objectives and goals, we are helping them to build the lifelong learning skills they will need after residency. Learners with some choices and control in building their individualized learning path will be better motivated to learn the topic. Self-determination theory encapsulates this well: learners must perceive some control or autonomy in order to have intrinsic motivation [21].

Practically speaking, there are a few ways to integrate opportunities to give learners control into didactic sessions. One approach we have used is to format a session a bit like a "choose your own adventure" book. For example, at our hands-on procedural practice sessions, we give learners two choices for groups of procedures to practice for the day. While we provide advice about which procedures are most relevant to different career paths, we ultimately allow each resident to decide how best to spend their time at the session. This allows each learner to consider their prior experiences/training, goals, and career plans in shaping their curriculum for the day. This same individualized approach can also be taken with a more typical didactic session that separates learners into two rooms: one that covers an introduction to a topic and one that takes on a more advanced approach to the same topic. Engaging learners with more experience to help take the lead in discussion or small groups can also be helpful.

Creating scholarly tracks or certificate programs is another way to create opportunities for learners to shape their own curriculum. For example, our program offers a Global Health Certificate which allows interested learners to further immerse themselves in the knowledge and skills necessary to work in global health [22].

Principle #6: Curriculum Development Is a Circle

Curriculum development is a circle and a circle has no end. The work of curriculum development is never finished. Certainly, there is new knowledge and changes in practice patterns to keep up with. But learners are also always changing and new tools and methods, such as AI, are being developed. The ideal session with perfectly suited instructional methods for one group of learners at a specific point in time may not be as effective as time passes. So, we as educators must always be evaluating and revising our curriculum. This is why all pictorial depictions of Kern's six steps of curriculum design depict the steps forming a circle and moving from the last step of curriculum evaluation back into the first step of needs assessment again [10].

With these guiding principles in mind, we will now turn to two examples of strategies that employ many of the best practices mentioned above.

The "How": Selected Teaching Strategies for GME

Educators have a wonderful opportunity to engage their creativity and step away from a typical lecture through a number of techniques. We will explore a Team-Based Learning exercise and approaches to Game-Based Learning. These interactive approaches can help to keep adult learners engaged and active in their learning.

Team-Based Learning

One example of Team-Based Learning is a group quiz learning activity as outlined in Fig. 14.2. The instructor creates a short multiple-choice quiz, somewhere between 5 and 10 questions. Individuals are first given protected quiet time to answer the questions. Plan about 1 min per question. Once individuals have completed their quiz, they form a small group and discuss amongst themselves and come to a consensus on the answer for each question. Finally, the instructor reviews each question. Prior to reviewing each question, the groups show their answer, either through digital polling or holding up a piece of paper with their answer choice. If the instructor notes that many participants answered the question correctly, they should explicitly state this and spend less time reviewing that content. They can then quickly move on to spend more time on content that most of the group answered incorrectly. This approach keeps all learners engaged and has several important benefits. First, the individual learner must complete the quiz and commit to what they believe is the correct answer. In this way, they receive a definitive knowledge check on the content area being delivered. Second, when the group reviews together, it provides an opportunity for peer-based teaching. This near-peer teaching can be very effective both for the teacher, who will secure their content knowledge through explaining it to another, and for the near-peer learner may benefit from instruction from someone with a similar experience level. Finally, the instructor gets real-time information about the level of content knowledge that the audience had prior to their session. This allows the instructor to tailor their teaching to the areas of greatest need, rather than reiterating content that is already secure for most attendees.

Game-Based Learning

As mentioned in the principles above, active learning and near-peer teaching can be powerful approaches to improving engagement. Game-based learning can be a useful approach to incorporate many of the key elements mentioned above. Game-based sessions can take many formats, from adapting a well-known game such as Jeopardy or Family Feud to a more complex

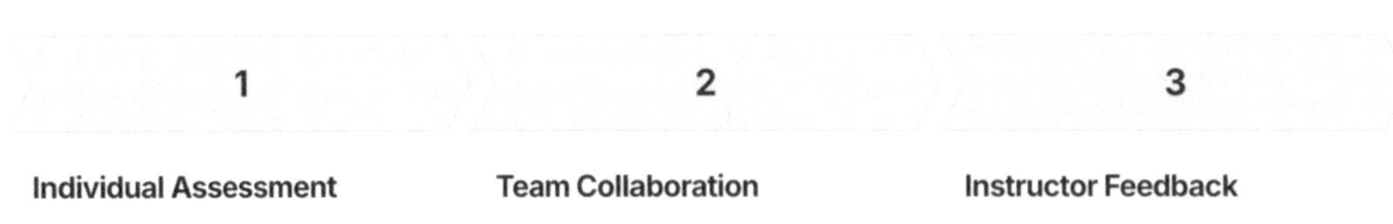

Fig. 14.2 General outline of a team-based learning approach using quizzing

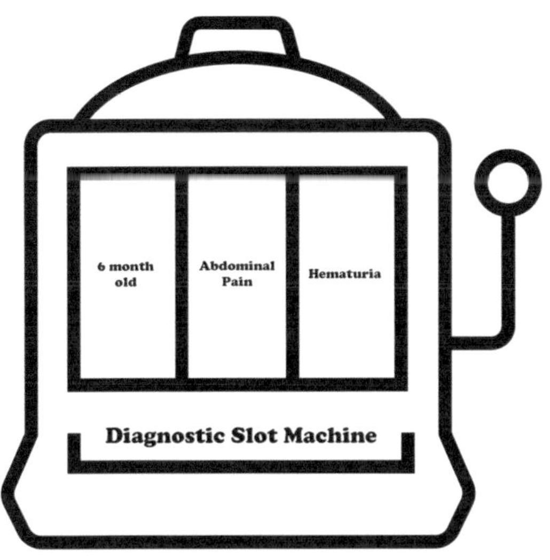

Fig. 14.3 Example of the combination of patient characteristics that could be generated during the Diagnostic Slot Machine learning exercise

game such as an escape room [23]. Educators should focus on games that can be collaborative and consider creative approaches where there isn't a single right answer [24].

Taking the approach of focusing on idea generation rather than a single correct answer is particularly important when helping trainees to build their diagnostic reasoning skills in a structured manner beyond the direct clinical learning environment. Case-based learning, often in a "morning report" format, is a traditional mechanism for building diagnostic reasoning skills. One trainee presents a case while others ask for information and go through the diagnostic process collectively. The Socratic method is common in this format. Program leaders should consider if other game-based formats might enable better engagement with other formats. One example is a "diagnostic slot machine" approach: there are three categories with multiple entries for each category, then participants draw from each category (electronically or from decks of notecards), which identifies a presentation of age, chief complaint, and sign or symptom [25] (Fig. 14.3). So, the group is then tasked to develop a differential diagnosis and work through pertinent history, physical exam, and diagnostic evaluation required to evaluate the "patient."

Example of slot machine case-based learning

Category 1: age (e.g., 4-week-old, 6-month-old, 30-month-old, 5-year-old, etc.)
Category 2: chief complaint (e.g., abdominal pain, headache, etc.)
Category 3: symptoms (e.g., hematuria, conjunctivitis, abdominal rash, etc.)
→ 6-month-old with abdominal pain and hematuria.

The "Who": Defining Roles for Structured Education Faculty and Staff

The program leadership team must take responsibility for developing curricular goals and ensure trainees have protected time for learning and curriculum outside the clinical learning environment. They should work to determine how to engage content experts while ensuring those delivering content are also equipped to be effective educators.

Program leaders might consider having education faculty among multiple specialties be members of a curriculum planning team, or multiple teams. The program and/or associate program director role would be to share curricular goals, available time, and be a resource for helping plan effective education.

It is more important to decide how to define the subsets of curricular needs than finding a single "right" way to do it. Local expertise and faculty interest may also shape some aspect of how structured curriculum is organized and delivered. Chief residents often play a key role in developing and implementing many aspects of the structured curriculum. Partnering with experts outside of the field of pediatrics can help to enhance teaching sessions and expand the roster of teachers. Collaborators include colleagues in family medicine, internal medicine, psychiatry, obstetrics-gynecology, dentistry, ophthalmology, pharmacy, and nursing.

Program leadership (director and/or associate program director) will likely need to provide guidance related to curriculum planning and is encouraged to utilize defined structures, for example, Kern's 6 steps of curriculum development, among other possibilities [10]. This guidance may be particularly important for teachers who are earlier in their careers, including chief residents. Dedicating time during chief resident orientation (and throughout the year) to skill building in curriculum design and delivery is recommended.

Logistic planning is another key to success. This includes content delivery modality, timing, space, and any necessary materials such as handouts, task trainers.

Program administrators need to be familiar with system resources, administrative contacts, and timelines for utilizing them. For example, a list of available conference rooms, capacity, and AV resources, along with who manages room reservation, how far in advance room reservations are needed/available, and consistent scheduling modalities, are helpful. Standing educational session times (e.g., every Friday afternoon) can offer consistency not only for participants and facilitators but also for space needs and administrative support responsibilities.

Program leadership should have a budget to mobilize departmental or other funding sources and share with session facilitators who may have specific needs for a particular session. Leadership should be aware of what, if any, expected involvement all faculty are to have in non-clinical education of GME trainees as part of their appointment and work with departmental leadership to align requests for faculty support within those expectations. Consider utilizing the support of those who already have protected academic time for education (e.g., associate program directors). Protected academic time for additional faculty members may be considered depending on the level/time of engagement. Available financial resources may partially dictate the frequency with which some sessions can be held. Some sessions, such as simulation or procedural skills, may be more expensive than other sessions.

Close coordination among program administrators, leadership, and facilitators is important so everyone understands their individual expectations. As shown in Fig. 14.4, the program might develop a checklist to be shared among all stakeholders for each session. Depending on session complexity, a "dry run" for session set-up may uncover unanticipated glitches and, after troubleshooting, enable a more successful synchronous session.

Another administrative support to consider utilizing is an artificial intelligence (AI) program, such as ChatGPT. This may be helpful in developing content outlines, presentation templates, and educational visual aids. AI platforms may relieve some of the administrative burden, however accuracy must be confirmed and they should not be considered a substitute for content experts. Some AI platforms were specifically developed for medical professionals and may be particularly supportive for GME curriculum development. For example, the newer tool OpenEvidence could be an adjunct for residents to use during an evidence-based medicine teaching session [26].

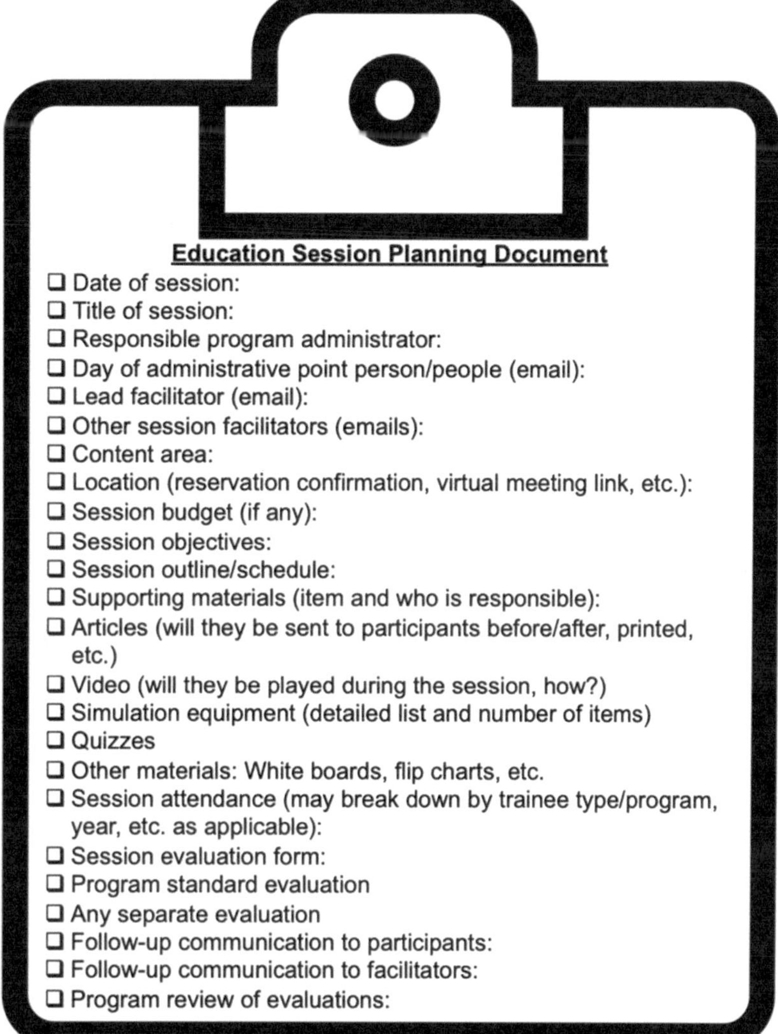

Education Session Planning Document

- ❑ Date of session:
- ❑ Title of session:
- ❑ Responsible program administrator:
- ❑ Day of administrative point person/people (email):
- ❑ Lead facilitator (email):
- ❑ Other session facilitators (emails):
- ❑ Content area:
- ❑ Location (reservation confirmation, virtual meeting link, etc.):
- ❑ Session budget (if any):
- ❑ Session objectives:
- ❑ Session outline/schedule:
- ❑ Supporting materials (item and who is responsible):
- ❑ Articles (will they be sent to participants before/after, printed, etc.)
- ❑ Video (will they be played during the session, how?)
- ❑ Simulation equipment (detailed list and number of items)
- ❑ Quizzes
- ❑ Other materials: White boards, flip charts, etc.
- ❑ Session attendance (may break down by trainee type/program, year, etc. as applicable):
- ❑ Session evaluation form:
- ❑ Program standard evaluation
- ❑ Any separate evaluation
- ❑ Follow-up communication to participants:
- ❑ Follow-up communication to facilitators:
- ❑ Program review of evaluations:

Fig. 14.4 Sample checklist to be used for education session planning

The "Where" and the "When": Academic Half-Days Versus Morning Reports Versus Noon Conferences

Determining the best setting and timing for structured education is a critical starting point when approaching a plan for didactic learning. Are morning conferences or lunch-time conferences better for your program? Do you want to consider an academic half-day model? Program leadership is encouraged to first consider an ideal educational format based on the topic to be covered. For example, diagnosis-based teaching and discussion of clinical reasoning based on recent admissions can be very high yield and may be best simultaneously or soon after trainees are caring for the patient. A brief session in the morning or at midday may work well for this type of learning. Alternatively, covering the pediatric rheumatology content specified by the ABP may involve sessions about the most common pediatric rheumatologic diseases, the rheumatology exam, approaches to ordering and interpreting rheumatology studies, and when to consult a pediatric rheumatologist. A longer session may be best for this content; for example, it could be a 3-h academic half-day session with sub-sections including didactic content, physical exam practice, case-based discussions, and a board review exercise. Many factors will influence the choice between an academic half-day predominant model versus a noon conference predominant model.

After identifying the best learning strategies, practical topics must also be considered. Common practical considerations about how and when to schedule protected education time include, but are not limited to:

- The number of trainees who will be gone from the clinical learning environment (all, PGY1 versus 2 versus 3 only, other subsets).
- The length and frequency of protected time.
- Who will cover resident patient-care duties while they are away (e.g., ICU attending, advanced practice provider, in basket unless urgent/emergent issue, etc.). This, in turn, requires ensuring those responsible have adequate bandwidth to cover these duties and provide safe patient care (i.e., if a resident is not on the wards and the attending is covering, the attending should not simultaneously have a full panel of clinic patients scheduled).
- Conflicting duties such as continuity clinic and attendance (or not) while scheduled for night shifts. For example, to start an academic half-day model, programs may need to modify continuity clinic timing.

When an educational session is required for all residents, program leadership will have to work closely with hospital leadership, particularly related to coverage of patient care duties typically covered by residents. This may present a minor challenge for a short morning or mid-day conference, and a much more complex set of considerations for a recurring academic half-day session. At times, clinical services may need to have additional clinical care support (another attending, an additional advanced practice provider) while residents are at educational sessions. Assurance should be made that tasks such as order entry and documentation are not "put on hold" until residents come back, but are accomplished over typically expected timeframes. For continuity clinic attendance, it may make sense for academic half-days to align with a day that no residents have continuity clinic or for the academic half-day to alternate days of the week (ensuring residents miss continuity clinic for academic half-days only once every 5 weeks). For Programs with X + Y scheduling, this may present an opportunity to be strategic about how academic half-days fit into certain portions of the schedule.

For programs with multiple clinical sites, program leaders will need to decide how they want to approach delivering the same content to all residents. One approach could be running concurrent sessions on the same topic (if there is adequate expertise at each site). For example, all sites could be assigned to have a talk on jaundice during the first week of a rotation. Offering hybrid sessions is another solution that can allow synchronized content delivery. Finally, bringing residents together to one site to learn may be the best approach for some topics. Programs will need to consider teaching expertise available at each of their training sites, and logistic considerations such as the capacity and type of rooms available, distance/length of travel for trainees and others between sites, and support staff availability. However, the educational content and value ideally receives more weight in determining among in-person, virtual, and hybrid formats [27].

Evaluation and Feedback

Curriculum evaluation and feedback are critical to determine whether curricula are meeting the goals and fulfilling session objectives and assist in iterative planning over time. Multiple evaluation methods, with considerations based on what facilitators and leaders seek to capture and measure [28]. At a minimum, evaluations should elicit whether a session has met objectives and have space for trainees to share formative/constructive feedback. Practical considerations include the evaluation format (e.g., paper versus online), length, and timing (e.g., completed during before the session versus emailed afterwards), tailored to program and trainee characteristics to maximize response rates and obtain more accurate results.

The program administrative team should be engaged to collate feedback and send a letter of appreciation and feedback report to facilitators. The importance of collating evaluations is for multiple reasons:

- Iterative program evaluation and planning.
- Individual faculty development, so they continue what they are doing well and improve on areas of constructive feedback.
- Encourage faculty to list sessions on their CVs and save feedback for their portfolios for promotion and tenure.

Appreciation for faculty involvement and positive encouragement from program leadership can include opportunities to meet, to review feedback, and provide coaching on educational best practices. Program leadership may consider planning department-wide faculty development opportunities with a focus on any common improvement areas.

Conclusion

Planning, implementing, and managing the structured curriculum for a residency program is a complex system. It is also an area where program leaders and faculty can exercise creativity and experience the joy of teaching. Engaging a broad team of stakeholders, including administrative team members, chief residents, program leaders, and many faculty is key to success. Program leaders should start with the end in mind: What core knowledge, skills, and attitudes do they want to ensure that all graduates of their program have? By using the curricular roadmaps available from ABP and ACGME, adhering to solid principles in education theory, and continually revising, a residency program can ensure a high-quality and engaging educational experience. Program leaders can continue to come back to the basic elements of who, what, where, when, and how to help guide continuous improvement of their structured educational offerings.

References

1. ACGME Pediatric Residency Requirements, effective July 1 2025.
2. American Board of Pediatrics, General Pediatrics Content Outline. For all examinations administered October 15, 2024 or after.
3. General Pediatric EPAs and curricular components, American Board of Pediatrics.
4. Ruedinger E, Olson M, Yee J, et al. Education for the next frontier in patient safety: a longitudinal resident curriculum on diagnostic error. Am J Med Qual. 2017;32:625–31. https://doi.org/10.1177/1062860616681626.
5. Olson ME, Borman-Shoap E, Mathias K, et al. Case-based simulation empowering pediatric residents to communicate about diagnostic uncertainty. Diagnosi. 2018;5:243–8. https://doi.org/10.1515/dx-2018-0025.
6. Ziemba JB, Berns JS, Huzinec JG, et al. The RCA ReCAst: a root cause analysis simulation for the interprofessional clinical learning environment. Acad Med. 2021;96:997–1001. https://doi.org/10.1097/ACM.0000000000004064.
7. Perdomo J, Tolliver D, Hsu H, et al. Health equity rounds: an interdisciplinary case conference to address implicit bias and structural racism for faculty and trainees. MedEdPORTAL. 2019:10858. https://doi.org/10.15766/mep_2374-8265.10858.
8. Sweller J, Ayres PL, Kalyuga S. Cognitive load theory. New York: Springer; 2011.
9. Young JQ, Van Merrienboer J, Durning S, Ten Cate O. Cognitive load theory: implications for medical education: AMEE guide no. 86. Med Teach. 2014;36:371–84. https://doi.org/10.3109/0142159X.2014.889290.
10. Thomas PA, Kern DE, Hughes MT, et al. Curriculum development for medical education: a six-step approach. Baltimore, MD: Johns Hopkins University Press; 2016.
11. Stuart J, Rutherford RJD. Medical student concentration during lectures. Lancet. 1978;312:514–6. https://doi.org/10.1016/S0140-6736(78)92233-X.
12. Burns RA. Information impact and factors affecting recall. Austin, TX; 1985.

13. Thaman RG. Effective use of pause procedure to enhance student engagement and learning. JCDR. 2014; https://doi.org/10.7860/JCDR/2014/8260.4691.
14. Ruhl KL, Hughes CA, Schloss PJ. Using the pause procedure to enhance lecture recall. Teach Educ Spec Educ. 1987;10:14–8. https://doi.org/10.1177/088840648701000103.
15. Snell YS, Linda S. Interactive lecturing: strategies for increasing participation in large group presentations. Med Teach. 1999;21:37–42. https://doi.org/10.1080/01421599980011.
16. Hew KF, Lo CK. Flipped classroom improves student learning in health professions education: a meta-analysis. BMC Med Educ. 2018;18:38. https://doi.org/10.1186/s12909-018-1144-z.
17. Roediger HL, Pyc MA. Inexpensive techniques to improve education: applying cognitive psychology to enhance educational practice. J Appl Res Mem Cogn. 2012;1:242–8. https://doi.org/10.1016/j.jarmac.2012.09.002.
18. Alexander SM, Dallaghan GLB, Birch M, et al. What makes a near-peer learning and tutoring program effective in undergraduate medical education: a qualitative analysis. MedSciEduc. 2022;32:1495–502. https://doi.org/10.1007/s40670-022-01680-0.
19. Poeppelman RS, Liebert CA, Vegas DB, et al. A narrative review and novel framework for application of team-based learning in graduate medical education. J Grad Med Educ. 2016;8:510–7. https://doi.org/10.4300/JGME-D-15-00516.1.
20. Van Melle E, Frank JR, Holmboe ES, et al. A core components framework for evaluating implementation of competency-based medical education programs. Acad Med. 2019;94:1002–9. https://doi.org/10.1097/ACM.0000000000002743.
21. Sawatsky AP, O'Brien BC, Hafferty FW. Autonomy and developing physicians: reimagining supervision using self-determination theory. Med Educ. 2022;56:56–63. https://doi.org/10.1111/medu.14580.
22. Pitt MB, Slusher TM, Gladding SP, et al. The Minnesota model: a residency global health track framework. Am J Trop Med Hyg. 2020;102:11–6. https://doi.org/10.4269/ajtmh.19-0463.
23. Friedrich C, Teaford H, Taubenheim A, et al. Escaping the professional silo: an escape room implemented in an interprofessional education curriculum. J Interprof Care. 2019;33:573–5. https://doi.org/10.1080/13561820.2018.1538941.
24. Pitt MB, Borman-Shoap EC, Eppich WJ. Twelve tips for maximizing the effectiveness of game-based learning. Med Teach. 2015;37:1013–7. https://doi.org/10.3109/0142159X.2015.1020289.
25. Kamra P, Borman-Shoap EC, Zhang L, Pitt MB. Gaming the system: creation of a random case-generating game for use in morning report. Acad Pediatr. 2018;18:234–6. https://doi.org/10.1016/j.acap.2017.09.009.
26. OpenEvidence. In: OpenEvidence. https://www.openevidence.com. Accessed 24 Nov 2024.
27. Zeldin ER, Charles SC, Tumin D, et al. Impact of a hybrid-virtual teaching model on the physical examination skills of fourth-year medical students. Am J Phys Med Rehabil. 2022; https://doi.org/10.1097/PHM.0000000000002032.
28. Li S-TT, Klein MD, Balmer DF, Gusic ME. Scholarly evaluation of curricula and educational programs: using a systematic approach to produce publishable scholarship. Acad Pediatr. 2020;20:1083–93. https://doi.org/10.1016/j.acap.2020.07.005.

15 Individualized Curriculum and Career Choice

Heather Howell and Lynn Thoreson

Background

The Accreditation Council for Graduate Medical Education (ACGME) intentionally designs the educational program requirements for pediatric residency training to provide foundational experiences, those experiences that all residents complete to develop the skills needed to succeed as a general pediatrician, and individualized experiences, experiences that are unique to each resident. Individualized curriculum (IC) is an essential component of pediatric residency training that allows residents to participate in experiences specifically tailored to meet their unique learning goals. The integration of IC in training is a response to the rapidly evolving field of pediatrics and the need for training to be sufficiently flexible to best prepare residents for increasingly differentiated careers [1].

The ACGME first required IC as part of pediatric residency programs in 2013. The initial requirement called for a minimum of 6 months. Beginning in July 2025, the new requirement will expand IC time to a minimum of 40 weeks, representing almost one-third of the total residency training time. Per the ACGME, the IC "must be determined by the learning needs and career plans of each resident and must be developed through the guidance of the program director or designee." IC experiences are distributed over all 3 years of training, with 20 weeks dedicated to elective clinical, scholarly, or other experiences [2]. The remaining 20 weeks are dedicated to additional subspecialty training, beyond the experiences utilized to meet the inpatient and outpatient requirements.

The integration of IC into pediatric residency strengthens the training experience in a number of important aspects of professional development. IC supports Professional Identity Formation (PIF), operationalizes adult learning theories in medical education, and promotes self-directed learning. This approach to trainee professional development aligns with the goals of Competency-Based Medical Education (CBME), as trainees progress on individual paths towards competence [3].

Cruess et al. describe physician PIF as "a representation of self, achieved in stages over time during which the characteristics, values and norms of the medical profession are internalized, resulting in an individual thinking, acting and feeling like a physician" [4]. Beginning in medical school and continuing throughout training and career, PIF is the process of enculturation into the actions, interactions, values, and norms of the medical profession [5]. There are multiple

H. Howell (✉)
New York University Grossman School of Medicine, New York, NY, USA
e-mail: Heather.Howell@nyulangone.org

L. Thoreson
Dell Medical School, The University of Texas at Austin, Austin, TX, USA

H. McPhillips et al. (eds.), *Graduate Medical Education in Pediatrics*, Excellence in Medical Education 3, https://doi.org/10.1007/978-3-032-12952-9_15

factors that influence the socialization process that ultimately shape a physician's professional identity (Fig. 15.1). IC incorporates a number of factors contributing to socialization, including interactions with mentors, self-assessment, and selection of learning environments and clinical experiences. Dedicating a portion of residency training to individualized learning experiences encourages a trainee to view themselves as unique and have ownership over their training experience, rather than participating in a one-size-fits-all training program. It supports the development of their distinct identity.

IC also operationalizes concepts of adult learning theory, most notably described by Knowles as a way to conceptualize how adults learn differently than children due to motivation, experience, and understanding of why learning is important. Evolving approaches to adult learning acknowledge that many theories can be used to describe adult learning principles, with much overlap, but the concepts of experience, self-direction, reflection, community, and motivation are essential to building a successful curriculum that promotes acquisition of knowledge, skills, and attitudes [6]. IC, as defined by the ACGME for pediatric trainees, highlights adult learning theory concepts in promoting experiences built upon learner goals with support from mentors. The process inherently promotes reflection and self-direction with socialization and feedback from a community, namely mentors, faculty, and program leadership. Initial literature supports the importance of self-direction in IC, as residents who selected their IC experiences (versus experiences selected by the training program) were more likely to report the experience as important to the next steps in their career [7].

With the rapidly changing medical environment, the acquisition of new knowledge, skills, and attitudes is essential to medical practice focused on patient outcomes. Acquisition and utilization of self-directed learning skills are essential for trainees to maintain continued learning into independent practice. The ACGME directs the teaching of this skill through competency in practice-based learning and improvement and the use of individualized learning plans (ILPs) during training [2, 8, 9]. Self-directed learning describes learner management of their learning process through identifying learning goals and strategies to achieve those goals. Self-directed learning in medical education (SDL-ME) acknowledges the complexity of self-directed learning in the medical environment as compared to a classroom setting, as decisions affect patient

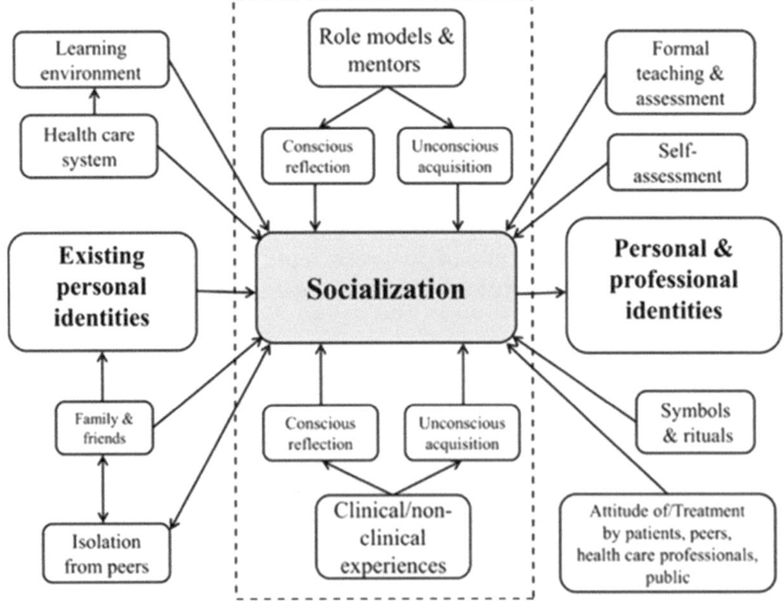

Fig. 15.1 A schematic representation of the multiple factors involved in the process of socialization in medicine. The large center box surrounded by the dotted line, which includes role models and mentors and experiential learning, indicates their importance to this process. The direction of the arrows from existing personal identities to personal and professional identities indicates the dynamic nature of this process [5]

outcomes and learning environments involve complicated systems processes for care delivery [10]. IC development is an opportunity to implement many strategies thought to support SDL-ME, specifically creating learning environments that support curiosity, explicit learner ownership of training/learning, and focused feedback on the process of learning using individual practice data [10]. Supporting IC through faculty mentorship in an environment created around supervision allows trainees to practice SDL skills while mitigating some of the potential adverse consequences to patient outcomes. Success in SDL during training may promote these behaviors in lifelong practice.

The integration of IC into pediatric training provides a structure by which residents can be evaluated by competency. CBME has been described as "an approach to preparing physicians for practice that is fundamentally oriented to graduate outcome abilities and organized around competencies derived from an analysis of societal and patient needs" [11]. The learner-centered approach is paramount in CBME as it seeks to emphasize the level of ability and individual development over the traditional time-based curricular design [11, 12]. Thus, IC is an essential component of CBME, allowing trainees with mentorship input to focus experiences on competencies that have yet to be obtained rather than assuming competence occurs because a time-limited rotation or training has been completed.

Approach to Individualized Curriculum

Curricular Structure

Despite the fact that IC has been part of ACGME requirements for more than 10 years, limited evidence supports an effective curricular structure or evaluation process. In an effort to better align curricular goals for the implementation and study of IC, Gifford et al. proposed a framework based on self-determination theory. The framework proposes three interconnected domains [13]. The first domain, relatedness, addresses how residents cultivate their professional identity through connecting with mentors, exploring career options, and finding their purpose within medicine. The second domain, autonomy, requires residents to identify their own learning needs and gaps and use that to inform the development of goals and a plan for how to accomplish the goals. The last domain, competence, emphasizes the development of knowledge and skills that prepare residents to advance in their career (Fig. 15.2). This framework helps resident and faculty understand the purpose of IC, supports the resident choosing meaningful experiences and provides clear metrics that the faculty can evaluate.

Rotation Structure

At present, there is no consistent approach for how to structure IC in pediatric training. With the implementation of different scheduling models, including X + Y, programs need to assess how IC fits into the framework of the rotation schedule. IC rotations should be viewed as separate experiences from core rotations, allowing the resident to have differentiated experiences, even if practicing in core rotation settings. IC also differs from electives, which is a separate requirement by the ACGME [2]. Electives are rotations chosen by residents that allow them exposure to sub-specialty interests or academic pursuits. Electives can include patient care and direct interaction with attending physicians. Residents often use elective time to enhance a particular interest or investigate a sub-specialty more deeply. Selectives are rotations required by the program to meet specific academic and/or workforce needs and provide educational content that the program wants experienced by all residents. While the structure of IC may vary from program to program, it is not meant to be simply additional elective or selective blocks, but rather a collection of experiences that is intentional in the purpose of meeting each resident's individual learning needs and career goals.

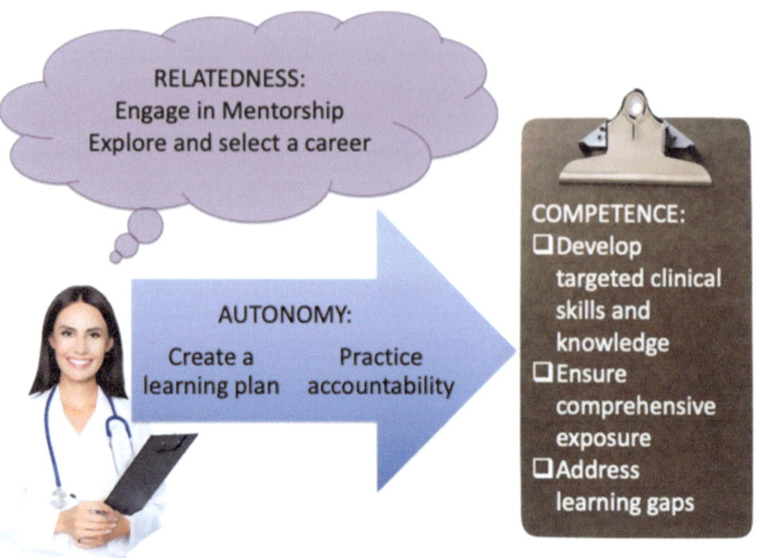

Fig. 15.2 Framework for the goals of individualized education structured using self-determination theory [13]

With no evidence to support an ideal structure, multiple approaches have been utilized. Programs may opt to use a single approach, combine strategies, or develop a new approach that aligns with ACGME requirements. Experiences can also be designed as one-time opportunities or a longitudinal exposure. Experiences requiring longer time frames for positive outcomes, like research or advanced continuity clinic sessions, benefit from longitudinal structures. Any approach should be coupled with mentorship from program leadership or faculty to ensure appropriate selection of educational experiences. Additional research studying the most effective IC rotation strategies is warranted.

Tracks

One approach is for programs to develop career-specific "tracks," providing experiences with optimal exposure for a resident's chosen career. Most commonly, tracks are divided between primary care, subspecialty/fellowship, and academic interests (e.g., academic medicine, global health, medical education, clinical research). Utilizing expert opinion from faculty in the careers, ideas for clinical and non-clinical experiences are gathered. These ideas can be used to design a "track" where residents all complete the same experiences, all complete required experiences and select options from a menu of choices, or develop their own track from a program provided menu of choices. Advantages of this approach are ease of scheduling as residents are more predictably available for clinical coverage, residents have options for rotation selection, and expert guidance in the career drives decision-making. Disadvantages include a lack of flexibility and resident experiences that too closely model required rotations. Limited evidence supports that the resident's ability to choose at least portions of the IC experience is important [7].

Resident Self-Design

Another approach is for residents to completely self-design experiences with the purpose of aiding in career decisions or to enhance knowledge, skills, or attitudes in an area of professional development or intended career path. IC blocks or longitudinal time is provided in the schedule, and residents select experiences to complete their schedule. Residents may select an entire IC schedule, select portions of their schedule, and/or create new IC experiences that meet a career or professional goal. Residents can practice goal writing by providing individualized goals for the experience to be used by faculty to understand their learning interests. Advantages include increased autonomy in schedule decisions for residents, the ability to focus on skill development for a struggling learner without peer recognition of an alteration in schedules, and the development of a new curriculum spurred by resident interests. Disadvantages include the scheduling time and complexity, need for consistent faculty mentorship, and faculty development for individualized curriculum goals.

Advanced Experience

Often used as a component of either of the abovementioned strategies, learners or programs will create an "advanced" rotation for further experience in a core rotation. When learners wish for more experience in a core rotation, a new structure can be considered that elevates the expectations, work structure, or exposures to meet an educational need. For example, a resident may choose a cardiology elective to meet their core subspecialty requirement and complete the goals and objectives that are standard for all trainees. Since they are considering a career in pediatric intensive care, the same resident opts for an IC cardiology experience with a focus on additional time observing cardiac surgery, following patients in the cardiac intensive care unit, and interpreting EKGs. Advantages include an experience directed towards career goals that is built on knowledge, skills, and attitudes gained in the initial rotation, and less program administration time in creating new experiences. Disadvantages include the faculty development to ensure the rotation is elevated above a standard experience and program time in coordinating the different experiences.

Given the time dedicated to IC, considering non-clinical experiences is important in maximizing the opportunities for professional development. Research time to focus on project development, research methodology, and biostatistics can be important for trainees planning to apply to a fellowship. Experiences in advocacy, community service, medical education, medical informatics, health equity, or leadership/administration can support additional career trajectories in addition to clinical work. Ideas for non-clinical rotations can be gleaned from faculty interests, FTE allocation, and community organizations that support the overall health of children in the practice area.

Resources

For IC to meet its intended purpose, there must be adequate preparation that engages the resident, faculty mentors, and the program leadership. Resources for IC development, implementation, and evaluation can be a barrier for programs. Capitalizing on existing program structures and personnel can ease some of the administrative burden of IC. Potential opportunities for resources are provided.

Program Leadership

Program leadership can find the implementation of IC to be challenging due to scheduling constraints due to required staffing minimums, limited faculty in numbers or expertise, faculty development in mentoring and coaching, and time. Identifying a program leader to oversee IC can be helpful to streamline scheduling and communication. Utilizing the coordinator and chief resident expertise can ease the scheduling and program administration challenges. Creating an IC guide with minimum expectations, explicit learner instructions, previous successful IC experiences, and appropriate IC experiences by career interest can help learners with self-direction. Focusing time in program evaluation committee (PEC) meetings to specifically address IC rotations and collect feedback can help resolve issues early and gain faculty buy-in for the rotation experiences. Asking the Clinical Competency Committee to provide a specific goal(s) for IC experiences can assist faculty mentors in aligning formative evaluation with next steps for education. Capitalizing on intern orientation to introduce the concepts of IC and self-directed learning sets the stage for the use of the IC during training.

Faculty

Faculty mentorship is key for residency training and is a crucial component of implementing successful IC. Utilizing existing faculty mentor, advisor, or coaching structures to incorporate IC mentorship prior to yearly scheduling can ease the burden on faculty time. Identifying IC champions amongst faculty can help engage new faculty and support ongoing faculty development.

Resident

IC experiences meet their intended goals if residents learn self-directed skills and self-assessment. The residents should use the process of ILPs for their IC experience, either as part of their required yearly ILP or as a brief ILP before each IC rotation. The ILP has been demonstrated to support skills for life-long learning [14, 15]. Components of ILP are (1) reflection on long term career goals and self-assessment of areas of strength and weakness, (2) goal generation, (3) development of plans/strategies to achieve the goal, (4) assessment of progress on goal, and (5) based on assessment, revising goal/plan or generating a new goal [16]. Aligning ILP completion with yearly scheduling, semi-annual feedback, and faculty mentor meetings can streamline the process for the program, faculty, and residents.

Evaluation

With any curriculum, a method of evaluation is needed to identify successful components and areas for improvement. Evaluation has been a unique challenge with IC due to the variability in structure, lack of outcome data, and potential goal discrepancies amongst stakeholders. Developing an evaluation strategy for IC is further complicated by the variability in each experience, which occurs at the program, rotation, and learner levels. Although program leaders recognize the importance of assessment in IC, no systematic process exists [17].

Program Assessment

Program evaluation regarding the effectiveness of IC should be rooted in principles of programmatic assessment [18, 19]. Utilizing existing program evaluation structures, such as end-of-rotation evaluations, the annual program review, and the program evaluation committee, can help formalize a routine review of the IC structure. Engaging stakeholders, including faculty mentors and trainees, in the feedback process provides information on whether IC is meeting its desired outcomes and reinforces the goals for IC in training. Another avenue for assessment is the use of a graduate survey. The program can gain data from graduates about the extent to which IC prepared them for their post-residency training position, either in independent practice or in a subspecialty fellowship training program. Graduates can also provide information about their competence with clinical management and procedural abilities that may directly link back to their IC goals. Lastly, graduates may provide insight into how successful the use of IC was toward creating skills for life-long learning [17].

Trainee Assessment

Assessment of the resident's progress with their IC can include data from self-assessment, mentor feedback, and program evaluation. As discussed earlier, the optimal ILP should incorporate learner self-assessment. The self-assessment should address if the resident was able to develop goals aligned with career exploration or career planning, utilize available resources, and sufficiently accomplish their pre-set goals. Since IC is a dynamic experience, self-reflection should also investigate circumstances when the pre-set goals were not met and how the resident can engage with mentors and identify different resources to restructure their action plan. In the event that the pre-set goals were met, the resident can build upon experiences to inform the development of new goals. Mentor feedback to the resident also provides an assessment of IC. The mentor could assess if the resident developed appropriate goals with feasible outcome measures and was accountable for their progress. Lastly, during the semi-annual review for the resident, the program should assess the resident's progress with their IC.

Best Practice Examples

Training Year Focused

IC can be structured to align with overarching programmatic goals for each training year. Designing IC based upon training year is ideal for residents who enter residency undifferentiated with regard to their post-training career plan. The training year focused approach starts with broad exposure in the first year and then gradually narrows as the resident moves towards a career decision. The goal for the first year of training is *Exposure and Exploration.* The program should provide a wide array of clinical and non-clinical experiences to sufficiently expose the intern to the vast possibilities for pediatric careers. Exposure is achieved through participating in the required inpatient, outpatient, and elective rotations and also through rotations dedicated to individualized career exploration. The first-year schedule should be sufficiently flexible to dedicate time to areas within pediatrics that the intern is considering for their career. The time should include clinical experiences for the intern to gain an understanding of the patient population and disease processes that are typical of a specific career. It may also include non-clinical endeavors to gain a broad picture of day-to-day life as a specific type of pediatrician. Early exposure ideally provides information to support the resident with their career decision. During intern year the goals for IC may be broad, such as deciding if they prefer an in-patient or out-patient clinical environment.

Intern Year should include blocks of subspecialty clinics that are intentionally designed to maximize exposure to pediatric subspecialty medicine. In addition, there should be dedicated blocks of career exploration where the intern chooses areas within pediatrics and works with the program leadership to create educational opportunities that are representative of a career in that field. For example, if an intern chooses to explore neonatology as a career, they may spend time in the neonatal intensive care unit (in addition to required time), but also shadow faculty as they do prenatal consults, participate in multidisciplinary fetal care meetings, see patients in the neonatal developmental care follow-up program, or participate in divisional educational conferences.

The second year of training is focused on *Expansion.* A resident may have narrowed down their career prospects to a few areas and can utilize the second year to build on experiences that will help them decide their ultimate path. Through reflection on the broad experiences during their first year, the residents can then select more specific clinical and non clinical experiences that will continue to help them hone in on the ideal career path. For example, a resident may conclude that they prefer inpatient medicine but are undecided between hospitalist medicine and critical care. During their second year, they may structure their IC time to spend additional time in each of those clinical environments, allowing for reflection on the aspects of each that align with their personal identity. Alternatively, if a resident has decided they enjoy both outpatient and inpatient medicine and want to pursue an organ-based subspecialty, they may design their IC time to work with specific divisions to identify the best fit. Additionally, the resident may pursue skills that will strengthen their clinical competency, such as learning ultrasound if they are considering emergency medicine or rotating with pediatric anesthesia to learn intubation skills if they are considering critical care. Lastly, the second year is an ideal time for residents to begin longitudinal scholarly pursuits, such as research studies, quality improvement projects, medical education curriculum development, or advocacy interventions.

The third and final year of training is dedicated to *Optimization.* Once a resident has decided on a post-graduation career plan, they can utilize IC to strengthen their knowledge and skills to prepare for a successful transition. The resident's goals will be more specific and aligned with their chosen area within pediatrics. IC experiences can be directly related to their chosen career or adjacent experiences. Those experiences may be in subspecialties that significantly overlap with their chosen career or may engage atypical experiences that will strengthen their knowledge about a related field. For example, a resident planning to pursue cardiology may rotate with genetics, with specific goals around understanding genetic syndromes that typically have congenital heart disease as an associated feature. A resident who plans to pursue a gastroenterology fellowship may utilize IC to rotate with a nutritionist to learn best practices for total parenteral nutrition (TPN) with a goal of learning how to account for various patient ages and diseases when providing TPN. And lastly, a resident who will be a general pediatrician with clinical time in the well-baby nursery may spend IC working with a lactation consultant with the goal of knowing how to counsel new mothers on methods for successful breastfeeding. The final year of training is also an ideal time for residents to utilize IC for advanced experiences.

Career Focused

IC may also be structured by career choice with a "menu" of options based on the planned career and academic interests. Programs can develop an approach that can be used by any subspecialty to build IC experiences, thus eliminating some of the administrative burden inherent in building rotation experiences.

An example of this approach is available for residents pursuing pediatric hospital medicine fellowship (PHM) [20, 21]). Utilizing content domains and Entrustable Professional Activities (EPAs) for PHM from the American Board of Pediatrics, and national survey information about gaps in fellowship preparedness, two residency programs created an IC elective for residents interested in PHM or additional hospital medicine exposure. A broad list of activities, including clinical work on non-teaching teams and the community hospital site, transport experience, and non-clinical experiences involving coding/billing, research, QI and leadership rounds is available for selection based on the resident's stated goals. Residents are sent a brief electronic survey and asked to identify 3–4 goals for a 2-week PHM experience. Based on the resident's goals, a 2-week calendar of activities is prepared and shared with the resident and participating faculty. The resident goals are shared with faculty prior to the experience and form the basis of feedback. At the conclusion of the experience, the resident completes a self-assessment based on the goals submitted and the faculty completes an evaluation based on the self-assessment and their own observations.

This model can be applied to IC development for any career choice. A group of interested trainees and faculty develop a list of specific knowledge, skills, and attitudes that are essential for practice in the specialty. Incorporating previously published research into curriculum and gaps in the subspecialty and fellowship preparedness, board content, and available content domains, EPAs for the specialty, and learner feedback from program surveys and group meetings can be helpful in broadly defining the needed content. A list of potential experiences, both clinical and non-clinical, is created for learners to review. Learners self-identify goals and meet with a faculty mentor or chief to design an IC experience. Utilizing learners' stated goals as the format for feedback and evaluation simplifies the assessment process and reinforces the concept of self-directed learning.

Future Directions

Pediatric training will continue to evolve to meet the AMSPDC Workforce Initiative goal to "improve the supply and distribution of pediatric subspecialists with the ultimate goal of meeting the health and wellness needs of the wide diversity of US children, adolescents, and young adults" And the new ACGME program requirements for individualized curriculum [2, 22]. The transition to a competency-based training and promotion system from a time-bound system necessitates the use of IC. As each learner enters training with different skills, learning styles, and trajectories, flexibility and individualized curricula help programs and learners address gaps, eliminate unnecessary redundancies in areas of competence, and align with adult learning theories. The administrative and faculty mentorship needed to achieve this structure remains a significant barrier. A new paradigm, precision education, which utilizes data and analytics at the learner, program, and organization level to support a continuous cycle of intervention and outcomes, is a promising concept to overcome the barriers [23]. Ultimately, IC allows for a customized journey during residency that will meet the specific needs of each learner and best prepare them for the next step of their career.

References

1. Jones MD Jr, McGuinness GA, Residency Review and Redesign in Pediatrics (R3P) Committee. The future of pediatric residency education: prescription for more flexibility [published correction appears in J Pediatr. 2009 Apr;154(4):629]. J Pediatr. 2009;154(2):157–8. https://doi.org/10.1016/j.jpeds.2008.10.040.
2. The Accreditation Council for Graduate Medical Education Program Requirements for Graduate Medical Education in Pediatrics. https://www.acgme.org/globalassets/pfassets/programrequirements/2025-prs/320_pediatrics_2025.pdf
3. Ross S, Hauer KE, van Melle E. Outcomes are what matter: competency-based medical education gets us to our goal. MedEdPublish. 2016;2018(7):85. Published 2018 Apr 12. https://doi.org/10.15694/mep.2018.0000085.1.
4. Cruess RL, Cruess SR, Boudreau JD, Snell L, Steinert Y. Reframing medical education to support professional identity formation. Acad Med. 2014;89(11):1446–51. https://doi.org/10.1097/ACM.0000000000000427.
5. Cruess RL, Cruess SR, Boudreau JD, Snell L, Steinert Y. A schematic representation of the professional identity formation and socialization of medical students and residents: a guide for medical educators. Acad Med. 2015;90(6):718–25. https://doi.org/10.1097/ACM.0000000000000700.
6. Taylor DC, Hamdy H. Adult learning theories: implications for learning and teaching in medical education: AMEE guide no. 83. Med Teach. 2013;35(11):e1561–72. https://doi.org/10.3109/0142159X.2013.828153.
7. Schumacher DJ, Frintner MP, Cull WL. Resident experiences with the individualized curriculum: current state and future opportunities. https://www.aap.org/en/research/pas-abstracts/resident-experiences-with-the-individualized-curriculum-current-state-and-future-opportunities/
8. The Accreditation Council for Graduate Medical Education Executive Summary Individualized Learning Plans. https://www.acgme.org/globalassets/pdfs/milestones/guidebooks/individual-learning-plans.pdf
9. The Accreditation Council for Graduate Medical Education Pediatric Milestones. https://www.acgme.org/globalassets/pdfs/milestones/pediatricsmilestones.pdf
10. Ricotta DN, Richards JB, Atkins KM, et al. Self-directed learning in medical education: training for a lifetime of discovery. Teach Learn Med. 2022;34(5):530–40. https://doi.org/10.1080/10401334.2021.1938074.
11. Frank JR, Mungroo R, Ahmad Y, Wang M, De Rossi S, Horsley T. Toward a definition of competency-based education in medicine: a systematic review of published definitions. Med Teach. 2010;32(8):631–7. https://doi.org/10.3109/0142159X.2010.500898.
12. Carraccio CL, Englander R. From Flexner to competencies: reflections on a decade and the journey ahead. Acad Med. 2013;88(8):1067–73. https://doi.org/10.1097/ACM.0b013e318299396f.
13. Gifford KA, Thoreson L, Burke AE, et al. Describing overarching curricular goals for individualized education. Teach Learn Med. 2021;33(3):282–91. https://doi.org/10.1080/10401334.2020.1835665.
14. Li ST, Paterniti DA, Co JP, West DC. Successful self-directed lifelong learning in medicine: a conceptual model derived from qualitative analysis of a national survey of pediatric residents. Acad Med. 2010;85(7):1229–36. https://doi.org/10.1097/ACM.0b013e3181e1931c.
15. Li ST, Paterniti DA, Tancredi DJ, Co JP, West DC. Is residents' progress on individualized learning plans related to the type of learning goal set? Acad Med. 2011;86(10):1293–9. https://doi.org/10.1097/ACM.0b013e31822be22b.
16. Li ST, Burke AE. Individualized learning plans: basics and beyond. Acad Pediatr. 2010;10(5):289–92. https://doi.org/10.1016/j.acap.2010.08.002.
17. Reed S, Picca A, Lockwood L, et al. A qualitative analysis of assessment and evaluation practices within the individualized curriculum. Acad Pediatr. 2023;23(5):1001–10. https://doi.org/10.1016/j.acap.2023.04.007.
18. Balmer DF, Rama JA, Simpson D. Program evaluation models: evaluating processes and outcomes in graduate medical education. J Grad Med Educ. 2019;11(1):99–100. https://doi.org/10.4300/JGME-D-18-01084.1.
19. Balmer DF, Riddle JM, Simpson D. Program evaluation: getting started and standards. J Grad Med Educ. 2020;12(3):345–6. https://doi.org/10.4300/JGME-D-20-00265.1.
20. Elster MJ, Cohen A, Herchline D, Chieco D, Hoefert J, Denniston S. The transition to pediatric hospital medicine fellowship: a national survey-based needs assessment. J Hosp Med. 2024;19(3):159–64. https://doi.org/10.1002/jhm.13278.
21. Emamian A, Pham Q, Rose-Kamprath J, Patel A, Thoreson L, Elster M. Yes, Chef! Cooking up a great PHM resident elective. Workshop, PHM 2024, Minneapolis, MN; 2024.
22. Vinci RJ, Degnon L, Devaskar SU. Pediatrics 2025: the AMSPDC workforce initiative. J Pediatr. 2021;237:5–8.e1. https://doi.org/10.1016/j.jpeds.2021.02.004.
23. Desai SV, Burk-Rafel J, Lomis KD, et al. Precision education: the future of lifelong learning in medicine. Acad Med. 2024;99(4S Suppl 1):S14–20. https://doi.org/10.1097/ACM.0000000000005601.

16 Interprofessional Education

Jennifer D. Baird, Glenn Rosenbluth, and Sandrijn van Schaik

Key Concepts and Definitions

The term *interprofessional education* is commonly used in describing different aspects of graduate medical education (GME) and should be differentiated from the related terms of interprofessional learning, and interprofessional collaborative practice. In this chapter, we use the World Health Organization's definition of interprofessional education (IPE) as educational experiences that "occur when students from two or more professions learn about, from, and with each other" [26]. This commonly used definition was actually adapted from a report by the Centre for the Advancement of Interprofessional Education, which defined IPE as, "Occasions when two or more professions learn from and about each other to improve collaboration and the quality of care" [8]. The attention to improving the quality of care is well-aligned with GME. Additionally, this slightly broader definition goes beyond students; in this chapter, we do the same and include learners of any level in the healthcare environment, including those who are postgraduate, advanced trainees, professionals orienting in the clinical environment, up through and including faculty who may be engaged in lifelong learning.

Interprofessional learning has been defined in the context of the clinical learning environment (CLE) by an ACGME collaborative team [24], as "the meaningful exchange of knowledge between diverse professionals that results in the integration of perspectives and expertise with the aim to improve outcomes and experiences." The CLE is distinguished from the nonclinical learning environment (e.g., classroom setting) and includes unstructured learning, which may occur between colleagues working together to care for patients. Finally, *interprofessional collaborative practice* (IPCP) is defined as "multiple health workers from different professional backgrounds working together with patients, families, caregivers, and communities to deliver the highest quality of care" [26].

It is important to acknowledge that the Accreditation Council for Graduate Medical Education (ACGME) Common Program Requirements (CPR) [1] put relatively little emphasis on true IPE, instead focusing their language on learning in the setting of interprofessional teamwork, which is akin to IPCP. The ACGME CPR (last updated in 2023) set an expectation for residents and fellows (heretofore referred to as GME learners) to provide care in an environment that is interprofessional, highlighting that "Optimal patient safety occurs in the

J. D. Baird
Children's Hospital Los Angeles, Los Angeles, CA, USA

G. Rosenbluth (✉) · S. van Schaik
University of California, San Francisco, San Francisco, CA, USA
e-mail: Glenn.Rosenbluth@ucsf.edu

H. McPhillips et al. (eds.), *Graduate Medical Education in Pediatrics*, Excellence in Medical Education 3, https://doi.org/10.1007/978-3-032-12952-9_16

setting of a coordinated interprofessional learning and working environment" [1]. Interestingly, patient safety and quality improvement activities are the only domains in which the ACGME provides this specific language regarding interprofessional learning activities. However, in the GME CLE, it is reasonable to assume that interprofessional education occurs and has significant benefits beyond simply those two domains of patient safety and quality improvement.

The ACGME Clinical Learning Environment Review (CLER) program[20] has outlined much more detailed expectations for interprofessional interactions by GME learners. All of the core domains of CLER pathways (Patient Safety, Healthcare Quality, Teaming, Supervision, Well-being, and Professionalism) include direct or indirect language guiding specific knowledge, skills, or behaviors. Even the Supervision domain, which does not explicitly use the term "interprofessional," sets an expectation for supervision by or of nonphysician staff members. The "Teaming" domain is almost entirely focused on interprofessional teamwork. The CLER Pathways document acknowledges the diversity of learner levels in the CLE, and "the importance of modeling optimal behaviors for early learners."

Interprofessional Education, Learning, and Collaborative Practice in the CLE

The GME Interprofessional environment is unique in that education takes place primarily within the CLE. Providers routinely work in interprofessional teams, and most learners are developing skills in their professions while concomitantly using these skills to deliver direct patient care. In the CLE, GME learners have opportunities to interact with learners and/or practitioners from different professions, at levels from novice to expert, all of whom can share expertise. The environment, therefore, has many opportunities for interprofessional education, learning, and collaborative practice.

At the most basic level, an Interprofessional team in healthcare is composed of members from multiple professions, as appropriate to the clinical setting and task at hand [6]. For example, in the setting of inpatient rounds, the bare minimum composition of an interprofessional team for a low acuity patient might be a physician, a nurse, and a parent/family member. If the patient had significant medical complexity, then that team might expand to include a pharmacist, social worker, child life specialist, respiratory therapist, dietician, and more.

The interprofessional team composition might also change based on the task at hand, and concomitantly, the role of educator may be specific to the task at hand as well. For example, a senior resident or fellow might be the appropriate educator for understanding the presentation of an illness and initial stabilization of a patient with severe pneumonia. Subsequently, a respiratory therapist and pharmacist might take on the educator role to help develop GME learners' next steps in management. In doing so, the respiratory therapist and pharmacist can provide content knowledge and also may provide teaching about their roles on the team.

IP Educators

In considering Interprofessional Education in Pediatric GME, it is important to think about who is doing the educating and how they embody their role as educators. Learning in GME occurs in different ways, sometimes characterized as the formal curriculum (intentionally created and formally offered), the informal curriculum (unscripted and ad-hoc, often in clinical learning environments), and the hidden curriculum, (the unwritten, unofficial, and often unintended lessons, values, and perspectives learners gain from their environment due to organizational structures and culture) [27]. Educators from different professions can contribute to both the formal and informal curriculum depending on their background, their experience level, and the structure of the GME program. Importantly, whether they contribute to informal and formal curriculum in large part shapes the hidden curriculum, as their inclusion (or exclusion) as educators of pediatric

GME learners sends a strong message of the value a program or institution puts on the importance of interprofessional learning and collaboration.

In this respect, Hafferty's assertion that the hidden curriculum often supersedes, and can even contradict, the formal curriculum is important to consider [27]. Any efforts to provide formal didactics on the importance of interprofessional collaboration can easily feel disingenuous if what trainees encounter in actual practice does not reflect such lessons. As long as there is ample evidence that the everyday experience of interprofessional teamwork in healthcare is still riddled with issues related to power, hierarchy, and conflict [38], formal curricula should take such issues into account [5, 49]. In addition, actively engaging members of the interprofessional team in both the formal and informal curriculum can help negate negative stereotypes, flatten hierarchies, promote and model interprofessional collaboration, and thereby set a different tone for the hidden curriculum.

So what does this look like in practice? Members of the interprofessional team can participate in the formal curriculum by giving lectures, facilitating simulation sessions, and providing hands-on training on equipment. To give a few examples: pharmacists are well-positioned to give talks about principles of pharmacotherapy, social workers can facilitate simulation sessions for learning about difficult conversations, and respiratory therapists can play a major role in demonstrating how ventilators and other respiratory support equipment work.

Engagement in the informal curriculum in the CLE can take multiple forms: ad-hoc learning from other professionals at the bedside or in clinic, shadowing others during their daily work, and getting feedback from other professionals. The role that members of other professions, particularly nursing, play in GME learners' workplace-based learning has been documented across specialties, [23, 31, 59] yet many of these studies also highlight how this informal learning is not always fully recognized or valued. Creating structured experiences for GME learners to shadow nurses and other healthcare professionals can help legitimize their role as educators. It can also help GME learners understand the tasks and responsibilities of these healthcare team members, which in turn can improve interprofessional communication [61]. Further legitimation of other healthcare professionals' roles as educators can come from attending physicians modeling interprofessional collaboration and inviting various team members to teach and share perspectives during rounds and team meetings.

Another opportunity for informal learning comes in the form of interprofessional feedback, as there are many opportunities for other healthcare professionals in both inpatient and outpatient settings to observe GME learners interact with patients and their families, in addition to experiencing GME learners' communication and teamwork skills directly. While GME learners appear to be open to receiving feedback from other professionals, in particular about communication and teamwork [45, 60], several studies highlight challenges related to institutional culture, hierarchy, and psychological safety [9, 45, 60]. For interprofessional feedback to be successful, structured approaches as well as education on effective feedback are needed, as well as close attention to the skill domains each profession can and should provide feedback on.

As discussed above, it is worth noting that the above examples for formal and informal learning from other healthcare professionals do not fully fit the WHO definition of interprofessional education, in which two or more learners from different professions "learn about, from and with" each other, since the "with" is missing from these examples unless trainees from other fields are also present. Not all pediatric residencies will have opportunities to include learners from other professions in formal or informal teaching, yet it may be possible to take a collaborative approach to teaching with two or more professions. Coteaching can model interprofessional collaboration, flatten hierarchies, elevate principles of equity, and facilitate discussions that promote perspective taking [64].

For all interprofessional educators, the importance of faculty development cannot be understated. Members from other professions will need to understand and embrace their roles as educators and be supported in the development of the necessary knowledge and skills to be successful in that role [19]. In this context, it is also important to discuss the role of learners themselves as educators. Learners from different professions may have much to offer to pediatric GME learners, and pediatric GME learners themselves can help teach learners from other professions. Yet, because learners are still mastering their own professional skills, they must be able to recognize their limits and self-regulate what they choose to teach and what they feel comfortable accepting from other learner-teachers.

Lastly, while we typically do not think of patients and their families as healthcare professionals, it is important to recognize their potential roles as educators for pediatrics GME learners [33]. Patients and families interact with GME learners directly and observe their performance, and can be a great resource for both formal and informal learning. In particular, for children with chronic conditions, parents and the children themselves, depending on their age and developmental stage, bring significant expertise about both the medical aspects of the condition and the experience of living with chronic conditions. Such expertise can be shared with GME learners as part of routine patient care or through specially constructed experiential learning activities [10, 41]. In addition, GME learners can learn from parents by eliciting their feedback on select skills as part of 360 feedback mechanisms [13]. Parents can also be included in the formal curriculum, for example, in workshops about conducting "difficult conversations" [62].

Selected Exemplars in GME-Based Interprofessional Education in GME

Patient- and Family-Centered Rounds

Patient and Family-Centered Rounding (PFCR), often referred to simply as Family-Centered Rounding (FCR), is a natural setting for interprofessional learning. Although only the family is called out, FCR is generally understood to include several members of the interprofessional team, including nurses, clinical pharmacists, child life specialists, social workers, and more [35]. FCR presents a unique opportunity for all team members to make active contributions; however, this requires the intentional creation of an inclusive environment. Because of the traditional hierarchies in healthcare, physicians tend to dominate rounds, and team members from other professions may need to be invited and even "activated" to participate. Effective activation can increase opportunities for interprofessional education because individuals may feel more empowered to share their knowledge, and also may be more receptive to learning [4].

For example, bedside nurses often have key observations and expertise to share that may not be obvious to learners. In addition to having the most up-to-date information, nurses may be invited to share their knowledge of care delivery systems as well as opportunities to improve care. Common examples include teaching GME learners about wound care, tube feeding, and medication administration, all of which are topics about which most physicians tend to defer to nursing expertise. When nurses are invited to share this type of information on rounds, GME learners have the opportunity to learn both from and about nursing as a profession. Similar teaching and learning may come from including pharmacists, respiratory therapists, and social workers on clinical rounds. By creating space for other team members, attending physicians can model for their GME learners mutual respect and equity in the CLE. Certainly, some of this learning could occur in one-on-one discussions, but the framework of rounds both broadens the audience and has the potential to increase the legitimacy of the teaching.

GME learners also have the opportunity to learn directly from patients and families when these patients and families are actively included in PFCR. Including patients and families in rounds has been shown to have significant safety benefits [36, 37], and these benefits can be specifically highlighted for GME learners. In addition, GME learners may learn about families' experiences of care [7]. Finally, patients and their families can be specifically prompted to share knowledge about their medical conditions, including the impact of both the condition and of any prescribed treatments. The Institute for Patient- and Family-Centered Care (IPFCC), describes roles of "patient and family advisors" and "patient and family faculty" [29]. By viewing and framing patients and families as professionals, GME faculty can provide a context for interprofessional education directly from and with patients and families.

Case Conferences and Safety Event Reviews

Interprofessional case conferences (ICC) have been defined as "interactive, facilitated, case-based group discussions that have specific educational goals and involve members of two, and ideally more, health professions working collaboratively to improve patient care" [48]. These case conferences are ideal settings for GME learners and faculty to participate in interprofessional education and practice.

ICCs may be standing daily or weekly conferences and may range in format from brief huddles with an operational focus to more clinically focused conferences to support individual patients. As is the case with all IP settings, establishment of structure and roles is key to success [48]. Frequently, an individual may be called upon to present cases for discussion and/or review. When a supervising resident takes on this role, they should be prepared with an orientation to the goals of the conference, the specific expectations of their role, and the roles of others. Learners who are new to these conferences may not have clear expectations of what they can learn from others. Providing a scaffolding, such as a script or checklist, to support interprofessional engagement can facilitate effective presentations. These supports may help ensure that the learners have expectations of what lessons to take away from the conferences, and also support the hidden curriculum of interprofessional collaboration. Facilitation of ICCs is most effectively performed by one or more team members who are familiar with the structure and the expectations. As noted above, having facilitators from two or more professions colead ICCs can enhance their impact by modeling interprofessional collaboration.

Safety Event Reviews are a specific form of ICC that can encompass important interprofessional collaboration and learning opportunities. Interprofessional safety event reviews for purposes of medical education are well-received by learners [65], especially if the GME learners were proximate to the safety event at hand [15]. Expanding the team to include professionals such as biomedical engineers and informatics experts can have added benefits [46]. These reviews can facilitate cross-talk between content experts who may be very familiar with existing systems and structures and frontline providers who may bring a fresh perspective to identifying improvement opportunities. Outcomes from safety event reviews may lead to additional opportunities for interprofessional collaboration to develop solutions, and GME learners should be included in this follow-up work whenever possible.

Interprofessional Simulations

Interprofessional simulation-based team training is a well-documented strategy to improve teamwork and as a result improve quality of care and patient safety [11, 22]. Such training often takes place in situ in actual clinical environments, focusing on clinical emergency situations, and are often known as "mock codes" [58]. Depending on the format and availability of participants, mock codes may include doctors, nurses, pharmacists, and respiratory therapists navigating simulated patient care scenarios together. Such scenarios are typically followed by a debriefing or facilitated group discussion, during which most of the learning from simulation takes place.

Interprofessional simulation-based team training offers opportunities for GME learners to practice essential teamwork skills together with members from other professions and to learn from and about those team members during the debriefing. As with interprofessional feedback, ensuring that interprofessional learning during simulation is truly impactful is not without challenges. Pediatric GME learners often lack experience compared to staff members and may therefore feel vulnerable and incompetent despite being assigned the role of team leader [52]. Making such complex dynamics visible and explicitly discussing the role of power and hierarchy during the debriefing of simulation scenarios has been suggested as a strategy to enhance learning [11, 49, 52]. This requires expert facilitation, and as with all interprofessional education, is best accomplished by an interprofessional team of educators trained to facilitate discussions about these topics [11, 34].

In Situ Improvement Work Within the Healthcare System

Resident-led improvement work within the healthcare system is a natural opportunity for collaboration with an interprofessional team [1]. The ACGME Pursuing Excellence Initiative identifies interprofessional learning and practice as a key driver in the integration of healthcare systems and GME, with a specific call out to interprofessional team-based quality and safety work. Collaboration with existing interprofessional unit-based leadership teams presents a unique opportunity for GME learners to work with and learn from professionals who are engaged in patient- or systems-focused improvement work [53]. Unit-based leadership teams often have expertise in improvement work, and team members can educate GME learners in practical and hands-on approaches to improvement science. Additionally, by working in interprofessional teams to complete improvement work, GME learners have opportunities to learn about different professions and how they contribute to practice [15].

A supportive institutional culture may be an important facilitator in resident engagement in interprofessional team-based improvement work. Intentional system design with specific roles for GME learners can support this engagement. If trainees have meaningful roles and are supported in these roles, they may place greater value on IP collaboration [15]. Alternatively, if they participate simply as observers, they may be less likely to carry learnings to other work. Dissemination of work in collaborative settings such as institutional improvement symposia can provide additional opportunities for trainees to learn with and about contributors to improvement work in the CLE [53].

Assessing Competency

Competency assessment starts with identifying the knowledge, skills, and attitudes that determine competency, and careful consideration of suitable assessment strategies. The Accreditation Council for Graduate Medical Education (ACGME) Milestones framework includes interprofessional collaboration and communication in two of its six competency domains for all GME learners: Systems-based Practice (interprofessional patient-centered care coordination) and Interpersonal and Communication Skills (interprofessional communication) [2]. Within these competencies, the ACGME delineates milestones to help educators assess a learner's developmental progress; the highest of 5 levels involves coaching others in interprofessional care coordination and communication. To assist with operationalization of competency assessment, the American Board of Pediatrics (ABP) has formulated Entrustable Professional Activities (EPA), defined as "observable, routine activities that a general pediatrician should be able to perform safely and effectively to meet the needs of their patients" [3]. The competencies related to interprofessional collaboration and communication map to several of these EPAs, most notably to EPA 15, "Lead an Interprofessional Health Care Team" (see Table 16.1).

While these competencies and activities outlined by the ACGME and ABP are likely what most pediatric GME educators will use to assess interprofessional collaboration skills of pediatric GME learners, it is worth noting that these were created from a physician-focused perspective. In contrast, the competencies for interprofessional

Table 16.1 ABP entrustable professional activity and IPEC competencies

ABP EPA 10: Leading interprofessional teams to provide collaborative, family-centered care	IPEC competencies
Establishing a shared vision, goals, expectations, and outcome measures Engaging other team members in a way that utilizes their specific roles and capabilities, eliciting and valuing the perspective and contributions of others Demonstrating situation awareness by: Monitoring individual team member's performance to enable oversight and management of Current and evolving situations Balancing autonomy and supervision of team members by assigning/delegating unsupervised work to team members that aligns with their knowledge, skills, and attitudes, and supervising the work of team members that is designed to expand these Monitoring team performance and providing feedback Recognizing and managing the social cues, emotional responses, as well as the personal and professional needs of team members Role modeling as the team leader	Values and ethics: Work with team members to maintain a climate of shared values, ethical conduct, and mutual respect Roles and responsibilities: Use the knowledge of one's own role and team members' expertise to address individual and population health outcomes Communication: Communicate in a responsive, responsible, respectful, and compassionate manner with team members Teams and teamwork: Apply values and principles of the science of teamwork to adapt one's own role in a variety of team settings

collaborative practice formulated by the Interprofessional Education Collaborative (IPEC) are the consensus product across health professionals. IPEC was formed in 2009 as a unique partnership of six health professions education associations with the American Association of Medical Colleges (AAMC) representing Medicine. Version 3 of the IPEC competencies was just published in 2023, and although there is some overlap between the IPEC competencies and the activities listed in the ABP EPA, there are also some differences [30].

Most notably, the ABP EPA assumes a leadership role for the physician, and puts the physician in a role of oversight, delegating and supporting other team members. The most recent version of the IPEC competencies [30], under the teams and teamwork domain, puts an emphasis on shared leadership, which they define as "a dynamic, interactive influence process among individuals in teams for which the objective is to lead, follow, and/or support one another to the achievement of team or organizational goals or both." High-quality empirical research studies have been limited thus far, but there is data to suggest that shared or collective leadership benefits team performance [32, 55]. Pediatric GME educators may want to consider this broader context when setting expectations and benchmarks for interprofessional collaboration.

After clarifying what constitutes competence, the next step is to select appropriate assessment strategies. The options are myriad and span the spectrum of testing knowledge to evaluating performance in clinical practice, using anything from self-assessments and multiple-choice tests to objective structured examinations. A detailed description of all possible assessment strategies is beyond the scope of this chapter, but there are a few important points to keep in mind when choosing the best strategy.

First, the purpose of the assessment will greatly influence the choice of assessment strategy. Summative assessment, used to make decisions about advancement and readiness for independent practice, will require approaches that have been rigorously tested with sufficient validity information to justify high-stakes decisions. Formative assessment, on the other hand, aims to help a resident understand where their growth edges and support further development of skills. Formative assessment, consequently, has lower stakes, making reliability less of an issue. Second, if an assessment tool is used, recognizing the limitations of such tools is important. There are numerous checklists and rating tools to assist with the assessment of interprofessional teamwork skills, but few have been validated for the pediatric GME context [63]. A few of these teamwork assessment tools are based on the IPEC competencies. Most are focused on teamwork in high-acuity settings and, therefore, grounded in principles of crisis resource management, with limited attention to the unique aspects of interprofessional collaboration. Since most pediatric GME learners will go on to practice in low-acuity settings such as community clinics, the relevance of such tools can be questionable [57]. Third, if a tool is used for assessment, training of evaluators is essential to ensure they understand the purpose of the assessment and use rating scales as intended, especially for summative assessment. Lastly, with any form of assessment, attention to implicit bias is essential, as it is increasingly recognized that biased assessments are common in medical education, with potentially negative consequences [39].

In discussing competency assessment, it is important to note that we cannot expect our trainees to gain competency in skills we do not teach or model. Both pediatric GME learners and program directors feel there is room to improve in this regard when it comes to interprofessional teamwork. On the 2024 ACGME resident survey, the mean rating across all pediatric residency programs for the item "Interprofessional teamwork skills modeled or taught" was 4.0, below the national average for all specialties (4.2). Only 76% of pediatric programs were in compliance on this item, compared to 80% for all specialties combined. A survey of pediatric residency program directors similarly showed that only 68% of program directors were satisfied with their IPE curriculum, although 85% reported having such a curriculum [28].

Challenges

In spite of the numerous potential benefits that IPE presents for the interprofessional team and for patients and families, there are significant challenges that have hindered or even prevented more widespread adoption [12]. On the surface, IPE sounds intuitive to many in GME, given the interprofessional nature of clinical practice and the dependency of professionals from different disciplines upon each other for the optimal delivery of care. However, the clinical learning environment is frequently not at a stage of IPCP that is ready to embrace and support curricula based on IPE [5]. Clinical care delivery remains a hierarchical system—perhaps more multiprofessional than interprofessional. Even domains such as quality improvement and patient safety, which may seem ripe for resident participation in interprofessional activities, are rarely actually viewed as interprofessional by GME learners and program faculty [40]. So while it is easy to imagine an ideal state in which clinicians practice and learn together harmoniously, benefitting from each other's unique perspectives and giving deference to differing types of expertise, most academic medical centers have not achieved this. As a result, those learners who are educated using principles of IPE may not find themselves in a familiar or inclusive learning environment when they enter practice.

Another key barrier to safe and inclusive learning environments for interprofessional education is a lack of equity among different professionals on the care team. Despite long-standing efforts to recognize and address hierarchies among the healthcare team, these hierarchies continue to exist and may be exacerbated by racial, gender, or other biases. These hierarchies and biases create power dynamics that can prioritize the perspectives and practices of a particular group or groups and undermine the safety of the learning environment for those with less perceived or actual power [17].

IPE often involves different levels of learners, particularly when it occurs in the clinical setting as a component of, or supplement to, regular clinical care delivery. Learners with less experience may be intimidated by the expertise of those who are more senior, and those with more experience may feel frustrated if basic information needs to be explained or reviewed. This imbalance of experience also crosses professions; in settings where career nurses may have more experience than GME learners, power dynamics may limit learning from or even about each other [52].

When the clinical team involves both trainees and practicing clinicians, the time spent on education may be perceived as detracting from the time needed for efficient clinical care delivery. All these scenarios can impact the safety of the learning environment. In the absence of a safe learning environment where learners are seen as peers, it can be difficult for those who feel less powerful, lower in the hierarchy, or less experienced to fully engage in learning, receiving, or giving meaningful feedback, thus depriving learners of some of the important benefits of IPE.

As described, the complexity of the CLE creates many *unstructured* opportunities for interprofessional learning. On the other hand, creating *structured* opportunities for traditional interprofessional education may be much more challenging. The relatively rapid rotation of trainees into and out of clinical services creates both logistical and workforce (i.e., teacher) challenges. When team members turn over rapidly, it may be harder to establish trusting relationships with colleagues. The result may be that individuals revert to more traditional approaches to work, such as working alongside each other without the full benefit of collaborative practice. Countermeasures to this reversion may include clearly defined roles and practices, such as having nurses speak first on rounds to share important clinical events, having pharmacists review medication plans, etc. Defining clear roles for all team members also presents GME learners with exemplars of what individuals from each profession may contribute to clinical care. Clarity of roles has the added benefit of helping individuals understand their own responsibilities, reducing hierarchies, and potentially reducing the pressure on GME learners, which may increase psychological safety in the learning environment.

The question of who can be considered as faculty is ongoing in IPE. Traditional or formal faculty members (i.e., those with university appointments in professional schools) can play an important role, particularly in the thoughtful planning of IPE activities, preparation of learners for optimal engagement, and evaluation of the quality of the learning activity and assessment of the learner's development. However, in some cases, they may not be the best teachers for the content needed. The ACGME recognizes and supports the engagement of other professionals with expertise to serve as faculty for GME learners, and has specifically encouraged faculty development for all professionals who may provide teaching in the CLE [16]. In fact, the ACGME Common Program Requirements provide a very inclusive definition of faculty, stating, "'Faculty' refers to the entire teaching force responsible for educating GME learners. The term 'faculty,' including 'core faculty,' does not imply or require an academic appointment" [1]. So while there are specific qualifications required for physician faculty (i.e., Board certification or other acceptable credentials), the clear intent is to have a much broader pool of educators included as "faculty."

Despite the common examples we have provided, patients and families are an often-overlooked group of "faculty" in IPE who can be engaged in formal educational settings, such as the classroom or simulation environment, to share their experiences with the healthcare system or deepen the fidelity of the simulation. They are also important teachers in the clinical environment, where they can provide real-time feedback on their care experience that can inform trainees' learning and help to shape their practice. Thoughtful engagement with patients and families in both formal education settings and the clinical learning environment is needed to ensure that they can meaningfully engage in a way that supports learning and is respectful of their roles. For example, families for whom English is not the preferred language and those who have responsibilities at work or at home that prohibit them from freeing up time may not easily get included in formal educational activities. The result of this passive exclusion is a disproportionate impact on opportunities to learn from families who traditionally are excluded and marginalized in other aspects of healthcare. As a result, GME learners may get a biased view of families' expectations and needs. An equity-oriented approach to including parents as educators is essential. This approach will require resources for interpreters and appropriate reimbursement of participants for their time, as well as cultural humility to ensure parents' boundaries are understood and respected.

Additional challenges are the time needed to engage in meaningful IPE, and payment for this time [49]. Making time for interprofessional classroom sessions or simulation activities may displace other curricular elements in existing training programs that already feel pressured to include too much content in too little time. Training programs may also operate on different calendars, so the alignment of learner schedules can be difficult. When IPE involves a mixture of trainees and practicing clinicians and happens away from the clinical setting (as when resident or fellow physicians engage in simulation with nontrainee clinical nurses), the clinicians may need coverage for patient care duties. The time away from patient care may also be considered nonproductive paid time for the clinicians, which has implications for budgeting and may restrict engagement of the full complement of team members necessary for an optimal learning experience.

Health systems that value interprofessional education must be prepared to compensate their employees for both teaching and learning time, and can expect some degree return on this investment in the form of care delivery improvements [11, 53] as well as improved attitudes toward collaboration [47]. Calculation of costs may be relatively straightforward for employees who receive an hourly wage based on an existing contract. For salaried faculty, the value of teaching hours frequently becomes more complicated. Models of educational value units have been implemented[51], but their success and sustainability varies[44]. If interprofessional teaching in the CLE is not explicitly valued, faculty from all professions may not receive appropriate compensation for their time, and subsequently, this teaching may not be counted toward promotion and/or advancement. In order for IPE programs to be sustained, institutions should create and maintain clear and robust incentives for faculty who participate in IPE programs.

Finally, as described above, assessment of the quality of IPE and its impact on learner competency development is complex, and consensus on how best to assess this is still emerging [56]. A variety of assessment tools exist, but questions remain about what should actually be measured and whether the tools have sufficient theoretical grounding to effectively evaluate the impact of IPE. The subject of the assessment is also a question—should evaluation of IPE be an assessment of the individual, the interprofessional team, or some combination of the two? Additionally, multiple potential assessors exist—is IPE best evaluated by faculty or the other clinical members of the team? When IPE is occurring in situ, could patients or families assist in the evaluation? The lack of consensus on these assessment elements makes it difficult to understand the overall impact of IPE, which may be a deterrent to broader adoption.

What Is Next in IPE?

Each of these identified challenges lends itself to additional research and/or identification of best practices as part of the ongoing development and evolution of the field and as we work to solidify both the theoretical foundations and the practical application of IPE. What interventions, for example, help to reduce perceived hierarchy and inequity among learners/team members and enhance the psychological safety of the learning environment? [11]. How do we leverage IPE to meaningfully address and ameliorate biases both among the interprofessional team and in clinical care delivery? Emerging work using nontraditional educational strategies such as improvisational theater [18] and visual art education[14] may offer insights on how best to address these issues. Additional work is also needed to address some of the identified logistical challenges, and to answer lingering questions about the best way to evaluate both the quality of IPE and learner/team outcomes associated with engagement in interprofessional learning activities [11, 34].

The rapidly evolving technology landscape also creates additional opportunities for IPE. Simulation programs are leveraging virtual reality (VR) to create immersive learning experiences that can be relatively easily modified to address specific learning needs and that help to overcome some of the logistical challenges associated with traditional IPE [42]. VR sessions, for example, can allow the learner to engage with avatars representing patients, families, and members of the interprofessional team without the need for those additional team members to be physically present, thus overcoming typical scheduling challenges and reducing the personnel cost associated with the learning activity [50]. Artificial intelligence (AI) is helping to enhance the fidelity of these simulations through the use of AI-enabled virtual reality simulations that can more effectively capture the nuanced role of members of the interprofessional team [43].

Accelerated deployment of AI-driven assistive technology in the clinical space is creating a need for adaptation of our clinical training curricula to prepare learners for the judicious use of these technologies [21]. Given the cross-functional application of much of the technology, the incorporation of AI into IPE learning activities can help to ensure that learners and the clinical care teams on which they work are equipped to effectively and appropriately capitalize on the benefits of AI. Educators should keep in mind that AI is based on predictive modeling, and there may be fewer examples of IP collaborative practice in existing training data sets. As such, AI may underrecognize opportunities for IPE and IPCP and may amplify existing biases.

The rapid evolution of virtual care delivery models creates an additional opportunity for IPE, as learners and practicing clinicians adapt to shifting norms around the physical composition and location of the team and develop best practices for interaction to support care delivery for patients and families. The growing use of virtual nursing in the inpatient setting [54], for example, requires the healthcare team to interact with the virtual nurse as an additional member of the team and necessitates modifications to existing communication patterns and workflows. As virtual care delivery models continue to evolve, it is likely that other members of the care team will be supported by or replaced with virtual counterparts, and each of these changes to the existing model will require adaptations to team workflows and accompanying IPE to support these adaptations.

Conclusions

As the US healthcare environment increasingly relies on interprofessional care teams, GME learners must be adequately prepared to learn from and work with colleagues from a variety of professions. While opportunities abound for exposure to IPCP, program directors may need to identify and support opportunities for true IPE. Clinical learning environments provide ample opportunities for GME learners to learn with, from, and about colleagues from other professions, but the success and sustainability of these IPE opportunities require explicit support for both curricula and faculty. As IPE programs continue to develop, program directors can directly address existing professional biases, hierarchies, and inequities to ensure that GME learners can maximally benefit from and contribute to these interprofessional care environments and be effectively prepared for their future careers.

References

1. Accreditation Council for Graduate Medical Education. Common program requirements. 2023. Retrieved August 6, 2024, from https://www.acgme.org/globalassets/pfassets/programrequirements/cprresidency_2023.pdf.
2. Accreditation Council for Graduate Medical Education (ACGME) Pediatrics Milestones Work Group. Pediatrics milestones. 2021, Implementation Date: July 1, 2021. Retrieved August 6, 2024, from https://www.acgme.org/globalassets/pdfs/milestones/pediatricsmilestones.pdf.
3. American Board of Pediatrics. Entrustable professional activities for general pediatrics. 2024,

Last updated on May 29, 2024. Retrieved August 6, 2024, from https://www.abp.org/content/entrustable-professional-activities-general-pediatrics.
4. Ashcraft LE, Asato M, Houtrow AJ, Kavalieratos D, Miller E, Ray KN. Parent empowerment in pediatric healthcare settings: a systematic review of observational studies. Patient. 2019;12:199–212.
5. Bainbridge L, Regehr G. Should there be an "I" in team? A new perspective on developing and maintaining collaborative networks in health professional care. In: Interprofessional client-centered collaborative practice: what does it look like. New York: Nova Publishers; 2015. p. 51–66.
6. Baird J, Ashland M, Rosenbluth G. Interprofessional teams: current trends and future directions. Pediatr Clin N Am. 2019;66(4):739–50.
7. Bardach NS, Stotts JR, Fiore DM, Sarkar U, Sharma AE, Boscardin WJ, Avina L, Peralta-Neel C, Rosenbluth G. Family input for quality and safety (FIQS): using mobile technology for in-hospital reporting from families and patients. J Hosp Med. 2022;17(6):456–65.
8. Barr H. Interprofessional education today, yesterday and tomorrow, Commissioned by The Learning and Teaching Support Network for Health Sciences & Practice from The UK Centre for the Advancement of Interprofessional Education. Learning & Teaching Support Network; 2001.
9. Bhat C, LaDonna KA, Dewhirst S, Halman S, Scowcroft K, Bhat S, Cheung WJ. Unobserved observers: nurses' perspectives about sharing feedback on the performance of resident physicians. Acad Med. 2022;97(2):271–7.
10. Blasco P, Kohen H, Shapland C. Parents-as-teachers: design and establishment of a training programme for paediatric residents. Med Educ. 1999;33(9):695–701.
11. Bochatay N, Ju M, O'Brien BC, van Schaik SM. A scoping review of interprofessional simulation-based team training programs. Simul Healthc. 2023;10:1097.
12. Bogossian F, New K, George K, Barr N, Dodd N, Hamilton AL, Nash G, Masters N, Pelly F, Reid C, Shakhovskoy R, Taylor J. The implementation of interprofessional education: a scoping review. Adv Health Sci Educ Theory Pract. 2023;28(1):243–77.
13. Brinkman WB, Geraghty SR, Lanphear BP, Khoury JC, del Rey JAG, DeWitt TG, Britto MT. Effect of multisource feedback on resident communication skills and professionalism: a randomized controlled trial. Arch Pediatr Adolesc Med. 2007;161(1):44–9.
14. Chang L, Mosher D. Interprofessional art rounds. AMA J Ethics. 2023;25(5):317–23.
15. Cheng MKW, Collins S, Baron RB, Boscardin CK. Analysis of the interprofessional clinical learning environment for quality improvement and patient safety from perspectives of interprofessional teams. J Grad Med Educ. 2021;13(6):822–32.
16. Choi LW, Moriates C, Payne AS, Varaklis K, Gonzales R, Baron RB. CLER pursuing excellence: faculty development innovations in quality, safety, equity, and value. J Grad Med Educ. 2021;13(5):746–52.
17. Chou E, Grawey T, Paige JB. Psychological safety as an educational value in interprofessional health education. AMA J Ethics. 2023a;25(5):338–43.
18. Chou E, LaDisa AG, Zelenski A, Lauck S. How to use improv to help interprofessional students respond to status and hierarchy in clinical practice. AMA J Ethics. 2023b;25(5):311–6.
19. Clay MA, Sikon AL, Lypson ML, Gomez A, Kennedy-Malone L, Bussey-Jones J, Bowen JL. Teaching while learning while practicing: reframing faculty development for the patient-centered medical home. Acad Med. 2013;88(9):1215–9.
20. CLER Evaluation Committee. CLER pathways to excellence: expectations for an optimal clinical learning environment to achieve safe and high-quality patient care, version 3.0. Chicago, IL; 2024.
21. Connolly C, Hernon O, Carr P, Worlikar H, McCabe I, Doran J, Walsh JC, Simpkin AJ, O'Keeffe DT. Artificial intelligence in Interprofessional healthcare practice education – insights from the home health project, an exemplar for change. Comput Sch. 2023;40(4):412–29.
22. Eppich W, Howard V, Vozenilek J, Curran I. Simulation-based team training in healthcare. Simul Healthc. 2011;6(7):S14–9.
23. Floren LC, Pittenger AL, Wilting I, Irby DM, Cate OT. Medical residents' informal learning from pharmacists in the clinical workplace. Med Sci Educ. 2023;33(3):701–10.
24. Foshee CM, Walsh H, Van der Kloot TE, Boscardin CK, Calongne L, Telhiard NS, Ullman C, Backus C, Peyre SE. Pursuing excellence: innovations in designing an interprofessional clinical learning environment. J Grad Med Educ. 2022;14(1):125–30.
25. Frenk J, Chen L, Bhutta ZA, Cohen J, Crisp N, Evans T, Fineberg H, Garcia P, Ke Y, Kelley P. Health professionals for a new century: transforming education to strengthen health systems in an interdependent world. Lancet. 2010;376(9756):1923–58.
26. Gilbert JH, Yan J, Hoffman SJ. A WHO report: framework for action on interprofessional education and collaborative practice. J Allied Health. 2010;39(Suppl 1):196–7.
27. Hafferty FW. Beyond curriculum reform: confronting medicine's hidden curriculum. Acad Med. 1998;73(4):403–7.
28. Herrmann LE, Goldman E, Ottolini M. Interprofessional education curricula in pediatric residency programs: survey of US pediatric program directors. J Interprofessional Educ Pract. 2018;12:33–9.
29. Institute for Patient- and Family-Centered Care (IPFCC). Prevalence and functioning of patients and families as educators in hospitals and academic medical centers: a national study. Institute for Patient- and Family-Centered Care (IPFCC); 2021.
30. Interprofessional Education Collaborative. IPEC core competencies for interprofessional collaborative practice. 2023, Published November 20, 2023. Retrieved August 6, 2024, from https://www.ipecol-

laborative.org/assets/core-competencies/IPEC_Core_Competencies_Version_3_2023.pdf.

31. Jansen I, Silkens ME, Galema G, Vermeulen H, Geerlings SE, Lombarts KM, Stalmeijer RE. Exploring nurses' role in guiding residents' workplace learning: a mixed-method study. Med Educ. 2023;57(5):440–51.
32. Janssens S, Simon R, Beckmann M, Marshall S. Shared leadership in healthcare action teams: a systematic review. J Patient Saf. 2021;17(8):e1441–51.
33. Jha V, Quinton ND, Bekker HL, Roberts TE. Strategies and interventions for the involvement of real patients in medical education: a systematic review. Med Educ. 2009;43(1):10–20.
34. Ju M, Bochatay N, Werne A, Essakow J, Tsang L, Nottingham M, Franzon D, Lyndon A, van Schaik S. Changing the conversation: impact of guidelines designed to optimize interprofessional facilitation of simulation-based team training. Adv Simul. 2024;9:1.
35. Katkin JP, Kressly SJ, Edwards AR, Perrin JM, Kraft CA, Richerson JE, Tieder JS, Wall L. Guiding principles for team-based pediatric care. Pediatrics. 2017;140(2)
36. Khan A, Coffey M, Litterer KP, Baird JD, Furtak SL, Garcia BM, Ashland MA, Calaman S, Kuzma NC, O'Toole JK, Patel A, Rosenbluth G, Destino LA, Everhart JL, Good BP, Hepps JH, Dalal AK, Lipsitz SR, Yoon CS, Zigmont KR, Srivastava R, Starmer AJ, Sectish TC, Spector ND, West DC, Landrigan CP, Allair BK, Alminde C, Alvarado-Little W, Atsatt M, Aylor ME, Bale JF Jr, Balmer D, Barton KT, Beck C, Bismilla Z, Blankenburg RL, Chandler D, Choudhary A, Christensen E, Coghlan-McDonald S, Cole FS, Corless E, Cray S, Da Silva R, Dahale D, Dreyer B, Growdon AS, Gubler L, Guiot A, Harris R, Haskell H, Kocolas I, Kruvand E, Lane MM, Langrish K, Ledford CJW, Lewis K, Lopreiato JO, Maloney CG, Mangan A, Markle P, Mendoza F, Micalizzi DA, Mittal V, Obermeyer M, O'Donnell KA, Ottolini M, Patel SJ, Pickler R, Rogers JE, Sanders LM, Sauder K, Shah SS, Sharma M, Simpkin A, Subramony A, Thompson ED Jr, Trueman L, Trujillo T, Turmelle MP, Warnick C, Welch C, White AJ, Wien MF, Winn AS, Wintch S, Wolf M, Yin HS, Yu CE. Families as partners in hospital error and adverse event surveillance. JAMA Pediatr. 2017;171(4):372–81.
37. Khan A, Spector ND, Baird JD, Ashland M, Starmer AJ, Rosenbluth G, Garcia BM, Litterer KP, Rogers JE, Dalal AK, Lipsitz S, Yoon CS, Zigmont KR, Guiot A, O'Toole JK, Patel A, Bismilla Z, Coffey M, Langrish K, Blankenburg RL, Destino LA, Everhart JL, Good BP, Kocolas I, Srivastava R, Calaman S, Cray S, Kuzma N, Lewis K, Thompson ED, Hepps JH, Lopreiato JO, Yu CE, Haskell H, Kruvand E, Micalizzi DA, Alvarado-Little W, Dreyer BP, Yin HS, Subramony A, Patel SJ, Sectish TC, West DC, Landrigan CP. Patient safety after implementation of a coproduced family centered communication programme: multicenter before and after intervention study. BMJ. 2018;363:k4764.
38. Kim S, Bochatay N, Relyea-Chew A, Buttrick E, Amdahl C, Kim L, Frans E, Mossanen M, Khandekar A, Fehr R. Individual, interpersonal, and organisational factors of healthcare conflict: a scoping review. J Interprof Care. 2017;31(3):282–90.
39. Klein R, Julian KA, Snyder ED, Koch J, Ufere NN, Volerman A, Vandenberg AE, Schaeffer S, Palamara K, From the Gender Equity in Medicine (GEM) Workgroup. Gender bias in resident assessment in graduate medical education: review of the literature. J Gen Intern Med. 2019;34:712–9.
40. Koh NJ, Wagner R, Newton RC, Kuhn CM, Co JPT, Weiss KB, o. b. o. t. C. E. C. a. t. C. Program. CLER national report of findings 2021. Chicago: Accreditation Council for Graduate Medical Education; 2021.
41. Kube DA, Bishop EA, Roth JM, Palmer FB. Evaluation of a parent led curriculum in developmental disabilities for pediatric and medicine/pediatric residents. Matern Child Health J. 2013;17:1304–8.
42. Liaw SY, Ooi SL, Mildon R, Ang ENK, Lau TC, Chua WL. Translation of an evidence-based virtual reality simulation-based interprofessional education into health education curriculums: an implementation science method. Nurse Educ Today. 2022;110:105262.
43. Liaw SY, Tan JZ, Lim S, Zhou W, Yap J, Ratan R, Ooi SL, Wong SJ, Seah B, Chua WL. Artificial intelligence in virtual reality simulation for interprofessional communication training: mixed method study. Nurse Educ Today. 2023;122:105718.
44. Maggio LA, Costello JA, Kolars JC, Cervero RM, Jackson KM, Durning SJ, Ma T. In search of a "metric system" for measuring faculty effort: a qualitative study on educational value units at U.S. medical schools. Acad Med. 2024;99(4):445–51.
45. Miles A, Ginsburg S, Sibbald M, Tavares W, Watling C, Stroud L. Feedback from health professionals in postgraduate medical education: influence of interprofessional relationship, identity and power. Med Educ. 2021;55(4):518–29.
46. National Patient Safety Foundation. RCA2 improving root cause analyses and actions to prevent harm. Boston: National Patient Safety Foundation; 2016.
47. Nicholson L, Ortiz MV, Wang Y, Walsh H, Ottolini MC, Agrawal D. Successful implementation of a novel collaborative Interprofessional educational curriculum for nurses and residents in a pediatric acute care setting. J Interprofessional Educ Pract. 2019;17:100284.
48. O'Brien BC, Patel SR, Pearson M, Eastburn AP, Earnest GE, Strewler A, Gager K, Manuel JK, Dulay M, Bachhuber MR, Shunk R. Twelve tips for delivering successful interprofessional case conferences. Med Teach. 2017;39(12):1214–20.
49. Paradis E, Whitehead CR. Beyond the lamppost: a proposal for a fourth wave of education for collaboration. Acad Med. 2018;93(10):1457–63.
50. Qiao J, Xu J, Li L, Ouyang Y-Q. The integration of immersive virtual reality simulation in interprofes-

sional education: a scoping review. Nurse Educ Today. 2021;98:104773.
51. Regan L, Jung J, Kelen GD. Educational value units: a mission-based approach to assigning and monitoring faculty teaching activities in an academic medical department. Acad Med. 2016;91(12):1642–6.
52. Robertson K, Ju M, O'Brien BC, van Schaik SM, Bochatay N. Exploring the role of power during debriefing of interprofessional simulations. J Interprof Care. 2022:1–9.
53. Rosenbluth G, Choi LW, Boscardin CK, Gonzales R, Green A, Hernandez A, Vidyarthi AR, Julian KA, Baron RB. Engaging GME learners in health system-aligned improvement work in the clinical learning environment. Am J Med Qual. 2024;39(1):33–41.
54. Savitz ST, Frederick RK, Sangaralingham LR, Lampman MA, Anderson SS, Habermann EB, Bell SJ. Evaluation of safety and care outcomes after the introduction of a virtual registered nurse model. Health Serv Res. 2023;58(5):999–1013.
55. Silva JAM, Mininel VA, Agreli HF, Peduzzi M, Harrison R, Xyrichis A. Collective leadership to improve professional practice, healthcare outcomes and staff well-being. Cochrane Database Syst Rev. 2022;10:CD013850.
56. Smeets HWH, Sluijsmans DMA, Moser A, van Merriënboer JJG. Design guidelines for assessing students' interprofessional competencies in healthcare education: a consensus study. Perspect Med Educ. 2022;11(6):316–24.
57. van Schaik SM, O'Brien BC, Almeida SA, Adler SR. Perceptions of interprofessional teamwork in low-acuity settings: a qualitative analysis. Med Educ. 2014;48(6):583–92.
58. van Schaik SM, Plant J, Diane S, Tsang L, O'Sullivan P. Interprofessional team training in pediatric resuscitation: a low-cost, in situ simulation program that enhances self-efficacy among participants. Clin Pediatr. 2011;50(9):807–15.
59. Varpio L, Bidlake E, Casimiro L, Hall P, Kuziemsky C, Brajtman S, Humphrey-Murto S. Resident experiences of informal education: how often, from whom, about what and how. Med Educ. 2014;48(12):1220–34.
60. Vesel TP, O'Brien BC, Henry DM, van Schaik SM. Useful but different: resident physician perceptions of interprofessional feedback. Teach Learn Med. 2016;28(2):125–34.
61. Walsh HA, Jolly Inouye AA, Goldman EF. Improving communication through resident-nurse shadowing. Hosp Pediatr. 2017;7(11):660–7.
62. Wilson A, Hurwitz CA, Smith M, Patino T, Kudalmana AS, Gallas M. Parents as teachers: teaching pediatrics residents the art of engaging in difficult conversations. J Grad Med Educ. 2019;11(1):60–5.
63. Wooding EL, Gale T, Maynard V. Evaluation of teamwork assessment tools for interprofessional simulation: a systematic literature review. J Interprof Care. 2020;34(2):162–72.
64. Zambrotta ME, Aylward P, Roy CL, Piper-Vallillo E, Pelletier SR, Honan JP, Heller N, Ramani S, Shields HM. Nurse-doctor co-teaching: a pilot study of the design, development, and implementation of structured interprofessional co-teaching sessions. Adv Med Educ Pract. 2021;12:339–48.
65. Ziemba JB, Berns JS, Huzinec JG, Bammer D, Salva C, Valentine E, Myers JS. The RCA ReCAst: a root cause analysis simulation for the interprofessional clinical learning environment. Acad Med. 2021;96(7):997–1001.

Advocacy 17

Michelle M. Barnes and Ana C. Monterrey

Introduction: Pediatricians as Advocates

Advocacy is at the heart of what it means to be a pediatrician—for young children, because they are not able to communicate their needs, and for older children, because they are not able to participate in the systems that create policy in their communities. That leaves those who care for children, including health care providers, to advocate for their needs and interests, particularly in those areas that most impact child health.

Pediatricians have often been called natural advocates. The field of Pediatrics focuses on health, prevention, and the overall well-being of *all* children. Pediatricians frequently work not only with children, but with the families and communities that support them. They advocate for the needs of the most vulnerable to reduce health disparities and promote health equity. Dr. Abraham Jacobi, the father of American Pediatrics, envisioned physicians as advocates outside the walls of hospitals and clinics.

> *It is not enough, however, to work at the individual bedside in the hospital. In the near or dim future, the pediatrician is to sit in and control school boards, health departments, and legislatures. He is a legitimate advisor to the judge and jury, and a seat for the physician in the councils of the republic is what the people have a right to demand.* [1]

As Dr. Jacobi once imagined, today's pediatricians work with schools, community organizations, governmental agencies, and lawmakers to improve the health of whole populations of children. Pediatricians have a long history of advocating for the highest level of health for their patients and the communities they serve. Physicians like Dr. Jacobi recognized the harm of raw milk for babies, and he himself was a strong advocate for breastfeeding and public health measures like boiling milk before these practices were widespread [1]. Long before the first laws on child restraints were passed in the USA in the late 1970s, pediatricians advocated for child automobile safety seats, citing higher rates of morbidity and mortality for children as passengers [2]. When Congress threatened cuts to Medicaid and caps on spending in 2017, pediatricians mobilized to action with the #KeepKidsCovered campaign, sharing stories about the importance of access to health care for children and gathering the attention of major media outlets and elected officials [3].

In fact, child health societies like the American Academy of Pediatrics (AAP) were founded out of a need to advocate for and advance the health of pediatric populations [1]. Many child health societies today continue to include advocacy

M. M. Barnes (✉)
University of Illinois College of Medicine at Chicago, Chicago, IL, USA
e-mail: mbarnes@UIC.EDU

A. C. Monterrey
Baylor College of Medicine, Houston, TX, USA

H. McPhillips et al. (eds.), *Graduate Medical Education in Pediatrics*, Excellence in Medical Education 3, https://doi.org/10.1007/978-3-032-12952-9_17

work as one of their major missions. The AAP, American Pediatric Society (APS), and Academic Pediatrics Association (APA) provide their members with resources and support to participate in advocacy work as part of their careers. Groups like the Pediatric Policy Council, a collaboration between various child health societies, have also been working on legislative advocacy efforts for decades to shape policies impacting the health and well-being of children.

Advocacy training, therefore, has an important role in medical training. Many physicians are drawn to medicine with the goal of helping others, and resident trainees may feel a social responsibility and desire to effect change not only for their individual patients but also on a larger scale. The Accreditation Council for Graduate Medical Education (ACGME) training guidelines require pediatric residency programs to teach residents how to advocate for individual patients within the health care system. They expect residents to learn how to provide patient-centered, compassionate, and equitable care while "incorporating consideration of the impacts of social determinants of health and advocating for social justice." The ACGME also expects residents to learn to advocate for the "promotion of health and the prevention of disease and injury" at the population level [4].

Furthermore, the American Board of Pediatrics (ABP) provides guidance to residency programs on competencies that all general pediatricians should demonstrate by the conclusion of their training. The ABP outlines various entrustable professional activities (EPAs) or "everyday pediatrician activities" that a pediatrician should be able to perform to meet the needs of their patients. Core EPAs for general pediatricians include using strategies that promote health and address underlying causes of inequities among pediatric populations (EPA 11). They recommend pediatricians *advocate* for policies and funding in upstream interventions that optimize health outcomes in all patient populations, including children with medical complexity (EPA 2) [5]. Physician advocacy has also been cited as a tool to help combat burnout, which is a growing concern among the physician workforce. Teaching residents how to affect positive changes in the populations they serve can increase feelings of personal accomplishment and career satisfaction [6] and ensure a future workforce of physicians dedicated to caring for children. Advocacy work is truly at the foundation of pediatrics, and residency programs need to implement educational activities that equip trainees with the knowledge and skills to carry out various forms of advocacy in their future careers.

Education: Curriculum, Learner Assessment, and Program Evaluation

"Pediatricians are advocates for children." In its updated Program Requirements for Pediatrics, which went into effect July 1, 2025, the ACGME introduces the specialty of Pediatrics, affirming that advocacy is central to the work of a pediatrician [4]. This makes advocacy a critical part of the curriculum for pediatric residency training, similar to adolescent medicine or pediatric critical care. Just as with most aspects of residency education, there is not a single formula for teaching advocacy that will work for all programs, faculty, or residents. So, where does a program director begin to determine how best to teach advocacy in their curriculum?

In describing the pediatric curriculum in general, the ACGME expects programs to "design and conduct the program in a fashion consistent with the needs of the community." The ACGME describes this further: "Programs must understand the structural and social determinants of health of the population they serve and incorporate them in the design and implementation of the program curriculum, with the ultimate goal of addressing those needs and eliminating health disparities" [4]. Inherent in the goal of addressing the needs of a population and eliminating health disparities is advocacy, reiterating advocacy as the backbone of pediatric training. The ACGME goes on to describe social determinants of health and the importance of pediatricians advocating for social justice. By describing advocacy as part of the overall expectations for residency training, the ACGME leaves programs to determine where and how to incorporate advocacy into their curriculum. This provides program directors with the opportunity to consider the strengths and needs of their program and determine where advocacy fits best. Although it allows flexibility, the ACGME requires the overall pediatric curriculum to include "a minimum of 40 weeks of primarily ambulatory experiences, including elements of community pediatrics and child advocacy," requiring that advocacy is incorporated into the ambulatory general pediatrics curriculum, though innovative programs might also include advocacy elsewhere in their program's curriculum.

Within the competency of Medical Knowledge, the ACGME expects pediatric residents to demonstrate knowledge of health care inequities experienced by patients and communities [4]. Further, in the domain of Systems-Based Practice, the ACGME expects pediatric residents to advocate "for the promotion of health and the prevention of disease and injury in populations," to "advocate for patients within the health care system to achieve the patient's and patients' families care goals," and to "collaborate with community organizations, including schools and/or leaders in health care systems, in order to improve health care and well-being of patients" [4]. Finally, in describing the scholarship required of pediatric residents, the ACGME includes health equity as a potential area of scholarship. The ACGME makes clear its expectation that pediatricians learn to be advocates throughout the educational curriculum, though experts agree this should include, but not be limited to, a discrete educational experience [7–9].

Where does this leave programs? Program directors should work with their educational leads to determine where advocacy naturally fits within their curriculum. The next step, then, is to figure out how to teach advocacy. While the ACGME provides the expectation that residents learn to be advocates, they leave programs to determine what the curriculum includes in terms of content and the teaching methods used. Through the Community Pediatrics Training Initiative (CPTI), AAP leaders have developed multiple tools to guide program directors in designing their advocacy curriculum. Most recently, they have developed COCHAT (Core Objectives for Community Health and Advocacy Training), a tool that includes a comprehensive set of goals and objectives for pediatric advocacy training and guides programs in mapping those goals and objectives to their existing curriculum [10]. Programs can use this mapping tool to identify gaps within their curriculum, as well as opportunities for incorporating advocacy through educational activities already in place.

Though the ACGME expects programs to determine where best to incorporate advocacy throughout the curriculum, it is clear that it must be included in the ambulatory general pediatrics curriculum, at least in part [10]. Leaders at CPTI recently revised COCHAT to focus on those goals and objectives best taught in a dedicated advocacy experience. In addition to including a more focused set of goals and objectives, the new Community Pediatrics and Advocacy Curriculum (CPAC) includes suggested educational activities to help trainees acquire the skills needed to become strong advocates [11].

What types of educational activities might a program consider including in its advocacy curriculum? Unlike many other aspects of medical training that focus on the acquisition of medical knowledge, advocacy also requires trainees to develop the skills and behaviors necessary to succeed. Skill development in this domain will require trainees to step out of the clinical setting and into their communities. Some programs include advocacy projects within their curriculum, and this facilitates active learning for residents as they identify a community need, collaborate with partners to develop a project, and conduct the project. CPTI's Project Planning Tool can be used to help faculty mentors guide residents through each step of the process, reinforcing critical skills throughout the project [12].

Advocacy curricula may also require that trainees engage in reflection or small group discussion about their experiences. Many advocacy curricula include visits with community-based organizations for residents to understand the resources available to patients in their community.

However, reflection is a critical aspect of these experiences as residents develop their skills in collaboration with community partners. Supervising faculty can facilitate reflection and discussion—and in doing so assist in skill acquisition and engage in learner assessment. Leaders in the Education Subcommittee of the Academic Pediatrics Association (APA) Task Force on Child Poverty developed five modules to teach residents about key areas in advocacy [13]. The modules include the Epidemiology of Child Poverty, Social Determinants of Health, the Biomedical Influences of Poverty, Taking Action to Address Child Poverty, and Medicaid. The modules include content for learners using readings, videos, and gamification, as well as facilitator guides to support faculty mentors as they engage their residents in reflection and discussion. More recently, advocacy educators have expanded on the APA Child Poverty modules to develop the TEACH (Trainee Education in Advocacy and Community Health) curriculum [14]. Through this curriculum, residents participate in self-guided and community-facing activities to enhance their knowledge, skills, and behaviors in advocacy. These are only some examples of the many curricular resources available to programs as they consider what activities best meet the needs of their residents and their patient population. Program directors might find additional resources or connect with other advocacy educators through organizations like the Association of Pediatric Program Directors (APPD) and their Community Health and Advocacy Training Learning Community and the APA's Advocacy Training Special Interest Group.

Learner assessment is a critical component of any educational curriculum. The nature of advocacy training, falling largely within the domain of Systems-Based Practice, allows programs the opportunity to develop innovative approaches to learner assessment. Some programs assess skill acquisition through educational products such as advocacy projects, advocacy-related presentations, or written reflections. Through materials such as COCHAT, programs can map their curriculum to identify where they will provide educational activities to meet a given objective and then consider how they will assess a trainee's competence in a given objective. The ACGME's Pediatric Milestones and the American Board of Pediatrics (ABP)'s Entrustable Professional Activities (EPA) for Pediatrics include language related to advocacy. Program leaders can incorporate elements of both the EPA's and the Milestones into assessment tools for advocacy activities, using language already familiar to faculty and residents. Assessment is an area of growth for advocacy curricula, with some programs starting to integrate simulation into advocacy activities and assessment, and others gathering multisource assessments of learners from interprofessional colleagues within their institution (i.e., social workers, community health workers) or outside of their institution (i.e., community partners at Head Start or WIC).

As program directors develop their advocacy curriculum, they should engage in program evaluation of the curriculum at least annually. Programs can use the COCHAT mapping tool to conduct an analysis of strengths and areas for improvement and compare that to the prior year. Program directors can review evaluations of the curriculum completed by residents, faculty, and external partners. Using their gap analysis and input collected from key stakeholders, programs can develop curricular goals for the upcoming year and implement changes needed in curricular activities, community partners, faculty supervisors, or other areas to meet those goals.

In addition to the APA's Advocacy Training SIG and the APPD's Community Health and Advocacy Training Learning Community, other resources exist to help programs build their advocacy curriculum. CPTI offers grants such as the Leonard P. Rome CATCH Visiting Professorship to support programs in expanding their advocacy curricula. Through the Rome Visiting Professorship, programs apply to host a visiting professor with expertise in some aspect of advocacy for 2–3 days at their institution. For many programs, Rome Visiting Professorships have served to springboard their curricula to more effectively meet the needs of their residents and the communities they serve.

Pediatric advocacy education leaders may also find support and guidance within their own community. Several states, including California, Texas, New Jersey, North and South Carolina, New York, Missouri, and Illinois, have developed collaboratives of pediatric advocacy educators within their state or region [15, 16]. This has helped to foster community among educators as their advocacy curricula evolve to meet the changing needs of their residents and their patients. The New Jersey Pediatric Residency Advocacy Collaborative (NJPRAC) was particularly active during the COVID-19 pandemic. At the onset of the pandemic, they worked together to transition their curricula to a virtual platform. Further, they developed a process to meet the needs of their community partners and the families they serve as they evolved during the pandemic. They were able to enhance components of each program's advocacy curriculum by sharing educational activities and innovations. They also shared resources such as time and faculty support, and in doing so, they met the needs of more residents. Most importantly, they supported more community members through their collaboration. Not only did this provide each program director in the NJPRAC with strategies to expand their curricula, but their residents were able to see the direct impact of advocacy within their communities.

The ACGME's expectations for pediatric residency training have evolved and expanded considerably over the last two decades. For many program directors, this means that advocacy may not have been part of their own pediatric education, leaving them feeling unsure of how to develop an advocacy curriculum. Through networks available through member organizations such as the AAP, APA, and APPD, resources available through CPTI and APA, and partnerships with local pediatric advocacy leaders, program directors can develop the tools needed to develop pediatric residents into the advocates that their patients and communities need.

Socio-Ecological Framework

Advocacy comes in many forms, and we can use a socio-ecological framework to consider the various roles pediatricians play in advocacy for child health. Through this framework, modeled after UNICEF's Social Ecological Model [17], among similar models, we consider the four levels that impact child health, the role of the pediatrician in advocating for health promotion at each level, and how programs might incorporate each level of advocacy into their curriculum (Fig. 17.1) [11].

Individual Level

During their residency training, pediatricians spend much of their time learning how to care for children, in both the inpatient and outpatient

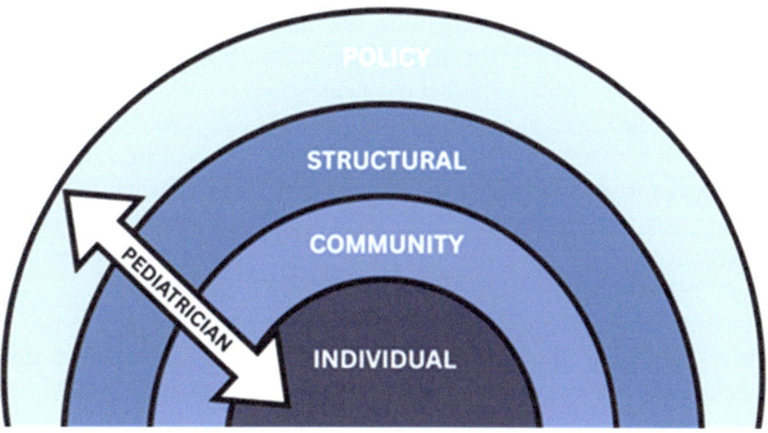

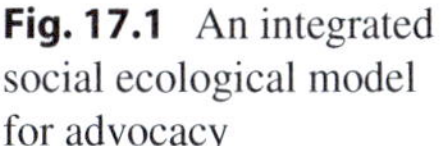
Fig. 17.1 An integrated social ecological model for advocacy

settings, and in primary and subspecialty care. They learn about the many disorders that a child can experience, and how to diagnose and treat them. Through this education, fundamental to the field of pediatrics, residents identify opportunities to advocate for their patients. This might include realizing their patient with poorly controlled asthma lives in a home with significant mold and helping the family to communicate the risk to the child's health to their landlord. This might also include recognizing that their patient's family is experiencing housing insecurity and connecting them to resources for temporary safe housing. While learning how to diagnose and treat children, pediatricians identify factors around the child that impact their health. In recognizing the factors that put their patient at risk for poor health outcomes and supporting the patient and their family to address those factors, pediatricians participate in advocacy at the *Individual* level [18]. This type of advocacy is inherent to the work of pediatricians in disease prevention and health promotion.

Community Level

Just as children exist within communities, so do pediatricians. Seeing patients regularly in their offices or in their hospital, pediatricians are on the frontlines in noticing trends among their patients. In her book, *What the Eyes Don't See*, Dr. Mona Hanna-Attisha, a pediatrician in Flint, Michigan, describes noticing that many of her patients' screening lead levels were returning with high values [19, 20]. This recognition made her ask important questions in her community to understand the factors at play. Dr. Hanna-Attisha worked with community leaders to understand the scope of the problem and to develop solutions to address the issues impacting child health in her community.

As pediatricians, we are scientists, and we learn through our medical training to recognize patterns and to question when what we are seeing does not align with what we had previously thought to be true. Children's health is impacted by their genetics and their family system, but it is also significantly impacted by the conditions in which they live, learn, work, and play, or the social drivers of health. When pediatricians identify patterns in their practices, they may turn to the community to understand if something has changed that has impacted their patients' health, just as Dr. Hanna-Attisha did. Although they may be on the frontlines in recognizing factors that affect child health in their communities, pediatricians are not alone in their goal of supporting children within their communities. They can work with community organizations to better understand the issues and to advocate for solutions to improve the health of children within their communities, thereby advocating at the *Community* level. Fundamental to community-level advocacy is working *with* community partners, recognizing the significant knowledge and expertise they have of the community served.

Structural Level

Child health is greatly influenced by the social drivers of health, which the Centers for Disease Control (CDC) define as economic stability, education access and quality, health care access and quality, neighborhood and the built environment, and social and community context [21, 22]. The structures in place within a community, often guided by local policy, determine how public systems function within the community. For example, public education systems vary significantly from one community to another, in terms of procedures, resources, and curricula, as they reflect the values of a community. Children spend much of their time in school and are thus impacted by the structure of public education within their community. During the COVID-19 pandemic, many pediatricians worked with their local public education systems to develop policies to keep children safe, such as those around return-to-school, masking, isolation, and immunization. Similarly, pediatric allergists may work with public school systems to develop policies and procedures around keeping children with food allergies safe in school, such as through decisions around where emergency epinephrine auto-injectors are stored throughout the school day and who is trained to use them. When they advocate for system-level change that promotes child health, pediatricians engage in advocacy at the *Structural* level.

Policy Level

In the United States, many decisions that impact child health are made at the legislative level—local, state, and federal. As experts in child health, it is critical that pediatricians serve as a resource to legislators as they develop policies that impact the health and well-being of children and families. Because they do not vote, children depend on the adults around them to create and support policies that promote child health. Some pediatricians influence policy by running for local, state, or federal office. However, there are many other ways to advocate for child health legislatively. Through organizations such as the American Academy of Pediatrics (AAP), which is committed to the optimal physical, mental, and social health and well-being for all infants, children, adolescents, and young adults, pediatricians can keep abreast of legislative issues related to child health [23]. They can contact their legislators to advocate for issues such as Medicaid reform or child passenger safety seat laws. Without the input of pediatricians as experts in child health, engaging in legislative advocacy at the *Policy* level, lawmakers may miss opportunities to develop policies that promote child health.

Advocacy at each level—individual, community, structural, and—is inherent to the work of pediatricians. However, not all pediatricians, or all pediatric educators, have experience with advocacy at each level. Extensive resources are available to help pediatric educators develop curricula around advocacy and to help residents enhance their skills in advocacy [12, 14, 15, 24].

Advocacy at the Individual Level

Advocacy for individual children is inherent to the work pediatricians do on a daily basis to promote health and prevent disease and injury. In providing direct care to children and families, they are witnesses to the many social determinants or social drivers of health that impact their patients' lives, such as food insecurity, poor housing conditions, community violence, or lack of health insurance. These social drivers have been found to influence health outcomes even more than direct healthcare or genetic factors [21]. Therefore, it is essential that pediatricians include advocacy in their work to truly improve health outcomes and address the underlying causes of health inequities for patients.

Residency programs should include education on social drivers of health in their advocacy curricula to help pediatricians better understand children within the context of their environments and recognize the root causes of the health disparities they observe. Learning about social drivers allows residents to identify potential ways to advocate for change when partnering with caregivers, schools, or childcare centers and the communities that support children. Addressing the individual social needs of patients is also an important way for residents to advocate at the individual level for the needs of their patients and fulfills competencies related to systems-based practice.

Screening for Social Drivers of Health

Screening for social drivers is already part of the routine well-child care training residents receive. Preventative care includes asking about mental and emotional health needs, access to nutritional foods, and environmental risks and exposures at home or in the child's surroundings [25]. However, pediatricians can screen more broadly for social drivers of health using comprehensive screening questionnaires [26]. These can provide pediatricians with more opportunities to connect families to resources with the goal of helping to improve health outcomes.

Teaching residents *how* to screen for social drivers of health is also an essential element of the curriculum. Pediatricians need to conduct screening and address social drivers in a sensitive manner with consideration for reducing stigma, avoiding stereotypes and bias, and respecting family autonomy. When done *inappropriately*, screening has the potential to cause further harm and can negatively impact the doctor-patient relationship [27]. Universal screening can help mitigate some of the potential bias or stigma patients perceive but requires knowledge about the patient population served to avoid further increasing inequities [28]. Therefore, the approach to screening is a vital component of teaching about social drivers of health. It should include education on framing screening questions to help normalize needs. For example, as many as 1 in 5 children nationally experience food insecurity [29], and hunger can influence not only health and growth, but also school performance. Introducing the Hunger Vital Sign [30] screening with this frame of reference can help caregivers understand the relevance of screening and how common food insecurity is. Next, discussing these issues without judgment and with transparency about resources available can help families feel more comfortable disclosing what is often sensitive information. Lastly, screening must always be done with careful consideration for personal implicit or explicit biases, and residents should be taught to avoid targeted screening that relies on assumptions about needs based on a family's race/ethnicity, education, or other demographic or physical apparent characteristics.

Screening Special Populations

Health disparities are common in certain populations of children, as they are more likely to have various health issues due to their social circumstances. Residency training curricula should therefore also include teaching about the needs of vulnerable populations of children. Children and families experiencing homelessness, children in foster care, children who are immigrants or refugees, and children with chronic health care needs or medical complexity are special groups to consider screening more specifically based on their risks or needs. For example, understanding the unique needs of vulnerable children allows residents to recognize the value of trauma screening for those in foster care or who are immigrants/refugees.

Addressing Social Drivers of Health

When addressing identified social drivers, pediatricians should use a strengths-based approach [26]. This involves recognizing assets within the family and their community structures, which can help mitigate adverse social circumstances. Teaching residents to consider protective factors like family attachment, social support networks, or spiritual and cultural communities can help them support families as they overcome obstacles to health. Additionally, respecting families' autonomy is essential to building trust and preserving a strong doctor-patient relationship. Residents must begin to reflect on the complexity of addressing social drivers and recognize that families have competing priorities in their lives. Allowing families to choose not to disclose social needs or decline referrals to resources is also valid and respects a family's right to make their own decisions.

Directly advocating for individual patients also includes teaching residents how to connect families to resources and benefits in the community. Providing knowledge about the services provided by local agencies and allowing trainees to become comfortable coordinating with community organizations on behalf of their patients is important. This can include helping families navigate their local school system by having a phone call with the school nurse about administration of prescription medications, writing a letter to assist families with necessary accommodations for their specific health needs, or helping families request learning evaluations for children struggling academically. Residents can also learn about the value of medical-legal partnerships, which help advocate for legal rights that impact health [31]—e.g., addressing poor housing conditions exacerbating asthma or preventing utility shut-offs that put the health of their patients with medical equipment at risk.

Lastly, residents should learn to advocate within the health systems where they work for the needs of individual patients. This may require them to contact health insurance providers to demonstrate or justify the need for services or benefits, medications, or therapies to be covered. This can also include coordinating care with other providers, multidisciplinary teams, or subspecialists in the inpatient, outpatient, or emergency settings.

Training residents to identify and address the social drivers of health impacting children's lives is at the root of advocacy at the individual level. Pediatricians should develop skills to screen for social needs effectively and compassionately and become comfortable referring to community organizations and collaborating with others to help address patient needs.

Advocacy at the Community Level

When a pediatrician realizes that more than one child might be experiencing or be at risk for an adverse outcome related to the factors within their community, such as access to child care, gun violence, access to immunizations, or safe places to play, they might consider community-level advocacy. Just as residents learn to work in interprofessional and multidisciplinary teams in the clinical setting, it is essential for them to develop the skills of community partnership.

Who might serve as a community partner? This depends on the child's health issue for which a pediatrician plans to advocate. Issues concerning schools in the community might lead pediatricians to partner with the local school board or school nurses. For questions related to immunization campaigns, pediatricians might contact the local public health department. Pediatric residents should learn to review the literature to identify examples of similar community-level efforts in other communities. This step is critical to learn what worked, and most importantly, what did not, and can help pediatricians understand what agencies and organizations they might seek out as potential partners. Identifying community partners is essential for several reasons: to develop a thorough understanding of the issues in the community, including their historical context; to understand the expertise that already exists within the community; and to engender trust within the community. At every step within community-level advocacy, pediatricians must ask themselves and their partners, "Who else should be at the table?" This ensures all voices are heard and all perspectives considered once the team has developed.

Fundamental to the pediatrician's role in community advocacy are partnership and collaboration. Inherent in partnership is the ability to ask questions, and more importantly, to listen. While pediatricians might be the experts on the team about children's physical health, and their voices are highly respected in many communities, they alone cannot understand all facets of an issue. Asking each partner, "Help me to understand the issue from your perspective," serves two purposes: to gain information from each partner and to demonstrate one's willingness to work together to develop solutions that work best for the whole community. Once again, a review of the literature can be helpful to enhance the pediatrician's understanding of the issue, an important part of knowing what questions to ask. When working with partners, individuals, or organizations, pediatricians should not assume that everyone shares their perspective on a particular issue. Potential partners might not agree that an issue is important, and even if they do, some partners may not have the capacity for collaborative efforts when approached. Differences of opinion are okay and will likely make the team stronger. If partners agree on the issue but are unable to commit the time to collaboration, pediatricians should ask if they can contact the partner later in the project to seek their input. With collaboration comes respect—for each other's opinions, experience, availability, and expertise in a given area. Partners who respect one another, particularly their differences, are more likely to demonstrate successful collaboration. Recognizing the importance of collaborative community partnerships, multiple resources have been developed to guide pediatricians and pediatric residents in building successful community partnerships [32–34].

Once the team has been established and everyone has a shared understanding of the issue, the next step is to conduct a needs assessment of the community related to the issue. Has this issue come up before? What efforts have been made to address it, and which of these have been successful? What barriers were identified? Is the time right to tackle this issue? These questions are essential to *understanding* the community and *working with* the community, not providing the pediatrician's expertise to the community.

Thus far, we have assumed that pediatricians have an issue in mind when planning to engage in community-level advocacy, as this is typically the case for practicing pediatricians. Designing and conducting a community-level advocacy project during training will enhance residents' knowledge, skills, and behaviors in community collaboration, while also increasing the confidence many pediatricians need to engage in this work as attendings. Some studies have shown that residents' attitudes toward community-level advocacy were positively influenced by conducting a community-advocacy project during their training [7, 8]. However, for some residents, it can be difficult to identify a topic for their community advocacy project. Asking them to reflect on the patients they have cared for in the last month—e.g., in continuity clinic, in the emergency department, or on their cardiology elective—might prime them to identify a topic. Other residents might draw on something from their own lives or something in the press that might affect their patients. Multiple resources exist to help advocacy educators, program directors, or residents themselves to narrow their focus and identify a meaningful project, such as the AAP Community Pediatrics Training Initiative Project Planning Tool [12] and the UCSF Center for Community Engagement Community Engagement Toolkit [35]. Residents might work together on projects, allowing them to learn from one another as they conduct their project, and they might use their advocacy project to meet their requirement for a scholarship during residency.

Once the team is assembled, the issue is clear, and the community's needs have been identified, the team should work together to develop a plan for their advocacy efforts. What is the goal of the advocacy effort, and what are the objectives for the project? Developing specific objectives at each stage of the project will help the team outline the steps needed to achieve the objectives. Determine who will serve in what role, what the time frame is, and how success will be measured. The team should plan to evaluate their progress at each step of the project to allow them to adjust their efforts as needed in an iterative manner. Part of this evaluation should include assessing how well the community's voice is represented. Having a shared understanding of the roadmap for the project, including the plan for evaluation, at the outset will help to maintain trust and cohesion among team members.

As medical professionals, pediatricians are trained to do, to act. When engaging in community-level advocacy, pediatricians must temper this instinct and spend a significant amount of time engaging, planning, preparing, and mobilizing their team. This includes having realistic expectations for how they define success and how long it might take to achieve. The importance of patience cannot be overstated. Similarly, the importance of celebrating success, including small wins, throughout the process is essential to maintain the team's momentum. All team members—individuals and organizations—should be recognized for their participation, no matter how small their role. This is a critical component to collaboration and helps to build long-lasting relationships with the potential for significantly impacting change within their communities.

Most practicing pediatricians and pediatric residents spend most of their professional time seeing patients, so how do they find the time and resources for successful collaboration within their communities? The AAP's Community Access to Child Health (CATCH) program [36] provides support for pediatricians to engage with community health partners on projects to advocate for child health-related issues outside of their medical institutions and within their communities. CATCH offers planning and implementation grants for both residents and practicing pediatricians to engage in community based collaborative projects with community partners. In addition to grant funding, CATCH provides resources and mentorship for grantees as they develop and conduct their projects. Residents who participate in CATCH grants during their training are more likely to engage in community-based advocacy as practicing pediatricians [37].

An important aspect to consider in community-based advocacy is whether the advocacy project will include a research component. This is by no means necessary, and as with all project components, it should be discussed at the outset of the project. In some cases, community partners may have restrictions that preclude them from participating in research. Team members may agree that research will take valuable time away from the project itself. In other cases, research might be an important consideration to demonstrate success to external stakeholders and thereby enhance the impact of the project's results. Community-based participatory research (CBPR) is described by the National Institutes of Health (NIH) as "collaborative interventions that involve scientific researchers and community members to address diseases and conditions disproportionately affecting populations experiencing health disparities… the community is involved in the CBPR program as an equal partner with scientists" [38]. A full review of CBPR is beyond the scope of this book; however, the fundamental component is the collaboration with community stakeholders at each phase of the project, and this is essential to maintaining trust between health care providers and community partners. Within child health, a systematic review showed the importance of CBPR in studying community-based interventions to address child health disparities, and particularly the importance of including children and young adults as stakeholders in the research process [39].

Community-based advocacy involves pediatricians stepping outside the walls of their clinic or hospital system to collaborate with community members to address issues related to child health. Engaging in advocacy and building community partnerships helps many pediatricians to reinvigorate their passion for child health and have a greater impact on the lives of the children and families they serve [22]. Particularly for pediatricians in training, developing these skills early in their careers may help them to maintain joy and meaning within their professional lives.

Advocacy at the Structural Level

Change within Healthcare Systems and Communities

In caring for individual patients and collaborating with communities, pediatricians become aware of common health problems affecting not just one, but many of their patients. Health disparities are health differences linked to social, economic, and/or environmental disadvantage [40]. Pediatric GME requires teaching about the promotion of health and the prevention of disease at the population level through an understanding of the systems in place that perpetuate health disparities [4]. Advocacy at the structural level allows pediatricians to think about health disparities and ways to reduce these differential health outcomes. Advocacy curricula, therefore, should include training on how to understand structures in place and changes that can be made at the structural level to impact large populations of children.

Pediatric residents should also be taught how to effect change within the health care systems and communities where they work. It is important for residents to become familiar with tools and resources to access patient data, review community health metrics, and analyze patterns in health outcomes, to then be able to communicate this to appropriate stakeholders and demonstrate the need for change [12]. Participating in scholarly projects, partnering with community organizations, or quality improvement work can allow residents to practice these skills. For example, residents may lead a quality improvement effort to screen for food insecurity after noting the rising number of children with obesity in their practice or community. Furthermore, they may choose to implement a food prescription program in partnership with the local food pantry or bring the food pantry into the clinic or hospital, recognizing transportation as a barrier driving this disparity. In doing this type of work, residents should also learn about developing outcome measures to demonstrate success and to monitor how interventions are impacting the target population.

Another area of advocacy at the structural level can involve serving the community by participating in advisory committees or as board members for nonprofit organizations. Their expertise on child health can impact the resources and services these organizations provide to the community. Learning about the local organizations working on different child health issues and gaining experience collaborating effectively with these groups can prepare residents for this role.

Lastly, the public school system is another common place for pediatricians to advocate, given the large amount of time children spend in this setting and the number of children impacted by school policies. Residents should learn about the role they can play, serving as consultants to school leadership. For example, pediatricians may be asked to educate school staff, students, and families on certain health issues. Their expertise may also be requested in the development of medical or emergency protocols or to assist school boards in making decisions that impact student health.

Media Advocacy

Media advocacy is also part of making changes at the structural level and involves communicating with the public to educate, spread awareness, and ultimately enact change. Teaching residents how to express their point of view, share their firsthand experiences with patients, and educate on health issues is a powerful way to reach a broad audience. Residency curricula can include teaching on how to write letters to the editor, opinion pieces, blog posts, or journal perspectives articles. Residents should learn the basic elements of advocacy writing, which typically include developing a case for an issue and making a call to action urging the general public or health professionals to make changes that will impact children [41]. Pediatricians are also sometimes asked to participate in media advocacy through television or radio segments to educate and spread awareness to the general public about health issues. Residency programs may include experiential activities like delivering educational talks in schools or community centers or participating in podcasts to help residents develop these skills. Social media is a platform used increasingly by physicians to participate in advocacy and should also be included in the curriculum. As trusted health experts, pediatricians can share accurate health information, dispel myths, and counter misinformation for their patient population and the general public. Teaching trainees how to use social media platforms responsibly, with consideration for patient privacy and respecting the institutions they represent, is essential [42]. Some programs may choose to use institutional social media accounts to have residents practice these skills. Physician societies also have resources for pediatricians who participate in media advocacy, including strategies for amplifying your voice, guidelines for writing opinion pieces (op-eds and letters to editors), and suggested child health topics to cover on social media [34].

Another important element of media advocacy work is collaboration with institutional government relations and public relations offices. Building relationships with both offices can be a great asset for residency programs since these experts can provide additional training to residents participating in media advocacy activities. They can provide guidance and editorial review to craft a strong message that appeals to a broad audience while still respecting patient confidentiality. They can coach pediatricians ahead of television or radio interviews to assist with talking points and provide techniques to enhance communication. They are often connected with faculty and child health experts doing advocacy work on various child health issues and can assist with networking and mentorship for residents. They may even help promote work after it is published to broaden its reach. Lastly, they can assist with defining a pediatrician's role and representation when participating in advocacy. Some child health topics may align with the institution's priorities, and governmental and public relations can provide clearance for sharing the pediatrician's institutional affiliation or may provide guidance on how to share messaging as an individual physician.

By advocating for upstream changes at the structural level, pediatricians have the opportunity to improve the health of entire communities of children and promote health equity. Teaching residents the skills to effectively impact change within healthcare systems and communities, as well as strategies to effectively communicate via media platforms, is an important part of advocacy education.

Advocacy at the Policy Level: Legislative Advocacy

Advocacy at the policy level is another important component of advocacy education. This type of advocacy has the potential to impact child health far beyond the local community. Since children cannot vote or participate in the legislative process, it falls to those who care about them to advocate for changes in public laws, policies, and regulations that affect their health and well-being. Teaching pediatric trainees the value of their voice as child health experts and how they can participate in the legislative process is essential for advocacy training.

Legislative advocacy involves participating in the electoral process and serving as a resource to lawmakers that prioritize child health issues. It can happen at the local, state, or federal level—by interacting with local school board members, meeting with city or state representatives, testifying at the state capitol, or traveling to Washington, DC to meet with members of the US Congress. Learning about the governmental structure at each of these levels can provide a basic understanding of civics and help residents identify methods they can use to be effective advocates. Additionally, teaching residents about the voting process, how laws are enacted, and skills to communicate with policymakers are some of the basic elements of legislative advocacy curricula.

There are various levels of interaction with legislators that can be highlighted for residents. Sending emails or making phone calls to an elected representative's office to share expertise on a certain issue is relatively easy and can collectively impact policy decisions. Social media platforms have also become an avenue for communicating with policymakers. Many elected officials have their own profiles on social media and have staff who monitor discussions, threads, or "hashtags" on current issues. Residents may feel comfortable sharing their expertise in these ways and may find social media an accessible option despite busy schedules with limited time. Other opportunities for communicating with policymakers can be more time-intensive but have the potential for greater impact. As trusted members of the medical community, pediatricians can meet and develop relationships with policymakers. Through ongoing and regular conversations, pediatricians can become valuable sources of accurate health information and inform lawmakers of relevant child health issues that need attention. They can provide advice directly to representatives or have opportunities to provide expert testimony on health issues being addressed by legislative committees.

Pediatricians often play a role in helping shape the policy and laws surrounding many public benefits and governmental programs. Understanding the structure of various programs like Medicaid, CHIP, food access (WIC, SNAP), and developmental and learning programs (early intervention, Head Start) is foundational to this work and should be a part of the residency curriculum. Pediatricians can provide guidance to lawmakers related to eligibility and access to these public benefits or serve in administrative roles to ensure all children, including those most vulnerable, are considered when creating policies and regulations.

Communicating with policymakers can seem intimidating to many residents and even some faculty; therefore, providing opportunities to practice is a valuable experience to include in advocacy curricula. Partnering with national societies and their respective state chapters can provide further training and opportunities to learn from experienced advocates and can help build advocacy networks for both trainees and faculty. These societies often develop legislative or policy priorities to guide pediatricians on current child health issues. They can provide talking points, template forms or letters to send to elected officials, guidance on testifying, and allow for networking with others who are passionate about similar issues. Many have resident and student advocacy days with programming focused on trainees and opportunities to meet and interact with elected officials under the guidance of experienced faculty or child health advocates. Local or regional nongovernmental organizations or advocacy groups focusing on specific child health topics can also be valuable partners. They can help inform residents on various issues, provide resources for communicating with representatives, and offer opportunities for group advocacy.

Lastly, it is essential to teach trainees how to participate in legislative advocacy while still following the rules and regulations of their employers. Residents should understand their role as part of an academic institution or health care system and receive guidance on participating in advocacy activities as individual citizens, without referencing affiliations to their member institutions unless they have received prior clearance. Active communication with the Governmental Relations Office can provide further guidance and ensure trainees follow any rules in place by their institutions or health care systems. The governmental relations and public relations teams are also valuable resources for training and support. They may have opportunities to participate in advocacy activities sanctioned by the institution on health issues that align with the institution's goals and priorities. They may also be able to provide talking points and coaching on certain child health issues.

Advocacy at the policy level is an important way for pediatricians to improve health outcomes for large populations of children. Teaching residents the power of their voice as child health experts empowers them to advocate for system changes and work toward reducing health inequities and promoting social justice.

Scholarship for Advocacy Educators

In the Pediatric Program Requirements that went into effect July 1, 2025, the ACGME's Pediatric Residency Review Committee states, "Pediatricians are advocates for children. They have a strong presence within communities, where they promote health and health equity in ways that build public trust in the profession" [4]. It is clear that the ACGME views advocacy as fundamental to the training of pediatric residents. Similarly, the American Board of Pediatrics (ABP), in its Entrustable Professional Activities (EPAs) required of all general pediatricians, states that all pediatricians are expected to be "advocating for the needs of individual patients and/or populations" [5]. Advocacy to improve child health outcomes is at the root of the discipline of pediatrics.

Given the expectation that pediatric residents are trained in advocacy and pediatricians participate in advocacy through their professional work, it is essential that pediatricians in academic institutions engage in advocacy. As academics, they are best positioned to study the impact of advocacy efforts on child health. Further, they are instrumental in developing and leading pediatric advocacy education efforts within graduate medical education (GME) at their institutions. For some pediatricians, advocacy is the basis for their academic scholarship, and it is a required component of pediatric residency training. Traditional academic systems, in which faculty promotion is dependent primarily on research products, do not provide space for academic pediatricians to document their advocacy-related efforts. In 2018, in response to the evolving requirements around advocacy in pediatric GME, pediatric advocacy leaders proposed the use of an Advocacy Portfolio

(AP) for advocacy educators to document their scholarship in advocacy [43].

Pediatric advocacy leaders responded to this proposal and worked with the AAP's Community Pediatrics Training Initiative (CPTI) to develop the Advocacy Portfolio (AP), modeled after the Educator Portfolio, increasingly used at academic institutions for faculty in medical education to document their scholarship through the promotion process. The AAP CPTI AP, developed in 2022, provides a model for academic pediatricians in advocacy to document their work in teaching advocacy, for scholarship around the impact of advocacy work, and for providing service to the community through their advocacy efforts in eight domains: the primary area(s) of concentration, the personal statement, advocacy engagement/knowledge dissemination, community engagement/outreach, advocacy teaching and mentoring, advocacy leadership and administration, products of advocacy scholarship, and advanced training in advocacy skills. Further, the authors call upon pediatric department leaders to identify leadership roles for those working in advocacy, such as vice chairs, and support professional development for junior faculty interested in pursuing scholarship in advocacy. These changes are important to recognize pediatric advocacy leaders within traditional academic medical hierarchies [44].

Within medical education, poster, oral, or workshop presentations at academic conferences are an important method to disseminate scholarly work. Advocacy-related medical education is no different. As directors of pediatric community health and advocacy develop new curricula, pediatric academic medical conferences such as those through the APA, the APPD, and the Council on Medical Student Education in Pediatrics (for undergraduate pediatric medical education) are an important venue for sharing these curricula. As with all curriculum development, evaluation is a key component of the process. If advocacy leaders study the impact of their curriculum as part of this evaluation (such as through outcomes related to pediatric residents), additional opportunities for scholarly dissemination of their work through research-related conferences arise. Advocacy educators can identify opportunities to collaborate on curriculum development or to study the impact of curricula through multi-institutional research, through communities of advocacy educators such as the APPD's Community Health and Advocacy Training Learning Community or the APA's Advocacy Training Special Interest Group. Further, leadership opportunities within local, regional, and national pediatric organizations such as the APPD, the APA, and AAP exist for advocacy educators. As key components of the traditional academic promotion process, curriculum development and dissemination, research on outcomes in advocacy-related medical education, collaboration across institutions, and leadership opportunities are important ways for academic pediatricians focusing on advocacy to demonstrate their academic efforts.

Elsewhere in this chapter, we discussed the importance of residents engaging in advocacy projects as part of their training. Community health and advocacy curriculum directors, or other faculty engaging in advocacy, may serve as faculty mentors for resident projects. The AAP CPTI AP provides guidance on how faculty might document such advocacy projects and mentorship through traditional promotion systems. Further, faculty might support residents in CBPR related to their advocacy projects, again providing opportunities for faculty to engage in scholarship (such as publications or presentations). The AAP's CPTI offers several community health and advocacy grants for residents, fellows, subspecialty and primary care faculty, residency programs, and learning collaboratives. In addition to CATCH grants, the Advocacy Training Grant supports resident/fellow-faculty pairs to engage in advocacy-related educational projects at their institution and to attend the annual AAP Advocacy Conference.

Finally, through national and state chapter AAP engagement, pediatric advocacy leaders can identify opportunities to collaborate on pediatric medical education and advocacy projects through participation in the various committees, councils, and sections in the AAP. Opportunities to contribute to AAP policy development, a clear example of pediatric advocacy, exist within many committees, sections, and councils, and these can translate to a scholarship (such as publication) that advocacy educators can include in their AP for promotion. In some states, such as New York, California, Missouri, New Jersey, and Illinois, collaboratives among community health and advocacy directors within nearby pediatric residency programs offer opportunities for collaboration on advocacy efforts and curriculum development [15, 16]. In some cases, collaboratives host annual conferences where residents and faculty can present advocacy-related scholarship.

Advocacy-related pediatric medical education is a relatively young field that is expanding rapidly as ACGME and ABP formalize their expectations of the role pediatricians play in advocating for child health. With this expansion, opportunities abound for pediatric advocacy educators to disseminate their scholarly work around curriculum development and advocacy efforts. Professional organizations such as the APPD, the APA, and AAP provide supportive environments for pediatric advocacy educators to identify opportunities for collaboration and leadership within medical education and advocacy.

References

1. Burke EC. Abraham Jacobi, MD: the man and his legacy. Pediatrics. 1998;101(2):309–12.
2. Bae JY, Anderson E, Silver D, Macinko J. Child passenger safety Laws in the United States, 1978–2010: policy diffusion in the absence of strong federal intervention. Soc Sci Med. 2014 Jan;100:30–7.
3. Ameenuddin N. Video campaigns highlight how pediatricians are natural advocates | AAP News | American Academy of Pediatrics [Internet]. 2018 [cited 2024 Dec 19]. Available from: https://publications.aap.org/aapnews/news/14662.
4. ACGME program requirements for graduate medical education in pediatrics [Internet]. Accreditation Council for Graduate Medical Education (ACGME); 2024 [cited 2024 Dec 19]. Available from: https://www.acgme.org/globalassets/pfassets/programrequirements/2025-prs/320_pediatrics_2025.pdf.
5. Entrustable Professional Activities for General Pediatrics | The American Board of Pediatrics [Internet]. [cited December 4, 2025]. Available from: https://www.abp.org/sites/public/files/pdf/epas-general-pediatrics-summary.pdf.
6. Coutinho AJ, Dakis KE. Incorporating advocacy training to decrease burnout. Acad Med. 2017;92(7):905.
7. Minkovitz CS, Goldshore M, Solomon BS, Guyer B, Grason H, On behalf of the community pediatrics training initiative workgroup. Five-year follow-up of community pediatrics training initiative. Pediatrics 2014;134(1):83–90.
8. Hufford L, West DC, Paterniti DA, Pan RJ. Community-based advocacy training: applying asset-based community development in resident education. Acad Med. 2009;84(6):765.
9. Shipley LJ, Stelzner SM, Zenni EA, Hargunani D, O'Keefe J, Miller C, et al. Teaching community pediatrics to pediatric residents: strategic approaches and successful models for education in community health and child advocacy. Pediatrics. 2005;115(Supplement_3):1150–7.
10. Hanson E, Sosa-Unguez C, Mogilner L, Barnes M, Sieplinga K, Hunter R. How to build an advocacy rotation: tips, tricks, and resources to start or enhance your program's advocacy training. Workshop presentation presented at: APPD annual meeting; 2024; Chicago, IL.
11. Bode S, Best D, Petrus-Jones M for the AAP Community Pediatrics Training Initiative (CPTI). Building an Effective and Sustainable Community Pediatrics and Advocacy Curriculum. August 2025. Cited December 4, 2025. https://www.aap.org/en/advocacy/community-health-and-advocacy/teach-community-health-and-advocacy/community-pediatrics-and-advocacy-curriculum/.
12. Hoffman BD, Rose J, Best D, Linton J, Chapman S, Lossius M, et al. The community pediatrics training initiative project planning tool: a practical approach to community-based advocacy. MedEdPORTAL. 13:10630.
13. Chamberlain LJ, Hanson ER, Klass P, Schickedanz A, Nakhasi A, Barnes MM, et al. Childhood poverty and its effect on health and well-being: enhancing training for learners across the medical education continuum. Acad Pediatr. 2016;13(3, Supplement):S155–62.
14. Falusi OO, Weisz J, Clarence I, Lichtenstein C, Coddington D, Avent G, et al. Leveraging e-learning and community assets to "TEACH" residents to address child poverty. Acad Pediatr. 2022;22(5):850–7.
15. Chamberlain LJ, Wu S, Lewis G, Graff N, Javier JR, Park JSR, et al. A multi-institutional medical educational collaborative: advocacy training in California Pediatric Residency Programs. Acad Med. 2013;88(3):314.
16. Traba C, Pai S, Bode S, Hoffman B. Building a community partnership in a pandemic: NJ Pediatric Residency Advocacy Collaborative. Pediatrics. 2021 Apr 1;147(4):e2020012252.
17. Mental Health and Psychosocial Support [Internet]. [cited 2025 Jan 13]. UNICEF's brief on the social ecological model. Available from: https://knowledge.

unicef.org/mental-health-and-psychosocial-support/resource/unicefs-brief-social-ecological-model
18. Carlisle S. Health promotion, advocacy and health inequalities: a conceptual framework. Health Promot Int. 2000;15(4):369–76.
19. Hanna-Attisha M. What the eyes don't see: a story of crisis, resistance, and hope in an American city. 1st ed. New York: One World, an imprint of Random House; 2018.
20. Hanna-Attisha M, LaChance J, Sadler RC, Champney SA. Elevated blood Lead levels in children associated with the flint drinking water crisis: a spatial analysis of risk and public health response. Am J Public Health. 2016;106(2):283–90.
21. CDC. About CDC. 2024 [cited 2024 Dec 19]. Social Determinants of Health (SDOH). Available from: https://www.cdc.gov/about/priorities/why-is-addressing-sdoh-important.html.
22. Tayloe D Jr. Advocacy and child health outcomes: do child health professionals realize their opportunities? Pediatr Rev. 2024;45(7):369–72.
23. About the AAP [Internet]. [cited 2024 Dec 19]. Available from: https://www.aap.org/en/about-the-aap/.
24. Hoffman BD, Barnes M, Ferrell C, Gellin C, Lichtenstein C, Donnelly J, et al. The community health and advocacy milestones profile: a novel tool linking community pediatrics and advocacy training to assessment of milestones-based competence in pediatric residency training. Acad Pediatr. 2016;16(4):309–13.
25. United States Department of Health and Human Services, Health Resources and Services Administration, Maternal and Child Health Bureau, Hagan JF, Shaw JS, Duncan PM. Bright futures: guidelines for health supervision of infants, children, and adolescents. Fourth edition. Elk Grove Village: American Academy of Pediatrics; 2017.
26. Gitterman BA, Flanagan PJ, Cotton WH, Dilley KJ, Duffee JH, Green AE, et al. Poverty and child health in the United States. Pediatrics. 2016;137(4):e20160339.
27. Garg A, Boynton-Jarrett R, Dworkin PH. Avoiding the unintended consequences of screening for social determinants of Health. JAMA. 2016;316(8):813–4.
28. Sokol R, Austin A, Chandler C, Byrum E, Bousquette J, Lancaster C, et al. Screening children for social determinants of health: a systematic review. Pediatrics. 2019;144(4):e20191622.
29. Child Hunger in America | Feeding America [Internet]. [cited 2024 Dec 19]. Available from: https://www.feedingamerica.org/hunger-in-america/child-hunger-facts.
30. Hager ER, Quigg AM, Black MM, Coleman SM, Heeren T, Rose-Jacobs R, et al. Development and validity of a 2-item screen to identify families at risk for food insecurity. Pediatrics. 2010;126(1):e26–32.
31. Medical-Legal Partnership [Internet]. [cited 2024 Dec 19]. National Center for Medical-Legal Partnership. Available from: https://medical-legalpartnership.org/.
32. Gborkorquellie T, Avent G, Falusi O, Barber A, Olujide M, Smiley Y, et al. Fostering community engagement to address racism: development and implementation of a service-learning curriculum for pediatric residents. Acad Pediatr. 2023;23(8):1496–9.
33. Greater New York Hospital Association. Improving Residency Program and Community-Based Organization Collaboration A Guide to Developing Innovative Partnerships [Internet]. 2018 [cited 2025 Jan 13]. Available from: https://www.gnyha.org/wp-content/uploads/2018/09/ImprovingResidencyTookit_WEB.pdf.
34. AAP Advocacy Guide [Internet]. [cited 2024 Dec 19]. Available from: https://www.aap.org/en/advocacy/aap-advocacy-guide/.
35. Community Engagement Toolkit [Internet]. [cited 2025 Jan 5]. UCSF Center for Community Engagement. Community Engagement Toolkit. Available from: https://communityengagement.ucsf.edu/welcome-community-engagement-toolkit.
36. Community Access to Child Health – American Academy of Pediatrics [Internet]. [cited 2024 Dec 19]. Available from: https://www.aap.org/en/advocacy/community-health-and-advocacy/community-access-to-child-health/.
37. Oettgen B, Ruch-Ross H, Barrett HA, Bennett-Tejes D, Palmer K, Hobson WL. The Community Access to Child Health (CATCH) program: a 25-year retrospective. Pediatrics. 2019;143(6):e20182551.
38. NIMHD [Internet]. [cited 2024 Dec 19]. Community-Based Participatory Research Program (CBPR). Available from: https://www.nimhd.nih.gov/programs/extramural/community-based-participatory.html.
39. Vaughn LM, Wagner E, Jacquez F. A review of community-based participatory research in child Health. MCN Am J Matern Child Nurs. 2013;38(1):48.
40. Health Equity in Healthy People 2030 - Healthy People 2030 | odphp.health.gov [Internet]. [cited 2024 Dec 19]. Available from: https://odphp.health.gov/healthypeople/priority-areas/health-equity-healthy-people-2030.
41. Gambill L, van der List L, Altillo B. Demystifying the Op-Ed: a practical guide to start writing. J Hosp Med [Internet]. 2024 Jun 22 [cited 2025 Jan 13]; Available from: https://pubmed.ncbi.nlm.nih.gov/38922795/.
42. Scott JT, Maryman J. Using social media as a tool to complement advocacy. Global journal of community psychology Practice 2016;1–22.
43. Nerlinger AL, Shah AN, Beck AF, Beers LS, Wong SL, Chamberlain LJ, et al. The advocacy portfolio: a standardized tool for documenting physician advocacy. Acad Med. 2018;93(6):860.
44. Bode SM, Hoffman BD, Chapman SH, Kaczorowski JM, Best DL, Shah AN, et al. Academic careers in advocacy: aligning institutional values through use of an advocacy portfolio. Pediatrics. 2022;150(1):e2021055014.

18 Incorporating Mental and Behavioral Health into Pediatric Training Programs

Elizabeth M. Chawla and Sue E. Poynter

The History of Behavioral and Mental Health Training for Pediatricians

Over the past four decades, there has been increasing recognition of the need to improve training in behavioral and mental health care for pediatric trainees. In 1978, the American Academy of Pediatrics Task Force on Pediatric Education published a report entitled "The Future of Pediatric Education" [1], which emphasized the need to enhance residency training in behavioral, developmental, and adolescent issues to ensure pediatricians in the United States would be prepared to meet the growing needs of youth in these areas. This was the first formal call to enhance training in Behavioral and Mental Health (BMH) for future pediatricians. In 1990, the ACGME established new requirements for pediatric residency training that included a requirement for "evidence of structured educational experiences in adolescent medicine, child development, child psychology, and the care of the handicapped child" [2], followed by the addition of a required rotation in Developmental-Behavioral Pediatrics (DBP) in 1997 [2]. In 2000, Johnson et al. published the Final Report of the Future of Pediatric Education II (FOPE II) Project, which again emphasized the increasing need for training in developmental and behavioral issues for general pediatricians [3]. At this time, a large proportion of developmental, cognitive, and behavioral concerns in children (e.g., oppositional behavior, hyperactivity, inattention, relational health, etc.) were managed by Developmental-Behavioral Pediatricians. In 2016, the ACGME program requirements added a mandate that each pediatric training program must have at least one faculty member who is certified in Developmental-Behavioral Pediatrics (DBP) with the goal of increasing exposure of pediatric trainees to this expertise. In 2025, the ACGME program requirements strengthened the emphasis on training pediatricians in mental health by adding a required rotation in pediatric mental health. In this chapter, we will describe the current training requirements for pediatric behavioral and mental health and common strategies to meet this educational mandate.

Growing Mental Health Needs

Even with this increased focus, the United States has seen an exponential growth in pediatric behavioral and mental health (BMH) concerns

E. M. Chawla
Medstar Georgetown University Hospital, Washington, DC, USA

S. E. Poynter (✉)
Cincinnati Children's Hospital Medical Center and University of Cincinnati College of Medicine, Cincinnati, OH, USA
e-mail: Sue.Poynter@cchmc.org

H. McPhillips et al. (eds.), *Graduate Medical Education in Pediatrics*, Excellence in Medical Education 3, https://doi.org/10.1007/978-3-032-12952-9_18

over the past several decades, which have only been exacerbated by the COVID-19 pandemic [4, 5]. Prior to the pandemic, studies estimate that at least one in five youth in America had a mental health condition [6], and current research shows these numbers have greatly increased during and after the global pandemic. An increasing number of children and adolescents are presenting to emergency departments for mental health concerns [7, 8], evidence of both an inadequate pediatric mental health care system and increasing acuity of BMH problems. Indeed, the suicide rate among people aged 10–24 has increased 62% from 2007 to 2021, and suicide remains the second leading cause of death among youth aged 10–14 in the United States [9]. In 2021, the American Academy of Pediatrics, the American Academy of Child and Adolescent Psychiatry, and the Children's Hospital Association issued a joint statement of national emergency in child and adolescent mental health [10] as hospitals and emergency rooms continued to fill with pediatric patients in mental health crisis.

Current Training Not Meeting Current Needs

Despite the advocacy by the AAP and the strengthening of requirements by the ACGME, residency training for future pediatricians has not been able to adequately prepare graduates to meet the growing needs of patients. In a survey by the American Academy of Pediatrics (AAP) published in 2013, 65% of responding primary care and specialty pediatricians indicated they "lacked training" in the treatment of children and adolescents with mental health problems, almost 40% lacked confidence in their ability to recognize those problems, and more than half lacked confidence in their ability to treat them [11]. These findings were more than a decade after the mandated DBP rotation. Although the majority of pediatric trainees agree that pediatricians *should be* competent in assessment, treatment, referral, and comanagement of common BMH conditions [12, 13], as recently as 2018, less than a third of residents reported competence in assessment skills, and only 19% reported competence in treatment skills at the time of graduation [12].

New ACGME Requirement as a Step Forward

Due to growing shortages of pediatric mental health providers in the US, less than half of youth in need of mental health (MH) services actually receive them [6]. This shortage has led pediatricians to fill the void despite a self-reported lack of training. In response to these evolving needs, the ACGME has once again added an additional training mandate. As of 2025, all residents are required to have a specific mental health rotation, in addition to the required rotations in developmental-behavioral pediatrics and adolescent medicine [14].

While there may have been a time when every child with a developmental or behavioral health concern could be referred to a DBP specialist or every child with a mental health concern could be referred to a MH provider, these experts are in very short supply and the needs are great. To overcome this lack of specialists, all pediatric providers in all clinical settings need to be part of the solution to ensure the emotional health needs of children are met at all levels of the emotional health continuum. As part of this network of care, the pediatrician of the present and the future needs training and expertise in all of these areas: developmental, behavioral, relational, emotional, and mental health. The training paradigm must adapt to prepare pediatric trainees to meet the changing needs of patients.

The Evolution of Behavioral/Mental Health Competence for Pediatricians

In 2013, the American Board of Pediatrics published the Entrustable Professional Activities (EPAs) for General Pediatrics, outlining competence for pediatricians doing "Everyday Pediatrician Activities" (see chapter on

Competency-Based Assessment for more details). This original set of 17 EPAs included an EPA defining the activities needed for a pediatrician to be competent to "Assess and manage patients with common behavioral/mental health problems" (EPA-9) [15]. Although mental health skills for pediatricians had previously been encouraged by the AAP through policy statements and practice guidelines, this was the first time "managing mental health issues" was officially included in the pediatrician's scope of practice by any certifying body. Primary care pediatricians have not always agreed on their role in treating patients with BMH concerns [16–19]. However, as stated in the BMH EPA, "mental health and behavioral issues are central to pediatric practice." Pediatric providers are in a unique position to address these needs as the first (or sometimes only) provider a patient has access to across clinical settings, and pediatricians play an integral role in the developmental, emotional, and mental health of patients across all stages from birth to young adulthood.

A pediatrician competent in behavioral and mental health should understand the foundations of emotional health situated within normal childhood development. Factors that promote early emotional health and healthy relationships, such as secure attachment, autonomy, perspective taking, problem solving, and the ability to self-regulate, can be reinforced and modeled in pediatric visits. A pediatrician should be able to guide families on how to support the development of these foundational skills as children grow. A pediatrician should be able to anticipate common behavioral challenges consistent with different developmental stages and ages, and counsel patients and families on how to manage these. They should recognize when behavioral concerns are outside the normal range for a patient's developmental stage, and when further evaluation is needed. These skills are integral to helping build strong and supportive families and can be important for early recognition and intervention if emotional health concerns do arise.

In addition, a pediatrician competent in BMH should be able to anticipate, recognize, evaluate, and manage common behavioral and mental health symptoms (e.g., low mood, inattention and impulsivity, disruptive behavior and aggression, anxiety, learning difficulty, substance use, suicidality, and social emotional issues in young children).

This would include the following skill sets:

- Be knowledgeable of evidence-based screening tools and diagnostic criteria for common conditions.
- Be knowledgeable of evidence-based treatments for these common problems.
- Know when each type of treatment would be indicated, including referral to the appropriate specialist or specific type of therapy as needed.
- Be able to initiate treatment, including pharmacotherapy for certain conditions when indicated (e.g., ADHD, depression, anxiety).
- Be able to monitor for side effects and treatment effects of any therapies or medications.
- Be competent in discussing treatment options with patients and families.

Like many other complex topics within medicine, competence in caring for patients with behavioral and mental health concerns requires more than simply knowledge acquisition. Despite more discussion in the public sphere in recent years, BMH concerns are often wrapped in stigma, misunderstanding, and sometimes shame, especially among certain communities. Being skillful at discussing these sometimes-sensitive topics with patients and families from all backgrounds requires practice over time. Learning by watching experts, experiential learning including observation and feedback, and personal reflection are all important to developing competence in addressing the BMH concerns of patients.

The Behavioral and Mental Health EPA includes other important skills as part of the pediatrician's scope of practice in caring for patients with BMH concerns. With the recognition that the pediatrician is part of a care network, knowledge of the other components of the network is integral to ensuring patients and families have access to the appropriate level of care and are supported in their communities (Fig. 18.1).

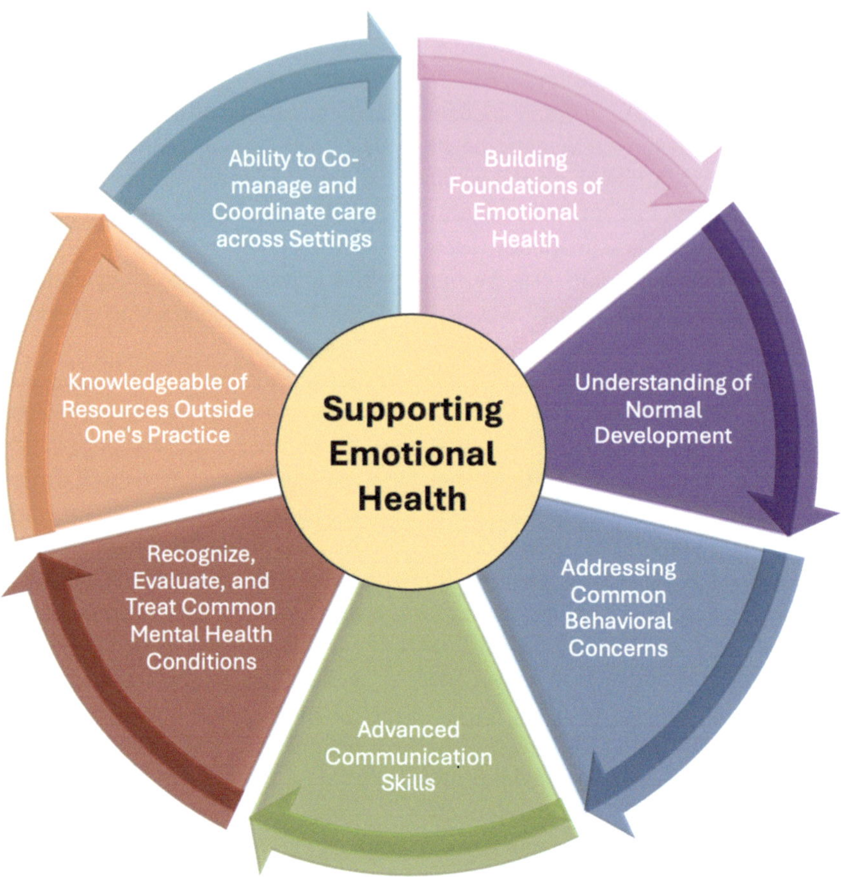

Fig. 18.1 Pieces of competence required for supporting the emotional health of pediatric patients

These additional skills include:

- Knowing the mental health resources available in one's community.
- Understanding which level of care is most appropriate for a patient's needs.
- Comanaging patients with the appropriate specialist(s) when indicated.
- The ability to coordinate care that includes resources outside one's practice.

"The coordination of an interprofessional team is essential to ensure inclusion of additional professionals, including mental health specialists, school and community resources, and support groups. A pediatrician must also provide culturally sensitive care relevant to a family's background, experience, and the developmental stage of the patient" (from the Behavioral and Mental Health EPA, scope of practice).

Common Approaches to Behavioral/Mental Health Education for Pediatric Trainees

In an effort to improve training in BMH care, many residency programs have added BMH curricula or training initiatives in recent years. While each of these initiatives is an improvement over what existed before (often very little BMH training), many of these strategies alone do not fully develop competency in BMH care. Here we will discuss some common approaches to behavioral/mental health education for pediatric trainees, highlighting some strengths and limitations to consider for each.

Behavioral/Mental Health Curricula

Many programs have started with knowledge acquisition, adding formal teaching on BMH topics to lecture schedules, academic half days, or the overall program curriculum. These are often taught by mental health providers, such as child psychiatrists or psychologists, or sometimes taught by pediatric faculty with experience or expertise in BMH topics. Some programs have created longitudinal curricula where the various topics are spaced throughout training and reinforced on various rotations. To give all residency programs access to standardized BMH education, the Association of Pediatric Program Directors (APPD) has created an internet-based BMH curriculum [the EMPOWER curriculum] based on the BMH EPA available to all pediatric trainees through APPD membership. These curricula are an important first step in ensuring pediatric trainees have access to the knowledge required for caring for patients with BMH concerns. In programs where trainees may have limited or sporadic exposure to patients with BMH concerns due to models of care or practice pathways that may not involve trainees, it is especially important to ensure a foundational level of content knowledge of BMH topics for all trainees. However, domain knowledge is only the first step. Without opportunities for trainees to also learn and practice domain skills in a longitudinal manner, it will be difficult for them to reach competence by the time of graduation.

Mental Health Track

Some programs have created a Mental Health Track to provide opportunities for trainees to gain additional exposure and practice caring for patients with BMH concerns. These can include additional time working with mental health experts or in clinical spaces where BMH care is provided, additional didactics or other curricula focused on BMH topics, and/or additional time in the outpatient pediatric clinic caring for patients within special BMH consult clinics that are often staffed by mental health providers. These additional experiences are a great addition to standard curricula focused on knowledge acquisition alone and can potentially offer trainees opportunities for learning and practicing domain skills. However, these additional experiences should not be offered only to those residents with an interest in BMH care or career goals within primary care. Pediatric providers encounter patients with BMH concerns in all clinical spaces: in pediatric ERs, on hospital wards, in subspecialty clinics, and in primary care. To ensure adequate training for all residents, regardless of future career plans, we should provide sufficient experiences for all future pediatric providers to reach competence in caring for patients with BMH concerns. Whether a patient presents to the clinic or the ER, or discloses a mental health need during a hospitalization or during a subspecialty visit, their provider should be adequately trained to respond to that mental health need competently.

Integrated Mental Health Clinics in Continuity Clinic

Integrating mental health services into primary care clinics has a long history within adult medicine and has gained momentum within pediatrics over the past several years. Different models of care exist, from colocation of providers to true integration of mental health providers within the flow of the clinic, with goals of improving access to mental health services for patients and improving the coordination of care between mental health providers and primary care providers [20]. Many residency programs have taken advantage of this unique arrangement to bring mental health providers into the continuity clinic teaching space or to bring trainees closer to mental health care. Workflows vary among programs, with some having the mental health provider physically present in the precepting space for real-time consultation and teaching, while others have the MH provider nearby and accessible as needed.

Using integrated clinics as an educational model has several advantages. The most notable is that any BMH evaluation or care being provided is for the trainee's own patient, increasing personal relevance. In addition, the BMH care is happening in the trainee's own patient care space as opposed to going to an "outside" clinical space to learn skills that should be within the pediatrician's own scope of practice. Providing the BMH care within the pediatrics continuity clinic also allows for the opportunity for the trainee to be part of any follow-up and continue to follow the patient longitudinally, which is integral for learning the life course of BMH issues as well as understanding the impact of treatment decisions.

However, given that residents are often busy and pressed for time in the continuity clinic space, there is a temptation to "hand off" the BMH concern to a nearby MH provider, removing the trainee from the care and thereby significantly reducing the opportunity for learning. Even when learning BMH within their own clinical spaces, such as a continuity clinic, residents will likely only learn what they have a chance to practice: if they only practice assessing and referring to in-house MH providers, they only learn how to assess and refer [19, 21]. This helps explain why, although integrating BMH providers within resident continuity clinics has shown promise as a potential educational model, the modest increases in self-rated competence are still quite low, with only about a third of pediatric trainees competent in assessment skills and less than a quarter competent in treatment skills at graduation [22].

For trainees to gain the most benefit from integrated clinic models, they must be given opportunities to provide the care for mental health concerns themselves, for their own patients, with coaching and support from the integrated MH provider. In clinics without resources for establishing this level of structured integrated clinic, a similar experience can be created by having the trainee call their state-level child psychiatry access program (https://www.nncpap.org/) for consultation, while maintaining ownership over the patient care when appropriate and within the scope of practice of primary care. In addition, trainees should have access to varied patient panels encompassing a variety of ages, including adolescents, and scheduling models should allow for follow-up with these same patients for continuity of the mental health care.

Dedicated Mental Health Rotation/Block

Although it was the ACGME 2025 requirements mandated a dedicated MH rotation, some pediatric training programs had recognized this gap in their curriculum and had already added this educational experience prior to the requirement. These types of rotations have taken on various shapes and sizes, with the majority consisting of a discrete 2- or 4-week block rotating within a department of child and adolescent psychiatry or with another type of MH provider within their own clinical space. Having opportunities to learn both domain knowledge and domain skills from an expert can be extremely valuable. Opportunities to practice skills are integral to the development of competence, yet opportunities for pediatric trainees to provide some of the BMH care within clinical spaces outside of general pediatrics are often limited. In addition, the level of BMH care needed for patients presenting to outside mental health services is often a higher level of need or complexity. While understanding the full spectrum of mental health needs is important, this should not be a trainee's only exposure to BMH care, as it is unlikely to be within their future scope of practice in subspecialty or general pediatrics. Exposure to patients with higher levels of mental health needs can be an important piece of their overall training if balanced with caring for mental health patients across the continuum in other clinical spaces.

Educational Strategies for Teaching BMH to Trainees

Experiential Learning

One of the most important educational strategies for learning complex tasks is the experiential learning cycle model, which is the practical application of Experiential Learning Theory as described by psychologist David Kolb and published in 1984 [23]. The Experiential Learning Cycle consists of four phases: Concrete Experience (having experience performing a task), Reflective Observation (reviewing or reflecting on how you did), Abstract Conceptualization (thinking about how you did in relation to best practice, learning from the experience), and Active Experimentation (planning how to adapt based on what was learned) (Fig. 18.2). This active learning and reflection inform and improve the next experience that the learner encounters. For complex tasks involved in caring for patients and families with BMH concerns, such as discussing a new diagnosis with a family affected by stigma, this method of iterative reflective practice can be very useful for improving skills and building competence. Subsequent experiences can occur in multiple clinical settings or additional rotations, if the trainee is intentional about the skills they are working on mastering. This model is appropriate for any level of learner and can also be continued for life-long learning even after training has ended. Although it is largely an internal process, the learning in this model can be significantly enhanced by the coaching of a skilled faculty member at various points, with or without direct observation.

For example, a trainee diagnoses a patient with ADHD based on multiple positive screeners and a careful history that confirms the patient meets diagnostic criteria. In discussing the diagnosis with the patient's caregiver, the caregiver expresses they do not believe in ADHD. Despite a long conversation including sharing the large evidence base for this diagnosis, the caregiver is not convinced. Both parties end the encounter feeling unsatisfied. Afterwards the trainee reflects on how the conversation went and why they were not successful. They discuss with a faculty mem-

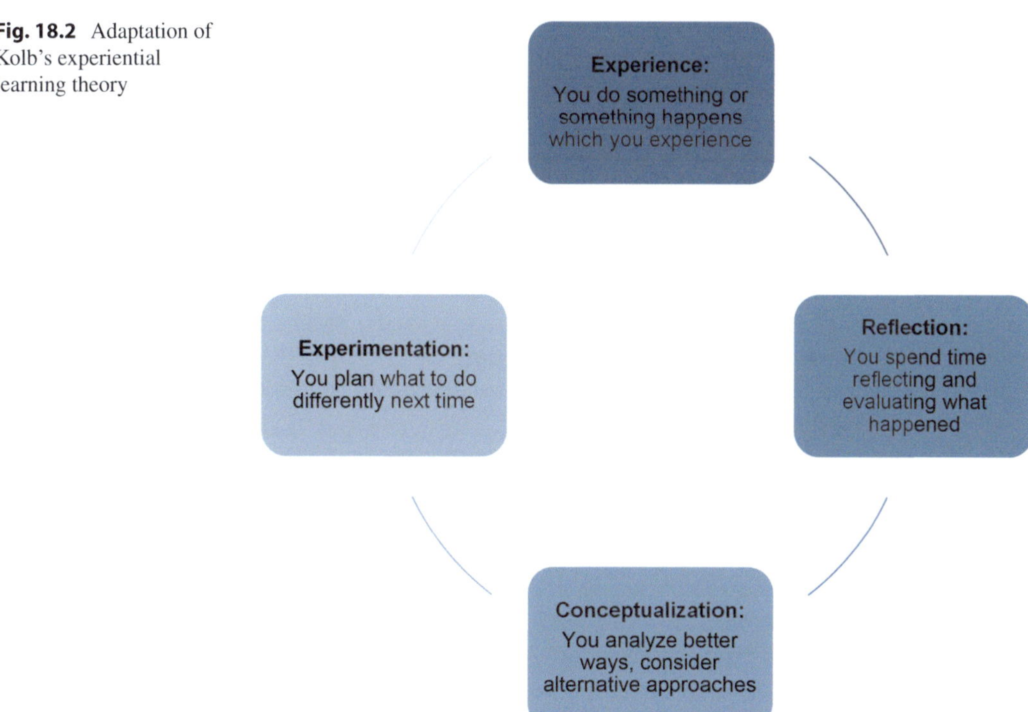

Fig. 18.2 Adaptation of Kolb's experiential learning theory

ber who helps the trainee realize through coaching that they didn't first take time to understand the caregiver's perspective of the problem or their understanding of BMH issues. The trainee realizes the importance of open dialogue, not just information sharing, and plans how they will approach the conversation differently next time. The following week, the trainee sees a patient with suicidal ideation in the ER who has a positive depression screen and tries a different approach by first exploring the patient's understanding of depression.

Observation of Experts with Shared Reflection

Experiential learning is not limited to internal processes. It may be difficult for a trainee, especially one who is still early in the process of learning BMH skills, to conceptualize how to adapt behavior or language to move their skills closer to best practice. Although trainees often express frustration with "observation only" learning experiences, observing expertise in practice can be extremely valuable for adding approaches and specific phrasing to their toolbox. The challenge is in helping the trainee to understand the learning opportunity in the observation—this can be fostered by shared reflection between the expert and the trainee following any observed encounter, and setting intentional learning goals for any observation experience.

For example, a trainee is assigned to attend the post-partum mental health clinic at the local women's mental health center as part of a BMH rotation. Given the nature of the visit, the providers at this clinic have decided it will be an observation-only learning experience for the pediatric trainee. However, learning goals for this experience are specifically stated on the course rotation schedule and include 'learn approaches for asking a post-partum mother about her own mental health'. During the observed encounter, the trainee is intentionally listening for how the expert opens the conversation and how they respond to any hesitancy the patient may have about disclosing any mental health symptoms. After the encounter, the mental health provider describes their approach to normalizing mental health symptoms in post-partum women and how to troubleshoot common barriers to disclosure. The trainee reflects on the encounter they just observed and relates this strategy to a phrase they heard the mental health provider use. The following week in continuity clinic, the trainee uses this same phrase with a parent of their 1-month-old patient which allows them to feel more comfortable in opening conversations about mental health with caregivers.

Situated Learning Theory

Situated Learning is a learning theory that emphasizes the importance of learning while performing tasks within the context the skill set is used and the social constructs within that context, first described by Jean Lave and Etienne Wenger in 1991 [24]. In Situated Learning Theory, the learning occurs by working with others in a community of practice, and what students learn is not always intentionally planned. It includes the knowledge and skills the learner acquires by performing the tasks, but also includes what they learn about roles, responsibilities, and social norms within that context. Situated Learning Theory illustrates why trainees will learn how to care for patients with BMH concerns best by caring for their own patients with BMH concerns, within the clinical spaces in which they usually work. Trainees learn through "legitimate participation" in the BMH care, learning not only how to provide the BMH care, but also understanding their role as part of the larger network of mental health care for children.

For example, a trainee rotates through an outpatient psychiatric clinic one afternoon as part of a mental health rotation, during which they see a 14-year-old patient with depression with the psychiatrist. During this encounter, they review the depression screener with the psychiatrist and then watch the psychiatrist discuss the diagnosis with the patient. They learn how to score and interpret depression screening tools and how those tools can help inform a diagnosis. In con-

trast, a different trainee sees a 14-year-old patient in continuity clinic who mentions symptoms of depression during the history. The trainee uses a depression screener to get more information, reviews the screener with their preceptor, and then uses it to help inform a more detailed history which confirms a diagnosis of depression. This trainee also learns how to score and interpret depression screening tools and how those tools can help inform a diagnosis. Additionally, this trainee also learns the importance of a pediatrician being able to recognize red flags in the history and being competent to respond and complete next steps during the encounter.

Common Challenges in Teaching Behavioral/Mental Health

The Hidden Curriculum

Not only is it important for trainees to learn skills within the clinical settings in which they will use them, but it is equally important for them to see those skills as part of their future scope of practice. This is often complicated by the "hidden curriculum"—unspoken norms that learners observe which are not openly intended. When pediatric trainees are taught by experts or faculty from other departments or when BMH patient care pathways do not involve trainees (e.g., in the ED), these unspoken realities can impact the trainees' perceived scope of practice. If they do not see a pediatric faculty member in their future career role performing mental health care, it may communicate that mental health care is not within the scope of practice for that type of clinician or is not valued.

There is a suggestion of this change in the perception of responsibility in a recent study of subspecialty fellows by Green et al. [13]. Of over 2000 pediatric subspecialty fellows surveyed, 56.4% reported a high level of interest in emotional and MH needs of children with complex medical conditions. Of these, 62.8% agreed that providers in their subspecialty should be responsible for the assessment of MH concerns. However, that perceived responsibility was significantly lower among second- and third-year fellows compared with first-year fellows, suggesting their perceived scope of practice changes from the time they enter fellowship to the time they finish.

It will be important to address this hidden curriculum while we focus on improving training for pediatric residents and fellows. Pediatric faculty, in all specialties and clinical practice areas, should be part of the movement toward improved training in BMH for future pediatricians. Faculty should voice support for the changing scope of practice for pediatric providers in caring for patients with BMH concerns. Faculty should model an interest in improving their own skills and should model the role a pediatric provider can play in improving a patient's access to BMH care at all levels of the continuum.

Faculty Development

This chapter began by describing the current gap between the mental health needs of patients and the current training for pediatricians. Considering this reality, it is not surprising that many current faculty across clinical settings do not feel confident or prepared for teaching these topics to trainees, and that 64% of pediatric program directors agree "a lack of experienced faculty" is a barrier to improving BMH training for residents [25]. Some programs are therefore relying on providers outside their core faculty to teach these topics to trainees, or using their own faculty who are constrained by their limited training out of necessity. As discussed earlier, it is imperative for trainees to see faculty within the role of their future career, including BMH within their scope of practice. This will require faculty development in every program and within every subspecialty division. Not only will faculty need training to improve their own BMH skills appropriate to their clinical practice area, but they will also need faculty development on the impact of their words and actions on culture change. In all clinical environments, trainees are watching and adopting, even the unspoken lessons.

Financial Barriers

Another major barrier to implementing widespread change in practice is the resources required, both time and financial. Organizing large-scale faculty development programming, planning, and implementing new curricula for trainees, as well as partnering with MH providers to assist with these pieces, requires a significant amount of effort and resources. At the same time, pediatric departments across the country are experiencing even tighter budgetary constraints because of the recent global pandemic and staffing changes needed to be in compliance with new ACGME requirements. The financial barrier has become a significant challenge for many programs across the country.

Fortunately, many other organizations, both national and local, have recognized the great BMH needs for children and adolescents and offer programming and resources to help. For example, state departments of health may offer grants or other types of one-time funding to support faculty development training programs or the creation of integrated clinics. Many state MAP (Mental Health Access Programs) programs across the country have an educational arm and can offer programming to faculty or trainees or both. Many mental health providers are overwhelmed with patient volumes and have begun to recognize the value in partnering with pediatric programs to provide some of the BMH care at the lower end of the spectrum—providing some education and coordination of care to streamline patient care. Finding ways that this type of partnership can benefit both parties can make partnering with mental health providers financially sustainable.

Resources Needed for Teaching BMH

Some training programs that lack existing BMH education and BMH experts may not know where to begin, but fortunately, these programs do not have to start from square one. In addition to the potential funding sources or partners listed earlier, many of the major national pediatric organizations offer resources for developing BMH skills at little to no cost. The APPD has created an online BMH curriculum [the EMPOWER curriculum] as part of its LESSON learning platform, which is provided to all trainees as part of APPD membership at no extra cost [26]. The modules can also be viewed by faculty as part of faculty development programming. The AAP has developed resources for practicing pediatricians, such as the Pediatric Mental Health Minute Series [27], which could also be used with trainees. The American Board of Pediatrics Foundation has created resources specifically to teach pediatric subspecialists to address emotional health in children with chronic medical conditions and their families [28], but these free educational resources are generalizable across specialties and clinical practice areas and can be used with trainees and faculty alike [29]. Programs such as the REACH Institute can be used for more robust faculty development [30], while several well-known pediatric blogs and podcasts offer discussion around BMH topics [31, 32].

BMH Program Evaluation and Assessment of Learners

One of the most important pieces of building any new curriculum or programming is evaluating the outcomes of that programming (see chapter on Curriculum Development for more details). But knowing which outcomes to measure can be complex when working to create culture change or designing programming to teach new areas historically not part of the pediatrician's scope of practice. How will we know what success looks like if it has not existed before? How will faculty be able to evaluate learners for competence when they themselves do not feel competent? Faculty often evaluates learners using themselves or their own skills as a frame of reference [33], but that task becomes complicated when the faculty assessor does not personally have the skill being assessed. In this case, faculty must look to standards set by pediatric organizations for guidance, such as the ABP BMH EPA [15] or the Mental Health Competencies as described by the AAP [34]. These resources provide an idea of the goal, even if the on-the-ground details of achieving the goal will take some time to understand. Faculty will need training in best practices for BMH care, not only to improve their own skills, but also to better assess trainees in these areas. This will be an iterative process, and in many cases, faculty and trainees will be learning together. Programs must move beyond simply checking a box of meeting the ACGME requirement for "4 weeks of a MH experience" and truly evaluate if their programming is moving trainees towards competence in BMH.

Future Directions

Although the pediatric community has recognized a need for improved BMH training for pediatricians since 1978, there is still much work to do. As patient needs in behavioral and mental health continue to grow, the pediatric education community must focus even more attention and resources on training pediatric providers to address the emotional health of their patients as a routine part of all encounters. An emphasis on strong emotional health development in the early years, supporting families and caregivers, anticipating emotional health needs during times of stress, transition, or physical health challenges, and being ready to respond to new or changing mental health needs from birth to young adulthood will be critical skills for the pediatrician of the future. Reaching this reality will require improved integration of BMH training in all clinical areas and pediatric specialties. Trainees will need to see BMH as part of the scope of practice for pediatric providers within all clinical areas, and faculty development will be needed to support this culture change. While leaders within the pediatrics education community are developing BMH workplace-based assessment tools to aid faculty in the evaluation of BMH skills, faculty will need training on BMH skills themselves to best use those tools. The Behavioral and Mental Health EPA has provided a detailed description of the end goal, but it will take all members of a training program—trainees, faculty, training directors, administrators, and pediatric faculty working in all departments, plus significant faculty development—to make that goal a reality.

References

1. American Academy of Pediatrics. Task Force on Pediatric Education. The future of pediatric education. Evanston: American Academy of Pediatrics; 1978.
2. Accreditation Council for Graduate Medical Education. ACGME program requirements for graduate medical education in pediatrics, background and archives. Available at: https://www.acgme.org/programs-and-institutions/programs/common-program-requirements/background-and-archives/.
3. Johnson RL, Charney E, Cheng TL, et al. Final report of the FOPE II education of the pediatrician workshop. Pediatrics. 2000;106:1175–98.
4. Bittner Gould J, Walter HJ, Bromberg J, Correa ET, Hatoun J, Vernacchio L. Impact of the coronavirus disease 2019 pandemic on mental health visits in pediatric primary care. Pediatrics. 2022 Dec 1;150(6):e2022057176. https://doi.org/10.1542/peds.2022-057176.
5. Cutler GJ, Bergmann KR, Doupnik SK, Hoffmann JA, Neuman MI, Rodean J, Zagel AL, Zima BT. Pediatric mental health emergency department visits and access to inpatient care: a crisis worsened by the COVID-19 pandemic. Acad Pediatr. 2022;22(6):889–91. https://doi.org/10.1016/j.acap.2022.03.015. Epub 2022 Mar 26. PMID: 35351651; PMCID: PMC8957359.
6. Whitney DG, Peterson MD. US national and state-level prevalence of mental health disorders and disparities of mental health care use in children. JAMA Pediatr. 2019;173(4):389–91. https://doi.org/10.1001/jamapediatrics.2018.5399. s
7. Lo CB, Bridge JA, Shi J, Ludwig L, Stanley RM. Children's mental health emergency department visits: 2007-2016. Pediatrics. 2020;145(6):e20191536. https://doi.org/10.1542/peds.2019-1536. Epub 2020 May 11.
8. Horowitz LM, Bridge JA. Upstream prevention strategies to prevent suicidal ideation-related ED visits. Pediatrics. 2022;150(6):e2022058151. https://doi.org/10.1542/peds.2022-058151. PMID: 36373283; PMCID: PMC9724168.
9. Curtin S. Deaths: Leading Causes for 2021. National Vital Statistics Reports; Vol 73. No 4. National Center for Health Statistics. April 8, 2024. Available at: https://www.cdc.gov/nchs/data/nvsr/nvsr73/nvsr73-04.pdf. Accessed 23 Sept 2024.
10. American Academy of Pediatrics. AAP-AACAP-CHA Declaration of a National Emergency in Child and Adolescent Mental Health. October 19, 2021. Available at: https://www.aap.org/en/advocacy/child-and-adolescent-healthy-mental-development/aap-aacap-cha-declaration-of-a-national-emergency-in-child-and-adolescent-mental-health/. Accessed 23 Sept 2024.
11. Horwitz SM, Storfer-Isser A, Kerker BD, Szilagyi M, Garner A, O'Connor KG, Hoagwood KE, Stein RE. Barriers to the identification and management

of psychosocial problems: changes from 2004 to 2013. Acad Pediatr. 2015;15(6):613–20. https://doi.org/10.1016/j.acap.2015.08.006. Epub 2015 Sep 26. PMID: 26409303; PMCID: PMC4639452.

12. Green C, Leyenaar JK, Turner AL, Leslie LK. Competency of future pediatricians caring for children with behavioral and mental health problems. Pediatrics. 2020;146(1):e20192884. https://doi.org/10.1542/peds.2019-2884. Epub 2020 Jun 19.
13. Green CM, Leyenaar JK, Tucker A, Leslie LK. Preparedness of pediatric subspecialty fellows to address emotional and mental health needs among children with chronic medical conditions. JAMA Pediatr. 2022;176(12):1266–8. https://doi.org/10.1001/jamapediatrics.2022.3451. PMID: 36190709; PMCID: PMC9531063.
14. Accreditation Council for Graduate Medical Education. ACGME Program Requirements for Graduate Medical Education in Pediatrics. ACGME-approved major revision: February 4, 2024; effective July 1, 2025. Available at: https://www.acgme.org/globalassets/pfassets/programrequirements/2025-prs/320_pediatrics_2025.pdf. Accessed 23 Sept 2024.
15. American Board of Pediatrics. Entrustable professional activities for general pediatrics, EPA-9. Revised 2021. Available at: https://www.abp.org/sites/abp/files/pdf/gen_peds_epa_9.pdf. Accessed 23 Sept 2024.
16. Imfeld SM, Darang DM, Neudecker M, McVoy MK. Primary care pediatrician perceptions towards mental health within the primary care setting. Pediatr Res. 2021;90(5):950–6. https://doi.org/10.1038/s41390-020-01349-7. Epub 2021 Feb 2.
17. Heneghan A, Garner AS, Storfer-Isser A, Kortepeter K, Stein RE, Horwitz SM. Pediatricians' role in providing mental health care for children and adolescents: do pediatricians and child and adolescent psychiatrists agree? J Dev Behav Pediatr. 2008;29(4):262–9. https://doi.org/10.1097/DBP.0b013e31817dbd97.
18. Horwitz SM, Caspary G, Storfer-Isser A, Singh M, Fremont W, Golzari M, Stein RE. Is developmental and behavioral pediatrics training related to perceived responsibility for treating mental health problems? Acad Pediatr. 2010;10(4):252–9. https://doi.org/10.1016/j.acap.2010.03.003. Epub 2010 Jun 2.
19. Ragunanthan B, Frosch EJ, Solomon BS. On-site mental health professionals and pediatric residents in continuity clinic. Clin Pediatr (Phila). 2017;56(13):1219–26. https://doi.org/10.1177/0009922816681136. Epub 2017 Jan 12.
20. Heath B, Wise Romero P, Reynolds K. A review and proposed standard framework for levels of integrated healthcare. Washington, DC: SAMHSA-HRSA Center for Integrated Health Solutions; 2013.
21. Garfunkel LC, Pisani AR, leRoux P, Siegel DM. Educating residents in behavioral health care and collaboration: comparison of conventional and integrated training models. Acad Med. 2011;86(2):174–9. https://doi.org/10.1097/ACM.0b013e318204ff1d. PMID: 21169773; PMCID: PMC4176864.
22. Green C, Leyenaar JK, Nuncio B, Leslie LK. Association of behavioral and mental health professionals in continuity clinic with resident-reported competence. J Pediatr. 2022;248:15–20.e1. https://doi.org/10.1016/j.jpeds.2022.05.012. Epub 2022 May 20.
23. Kolb D. Experiential learning: experience as the source of learning and development. Prentice-Hall; 1984.
24. Lave J, Wenger E. Situated learning: legitimate peripheral participation. Cambridge University Press; 1991.
25. Chawla E, Poynter S, Burke A, Ponitz K, McNeal-Trice K, "[State of the onion]: the many layers of pediatric mental health training in the US, a national needs assessment of pediatric residency programs", abstract presented at Association of Pediatric Program Directors National Meeting, San Diego, CA, May 2022.
26. APPD LESSON: Longitudinal Educational Software Solutions and Outcomes Network. Available at: https://www.appd.org/appd-lesson/ Accessed 21 Oct 2024.
27. American Academy of Pediatrics. Pediatric mental health minute series. Available at: https://www.aap.org/en/patient-care/mental-health-minute/?srsltid=AfmBOoqqEiDXMra13X2HGQtepn96-In08IcgA9HTHY2oI_wiODySifOA. Accessed 21 Oct 2024.
28. American Board of Pediatrics Foundation. The roadmap project. Available at: https://www.roadmapforemotionalhealth.org/. Accessed 21 Oct 2024.
29. Chawla EM, Schuler CL, Barnhardt EW, Herbst LA, Sarkissian A, McNeal-Trice K, Newmeyer A, Perry M, Poynter SE, Lannon C. Integrating education for clinical practice change. Clin Teach. 2024;21(4):e13753. https://doi.org/10.1111/tct.13753. Epub 2024 Feb 29.
30. The REACH Institute. Available at: https://thereachinstitute.org/. Accessed 21 Oct 2024.
31. Fallucco E. PsychEd4Peds: empowering and supporting pediatric clinicians. Available at: https://psyched4peds.com/ and on Apple Podcasts, Spotify, and Amazon Music. Accessed 21 Oct 2024.
32. American Academy of Pediatrics. Pediatrics on call podcast: the official podcast of the American Academy of Pediatrics. Available at: https://www.aap.org/en/pages/podcast/ and on Apple Podcasts, Spotify, and Amazon Music. Accessed 21 Oct 2024.
33. Kogan JR, Conforti L, Bernabeo E, Iobst W, Holmboe E. Opening the black box of clinical skills assessment via observation: a conceptual model. Med Educ. 2011;45(10):1048–60. https://doi.org/10.1111/j.1365-2923.2011.04025.x.
34. Foy JM, Green CM, Earls MF, Committee on Psychosocial Aspects of Child and Family Health, Mental Health Leadership Work Group. Mental health competencies for pediatric practice. Pediatrics. 2019;144(5):e20192757. https://doi.org/10.1542/peds.2019-2757. Epub 2019 Oct 21.

19 Procedures and Simulation

Amanda J. Rogers and Adrian D. Zurca

Introduction and History

Simulation-based medical education (SBME) is the use of educational activities to replace or amplify real patient experiences with scenarios designed to replicate real health encounters, using lifelike manikins, physical models, standardized patients, or computers [41].

The use of SBME has its origins in the military and aviation fields [15]. Its role in medical education has expanded rapidly over the past century as medicine transitioned away from primarily an apprenticeship model and as there has been an increasing focus on patient safety. Early uses of SBME focused on anatomic models and standardized patients. As technology advanced and became more readily available, the use of SBME has continued to evolve. It is currently commonplace in most pediatric residency programs. A recent survey of pediatric residency programs showed a wide range of current common uses within pediatric residency training, including for procedural simulations, mock codes/urgent situations, and communication training, as well as emerging additional uses, including competency assessment, contingency planning, and crisis resource management skill development [25].

The use of SBME has become an increasingly important element of pediatric resident education for multiple reasons. With the increasing focus on patient safety following the Institute of Medicine's "To err is human" report [69], there was a need for interventions to improve patient safety systems. SBME has played an important role in those efforts, providing a controlled environment to practice key clinical skills and procedures without compromising patient safety. This is especially true within pediatric training, where code events and select procedures are relatively rare, and it is essential to have alternative opportunities for trainees to experience those high-stakes/low-frequency events. Residency duty hour restrictions have also impacted clinical exposure during residency and led to an increased need for standardized experiences to ensure trainees have sufficient exposure to key clinical skills. Advancements in the interprofessional nature of medicine have altered the types and volumes of procedures performed by residents. Advancements in assessment requirements, including the implementation of Milestones [1] and subsequently Entrustable Professional Activities [68], have also highlighted gaps in what required assessments can be reliably completed from clinical exposure alone [45]. SBME can provide a valuable supplement to fill those gaps.

A. J. Rogers (✉)
Medical College of Wisconsin and Children's Wisconsin, Milwaukee, WI, USA
e-mail: arogers@mcw.edu

A. D. Zurca
Northwestern University Feinberg School of Medicine, Chicago, IL, USA

H. McPhillips et al. (eds.), *Graduate Medical Education in Pediatrics*, Excellence in Medical Education 3, https://doi.org/10.1007/978-3-032-12952-9_19

Benefits/Efficacy

Prior work has demonstrated the impact of SBME within medical education in general as well as specifically within pediatric medical education. Pediatric studies have shown improvement in learner knowledge, performance in simulated settings, behavior with patients, and time to task completion following clinical scenario-based SBME [16, 17, 19, 51]. Studies assessing the impact of SBME on procedural training have also shown improvement in confidence and performance in simulated settings with mixed results related to actual performance in the clinical setting [51]. Communication training has similarly demonstrated improvements in confidence and behavior in simulated settings with limited and mixed results focused on patient outcomes [10]. Current literature suggests an opportunity for future work to assess the impact on patient-level outcomes and the optimal approach to using SBME within pediatric medical education, which will be outlined later in this chapter.

Limitations/Overcoming Challenges

Despite the benefits of SBME, there are limitations to the use of SBME in pediatric medical education that should be considered when developing and implementing a simulation program/curriculum within pediatric residency education.

SBME is not meant to replace clinical experience and is not the solution to all gaps within pediatric residency education. It is important for programs to consider both when simulation should and should not be used within their broader curriculum. SBME is best suited for high-stakes/low-frequency events. Given the resources required to conduct this educational method, it may not be best to utilize it for events that trainees can get regular exposure to in the clinical setting. In addition, certain skills and competencies may be less amendable to SBME [45]. It is beneficial for residency leadership to partner with simulation experts to determine where there is a need to supplement current clinical education in areas that are also well-suited for SBME.

SBME can play an important role in both formative and summative assessments. There are important considerations, however, that programs should consider related to the use in summative assessments. The International Nursing Association for Clinical Simulation and Learning (INACSL) Standard of Best Practice outlines specific factors to consider when using simulation for more summative assessments, including sufficient pilot testing of scenarios, determining the validity and reliability of assessment tools, and ensuring appropriate training for the evaluators [59]. A fundamental element of ensuring psychological safety within simulation is transparency regarding the confidentiality of performance during the simulation. This is not to say that everything with simulation must remain confidential, but it is essential that programs are clear with trainees about what their performance during a simulation will and will not be used for, and also recognize the impact that this may have on their performance during the simulation.

There is also a risk of negative learning within SBME. Gaps in simulation scenarios or equipment may lead to learners skipping key steps, which can translate to problems in their clinical performance. For example, if manikins lack the ability to portray changes in skin color or tone, learners may become accustomed to not assessing for those factors or recognizing their clinical significance. In addition, skipping key steps in procedures such as obtaining informed consent or using proper personal protective equipment may lead to similar shortcuts with actual patients. It is important for educators to consider the goals and objectives of their simulation and ensure all essential elements are addressed to meet those goals in order to avoid reinforcing poor behaviors [76].

SBME is also a resource-intensive educational strategy that can impact its feasibility and sustainability [25]. Required assets to consider include [43]:

1. *People*: This includes both the availability of trained facilitators able to develop and conduct SBME as well as the availability of learners to participate in SBME. This can be particularly challenging within graduate medical education/residency training, where protected time for educational activities may be more limited due to competing clinical and educational requirements.
2. *Time*: This should include both the time to properly plan, conduct, and evaluate the SBME. When considering the time needed to conduct SBME, it is important to factor in not only the time of the simulation scenario itself but also sufficient time to properly debrief the simulation. A general rule of thumb is that the debrief should be two to three times the length of the simulation.
3. *Resources*: There is a variety of supplies and equipment needed, depending on the modality of the simulation that will be discussed later in this chapter. Considerations include sufficient access to manikins, task trainers, and additional procedural supplies. It should also be determined what space will be utilized, which could involve additional cost considerations for possible fees to utilize simulation centers.

There is a wide spectrum of resources available across programs. Some programs have access to extensive assets through institutional simulation centers, while other programs rely heavily on grassroots efforts from chief residents. Even centers with theoretical access to extensive local resources may have limited realistic access to those resources due to cost-prohibitive fees and/or competition from other programs and learners. It is therefore important for programs to consider ways to implement their SBME in a way that is practical and sustainable for their specific local needs and resources.

One way to overcome challenges related to resource access is through collaboration with other groups across institutions. Partnering with other specialties or disciplines may provide access to additional resources or the opportunity to pool funds to benefit both teams. This also opens the door for interprofessional simulations, which can help expand resources as well as provide invaluable opportunities to include interprofessional education in the simulation curricula.

There are also opportunities to make use of publicly available resources to limit the time and resources required to develop SBME. For example, AAMC MedEdPortal provides open access to many peer-reviewed simulation scenarios, so programs do not need to develop those internally. The American Academy of Pediatrics also created Peds Vitals, a free app to use as a pediatric patient monitor to display vital signs during simulations, which can be beneficial for programs lacking access to related technological resources.

It is also important to recognize that there are ways to be more cost-effective and resource-sparing without necessarily harming the educational impact of the simulation. Low-technology simulations can still provide high educational value. Programs should be cognizant of when more cost-effective methods could be used to best allocate available resources. For procedure-based training, many educators have found creative alternatives to high-cost task trainers to be able to provide impactful training without significant cost. Examples include the use of polenta and paintballs to replicate a superficial soft tissue abscess on ultrasonographic examination, the use of chicken in training peripheral IV placement, and the use of bananas in practicing suture techniques [4, 61, 63, 80].

Finally, there are opportunities to explore additional funding, including the Association of Pediatric Program Directors Special Projects funds, Grants & Special Projects—Association of Pediatric Program Directors (appd.org), International Network for Simulation-based Pediatric Innovation, Research and Education funding awards, and the Society of Simulation in Healthcare SSH Early Career Mentored Research Award.

An additional challenge to SBME is ensuring the education is high-quality and standardized across learners. Adhering to SBME best practices can help address those concerns and is important for residency programs to consider when implementing SBME within their curriculum. One help-

Table 19.1 International Nursing Association for Clinical Simulation and Learning (INACSL) healthcare simulation standard of best practice [75]

Standards of Best Practice	Details
Professional Development	Initial and ongoing professional development supports the simulationist across their career. As the practice of simulation-based education grows, professional development allows the simulationist to stay current with new knowledge, provide high-quality simulation experiences, and meet the educational needs of the learners.
Prebriefing	Prebriefing is a process that involves preparation and briefing. Prebriefing ensures that simulation learners are prepared for the educational content and are aware of the ground rules for the simulation-based experience.
Simulation Design	Simulation-based experiences are purposefully designed to meet identified objectives and optimize achievement of expected outcomes.
Facilitation	Facilitation methods are varied, and the use of a specific method is dependent on the learning needs of the learner and the expected outcomes. Facilitation provides the structure and process to guide participants to work cohesively, to comprehend learning objectives, and to develop a plan to achieve desired outcomes.
The Debriefing Process	All SBE activities must include a planned debriefing process. This debriefing process may include any of the activities of feedback, debriefing, and/or guided reflection.
Operations	All simulation-based education programs require systems and infrastructure to support and maintain operations.
Outcomes & Objectives	All simulation-based experiences originate with the development of measurable objectives designed to achieve expected behaviors and outcomes.
Professional Integrity	Professional integrity refers to the ethical behaviors and conduct that are expected of all involved throughout simulation-based experiences: facilitators, learners, and participants.
Simulation-Enhanced-IPE	Simulation-enhanced interprofessional education (Sim-IPE) enables learners from different healthcare professions to engage in a simulation-based experience to achieve linked or shared objectives and outcomes.
Evaluation of Learning and Performance	Simulation-based experiences may include evaluation of the learner.

ful resource to be aware of is the International Nursing Association for Clinical Simulation and Learning (INACSL) Standard of Best Practice [75] that is intended to guide the integration, use, and advancement of simulation-based experiences within academia, clinical practice, and research. It provides evidence-based guidelines and best practices for ten standards related to SBME (Table 19.1).

Simulation Formats

There are various aspects of simulation that should be considered when implementing this educational strategy into pediatric residency education, including modality, fidelity, and location.

Modalities There are a variety of modalities that can be considered when developing a simulation. Modality refers to the type(s) of simulation being used as part of the simulation activity [41]. The optimal choice depends both on the goals and objectives of the session as well as what is locally available and feasible for the training program (Table 19.2).

Fidelity Fidelity refers to the degree to which the simulation replicates the real event and the ability of the simulation to reproduce the reactions, interactions, and responses of the real-world counterpart [41]. There are various elements of fidelity that are important to consider when developing and implementing SBME, which include but are not limited to:

- *Conceptual fidelity*: The degree to which all elements of the scenario relate to each other in a realistic way so that the case makes sense as a whole to the learner(s) (e.g., vital signs are consistent with the diagnosis).

Table 19.2 Modalities in simulation-based medical education

Modality	Definition [41]	Examples
Manikin	A life-sized simulator representing a patient for health care simulation and education	A pediatric manikin with realistic exam features and physiological responses to use in a clinical scenario on the management of sepsis
Task trainers	A device designed to train in just the key elements of the procedure or skill being learned, such as lumbar puncture, chest tube insertion, and central line insertion	Lumbar puncture model for learning the steps to procedural skills
Standardized patients	Simulation using a person or persons trained to portray a patient scenario or actual patient(s) for health care education	An actor portraying a parent in a scenario focused on delivering difficult news
Remote simulation/ telesimulation	Utilizes communications technology to provide … simulation education between learners and instructors located remotely from one another	Off-site learners interact with an instructor in a simulation center via a video conferencing platform to walk through the management of a pediatric code event
Augmented reality	An interactive experience of a real-world environment where the objects are enhanced by computer-generated perceptual information	Learner wears augmented reality glasses that overlay an anatomical model on a physical simulation manikin
Virtual reality	Use of computer technology to create an interactive three-dimensional world in which the objects have a sense of spatial presence	Using a head-mount display to visualize the insertion of an umbilical venous catheter and walk through the required steps
Hybrid	The union of two or more modalities of simulation with the aim of providing a more realistic experience.	A standardized patient wearing a peripheral IV insertion task training for a simulation focused on procedural skills as well as communication with the patient during the procedure

- *Physical fidelity*: The degree to which the simulation looks, sounds, and feels like the actual task (e.g., the room set-up and equipment align with the learner's clinical environment).
- *Psychological fidelity*: The extent to which the simulated environment evokes the underlying psychological processes necessary in the real-world setting. (e.g., incorporating alarms or other background noises from a busy emergency department setting may help to better replicate the stress and pressure experienced by the provider during an actual clinical scenario).

It is important to note that "high-fidelity" does not always equate with high technology, as it is possible to achieve a highly realistic simulation with both high and low technology equipment, depending on how the scenario is designed and its learning objectives. For example, simulations focused on handoffs or other communication skills may be most effective and realistic utilizing standardized patients and a low-technology manikin to represent the patient. Having overly technologically complex manikin features in such a scenario may, in fact, distract the participant from the objectives of the session, making it seem less realistic, and decreasing the fidelity of the simulation.

It is also important to note that high-fidelity SBME does not always lead to higher levels of learning. The INACSL Standards of Best Practice [34] does not recommend a specific level of fidelity but rather that the level of realism should be what aligns best with the learning objectives of the simulation [39]. For example, for a simulation on peripheral IV insertion, a simple arm task trainer may be best for focusing on supplies needed or identifying landmarks, while a more advanced life-like manikin may be less well suited for practicing the intended procedure.

Location There are also various locations where SBME can take place, with their own respective benefits and limitations. It is again important to match the location to both the objectives of the session as well as the practical resources for the program.

1. In situ simulations: Simulations that take place in the actual patient care setting/environment [41]. Benefits of this format include enhanced fidelity or realism in the actual clinical setting, potential cost savings without the need to pay fees associated with simulation centers, and potential time savings without the need to relocate the learners. Challenges to this format to consider include safety factors to ensure simulation equipment does not get mixed in with actual patient care equipment.
2. Center-based simulations: Simulations that take place in facilities explicitly designed for training purposes. Benefits of this format include the ability to modify the environment to meet the needs of the session and the potential to enhance psychological safety by having a distinct location for SBME separate from the clinical environment, which can support confidentiality and focus. Challenges to this location include limitations in sufficiently mimicking the clinical environment and potential cost considerations for any fees for utilizing the space.
3. Computer-based simulations: The modeling of real-life processes with inputs and outputs exclusively confined to a computer [41]. Benefits of this format include the ability to standardize and replicate the learning experience, include remote learners, and conduct asynchronous simulations, which could help address time limitations. Challenges to this format include the lack of hands-on skills as well as the potential limited realism of the session.

Debriefing

High-quality debriefing is imperative in SBME. There is a saying in simulation that simulation is an excuse to debrief, highlighting the invaluable role the debriefing stage plays in the educational impact of SBME. There are a variety of debriefing techniques that can be utilized within pediatric residency simulation education [22, 60]. Some commonly referenced formats include Plus-Delta [18], GAS (gather, analyze, summarize), and Debriefing with Good Judgement [58]. Most models include three phases: the reaction phase, where learners are allowed to explore their own reactions and emotions following the simulation, the analysis phase, which focuses on what the learners did and thought during the simulation and why, and the summary phase which focuses on applications from what was discussed in the analysis phase and how it connects back to the clinical setting.

Regardless of technique, essential elements of debriefing have been outlined [60], including

1. Things to do prior to the debrief:
   - Ensuring psychological safety: Psychological safety is defined as a feeling within a simulation-based activity that participants are comfortable participating, speaking up, sharing thoughts, and asking for help as needed without concern for retribution or embarrassment [41]
   - Basic assumption [14]: A core value within SBME to help promote psychological safety based on the belief that everyone participating is intelligent, capable, cares about doing their best, and wants to improve
   - Establishing rules such as expectations on participation and maintaining confidentiality
2. Things to do during the debrief:
   - Establishing a shared mental model, reviewing the events to ensure a shared understanding of what occurred
   - Addressing learning objectives
   - Asking open-ended questions
   - Using silence

Ensuring sufficient training for simulation debriefers is essential to providing high-quality, effective SBME. While there are a variety of training resources available, they can be both cost and time-prohibitive. Programs should assess what training may be available to them locally as well as externally. An additional resource to be aware of is the PEARLS framework [7], a tool intended to fill this need for educators learning to facilitate SBME debriefs that integrates three common educational strategies and serves as a cognitive aid for debriefing.

Simulation Societies/Networks/ Collaborations

There are numerous organizations and networks focused on SBME and pediatric simulation education specifically. These organizations can be beneficial resources for pediatric residency programs looking to advance their simulation training, as well as looking for opportunities for collaboration and research within pediatric simulation education (Table 19.3).

Table 19.3 Overview of common organizations/groups related to pediatric simulation-based medical education

Group	Goal/mission	Website
American Academy of Pediatrics Section on Simulation and Innovative Learning Methods (SOSILM)	Supports the education and research interests of American Academy of Pediatrics members engaged in simulation and innovative learning in order to attain optimal physical, mental, and social health and well-being for all infants, children, adolescents, and young adults	https://www.aap.org/en/community/aap-sections/simulation-and-innovative-learning-methods/
Association of Pediatric Program Directors Healthcare Simulation in Pediatrics Learning Community	Serve as a resource in simulation for residency and fellowship programs to help advance everyone's work in simulation, regardless of level of expertise	https://www.appd.org/community/healthcare-simulation-in-pediatrics/
International Meeting on Simulation in Healthcare (IMSH)	Scientific conference that explores the latest innovations and best practices in healthcare simulation and provides the tools and resources healthcare professionals need to advance their skills, impact change in delivery systems and practice, and, ultimately, to improve patient safety	https://imsh2024.org/
International Network for Simulation-based Pediatric Innovation, Research, & Education (INSPIRE)	Collaborative group of simulation experts, clinicians, educators, investigators, statisticians, human factors researchers, and psychologists who have one common goal & mission to serve as a global community that catalyzes discoveries and promotes collaboration in simulation-based research, scholarship, and innovation	https://inspiresim.org/
International Pediatric Simulation Society (IPSS)	Global community of pediatricians, pediatric subspecialists, pediatric nurses, advanced practice providers, educators, and other allied health professionals from over 30 countries, all dedicated to improving the care of infants and children worldwide through multidisciplinary, simulation-based education, training, and research in pediatric simulation	https://www.ipss.org/
Society for Simulation in Healthcare	The Society for Simulation in Healthcare serves members by fostering education, professional development, and the advancement of research and innovation, promotes the profession of healthcare simulation through standards and ethics, and champions healthcare simulation through advocating, sharing, facilitating, and collaborating	https://www.ssih.org/

Specific Uses of SBME in Pediatric Residency

Simulation Education for Procedures

Procedural education expectations for pediatric residents are fluid and changing, with pediatric residencies often having different expectations for demonstration of competence. Discussions with pediatric residency program directors demonstrate evidence that all programs struggle to ensure adequate training in procedural skills for pediatric residents, with varying strategies and challenges defining competency and standardizing expectations for their residents [23]. Simulation has been increasingly used as an important resource to fill gaps in residents' clinical exposure to procedures [51]. Surveys of pediatric program directors have indicated that while simulation can be used to teach many pediatric procedures, program directors believe simulation is especially helpful to teach bag-mask ventilation, neonatal intubation, intraosseous line placement, and defibrillation [26]. The 2025 ACGME requirements significantly moved away from providing a long list of predefined procedures for all pediatric residents to learn during their training. Procedures that remain in the 2025 General Pediatric Residency requirements are: bag-mask ventilation, lumbar puncture, neonatal delivery room stabilization, peripheral intravenous catheter placement, and simple laceration repair. Programs are also required to provide opportunities for residents to perform other procedures, as applicable to each resident's future career plans [2]. Programs must also balance providing additional time for residents to have access to procedures that they will further hone during future fellowship training, with ensuring they leave residency with the necessary general pediatrics knowledge to safely care for pediatric patients in their future clinical environments. Residents planning to practice in areas where they will have access to fewer subspecialty resources may need to spend additional time developing competence in procedures necessary to stabilize neonates and children for transport to higher levels of care.

Practical Considerations for Simulation-Based Procedural Training

In general, learning objectives for procedural training should be concrete and observable. Early objectives often require knowledge of the necessary equipment and the different steps of a procedure, with a focus on the how. Task trainers are readily available for various procedures, including lumbar puncture, bag-mask ventilation, intravenous catheter placement, and laceration repair; however, there is significant variation in the quality and fidelity of each of these task trainers. Additionally, commercially available task trainers are not always produced in infant or smaller child sizes, so educators wishing to use commercially available task trainers may need to settle for using ones designed to replicate adult patients. Various types of "homemade" task trainers have also been described, including some using fruit, animal products, or household items to replicate certain procedures. Thus, educators wishing to teach a specific task would be recommended to not only consult with local simulation experts but also potentially conduct a search for techniques when planning their sessions.

Given the variability in task trainers, it is recommended that educators spend time practicing on the trainer they are planning to use so they understand the intricacies of the trainer and know how to troubleshoot it. Compared to simulations designed to teach medical management or communication-focused skills (see below), procedural education likely benefits from smaller learner-to-facilitator ratios and requires that each learner get time for hands-on practice. Facilitators may also find that rather than writing a longer script and waiting for residents to complete the entire scenario, residents will likely most benefit from coaching with frequent stops for feedback and to practice specific steps. Finally, since procedural education is often focused on the hands-on skills of performing the procedure, educators may need to deliberately incorporate information about not only how to do the procedure but also when and why—i.e., the indications, contraindications, and complications for each procedure. A related step, which may or may not be incorporated into the same educational session, is ensuring residents practice obtaining informed consent for procedures. The approach to using simulation to obtain informed consent is generally more similar to other communication-focused educational activities (see below).

Studies have demonstrated the positive impact of incorporating simulation-based video-recorded formative assessments, including direct and indirect feedback, on senior pediatric residents' perceptions of their own procedural knowledge, skills, and confidence, with an association with increased procedural engagement [29]. However, educators should be warned that while simulation can be used for exposure and has been shown to impact residents' self-confidence and perceived competence in individual skills, care should be taken to consider how to best measure or evaluate procedural performance in the simulation and clinical environments [5, 44, 49]. Many existing published assessments of procedural competence use checklists to ensure residents are completing all the necessary steps of a procedure, including considerations about obtaining consent and following sterile technique. However, educators should note that these checklist-based assessments can help ensure learners know the various steps of a procedure, but are not designed to assess proceduralists' understanding of the nuances of procedures, including positioning and troubleshooting, which can be the difference between a successful and unsuccessful procedure. Thus, competence in knowing the steps of a procedure or even successful completion of any one procedure does not guarantee future success, and educators may want to provide feedback during training that focuses not only on performing the procedure but also on discussions of what to do when procedures do not go smoothly and how to approach more challenging scenarios.

Bag-Mask Ventilation

Bag-mask ventilation is commonly referred to as the most important life-saving skill for pediatricians, as most pediatric cardiac arrests are secondary to respiratory arrest or failure. Residents are generally expected to become certified in the Neonatal Resuscitation Program (NRP) and Pediatric Advanced Life Support (PALS), which heavily relies on simulation to teach hands-on skills. Given that NRP and PALS certification is expected to be renewed every two years, most pediatric residents will need to renew their training at least once during their three years of training. However, evidence exists that relying on refresher training every two years is not enough to maintain competence in resuscitation skills and knowledge [51]. Very few to no studies have specifically and rigorously evaluated or even attempted to define competence in bag-mask ventilation; however, tools do exist to assist educators in rating pediatric residents' proficiency in performing airway skills in the simulated environment [77].

There is significant variability between airway manikins, with variability in fidelity, and no commercially available manikin completely realistically mimicking real-life human skin and soft tissues and the nuances of how to position patients to optimally provide respiratory support. Educators must also consider how different hospitals use different airway equipment, with some hospitals primarily using flow-inflating bags and others using self-inflating bags. Thus, educators should strive to adjust their learning sessions to ideally use locally available equipment; depending on the learner level and objectives of the session, they may also want to provide exposure to other equipment. While simulation-based interventions have been associated with increased resident confidence in bag-mask ventilation [28, 66], it is not clear if simulation-based training in bag-mask ventilation directly translates to residents' skills in actual practice, especially when considering the spectrum of pediatrics and how the pediatric airway changes from premature infants to older adolescents. Finally, it is unclear how often pediatric residents in the modern era are getting the opportunity to practice bag-mask ventilation on real patients; a review of a multi-institutional database describing pediatric endotracheal intubations indicates that pediatric residents are rarely the first-attempt providers in the emergency department and intensive care unit [13]. Thus, while simulation-based training is an important first step for developing competence in bag-mask ventilation, given the limitations in simulators, programs may need to spend additional effort to ensure residents have access to this skill in real patients. There is also an opportunity for the potential development of new, more realistic bag-mask ventilation trainers or the incorporation of video to help residents gain airway skills [50].

Lumbar Puncture

Lumbar puncture is a commonly performed diagnostic procedure as part of standard evaluation for neonatal sepsis, as well as a diagnostic and therapeutic modality for patients across the age spectrum with primary neurologic diseases. However, advances in vaccines have led to changes in the microbiology of neonatal sepsis and decreased incidence of neonatal meningitis; consequently, iterative studies have worked to evaluate and redefine protocols for evaluating infants with fevers, such that current pediatric trainees perform fewer lumbar punctures compared to prior generations of pediatricians. Studies have demonstrated that pediatric residents are often unsuccessful in performing lumbar punctures in both the simulated [55] and real clinical environments [37, 65]. Simulation-based training has had mixed effects, with one study indicating a decrease in residents' anxiety and improvement in their competence with the procedure [48], but another study demonstrating greater adherence to certain steps of the procedure but no change in first-attempt success [37].

Lumbar puncture task trainers exist, with variability in size/age of patient and also quality or fidelity of the trainer; nonetheless, any trainer can be used to help pediatric residents learn and practice the steps of the procedure. As with bag-mask ventilation, educators should seek to use the same lumbar puncture kits or equipment that are used in the actual clinical environment. Various checklist-based assessment tools have been created to assist educators in evaluating whether residents perform the various steps of the procedure [27, 35, 38]. A very important step in lumbar puncture is positioning the patient, which may be glossed over when using a task trainer since these are often manufactured to be in either the lateral recumbent or upright position, and so residents do not need to go through the process of positioning the simulated patient in the same way that they would need to do for real patients. Thus, educators should pay special attention to ensuring residents discuss and demonstrate positioning when training them using existing lumbar puncture trainers. Simulation facilitators may also want to consider how or when to have residents practice obtaining opening pressures when performing a lumbar puncture. Finally, specific training may be needed to ensure residents know how to properly obtain informed consent for lumbar punctures [52].

Other ACGME-Mandated Procedures

While listed as a procedure by the ACGME, neonatal delivery stabilization is a type of resuscitation that involves a combination of skills, procedures, and knowledge, and will be discussed in more detail in the next section. Less has been published about the impact and use of simulation for teaching pediatric residents, peripheral intravenous catheter placement, and simple laceration repair. However, trainers exist for both procedures and thus both are amenable to simulation-based education, with similar caveats discussed above regarding the limitations of trainer-based simulations. Interest is increasing in the use of ultrasound to place peripheral intravenous catheters, although there is likely significant variability between programs in whether or how this skill is taught to pediatric residents, and there is a dearth of trainers available that can represent the full range of pediatric patients. Scales and checklists exist to assist educators in teaching and evaluating pediatric residents performing laceration repairs [64], and multiple techniques exist for low-cost fruit- or animal-based trainers.

Other Non-mandated Procedures

Pediatric residents may also benefit from exposure to other procedures, all of which are amenable to simulation-based training. A Delphi study of a group of experts in pediatric simulation-based medical education indicated that the following procedures were important to teach pediatric residents using simulation-based education: placement of an intraosseous line, management of tracheostomy tubes (suctioning, exchange), changing a gastrostomy tube, needle decompression of a pneumothorax, splinting of fractures, incision and drainage of an abscess, and bladder catheterization [33]. It would be difficult for any one program to seek to ensure each of their residents has exposure, let alone demonstrates competence, to each of these procedures; however, program leadership should be aware that these procedures are all amenable to simulation-based training and can consider how to make these educational experiences available for residents who either have an interest in them or require them for their careers after residency.

Simulation Education for Medical Knowledge and Clinical Decision-Making

In general, simulation for the purpose of helping pediatric residents learn or practice the management of certain disease presentations can be performed with larger groups of learners compared to simulation for procedural training. Learning objectives for these types of simulations may also include some hands-on or procedurally focused objectives, but more often include objectives that focus on team functioning or communication, medical decision-making, and developing or practicing patient care algorithms. These types of simulations can occur in both the simulation lab environment and in situ in the clinical environment. Educators should also consider the composition of their learner groups—whether they are composed of residents of the same or a mix of levels of training, or if nonphysician healthcare providers should also take part in the simulation. Simulation has also increasingly been used to assess and inform pediatric quality and safety initiatives, which also directly impact residents' clinical environments.

Since the learning objectives are generally more focused on the diagnosis and management of certain disease processes, high-fidelity manikins are often used for these types of simulations that allow for the ability to display vital signs and administer medications or other therapies to the simulated patient; however, simulation using low-fidelity manikins can also yield similar learning outcomes. Simulation scenarios for these types of sessions should be tailored to the expected actions and knowledge of each learner group. Practically, while the learner group may be bigger, the facilitator-to-learner ratio may still be similar to procedural training. It is often helpful to have one educator designated as the main facilitator and dedicated to observing the scenario, while other persons may function as either embedded participant(s) (i.e., playing the roles of a nurse or parent), and a third person focusing on adjusting vital signs in real-time in response to learners' actions. Regardless of the composition of the educator team, facilitators should ensure that at least half of the simulation time is reserved for debriefing.

Resuscitation

As noted above, residents are taught pediatric cardiac arrest protocols during NRP and PALS; however, since these courses are only renewed every two years and these types of cardiac arrest scenarios are relatively rare in pediatrics, it is common for resuscitation skills and knowledge to decay in the months after training. Various studies have demonstrated a favorable impact of simulation-based resuscitation training (outside of NRP or PALS) on residents' resuscitation skills and confidence with those skills, often in the pediatric intensive care unit, neonatal intensive care unit, or pediatric emergency department environments [20, 30, 57, 67, 70]. Studies have also demonstrated how simulation-based training can help residents learn more about the equipment necessary during emergent situations [79] and assist with residents' feelings of self-confidence and preparedness for these situations [32]. It is important to note that while resuscitation events may take longer, simulation sessions designed for pediatric residents may want to focus on the first five minutes of resuscitation events—i.e., the recognition, call for help, and initial management—as in most clinical situations, additional assistance would have arrived after five minutes [78].

Clinical Management and Skills

Published scenarios and simulation-based curricula exist for a large variety of noncardiac arrest scenarios, and simulation has been utilized to help teach disease processes affecting every organ system and in most clinical environments. Simulation-based medical education experts have recommended a long list of topics that are important to teach pediatric residents using simulation-based education (Table 19.4), although educators should not feel constrained to these topics. Efforts should be made to maximize fidelity and spend time orienting learners to the simulation environment, including what the manikin can and cannot do, as well as where learners should look for information not obtainable in the simulation environment. For example, neurologic function and abdominal exams are often difficult to simulate with commonly available manikins. Doing so should minimize the amount of time learners spend confused or misled by artifactual elements native to the simulation environment. As noted above, facilitators should ensure there is sufficient time to fully debrief the scenario. Educators may also choose to set aside time to repeat parts of the scenario, especially if the learning objectives revolve around the deployment of certain algorithms.

Communication within the medical team and team leadership are important components of medical management. PALS does include components that discuss team communication, with an emphasis on closed-loop communication; however, the majority of PALS focuses on understanding and applying clinical algorithms. While the majority of simulation-based curricula include objectives that focus on residents' medical management of patients requiring either urgent or emergent intervention, relatively few studies have evaluated the impact of these scenarios on pediatric residents' leadership and communication. Nonetheless, objectives focusing on leadership, communication, and shared decision-making can often be included in the same scenarios that focus on clinical management and skills. Educators wishing to help residents learn or practice communication or leadership skills should build in time specifically for this purpose and may consider using less complicated or challenging scenarios so that residents can focus on the nonmedical knowledge aspects of the experience. Some studies have also begun exploring the impact of the relatively simple intervention of blindfolding team leaders on

Table 19.4 Disease processes (diagnosis and management) teachable using simulation

Respiratory distress (Newborn)	Pulseless electrical activity
Respiratory Failure (Child)	Asystole
Sepsis	Supraventricular Tachycardia
Seizures/Status Epilepticus	Ventricular Tachycardia (no Pulse)
Pediatric Trauma	Ventricular Fibrillation
Asthma Exacerbation/Wheezing	Bradycardia
Allergic Reaction/Anaphylaxis	Cardiogenic Shock
Suspected Child Abuse	Uncompensated Shock
Increased Intracranial Pressure	Hypovolemic Shock
Upper Airway Obstruction	Neurogenic Shock/Spinal Cord Injuries
Pneumothorax	Acute Hemorrhage
Cyanotic Congenital Heart Lesion	Hyperkalemia/Electrolyte Disturbances
Altered Mental Status	Severe Hypertension
Disordered Control of Breathing	Heart Failure
Hypoglycemia	Stroke
Foreign Body Aspiration	Traumatic Brain Injury
Transfusion Reaction	Oncologic Emergencies

Adapted from: Huber et al. [33]

team communication characteristics, with promising results [12, 42, 62].

Simulation for Assessment of Residents' Clinical Progress

Some pediatric residency programs are using simulation not only as a component of their educational delivery but also as a way of assessing residents' clinical skills. A survey of pediatric simulation experts and pediatric program directors asking about current use of simulation for assessment demonstrated that few use simulation for summative assessment, with respondents indicating that subcompetencies relating to interprofessional teamwork, clinical decision-making, and effective communication are ones most suitable for assessment using simulation [45]. There is also a published example of how a pediatric program developed formative and summative simulation cases, and demonstrated a significant relationship between scores on the summative cases and Pediatric Milestones' scores as determined by the program's clinical competency committee [24]. While more work needs to be done in this area, observed simulated clinical encounters for use with pediatric residents have been published and are available for programs interested in adding simulation-based clinical assessments to their educational programs [9, 36, 46].

Simulation Education for Interpersonal and Communication Skills

As opposed to simulation being performed for procedural skills or medical management purposes, simulation education designed to improve residents' interpersonal communication skills with patients or families is generally best performed using standardized patients. Working with standardized patients can, over time, be more costly than a one-time purchase of a task trainer or manikin; however, current technology is generally not available to replicate the experience of practicing communication skills with another human. For ease or financial purposes, educators may also consider having either faculty or peers play the role of a parent or patient; doing so should be balanced with an understanding of the limitations of potentially interfering with the realism of the scenario due to participants either working with someone they know or with someone who does not have adequate training to play the role. Communication-focused simulations generally benefit from having one-on-one feedback from facilitators to learners, although some models also employ having other learners observe and provide feedback to their peers.

In general, rather than writing scenarios that include vital signs or significant medical information, scenarios for communication-focused skills should include some general information about the patient and the current situation for the learner to know. Whoever is playing the role of the parent or patient should also be provided with a script to guide them in how they may want to react or respond to certain pieces of information. This is especially important to maintain some amount of standardization of residents' experiences. Facilitators may also want to employ components of rapid cycle deliberate practice, with the ability for learners, standardized patients, or facilitators to call for a pause to discuss particularly challenging aspects of the conversation before returning to the simulated scene and potentially allowing the learner to immediately apply certain concepts or practice certain ways of phrasing information.

Challenging Conversations with Parents/Families

Multiple studies have been done to evaluate the impact of communication-focused simulation interventions on healthcare professionals' communication skills. A 2018 review of the impact of simulation-based education on healthcare providers' communication skills found that most research at that time explored benefits only at lower levels of evaluation (reaction and learning), with limited understanding of the long-term impacts of these educational interventions or how to best deliver them [10]. Nonetheless, individual studies of communication-focused simulation-based interventions have demonstrated improvements in pediatric residents' self-perceived skills, preparedness, and competence in delivering difficult news and end-of-life discussions [3, 47, 53]. "SPIKES" is a common mnemonic used to help learners deliver difficult news [6]. While standardized patients are currently most utilized, advances in technology may eventually assist in helping medical trainees practice these skills. As an example, a novel study utilized virtual reality to teach pediatric residents communication skills when discussing influenza vaccine hesitancy and found that residents who had undergone the virtual reality intervention had significantly fewer vaccine refusals among their actual patients in the months following the intervention, compared to residents who had undergone standard training [56].

Simulation: Optimizing Equity and Mitigating Bias

Despite increased attention to the historical and systemic underpinnings of health inequities and the widespread acknowledgment of the prevalence of bias within medicine, these topics are often difficult to discuss and address. Simulation provides an opportunity for healthcare providers to practice recognizing and proactively addressing situations where biased behavior is impacting a patient, family member, colleague, or other healthcare worker. Simulation has been used to evaluate the influence of sociodemographic characteristics on medical decision-making and identify biases [11, 40, 71], as well as help healthcare providers learn how to identify biased care in themselves and others [8, 31, 73].

When writing simulation cases, educators should also be mindful of how and when sociodemographic information is included and monitor for anchoring biases, as well as be cognizant of potential biases that may exist among faculty and facilitators [72]. Accordingly, using standardized checklists and objective measures for evaluation of trainees—especially if simulation is being used as a formative assessment—may help mitigate biases that may exist against trainees of certain backgrounds. Simulation involving standardized patients can also involve biases [54], and training has even been described for teaching standardized patients who work in healthcare simulation to be less biased in their own work [74]. Educators wishing to use simulation to teach residents behavioral skills related to equity, diversity, and inclusion are recommended to review existing literature [21] and consult with local experts in equity.

Next Steps/Future Opportunities

Looking forward in the field of SBME in pediatric training, there are multiple areas warranting additional focus and exploration.

There is a need for future work to further advance the impact of SBME on higher-level outcomes, including learner behaviors and patient outcomes, and comparative studies identifying optimal types and characteristics of impactful SBME [51]. In addition, there are opportunities for further work developing validated assessment tools to use within SBME to better understand the impact of the education as well as the performance of trainees.

As technology continues to develop, there are opportunities to incorporate new and innovative emerging tools into pediatric SBME. The fields of virtual reality/augmented reality are continuing to expand, with a need to better understand their use and impact within pediatric residency training.

The use of SBME for assessment will also likely continue to expand with the additional requirement to report on Entrustable Professional Activities.

There is also value in continuing to enhance the quality of SBME provided within pediatric residency education through the implementation of best practices and professional development training for facilitators. And to standardize training through a potential standard curriculum across programs [33].

Conclusion

SBME is a rapidly evolving and increasingly essential element of pediatric residency training. There is currently a wide array of uses within pediatric residency that helps programs to meet various requirements and supplement elements of their clinical and educational experiences. There are future steps to be taken to continue to optimize its integration within pediatric residency and better understand its impact on patient-centered outcomes.

References

1. Accreditation Council for Graduate Medical Education (ACGME). Pediatric Milestones [WWW Document]. 2021. https://www.acgme.org/globalassets/PDFs/Milestones/PediatricsMilestones.pdf. Accessed 8.9.2024.
2. Accreditation Council for Graduate Medical Education (ACGME). ACGME program requirements for graduate medical education in pediatrics. 2025.
3. Asuncion AM, Cagande C, Schlagle S, McCarty B, Hunter K, Milcarek B, Staman G, Da Silva S, Fisher D, Graessle W. A curriculum to improve residents' end-of-life communication and pain management skills during pediatrics intensive care rotation: pilot study. J Grad Med Educ. 2013;5:510–3. https://doi.org/10.4300/JGME-D-12-00148.1.
4. Augenstein JA, Yoshida H, Lo MD, Solari P. A readily available, inexpensive, and reusable simulation model for teaching ultrasound-guided abscess identification and drainage. J Emerg Med. 2016;50:462–5. https://doi.org/10.1016/j.jemermed.2015.12.020.
5. Augustine EM, Kahana M. Effect of procedure simulation workshops on resident procedural confidence and competence. J Grad Med Educ. 2012;4:479–85. https://doi.org/10.4300/JGME-D-12-00019.1.
6. Baile WF, Buckman R, Lenzi R, Glober G, Beale EA, Kudelka AP. SPIKES—A six-step protocol for delivering bad news: application to the patient with cancer. Oncologist. 2000;5:302–11. https://doi.org/10.1634/theoncologist.5-4-302.
7. Bajaj K, Meguerdichian M, Thoma B, Huang S, Eppich W, Cheng A. The PEARLS healthcare debriefing tool. Acad Med. 2018;93:336. https://doi.org/10.1097/ACM.0000000000002035.
8. Barber Doucet H, Wilson T, Vrablik L, Wing R. Implicit bias and patient care: mitigating bias, preventing harm. MedEdPORTAL. 2023:11343. https://doi.org/10.15766/mep_2374-8265.11343.
9. Ben-Isaac E, Zipkin R, Thompson M. Modified objective structured clinical examinations for PL-3 pediatric residents. MedEdPORTAL. 2016:10382. https://doi.org/10.15766/mep_2374-8265.10382.
10. Blackmore A, Kasfiki EV, Purva M. Simulation-based education to improve communication skills: a systematic review and identification of current best practice. BMJ Simul Technol Enhanc Learn. 2018;4:159–64. https://doi.org/10.1136/bmjstel-2017-000220.
11. Brand G, Bonnamy J, Dix S, Morphet J, Molloy R, Davis J, Challis H, Watts A, Daniel M, D'Astoli P, Wise S, Sevenhuysen S. 'You don't see what I see': co-designing simulation to uncover and address cognitive bias in healthcare. Med Teach. 2024;46:885–8. https://doi.org/10.1080/0142159X.2024.2313581.
12. Buyck M, Manzano S, Haddad K, Moncousin A-C, Galetto-Lacour A, Blondon K, Karam O. Effects of blindfold on leadership in pediatric resuscitation simulation: a randomized trial. Front Pediatr. 2019;7:10. https://doi.org/10.3389/fped.2019.00010.
13. Capone CA, Emerson B, Sweberg T, Polikoff L, Turner DA, Adu-Darko M, Li S, Glater-Welt LB, Howell J, Brown CA, Donoghue A, Krawiec C, Shults J, Breuer R, Swain K, Shenoi A, Krishna AS, Al-Subu A, Harwayne-Gidansky I, Biagas KV, Kelly SP, Nuthall G, Panisello J, Napolitano N, Giuliano JS, Emeriaud G, Toedt-Pingel I, Lee A, Page-Goertz C, Kimura D, Kasagi M, D'Mello J, Parsons SJ, Mallory P, Gima M, Bysani GK, Motomura M, Tarquinio KM, Nett S, Ikeyama T, Shetty R, Sanders RC, Lee JH, Pinto M, Orioles A, Jung P, Shlomovich M, Nadkarni V, Nishisaki A, for the National Emergency Airway Registry for Children (NEAR4KIDS) Investigators, Pediatric Acute Lung Injury, Sepsis Investigators (PALISI). Intubation practice and outcomes among pediatric emergency departments: a report from National Emergency Airway Registry for Children (NEAR4KIDS). Acad Emerg Med. 2022;29:406–14. https://doi.org/10.1111/acem.14431.
14. Center for Medical Simulation. 2004. https://harvardmedsim.org/resources/the-basic-assumption/
15. Cheng A, Duff J, Grant E, Kissoon N, Grant VJ. Simulation in paediatrics: an educational revolution. Paediatr Child Health. 2007;12:465–8. https://doi.org/10.1093/pch/12.6.465.
16. Cheng A, Hunt EA, Donoghue A, Nelson-McMillan K, Nishisaki A, LeFlore J, Eppich W, Moyer M, Brett-Fleegler M, Kleinman M, Anderson J, Adler M, Braga M, Kost S, Stryjewski G, Min S, Podraza J, Lopreiato J, Hamilton MF, Stone K, Reid J, Hopkins J, Manos J, Duff J, Richard M, Nadkarni VM, Express Investigators FT. Examining pediatric resuscitation education using simulation and scripted debriefing: a multicenter randomized trial. JAMA Pediatr. 2013;167:528. https://doi.org/10.1001/jamapediatrics.2013.1389.
17. Cheng A, Lang TR, Starr SR, Pusic M, Cook DA. Technology-enhanced simulation and pediatric education: a meta-analysis. Pediatrics. 2014;133:e1313–23. https://doi.org/10.1542/peds.2013-2139.

18. Cheng A, Eppich W, Epps C, Kolbe M, Meguerdichian M, Grant V. Embracing informed learner self-assessment during debriefing: the art of plus-delta. Adv Simul. 2021;6:22. https://doi.org/10.1186/s41077-021-00173-1.
19. Cook DA, Hatala R, Brydges R, Zendejas B, Szostek JH, Wang AT, Erwin PJ, Hamstra SJ. Technology-enhanced simulation for health professions education: a systematic review and meta-analysis. JAMA. 2011;306 https://doi.org/10.1001/jama.2011.1234.
20. Couloures KG, Allen C. Use of simulation to improve cardiopulmonary resuscitation performance and code team communication for pediatric residents. MedEdPORTAL. 2017:10555. https://doi.org/10.15766/mep_2374-8265.10555.
21. Daya S, Illangasekare T, Tahir P, Bochatay N, Essakow J, Ju M, van Schaik S. Using simulation to teach learners in health care behavioral skills related to diversity, equity, and inclusion: a scoping review. Simul Healthc J Soc Simul Healthc. 2023;85:312–20.
22. Duff JP, Morse KJ, Seelandt J, Gross IT, Lydston M, Sargeant J, Dieckmann P, Allen JA, Rudolph JW, Kolbe M. Debriefing methods for simulation in healthcare: a systematic review. Simul Healthc J Soc Simul Healthc. 2024;19:S112–21. https://doi.org/10.1097/SIH.0000000000000765.
23. Forson-Dare Z, Du NR, Ocran A, Tiyyagura G, Bruno CJ, Johnston LC. How good is good enough?: current-day pediatric residency program directors' challenges in assessing and achieving resident procedural competency. Acad Pediatr. 2023;23:473–82. https://doi.org/10.1016/j.acap.2022.11.005.
24. Frey-Vogel AS, Scott-Vernaglia SE, Carter LP, Huang GC. Simulation for milestone assessment: use of a longitudinal curriculum for pediatric residents. Simul Healthc J Soc Simul Healthc. 2016;11:286–92. https://doi.org/10.1097/SIH.0000000000000162.
25. Frey-Vogel A, Rogers A, Sparger K, Mehta R, Mirchandani-Shah D, Mangold K, Mitchell D, Wood A, 2020. Taking the pulse on pediatric simulation: a national survey of pediatric residency programs' simulation practices and challenges. Pediatr Emerg Care. Publish Ahead of Print. https://doi.org/10.1097/PEC.0000000000002013
26. Gaies MG, Landrigan CP, Hafler JP, Sandora TJ. Assessing procedural skills training in pediatric residency programs. Pediatrics. 2007;120:715–22. https://doi.org/10.1542/peds.2007-0325.
27. Gerard JM, Kessler DO, Braun C, Mehta R, Scalzo AJ, Auerbach M. Validation of global rating scale and checklist instruments for the infant lumbar puncture procedure. Simul Healthc J Soc Simul Healthc. 2013;8:148–54. https://doi.org/10.1097/SIH.0b013e3182802d34.
28. Goldman MP, Bhatnagar A, Nagler J, Auerbach MA. Advanced pediatric emergency airway management: a multimodality curriculum addressing a rare but critical procedure. MedEdPORTAL. 2020:10962. https://doi.org/10.15766/mep_2374-8265.10962.
29. Goldman MP, Rudd AV, Baum SC, Nagler M, Weiss DL, Gross IT, Auerbach MA. Formative assessments promote procedural learning and engagement for senior pediatric residents on rotation in the pediatric emergency department. MedEdPORTAL. 2022;11265:10.15766/mep_2374-8265.11265.
30. Harwayne-Gidansky I, Askin G, Fein DM, McNamara C, Duncan E, Delaney K, Greenberg J, Mojica M, Clapper T, Ching K. Effectiveness of a simulation curriculum on clinical application: a randomized educational trial. Simul Healthc J Soc Simul Healthc. 2022;17:71–7. https://doi.org/10.1097/SIH.0000000000000598.
31. Holm AL, Rowe Gorosh M, Brady M, White-Perkins D. Recognizing privilege and bias: an interactive exercise to expand health care providers' personal awareness. Acad Med. 2017;92:360–4. https://doi.org/10.1097/ACM.0000000000001290.
32. Holzemer NF, Pomeranz ES, Tomlinson S. Improving the pediatric emergency department learning experience: a simulation-based orientation for pediatric PGY 1 residents. MedEdPORTAL. 2020:10919. https://doi.org/10.15766/mep_2374-8265.10919.
33. Huber L, Good R, Bone MF, Flood SM, Fredericks R, Overly F, Tofil NM, Wing R, Walsh K. A modified Delphi study for curricular content of simulation-based medical education for pediatric residency programs. Acad Pediatr. 2024;24:856–65. https://doi.org/10.1016/j.acap.2024.04.008.
34. INACSL standards of best practice: Simulation SM debriefing. Clin Simul Nurs. 2016;12:S21–S25. https://doi.org/10.1016/j.ecns.2016.09.008
35. Iyer MS, Santen SA, Nypaver M, Warrier K, Bradin S, Chapman R, McAllister J, Vredeveld J, House JB. Assessing the validity evidence of an objective structured assessment tool of technical skills for neonatal lumbar punctures. Acad Emerg Med. 2013;20:321–4. https://doi.org/10.1111/acem.12093.
36. Joorabchi B. objective structured clinical examination in a pediatric residency program. Am J Child. 1991;145(7):750–4.
37. Kessler D, Pusic M, Chang TP, Fein DM, Grossman D, Mehta R, White M, Jang J, Whit T. Impact of just-in-time and just-in-place simulation on intern success with infant lumbar puncture. Pediatrics. 2015;135:e1237–e124635.
38. Kessler DO, Chang TP, Auerbach M, Fein DM, Lavoie ME, Trainor J, Lee MO, Gerard JM, Grossman D, Whitfill T, Pusic M. Screening residents for infant lumbar puncture readiness with just-in-time simulation-based assessments. BMJ Simul Technol Enhanc Learn. 2017;3:17–22. https://doi.org/10.1136/bmjstel-2016-000130.
39. Kim J, Park J-H, Shin S. Effectiveness of simulation-based nursing education depending on fidelity: a meta-analysis. BMC Med Educ. 2016;16:152. https://doi.org/10.1186/s12909-016-0672-7.
40. Lebo C, Souza M, Atkins R, Woods L, Perron T, Jakubowski T, Brown N., n.d. Development of tele-

medicine simulations addressing social determinants of health. J Nurs Educ 2023 6(2):158-161.
41. Lioce L, editor. Healthcare simulation dictionary. 2nd ed. Agency for Healthcare Research and Quality; 2020. https://doi.org/10.23970/simulationv2.
42. Lopez De Alda JX, Patel N, McNinch N, Ahmed RA. A blindfolded pediatric trauma simulation and its effect on communication and crisis resource management skills. Cureus. 2021; https://doi.org/10.7759/cureus.19484.
43. Lopreiato JO, Sawyer T. Simulation-based medical education in pediatrics. Acad Pediatr. 2015;15:134–42. https://doi.org/10.1016/j.acap.2014.10.010.
44. Maleknia L, Boshuizen V, Caputo H, Shah R. Improving procedural skill confidence in pediatric residents: a longitudinal simulation-based workshop curriculum. MedEdPORTAL. 2023:11322. https://doi.org/10.15766/mep_2374-8265.11322.
45. Mallory LA, Calaman S, Lee White M, Doughty C, Mangold K, Lopreiato J, Auerbach M, Chang TP. Targeting simulation-based assessment for the pediatric milestones: a survey of simulation experts and program directors. Acad Pediatr. 2016;16:290–7. https://doi.org/10.1016/j.acap.2015.09.007.
46. Mangold KA, Jeffers JM, Burns RA, Trainor JL, Unti SM, Eppich W, Adler MD. An objective structured clinical examination to improve formative assessment for senior pediatrics residents. J Grad Med Educ. 2015;7:470–4. https://doi.org/10.4300/JGME-D-14-00777.1.
47. Marsh MC, Reed SM, Mahan JD, Schneider L, Fernandes AK, Liao N, Spears I, Lauden S. Advanced multimodal communication curriculum for pediatric residents. J Med Educat Curri Develop. 2021;8:238212052110352. https://doi.org/10.1177/23821205211035239.
48. McMillan HJ, Writer H, Moreau KA, Eady K, Sell E, Lobos A-T, Grabowski J, Doja A. Lumbar puncture simulation in pediatric residency training: improving procedural competence and decreasing anxiety. BMC Med Educ. 2016;16:198. https://doi.org/10.1186/s12909-016-0722-1.
49. Meerkov MS, Fischer JB, Saba TG. A simulation procedure curriculum to increase pediatric resident exposure to procedures rarely performed in clinical practice. Med Educ Online. 2019;24:1611305. https://doi.org/10.1080/10872981.2019.1611305.
50. Miller KA, Monuteaux MC, Aftab S, Lynn A, Hillier D, Nagler J. A randomized controlled trial of a video-enhanced advanced airway curriculum for pediatric residents. Acad Med. 2018;93:1858–64. https://doi.org/10.1097/ACM.0000000000002392.
51. Mills DM, Williams DC, Dobson JV. Simulation training as a mechanism for procedural and resuscitation education for pediatric residents: a systematic review. Hosp Pediatr. 2013;3:167–76. https://doi.org/10.1542/hpeds.2012-0041.
52. Omoruyi EA, Guardiola A, Barratt MS. Are incoming pediatric interns ready to obtain the essential components of an informed consent for lumbar puncture? Acad Pediatr. 2019;19:410–3. https://doi.org/10.1016/j.acap.2018.11.011.
53. Peterson EB, Porter MB, Calhoun AW. A simulation-based curriculum to address relational crises in medicine. J Grad Med Educ. 2012;4:351–6. https://doi.org/10.4300/JGME-D-11-00204.
54. Picketts L, Warren MD, Bohnert C. Diversity and inclusion in simulation: addressing ethical and psychological safety concerns when working with simulated participants. BMJ Simul Technol Enhanc Learn. 2021;7:590–9. https://doi.org/10.1136/bmjstel-2020-000853.
55. Pruden CM, Kerrey BT, Mittiga M, Del Rey JG. Procedural readiness of pediatric interns: defining novice performance through simulation. J Grad Med Educ. 2010;2:513–7. https://doi.org/10.4300/JGME-D-10-00092.1.
56. Real FJ, DeBlasio D, Beck AF, Ollberding NJ, Davis D, Cruse B, Samaan Z, McLinden D, Klein MD. A virtual reality curriculum for pediatric residents decreases rates of influenza vaccine refusal. Acad Pediatr. 2017;17(4):431–5.
57. Ross JC, Trainor JL, Eppich WJ, Adler MD. Impact of simulation training on time to initiation of cardiopulmonary resuscitation for first-year pediatrics residents. J Grad Med Educ. 2013;5:613–9. https://doi.org/10.4300/JGME-D-12-00343.1.
58. Rudolph JW, Simon R, Rivard P, Dufresne RL, Raemer DB. Debriefing with good judgment: combining rigorous feedback with genuine inquiry. Anesthesiol Clin. 2007;25:361–76. https://doi.org/10.1016/j.anclin.2007.03.007.
59. Sando CR, Coggins RM, Meakim C, Franklin AE, Gloe D, Boese T, Decker S, Lioce L, Borum JC. Standards of best practice: simulation standard VII: participant assessment and evaluation. Clin Simul Nurs. 2013;9:S30–2. https://doi.org/10.1016/j.ecns.2013.04.007.
60. Sawyer T, Eppich W, Brett-Fleegler M, Grant V, Cheng A. More than one way to debrief: a critical review of healthcare simulation debriefing methods. Simul Healthc J Soc Simul Healthc. 2016;11:209–17. https://doi.org/10.1097/SIH.0000000000000148.
61. Sawyer T, Gray M, Hendrickson M, Jacobson E, Umoren R. A Real human umbilical cord simulator model for emergency umbilical venous catheter placement training. Cureus. 2018; https://doi.org/10.7759/cureus.3544.
62. Scicchitano E, Stark P, Koetter P, Michalak N, Zurca AD. Blindfolding improves communication in inexperienced residents undergoing ACLS training. J Grad Med Educ. 2021;13:123–7. https://doi.org/10.4300/JGME-D-20-00620.1.
63. Selame LA, Risler Z, Zakaria SJ, Hughes LP, Lewiss RE, Kehm K, Goodsell K, Kalwani R, Mirsch D, Kluger SB, Au A. A comparison of homemade vascular access ultrasound phantom models for peripheral intravenous catheter insertion. J Vasc Access. 2021;22:891–7. https://doi.org/10.1177/1129729820961941.

64. Seo S, Thomas A, Uspal NG. A global rating scale and checklist instrument for pediatric laceration repair. MedEdPORTAL. 2019:10806. https://doi.org/10.15766/mep_2374-8265.10806.
65. Shafer S, Rooney D, Schumacher R, House JB. Lumbar punctures at an academic level 4 NICU: indications for a new curriculum. Teach Learn Med. 2015;27:205–7. https://doi.org/10.1080/10401334.2014.979185.
66. Smolcich A, Joseph Resch, Amanda Rogers, Robert Treat. The use of direct observation and an individualized simulation workshop is associated with improved resident confidence in bag mask ventilation and intubation skills. Acad Pediatr. n.d.;18:e5–6.
67. Surcouf JW, Chauvin SW, Ferry J, Yang T, Barkemeyer B. Enhancing residents' neonatal resuscitation competency through unannounced simulation-based training. Med Educ Online. 2013;18:18726. https://doi.org/10.3402/meo.v18i0.18726.
68. The American Board of Pediatrics. 2024. Entrustable professional activities.
69. To err is human: Building a safer health system. National Academies Press, Washington, DC; 2000. https://doi.org/10.17226/9728
70. Tofil NM, Benner KW, Zinkan L, Alten J, Varisco BM, White ML. Pediatric intensive care simulation course: a new paradigm in teaching. J Grad Med Educ. 2011;3:81–7. https://doi.org/10.4300/JGME-D-10-00070.1.
71. Tucker Edmonds B, McKenzie F, Fadel WF, Matthias MS, Salyers MP, Barnato AE, Frankel RM. Using simulation to assess the influence of race and insurer on shared decision making in periviable counseling. Simul Healthc. 2014;9(6):353–9.
72. Vora S, Dahlen B, Adler M, Kessler DO, Jones VF, Kimble S, Calhoun A. Recommendations and guidelines for the use of simulation to address structural racism and implicit bias. Simul Healthc J Soc Simul Healthc. 2021;16:275–84. https://doi.org/10.1097/SIH.0000000000000591.
73. Ward-Gaines J, Buchanan JA, Angerhofer C, McCormick T, Broadfoot KJ, Basha E, Blake J, Jones B, Sungar WG. Teaching emergency medicine residents health equity through simulation immersion. AEM Educ Train. 2021;5 https://doi.org/10.1002/aet2.10680.
74. Ward-Gaines J, Coyle T, Miller SK, Basha E, Jensen D, Lee R, Roosevelt G, Pierce C, Rustici M, Neumeier A. Creation and evaluation of a health equity certificate program for standardized patients. Acad Med. 2023;98:S190–1. https://doi.org/10.1097/ACM.0000000000005403.
75. Watts PI, Rossler K, Bowler F, Miller C, Charnetski M, Decker S, Molloy MA, Persico L, McMahon E, McDermott D, Hallmark B. Onward and upward: introducing the healthcare simulation standards of best PracticeTM. Clin Simul Nurs. 2021;58:1–4. https://doi.org/10.1016/j.ecns.2021.08.006.
76. Weller JM, Nestel D, Marshall SD, Brooks PM, Conn JJ. Simulation in clinical teaching and learning. Med J Aust. 2012;196:594. https://doi.org/10.5694/mja10.11474.
77. Wing R, Baird J, Duffy S, Brown L, Overly F, Kelley MN, Merritt C. Pediatric airway assessment tool (PAAT): a rating tool to assess resident proficiency in simulated pediatric airway skills performance. MedEdPORTAL. 2020:10997. https://doi.org/10.15766/mep_2374-8265.10997.
78. Wing R, Tsao HS, Toomey V, Mercurio L, Carillo M, Brown LL, Kelley MN. Excellence in communication and emergency leadership (ExCEL): pediatric first 5 minutes workshop for residents. MedEdPORTAL. 2020:10980. https://doi.org/10.15766/mep_2374-8265.10980.
79. Wing R, Tsao HS, Carillo M, Mercurio L, Beucher M, Brown L, Kelley MN. Excellence in communication and emergency leadership (ExCEL): pediatric critical care resource utilization workshop for residents. MedEdPORTAL. 2022:11268. https://doi.org/10.15766/mep_2374-8265.11268.
80. Wong K, Bhama PK, d'Amour Mazimpaka J, Dusabimana R, Lee LN, Shaye DA. Banana fruit: an "appealing" alternative for practicing suture techniques in resource-limited settings. Am J Otolaryngol. 2018;39:582–4. https://doi.org/10.1016/j.amjoto.2018.06.021.

20 Using Technology in Curriculum

Linda Waggoner-Fountain and Alan Chin

Evolution of Trends in Learners and Safety Expectations

Changes in Learners

The demographics of pediatric residents are shifting, with an increasing number of residents from diverse backgrounds. This diversity necessitates inclusive educational practices that address the unique learning needs of different groups. The use of inclusive multimodal teaching allows teachers to better educate all learners. Studies indicate that diverse learning environments can improve educational outcomes and better prepare all trainees for the diverse populations they will serve [1].

Residency training is challenging at baseline, often taking a toll on the mental health of learners, program leadership, and teaching faculty. In the past, these mental health challenges were frequently not acknowledged or addressed. Technology can enhance the well-being of our learners by providing resources and tools for stress management and well-being. The COVID-19 pandemic had a substantial impact on the well-being of residents and pediatricians, partly due to isolation and lack of socialization [2] and it created an opportunity to improve mental health care access for physicians. It has been a challenge for many trainees to receive confidential mental health care at the institutions where they work. The rapid advancements in virtual therapy have made an obtainable reality by making confidential mental health resources more accessible. For example, the META app in the USA provides mental health resources and connects users with therapists and counselors. Both the USA and Canada have integrated wellness awareness and curricula into residency training programs to support trainee mental health [3].

Changes in Safety/Quality Experience

The days of "see one, do one, teach one" are past, with significantly increased direct and indirect supervision of our trainees. Equally important, technological advancements have improved safety and quality in both medical care and medical training. Simulation tools and virtual reality (VR) environments allow residents to practice procedures in risk-free or low-risk settings, enhancing both their skills and confidence. Both low and high-fidelity simulation tools are used in medical school, residency, and fellowship training. Simulation allows the learner to decrease their cognitive load by focusing on the germane

L. Waggoner-Fountain (✉)
University of Virginia School of Medicine, Charlottesville, VA, USA
e-mail: LAW4Q@uvahealth.org

A. Chin
UCLA Mattel Children's Hospital, Los Angeles, CA, USA

H. McPhillips et al. (eds.), *Graduate Medical Education in Pediatrics*, Excellence in Medical Education 3, https://doi.org/10.1007/978-3-032-12952-9_20

portions of the task at hand and rehearsing this to allow for success when additional external factors are added in the clinical environment. In addition to decreasing cognitive load, simulation also allows novice learners to practice challenging skills in both a mentally and physically safe environment. The opportunity to practice these skills in increasingly demanding situations allows the learner to demonstrate advancing proficiency prior to performing procedures and care on patients [4].

Technological Trends

AI/Machine Learning/Deep Learning

Artificial intelligence (AI) and machine learning can help advance medical education. In this context, AI is defined as an approach to data analysis on large data sets utilized to synthesize new information. Machine learning, also known as "deep learning," is a branch of AI that focuses on using data and algorithms to enable AI to imitate the way that humans learn, gradually improving AI accuracy. These technologies can analyze large datasets to provide insights into patient care. AI is being used to personalize learning experiences and improve diagnostic accuracy in medical training. Machine learning is being utilized to improve diagnostic accuracy, especially in visual pattern recognition, such as interpreting radiographs or examining blood smears. There is a growing use of AI in medical education to enhance diagnostic skills and personalize learning experiences [5]. Additional features of AI will be addressed later in this chapter.

Flexible Learning

The flexibility of synchronous and asynchronous learning allows residents to access educational content at their own pace. Online modules, webinars, and virtual classrooms enable continuous learning, accommodating diverse schedules and learning preferences [6]. Learning management systems, the internet, online medical library resources, and various platforms offer medical information that can be accessed anytime by learners in a variety of settings. Studies have shown that asynchronous learning modules can significantly improve knowledge retention and learner satisfaction [7]. This rapid access to medical information is beneficial to both the learner and their patients; however, due to the vast quantity of these materials, educators need to consider what is the best format for the delivery of this information and how to teach learners how to analyze this large amount of information in an efficient and effective manner.

Push Learning Versus Retrieval Learning

With the easy access to large quantities of medical information, technology can enhance the use of just-in-time learning. Push learning involves delivering information to learners proactively, whereas retrieval learning emphasizes the active recall of information. Technology facilitates both approaches, offering personalized learning experiences that enhance knowledge retention. In the USA, educational platforms use AI to push relevant content to learners based on their progress and needs. Many hospitals have a rudimentary form of push learning embedded into their electronic medical records (EMR) with pop-up reminders appearing when a physician prescribes a particular drug, providing education about side effects, alternative therapies, and/or cost before being allowed to prescribe the medication. Another circumstance where personalized learning is routinely used by residents is when they are preparing for standardized tests using standardized practice questions via third-party proprietary review materials. Initial questions would be classified as examples of retrieval learning. When a learner answers an initial question incorrectly, that question is asked again to the same learner. This emphasizes both active recall, but this sequence of asking the same question again is pushing challenging subject matter to the top of a review list for the learner. These programs will continue to repeat question content for residents when they answer the question incorrectly. This type of spaced learning has been shown to be effective and is utilized by the American Board of Pediatrics in their Maintenance of Certification examination questioning for practicing pediatricians as well [8].

Personalized Learning

Personalized learning refers to instruction in which the pace of learning and the instructional approach are optimized for the needs of each learner. The definitions of personalized learning vary depending on the framework of the author; however, common themes that describe personalized learning are a learner-centered approach, learner agency, flexible learning, demonstrated mastery of competencies, and a holistic perspective to the learner [9]. With personalized learning, learning objectives, instructional approaches, and instructional content and their sequencing all may vary based on the learner's needs. The learning activities used with personalized learning in adult learners are typically relevant to the learners, driven by their interests, and often are self-initiated. (U.S. Department of Education, 2017, page 1) [10]. Within a pediatrics residency training program, there are certain, well-defined topics that must be learned by each resident. The care of patients is one major way this curriculum is taught, but all learners will require augmentation of this clinical learning to gain true competence in the field of pediatrics. Broadly construed, personalized education refers to the adaptation of instruction to a specific learner and is juxtaposed with "traditional" instruction that is targeted at entire groups of learners. By changing the mode, content, or rate of instruction in accordance with some characteristic of the learner, it is suggested that individual shortcomings of learners can be addressed, and their resources leveraged [11].

The goal of personalized learning is to engage learners in the process, building on their interests, aptitudes, and strengths, thus creating intrinsic motivation for achievement and success. Residents feel empowered when involved in their own goal-setting and decision-making processes. This also sets up a foundation for developing the skills needed for a lifetime of learning within pediatrics. In general, personalization is most successful when relevant learner characteristics are measured repeatedly during the learning process and when these data are used to adapt instruction in a systematic way. Residency program administrators and resident coaches can review these data and help residents create their individualized learning plan. Residency programs need to help our educators assume the role of coaches or facilitators rather than all-knowing providers of information.

Individual personalized learning can occur in a variety of settings and formats, with technology providing greater opportunities and media for meeting learner needs. The use of videos for educational tutorials on many medical topics is an example of using technology to change the availability of learning opportunities. As the basic knowledge for the diagnosis and management of medical illnesses is increasingly exponential, this emphasizes the need for residents to develop into lifelong learners. Educators and trainees need to focus on information finding and problem-solving abilities that will utilize the vast amount of readily available data, rather than memorizing large quantities of data.

The concept of microcredentials evolved from digital badges and can be described as bite-sized learning activities of professional development experiences that can often be stacked to create a tower of knowledge or expertise. These mini "certifications" can push the resident to learn a small amount of information about a given medical topic that can be subsequently applied in clinical experiences. This can be related to an opportunity for personalized learning on a topic of interest or meaning to the learner, thus increasing internal motivation and agency. A simple example of this could be neonatal resuscitation training that is undergone by each pediatric resident. Neonatal resuscitation training includes review of didactic information, bedside teaching, and demonstration of skills on mannequins. The microcredential includes invoking the learner's intrinsic motivation, exposure to new knowledge, support for skill development, and reflection on the process.

Changes for Future Work and Skills

The medical field is evolving, requiring new skills and competencies for all physicians, including pediatricians. The ACGME recently revised the core pediatric residency curriculum to address the patient care needs for the next generation of children. One portion of this curriculum overhaul specifies that each resident must have at least 40 weeks of individualized curriculum to help prepare them for their career. As pediatric medicine evolves to include complex chronic conditions, such as caring for children and adolescents with behavioral and mental health diagnoses, as well as other children with medical complexity, the landscape of what type of providers care for certain groups of children may change. Pediatricians need to be prepared to care for children with both simple and highly complex medical issues, depending upon where they practice and what additional resources are available to their patients. Medical schools have incorporated digital health and informatics into their curricula to prepare future physicians, and this must be further advanced during pediatric residency education. The political landscape has impacted both medical education and pediatric care, with varying state regulations influencing the content and scope of training. In the USA, differing state policies on healthcare and education create challenges for programs to deliver consistent curricula about perceived political topics such as gender-affirming care, violence prevention, and equity in healthcare [12]. Technology can offer educational resources that may not be available in certain clinical settings.

Economic Trends

The cost of both undergraduate and graduate medical education continues to grow and is a significant concern. Technological solutions, such as online learning platforms and digital resources, can help reduce expenses while maintaining high-quality training. In the USA, the high cost of medical education has led to the adoption of cost-effective digital learning tools. The use of technology in education has been shown to reduce costs by minimizing the need for physical resources and allowing for scalable educational content [13]. It is important for educators to carefully assess which technology is helpful with resident education and which education needs to stay "low-tech" or "no-tech" and make an assessment based on educational value rather than simply on economic value.

Use of Technology to Deliver Educational Content

In this section, we will share practical considerations when using technology in pediatric GME. Specifically, we will address how technology can be used to enhance in-person education, allow asynchronous learning, and connect to or reach additional learners.

Use of Technology to Enhance In-Person Learning

The important considerations when using technology to enhance in-person learning align with principles of adult learning theory in general: create an effective learning climate, allow for learners to have agency in their education, and promote understanding and retention. When choosing to use technology for in-person education in pediatric GME, you should consider how technology addresses one or more of the above principles.

One common tool is presentation software, such as Microsoft PowerPoint, Apple Keynote, Google Slides, etc. Presentation software is a tool that helps organize material, reinforce concepts, emphasize important content, and integrate multiple types of media. In general, these applications use digital slide decks to organize information and are presented in a predetermined order to cover the planned educational content.

One pitfall when using presentation software is when the slide deck is mostly text that is read to the learners—essentially, reading a textbook out loud to learners. There is limited interactivity, and the presentation software is not used to its full potential to engage learners with the material. To avoid this, when preparing a slide deck for a presentation, an educator must consider ways in which to engage learners and highlight important learning points for clarity. For example, consider if a visual, figure, or video may more effectively transmit the concept to your learners; transition the text content to lecturer notes that you convey in-person to explain the media that is shared in the presentation. If you choose to use a text-based slide, consider what information is included on-screen, and what content can be spoken by the lecturer. Consider using text animations, colors, or other visuals to summarize and emphasize key concepts. A simple rule of thumb—if the amount of text on screen is hard to read, then it is too much text.

An advanced way to provide more agency to the learner is to utilize the prepared slide deck as a type of reference material for the in-person presentation and utilize it in a nonlinear fashion. For example, you can create a comprehensive slide deck about neonatal hyperbilirubinemia, but tailor what is presented based on the learner group that you have. If teaching early learners, then the presentation can start with sections on epidemiology and pathophysiology of how hyperbilirubinemia develops in the neonate. For more advanced learners, pathophysiology sections of the larger presentation can be skipped to focus on complicated situations and discussions, such as when treatment should be initiated in an ICU setting because of the possible need for exchange transfusion. Because the slide deck is digital, the teacher is able to adapt their presentation "on-the-fly" to the needs of the learner.

Additional educational technologies can be integrated with presentation software. One common application is audience response software (ARS), such as Poll Everywhere, Slido, Zoom Polls, Mentimeter, etc. ARS is used to obtain information from your learners during the presentation. Learners will join the polling system—usually via text message, website, or app—and respond to questions. Their responses are collected, either as numbers or percentages of responses for multiple choice or word clouds and lists for free response, and can be integrated into presentations to share those responses with the learners. The application of ARS can vary. Examples include using ARS to assess learners' understanding of the topic before a presentation; ideally, used to then adapt the presentation to the learners. ARS can be used to increase the engagement of the learners during the presentation by having them actively reflect on the information shared. At the end of presentations, ARS can be used to check for understanding and to reinforce key concepts.

One logistical consideration about the learning environment when using presentation software is whether there is supporting technology necessary for the presentation itself—is there a large enough screen to display the presentation for the target learner audience? If audio and video are included, will there be a speaker system integrated with the display you are using? If accessing the presentation online or playing media from an internet-based source, will you have access to an internet connection on the display system? Understanding what technology needs you will have for a presentation can ensure that you are prepared and create the effective learning environment required for your presentation—you can review the presentation venue or ask for specific resources that are needed ahead of time.

Another type of in-person learning where technology can be helpful is in educational games. By integrating educational content into a game format, an educator can increase engagement and active participation in the educational session. If there are multiple topics in the medical education game, this also provides learners with agency in what they want to learn during the session. Software or online app-based quiz programs include Kahoot!, Quizlet, Padlet, etc. You can also consider templates built into presentation software based on popular game shows, such as Jeopardy, Family Feud, and Who Wants to Be A Millionaire. In each of these examples, educators create questions for the learners to answer, followed by the correct response with an explanation. Points are awarded for correct answers, and in some cases, for how quickly the learner reaches the correct answer. Learners compete in a positive, friendly environment to win the game. While technology is a helpful tool, it is important for the educator to remember that the explanations and discussion that follow the question are the most important part of learning. If a learner picks the incorrect response, an educator can check for understanding and fill in knowledge gaps. If a learner picks the correct response, an educator can ask the learner for their thought process to reinforce understanding.

Use of Technology for Asynchronous Learning

Educational technology has seen significant growth in use for asynchronous learning. In this context, asynchronous learning is any time in which the educator creates a curriculum to be completed by the learner when the educator does not present the information in real-time.

The flipped classroom has become a popular approach to asynchronous learning. In the flipped classroom approach, foundational content materials are studied by the learner independently through preclassroom activities, such as reading an article or textbook chapter, watching a multimedia presentation, or listening to a lecture in advance of classroom time. The classroom is reserved for applying foundational content knowledge in small group discussions to promote higher-order thinking and active learning [14]. Technology has increasingly been used for these preclassroom activities. Early tools were focused on sharing digitized content to learners, such as scanned or online textbook chapters and PDF versions of articles. Technology tools have progressed to include audio presentations, such as podcasts or recorded lectures, multimedia presentations, such as video or recorded presentations, and interactive learning modules. While these tools can be used for a flipped classroom approach in preclassroom activities, they are also used in primary delivery of asynchronous learning, and each will be addressed in this section.

Audio presentations can be used to provide asynchronous education to learners. One significant benefit of the audio format is the accessibility for the learner. A learner can listen to an audio presentation on their own time, can adjust speed, listen on multiple devices, and can integrate it into other daily activities, such as during commutes or with exercise. There are disadvantages to the audio format, including that it is generally a passive learning modality, which may affect attention and knowledge retention, and does not allow for visual content that may enhance understanding. Audio presentations can be simple audio recordings of presentations or lectures. Audio content can be purposefully recorded in the audio format by the educator, or audio can be extracted from a video recording of a presentation or lecture. With the increased usage of teleconferencing technology during the COVID-19 pandemic, there has been a concurrent increase in the availability of recording devices through webcams and microphones on a variety of devices for educators to use to make recordings. To improve attention and engagement with audio content, the podcast format has also been used to deliver audio education. Generally, podcasts adapt educational content for a discussion between two or more speakers; usually, a "host" that has some knowledge on the topic facilitates the discussion with a "guest" content expert. Due to the integration of multiple speakers in a podcast, attention must be paid to how each speaker will be recorded, such as whether there needs to be multiple microphones to improve audio quality for both the host and the guest. However, the discussion format of a podcast can increase the depth of content presented and may help maintain a learner's attention in an otherwise passive audio presentation. Specifically, in a study of Emergency Medicine trainees, residents felt that podcasts that featured *multiple voices* were effective in highlighting expert clinicians' nuanced variations in diagnosis, management approaches, or treatments [15].

Video presentations, which integrate visual and audio content, have increasingly been used for asynchronous learning. With improved technology to simultaneously record audio and video content and increasing capacity of online storage for learners to access these multimedia recordings, video is quickly becoming the most popular way to provide learners with prerecorded content. The most common type of video used in asynchronous learning records the educator giving a lecture and focuses the visual attention of the learner on presentation software slides, whereas audio recording availability and tools for recording video have significantly increased since the COVID-19 pandemic. While previous applications to record video, including directly through presentation software, have been cumbersome and difficult to use, the advent of teleconferencing technology has lowered the barrier for recording video. In general, an educator will need a computer, webcam, microphone, and teleconferencing software—with these tools, an educator will be able to record a video presentation, the same as they would "share screen" during a teleconference. In addition to recording a slide presentation, educators can use recorded video to share animations, alternate between slides, and have the presenter demonstrating a procedure or process on camera, or other alternatives to slide presentations. Benefits to the learner include being able to watch the video presentation at their own time, adjusting the playback speed, viewing on multiple devices, and learning from both audio and visual content presented. Disadvantages include that video is a passive learning format, and focused attention is usually required to view the visual & audio content—i.e., it is not recommended to watch a video while driving a vehicle.

Often, asynchronous learning occurs in short bursts that are significantly shorter than traditional audio or video lectures. This has led to educators utilizing social media applications, such as Twitter/X, TikTok, Instagram, etc., to share quick "teaching pearls" with learners. With smartphones ubiquitous in the GME clinical environment, learners have consistent access to these social media applications, making them appealing modalities to share learning points. Social media posts are able to share text, images, audio, and video, and link to other online resources. Posts can be shared in real-time by the educator or scheduled for a specific date and time. The disadvantages include limitations to the amount of content that can be shared in each post and limited control over the distribution of the social media post, with most of the platforms supporting public posts as well as comments, which may lead to unrelated content or misinformation being shared in response to the educator's original post.

Lastly, we will briefly discuss interactive learning modules presented through Learning Management Systems (LMS)—a technology tool used in asynchronous learning that can present multiple formats of content and integrate assessment into the learning module. LMS used in medical education have included Canvas LMS, Oasis LMS, Cornerstone, Blackboard Learn, Moodle, and Google Classroom. In general, these systems have been designed to support traditional college and university courses and are able to integrate learning content and assessment tools into a single learning module. For example, an interactive learning module can play a video lecture that you previously recorded on the topic, transition to an interactive screen in which key points are summarized through hyperlinked buttons, followed by a knowledge assessment quiz that is scored, and ends with links to references. The benefits of an LMS are the variety of different content modalities that can be used, the addition of interactive elements, such as interactive buttons and knowledge assessments, and LMS allow to track/monitor learner performance. The disadvantages include financial cost in licenses and subscriptions to the LMS, and faculty development needed to effectively create an interactive learning module in each LMS. These disadvantages generally lead educators to utilize the LMS system supported by their institution, regardless of whether the specific LMS has the functions desired by the educator. In addition to institutions, national organizations have also utilized LMS to deliver educational content to their members. For example, the Association of Pediatric Program Directors (APPD) utilizes an LMS to house its Longitudinal Educational Software Solutions and Outcomes Network (LESSON), where curricula for pediatric residents and fellows have been developed and distributed to learners in areas such as mental health, telehealth, and hospital medicine.

Use of Teleconferencing Technology

With the need to transition to remote learning during the COVID-19 pandemic and the subsequent increase in availability of teleconferencing technologies, educators should consider whether to incorporate remote learners into their educational sessions. Considerations include the hardware required, such as a webcam/microphone, smartphone, or personal smart device, and/or conference room systems, and software used, such as Zoom, Microsoft Teams, Google Meet, Webex, etc. With the prerequisite hardware and software, learners can join sessions from almost any location with internet access. While there are specific issues with every teleconferencing software that can be used, in general, each allows an educator to "share screen" while presenting their lecture through connected audio and/or video. As we discussed previously, this same technology can be used to easily record video presentations for future use. Learners can join the teleconference and see the shared video—usually of both the presentation slides and the presenter. Learners can interact with the lecture through text chat, reactions, and their own audio and video. There are specific considerations when using teleconferencing technologies. For example, access to the presentation must be a balance between ease of connection for the learner and protection against uninvited attendees interrupting the session. Most teleconference software has specific security controls, such as an attendee "waiting room" or password-protected links, which educators should be aware of. In addition, ease of access to the teaching session via teleconference should be balanced with the loss of in-person interaction. There may be topics or educational sessions that may not be as effective in the virtual format, and may be more effective in-person, even if that means the number of learners is less. Lastly, educators should consider hybrid formats—where some learners are in-person and others join remotely with teleconferencing software. While this can increase the number of learners in the session, there is a discrepancy in engagement between in-person learners and remote learners. Additionally, most teleconferencing rooms where the in-person learners will be located are not designed to allow easy interaction between an individual in-person and an individual joining remotely. These all need to be considered when deciding whether an educational session should be in-person, hybrid, or remote/virtual.

Changes in Learning (Instructional) Design

To keep up with the advancements in technology, it is important to consider the pedagogy one plans to use to teach different elements of pediatric medicine. Technology should be used to enhance education, and simply because a technology is available does not necessarily mean that it is the best way to teach that subject. It is important for educators to implement design thinking and consider backwards construction of their pedagogy. The faculty member should consider what they want the trainee to gain competence in doing and what educational techniques a teacher or coach could use to help the trainee gain this expertise. Often, technology allows educators the ability to augment a primary methodology of teaching rather than totally replace it. The educator also needs to coordinate the use of new technology with active learning to increase overall learning.

Design Thinking

In education, design thinking is sometimes referred to as "design-based learning." It is a problem-solving approach dealing with the solutions to everyday problems. This approach is a nonlinear process that can help understand learners, challenge previous assumptions, redefine problems, and create innovative learning plans to test. Learning and knowledge creation in design thinking education are based on highly iterative processes, which can be described with Kolb's experiential learning theory [16] (Fig. 20.1). It is useful for teachers to utilize Kolb's learning theory to examine the material their learners need to master and propose different methods to teach this material.

Increasing Learner Engagement and Centering on the Learner

The two major reasons to consider an increase in the use of technology in instructional design are to (1) increase learner engagement and (2) focus the center of learning on the learner. Some aspects

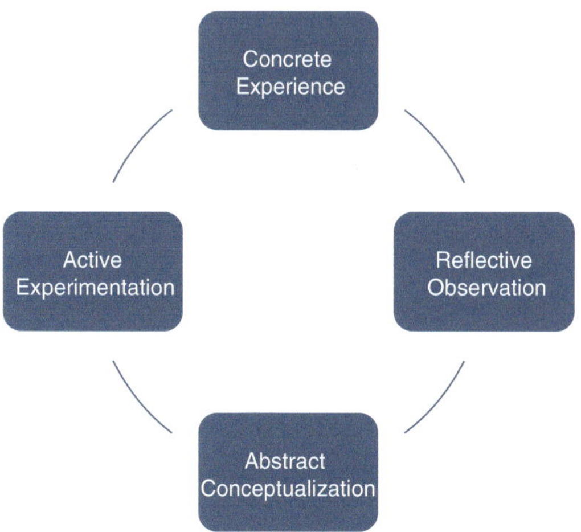

Fig. 20.1 Kolb's cycle of experiential learning

of pediatrics have remained largely unchanged since its inception, while many others have evolved significantly. When considering learner engagement, it is clear that residents are drawn to pediatrics because they want to make a meaningful impact on the health of children and future generations. While this core motivation remains unchanged, today's learners have evolved—shaped by their unique educational journeys and the social and demographic factors that have influenced them before entering residency. Educators must acknowledge that the teaching methods that worked for them may not necessarily be the most effective for today's trainees. Instead, faculty should thoughtfully assess the experiences residents bring to their training and adapt pedagogical approaches to best support their learning.

The other significant reason to consider the use of technology is to shift the focus of learning to the learner. Everyone in medicine understands that the patient always comes first, but the second most important element in caring for patients with graduate medical trainees is the education of the residents. The faculty member needs to recognize that they will continue to be the expert in some aspects of pediatric medicine; their experiences and wealth of knowledge are critical as we continue to teach and learn medicine with the apprenticeship model; however, technology can aid in helping augment learning that is centered on the resident's individual needs. An important part of this process is coaching and instructing the residents in how to assess their own learning needs on a continuous basis—to build habits of inquiry as an everyday professional activity. The educational faculty also needs to consider the use of adaptive technology to be used in coordination with active learning, which will increase the residents' learning.

Educator's Skills and Knowledge Related to Technology

The integration of technology in healthcare education requires educators to understand the potential pros and cons of using the various technologies, both in the classroom and healthcare practice, and to communicate this to the learners.

It is important to educate faculty on how to use these new technologies and new educational approaches. Something as simple as an audience response system can feel as complex as solving a quantum mechanics problem when the technology is new or not working in the assigned educational space. The teacher is frustrated, the learner quickly becomes disinterested, the teaching time disappears, and trust is often lost. Institutions need to provide access to relevant training so that educators can learn how to use the technology effectively and develop the necessary skills to conduct based troubleshooting [17]. Furthermore, healthcare educators must be mindful of technological developments [18] and continually "upgrade their technical skills" [19]. Three common barriers that need to be considered when implementing new technology tools include (1) resistance to change by teachers and students, which can pose a barrier for the adoption of new technologies, (2) the cost of acquiring and maintaining the new technologies, and (3) data privacy and security concerns related to patient and learner sensitive information. It is also critical that learners understand the importance of maintaining digital professionalism and confidentiality [20].

Scott et al. [21] note that mobile devices have the potential to become a distraction in the classroom or clinical setting and disrupt normal healthcare practice as the "devices allow information to permeate everywhere." It is therefore essential that healthcare educators advise their learners about the appropriate use of mobile devices in both settings and ensure that their learners can practice competently without always relying on the technology [18].

The literature also indicates that healthcare educators need to be aware that the experience of e-learning can be isolating for some learners [19]. This lesson was reinforced yet again by the individualized learning that was required during the peak of the pandemic. Programs and educators need to provide regular opportunities for residents to have learning interactions with others to allow trainees to refine their understanding through discussion, develop strong communication skills, share diverse perspectives, be held accountable for learning, handle more complex clinical problems than they could individually, and become part of a learning community of pediatricians in training.

Use of Technology in Pediatric Resident Learner Assessment

The integration of technology into pediatric resident assessment has revolutionized how educators identify and support learners. Learning Management System (LMS) analytics enable educators to track residents' progress, highlighting those who are excelling in core skills and knowledge. Additionally, LMS-based question repositories can help predict which residents are likely to pass or may be at risk of failing the American Board of Pediatrics (ABP) certifying exam. This generation of learners has become accustomed to using third-party online proprietary question banks and platforms as a primary resource for standardized exam preparation, including the SAT, ACT, MCAT, USMLE, and COMLEX. These practice questions allow the learners to test their knowledge in a low-pressure environment. The learners benefit from the personalization of feedback for missed questions, identifying areas where they need further study. Residents often use these question databases as a method of spaced repetition learning. These same principles can be used for resident remediation and individualization of the curriculum if data are collected on an ongoing basis.

LMS Analytics for Identifying Student Performance

Learning Management Systems (LMS) have become invaluable tools in medical education, providing a wealth of data that can be used to monitor and assess student performance. Common examples of LMS include Blackboard Learn, Canvas, Moodle, and Google Classroom. The Association of Pediatric Program Directors

(APPD) utilizes an LMS to house its Longitudinal Educational Software Solutions and Outcomes Network (LESSON), which produces meaningful educational materials that advance the training of pediatric residents and fellows for the purpose of improving the health and well-being of children. LESSON is designed to advance pediatric graduate medical education through the assistance of educational technology, outcome-based EPA curriculum development, and learner assessment. LMS analytics can track various metrics such as login frequency, time spent on learning materials, quiz scores, and participation in discussion forums. By analyzing these data points, educators can identify patterns that indicate which residents are excelling and which are at risk of not progressing through residency training or passing the certifying examination at the completion of residency.

Personalization of Feedback for Remediation and Individualization of Curriculum

Bloom advocated for one-on-one tutoring, emphasizing that a personal tutor can better assess a learner's unique characteristics and tailor instructional methods and materials accordingly—such as identifying the zone of proximal development [22] (Fig. 20.2) and selecting tasks within it. While an LMS cannot independently determine a learner's zone of proximal development, it can provide valuable data and resources to support educators in making these assessments. For example, an LMS can track performance trends and suggest targeted learning activities, such as individualized online videos on a specific pediatric topic, additional clinical sessions with a nephrologist, extra patient encounters in the emergency department, or extended time in the simulation lab to practice recognizing worrisome cardiac rhythms [23]. This approach aligns well with the ACGME requirement for six months of individualized curriculum in pediatric residency training.

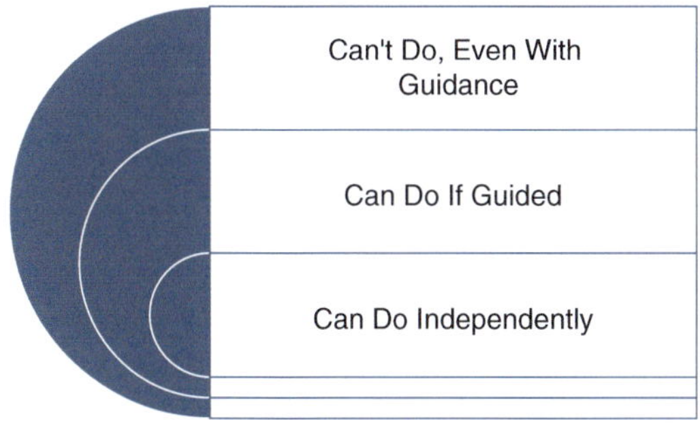

Fig. 20.2 Vygotsky's zone of proximal development & scaffolding theory

Intelligent tutoring systems can increase learning gains when compared with regular instruction. These systems have two defining features: (1) student modeling, i.e., the assessment of several specific learner characteristics through direct measure (e.g., correct or incorrect responses to tasks) or indirect measures (e.g., logfiles of clicking behavior), and (2) the subsequent adaptation of instruction.

The use of technology in medical education should be to support learning; it should not be a replacement for face-to-face learning. Educators must still focus on the principles of teaching, not on the specific technologies. Technologies are just one tool in the educational toolbox. The task of medical educators is to use these new technologies effectively to transform learning into a more collaborative, personalized, and empowering experience.

Use of Generative Artificial Intelligence (AI) in Pediatric GME

The goal of this section is to introduce general concepts in the use of generative AI tools in pediatric graduate medical education. We will define key terms, propose scenarios in which generative AI tools can be utilized, and outline current understanding of benefits and complications in each context.

We recognize that innovations in generative AI tools, such as OpenAI ChatGPT, Google Gemini, Microsoft Co-Pilot, etc., are rapidly evolving. Therefore, we will avoid discussing any specific tool but instead discuss general contexts in which generative AI tools will likely be used in pediatric medical education.

Definitions

Artificial Intelligence (AI) in this context is not one method but rather an approach to data mining and analysis using a wide range of statistical techniques on large and often complex data sets [24].

Machine learning is a branch of AI and computer science that focuses on using data and algorithms to enable AI to imitate the way that humans learn, gradually improving AI accuracy [25].

Natural language processing is a subfield of computer science and AI that uses machine learning to enable computers to understand and communicate with human language [26].

Generative AI is a type of AI that uses machine learning algorithms to create new content based on existing data, often generating high-quality text through natural language processing, images, and other content based on the data they were trained on [27].

AI Hallucination—most generative AI tools create responses based on the most likely and frequent words and statements that follow each other from their dataset. This means generative AI tools may create well-written text with citations or references that do not actually exist or create content that is incorrect from a factual perspective. This illustrates the importance of verifying and checking important information when using generative AI.

Summarization of Content and Text Analysis

The volume of health information continues to increase at a rapid pace—so much so that it has increased beyond the capacity of humans to sift and digest. Due to the high volume of information that needs to be reviewed, generative AI tools are an attractive way to support the education of resident trainees [28]. One potential benefit of generative AI tools is their use in natural language processing to review the overwhelming amount of data into easily understandable summaries. For trainees who are required to learn an incredible amount of information in a short time, these tools provide immediate access to medical knowledge, research studies, and clinical guidelines [29]. Very similar to previous technological advances, such as web search and searchable online clinical references, educators will need to provide guidance regarding the appropriate use of generative AI tools, including verifying the accuracy of the summaries produced by these AI tools and ensuring the selection of high-quality source materials as inputs to the generative AI tool.

Generation of Education Materials

Many of these generative AI tools have demonstrated competence in multiple standardized clinical exams, potentially making them a valuable reference for trainees and educators. These AI models can provide physician trainees with realistic clinical scenarios and feedback, thus enhancing clinical education [29, 30].

Generative AI tools can interact with trainees and provide educational guidance based on the trainee's questions and needs. For example, AI tools can offer additional explanations, examples and case studies, exercises, and questions, and visual aids to help trainees gain a deeper understanding of clinical concepts and principles [30]. Learners can then focus on understanding and problem-solving rather than rote memorization.

In addition, generative AI tools can help trainees and educators by improving writing style and formatting for clarity and coherence, while also providing appropriate language and terminology for writing accuracy. This can make for more effective educational materials and support the development of clinical curricula. Viewed from an equity perspective, these tools can be used by those with limited English proficiency or those who have limited resources for review and revision of scholarly work—potentially "leveling the playing field" and improving the educational process across a variety of contexts.

Importantly, there are limitations of generative AI tools that GME leaders should be aware of—including variability in response, "AI hallucination," AI detection, and developing policies on AI usage in the academic community.

When using AI, there is a wide variability in the responses generated by the AI tools. The information provided to the learner is highly dependent on the "prompt" that the user submits to the AI tool—for example, the response to "tell me how to treat pneumonia" versus "tell me how to treat pneumonia with references" creates different responses, the latter with antibiotic doses but less general explanation. Repeating the same prompt may elicit varied responses, and the resources that the generative AI tool uses to create the response may differ each time, not to mention the differences in responses generated by different AI tools.

As generative AI tool use has increased, academic communities have moved to respond to potential issues, including concerns regarding plagiarism, inauthenticity, and other ethical considerations. Many respected peer-reviewed journals have developed policies that either prohibit or limit the use of generative AI tools in their submissions. Universities have also developed policies to address generative AI tool use for class assignments, including appropriately citing AI tools if used.

Example Citation: Generated using [AI Tool Name], Date of Query, "[Prompt submitted]," [AI Tool Name], [URL Link to AI tool]

With AI being prohibited in some contexts, there has been the development of AI detection software. AI detection software analyzes submitted text and reviews it against a dataset of generative AI-created text, providing a likelihood of the text having been created using an AI tool. While imperfect, GME leaders and trainees should have a basic understanding of AI detection software.

Implications in the Clinical Learning Environment

Many healthcare institutions are integrating generative AI tools into the clinical environment. Examples have included generating responses to patient communication in the electronic medical record, using machine learning to develop clinical decision support in medical imaging, and using natural language processing to take locally recorded patient encounters to generate clinical notes. While detailing all the various applications of generative AI in the clinical setting is beyond the scope of this chapter, it is important that GME leaders understand the tools that may be used by their trainees, now or in the future. As generative AI tools continue to be integrated into clinical practice, it is important to ensure patient privacy and confidentiality. Most generative AI tools integrated into clinical practice are either processed locally within the healthcare institution or in HIPAA-compliant, encrypted cloud services. There are two implications to this that are important for medical educators.

First, it is important to let learners and trainees know that the generative AI tools used in the clinical setting may create different responses than expected from publicly available AI tools. Whether due to more limited references accessed during the response generation or limited processing resources, the responses may not be what the trainee expects and should be reviewed and verified before use.

Second, with the many exciting innovations in generative AI, learners and trainees may be tempted to use publicly accessible tools to assist in their clinical work. However, GME leaders should emphasize that private health information (PHI) should not be transmitted to non-HIPAA-compliant tools. For example, a trainee may want to improve the clarity of their progress notes by reviewing them in a publicly available generative AI tool; however, the trainee may not realize that if patient identifiers are not removed prior to review, they have sent PHI into a non-HIPAA-compliant tool. Educators should understand and convey the difference between approved and vetted generative AI tools in the clinical setting versus the AI tools available for public and commercial use.

Implications for GME Recruitment

Because of the widespread use of generative AI, applicants to GME programs may consider using

AI tools to help write personal statements, activity descriptions, or other areas of residency applications. AI tools can assist in writing efficiency, help with brainstorming, improve communication for those for whom English is a second language, and can improve equity in access to application assistance resources [31]. Faculty may consider using AI tools to generate letters of recommendation and/or summarize applications. Program leaders may consider using generative AI tools for application analysis and screening.

For GME applicants and faculty letter writers, we recommend these guidelines adapted from Mangold et al. [31]:

- Follow and respect program-specific guidelines for AI use—review any program guidelines for AI use prior to submission.
  - Similar to some peer review journals, programs may consider setting expectations for AI use during recruitment—e.g., "we wish to learn about your authentic self, so we ask that generative AI tools not be used in applications to our program."
- Be aware of plagiarism and maintain authenticity.
  - Utilizing AI to create materials may qualify as plagiarism. Authenticity is important for all materials created for GME recruitment, but especially letters of recommendation, personal statements, etc.
- Disclose AI use clearly if generative AI tools are utilized.
- Proofread drafts created by generative AI tools and ensure errors are corrected.

In regard to the use of AI tools in application analysis and screening, there are benefits to a tool that can efficiently review the ever-increasing number of applications that programs need to review, and AI tools can bring some consistency to a process that is fairly subjective. Many of these AI tools for residency application review are already in use or in development. Most require that program leaders provide examples of what they value in applicants, pointing to specific areas in the example applications to the AI tool as part of the machine learning process. GME leaders need to be aware that this process may exacerbate or perpetuate bias in the application review process—essentially codifying implicit (or explicit) bias when training the AI tool. Also, because the machine learning algorithm is not explicitly observable once trained, it is very difficult to change in the future. GME leaders who choose to use AI tools for application review and screening should be aware of these limitations.

The AAMC has provided this framework for the use of AI tools in medical education admissions and recruitment [32]:

1. Balance Prediction and Understanding. Ensure that AI tools deliver insights that improve prediction and efficiency while being comprehensible and usable by the institution, aligning with its objectives and needs.
2. Protect against Algorithmic Bias. Rigorously assess and manage biases arising from historical data to ensure fair AI processes and outcomes.
3. Provide Notice and Explanation. Maintain transparency by informing applicants how AI is used and how it affects the assessment of their application.
4. Protect Data Privacy. Safeguard information with the utmost care, maintaining confidentiality at every step.
5. Incorporate Human Judgment. It is crucial to strike the appropriate balance between technology and the irreplaceable value of human judgment and ethical standards.
6. Monitor and Evaluate. Assess the outputs and outcomes of the AI system to ensure they remain fair, accurate, and aligned with institutional goals.

Conclusion

Technology has become an integral part of pediatric graduate medical education, driving significant changes in how pediatric residents are trained. By embracing technological advancements and addressing social, content, and economic trends, educators can enhance the learning experience and better prepare pediatricians for the future. As the field of pediatrics continues to evolve, ongoing adaptation and innovation in educational practices will be essential to meet the needs of both pediatric resident learners and their future patients. By leveraging these technological tools, educators can create a more effective and supportive learning environment, ultimately improving learner outcomes and ensuring that future pediatricians are well-prepared for their careers.

References

1. Wallihan R, Smith KG, Hormann MD, Donthi RR, Boland K, Mahan JD. Utility of intermittent online quizzes as an early warning for residents at risk of failing the pediatric board certification examination. BMC Med Educ. 2018;18:1–7.
2. Kesselheim JC, Althouse LA. The impact of COVID-19 on pediatric training. J Grad Med Educ. 2021;13(4):519–23.
3. Fischer JL, Zinsmeister AR. Integrating wellness into medical education. Acad Pediatr. 2019;19(1):10–3.
4. Cook DA, Hatala R. Simulation-based education in medical schools. JAMA. 2011;306(9):978–88.
5. Kolachalama VB, Garg PS. Machine learning and medical education. PLoS One. 2018;13(3):e0193426.
6. Masters K, Ellaway R. e-Learning in medical education Guide 32 Part 2: technology, management and design. Med Teach. 2008;30(5):474–89. https://doi.org/10.1080/01421590802108349.
7. Pei L, Wu H. Does online learning work better than offline learning in undergraduate medical education? Med Educ Online. 2019;24(1):1–13.
8. Larsen DP, Butler AC. Repeated testing improves long-term retention relative to repeated study: a randomized controlled trial. Med Educ. 2013;47(7):718–26.
9. DeMonte J. Personalized learning: what it is and why it matters. 2019. Unpublished manuscript, cited in Randi, J., & Corno, L. (2020). Individual personalized learning. Educ Consider 46(2):4. https://files.eric.ed.gov/fulltext/EJ1275355.pdf
10. U.S. Department of Education. Office of Educational Technology. Reimagining the role of technology in education: 2017 National Education Technology Plan Update. 2017.
11. Dockterman D. Insights from 200+ years of personalized learning. npj Sci Learn. 2018;3:15. https://doi.org/10.1038/s41539-018-0033-x.
12. Romanelli RJ, Martinez RG. Political determinants of health in medical education. Acad Med. 2019;94(6):840–4.
13. Heitz C, Prusakowski M. Cost-effectiveness of online learning platforms in medical education. J Med Internet Res. 2018;20(8):e242.
14. King AM, Gottlieb M, Mitzman J, Dulani T, Schulte SJ, Way DP. Flipping the classroom in graduate medical education: a systematic review. J Grad Med Educ. 2019;11(1):18–29. https://doi.org/10.4300/JGME-D-18-00350.2.
15. Riddell JC, Robins L, Sherbino J, Brown A, Ilgen J. Residents' perceptions of effective features of educational podcasts. West J Emerg Med. 2020;22(1):26–32. https://doi.org/10.5811/westjem.2020.10.49135.
16. Kolb DA. Experiential learning: experience as the source of learning and development. Englewood Cliffs, NJ: Prentice-Hall; 1984.
17. Lai JWM, Bower M. Evaluation of technology use in education: findings from a critical analysis of systematic literature reviews. J Comput Assist Learn. 2020;36:241–59. https://doi.org/10.1111/jcal.12412.
18. Masters K, Ellaway RH, Topps D, Archibald D, Hogue RJ. Mobile technologies in medical education: AMEE Guide No. 105. Med Teach. 2016;38(6):537–49. https://doi.org/10.3109/0142159X.2016.1141190.
19. Lee Y-H, Waxman H, Wu J-Y, Michko G, Lin G. Revisit the effect of teaching and learning with technology. Educ Technol Soc. 2013;16(1):133–46.
20. Ellaway R, Masters K. AMEE Guide 32: e-learning in medical education part 1: learning, teaching and assessment. Med Teach. 2008;30(5):455–73. https://doi.org/10.1080/01421590802108331.
21. Scott KM, Nerminathan A, Alexander S, Phelps M, Harrison A. Mobile devices for learning in clinical settings. Br J Educ Technol. 2017;48(176–190):190. https://doi.org/10.1111/bjet.12352.
22. Rieber RW, Carton AS, eds. The collected works of L. S. Vygotsky: problems of general psychology, including the volume thinking and speech. Vol. 1. New York, Springer; 1987. https://doi.org/10.1007/978-1-4613-1655-8.
23. Colbert CY, Foshee CM, Prelosky-Leeson A, Schleicher M, King R. Differentiated instruction as a viable framework for meeting the needs of diverse adult learners in health professions education. Med Sci Educ. 2023;33(4):975–84. https://doi.org/10.1007/s40670-023-01808-w. PMID: 37546185; PMCID: PMC10403478.
24. Tolsgaard MG, Pusic MV, Sebok-Syer SS, et al. The fundamentals of Artificial Intelligence in medical education research: AMEE Guide No. 156. Med Teach. 2023;45(6):565–73. https://doi.org/10.1080/0142159X.2023.2180340.
25. What is Machine Learning (ML)? IBM Explainers. https://www.ibm.com/topics/machine-learning. Accessed 16 Jul 2024.

26. What is NLP (natural language processing)? IBM Explainers. https://www.ibm.com/topics/natural-language-processing. Accessed 16 Jul 2024.
27. What is generative AI? IBM Research Blog. https://research.ibm.com/blog/what-is-generative-AI. Accessed 16 Jul 2024.
28. Sullivan GM, Simpson D, Yarris LM, Artino ARJ. Residents, faculty, and artificial intelligence: brave new world or utopia? J Grad Med Educ. 2023;15(5):517–9. https://doi.org/10.4300/JGME-D-23-00534.1.
29. Lucas HC, Upperman JS, Robinson JR. A systematic review of large language models and their implications in medical education. Med Educ. 2024; https://doi.org/10.1111/medu.15402.
30. Shang L, Li R, Xue M, Guo Q, Hou Y. Evaluating the application of ChatGPT in China's residency training education: an exploratory study. Med Teach. Published online July 12, 2024:1–7. https://doi.org/10.1080/0142159X.2024.2377808.
31. Mangold S, Ream M. Artificial intelligence in graduate medical education applications. J Grad Med Educ. 2024;16(2):115–8. https://doi.org/10.4300/JGME-D-23-00510.1.
32. Principles for Responsible AI in Medical School and Residency Selection. AAMC - Medical Education. https://www.aamc.org/about-us/mission-areas/medical-education/principles-ai. Accessed 30 Jul 2024.

Part V

Assessment and Program Evaluation

21 Competency-Based Assessment

Katherine Nowicki and David A. Turner

Introduction

The modern paradigm of graduate medical education in pediatrics is described as competency-based, but in most circumstances, the full potential of a competency-based approach to education and assessment has not been realized. A competency-based medical education (CBME) system should focus on specific and pre-defined outcomes to determine a trainee's progress and readiness for their next phase of practice rather than simply the passage of time through training. CBME represents a philosophical approach to education and assessment that "begins with the end in mind" and involves implementation of education and assessment that is patient-focused and learner-centered. When organizing a training program to embrace a CBME philosophy, there are five generally accepted core components, which include (1) an outcome competency framework, (2) sequenced progression of learning, (3) tailored learning experiences, (4) competency-focused instruction, and (5) programmatic assessment [41]. In this chapter we will emphasize that "assessment is an educational design problem that needs a programmatic approach," meaning that assessment should be considered throughout the process of designing a curriculum and not be an afterthought or simply be based on regulatory requirements [40].

For a CBME system to be effective, each of the five core components, referenced above, is essential. The first component is foundational and includes developing a clear definition of the desired outcomes expected for an individual learner, which should be based on the needs of patients. In this way, CBME is first and foremost patient-centered. The pediatric community has defined our outcomes framework using the Entrustable Professional Activities (EPAs) [2]. EPAs describe the activities expected in practice by all pediatricians and pediatric subspecialists, and they integrate a wide range of competencies, including the knowledge, skills, attitudes, and behaviors needed by an individual to execute the activities that are essential for optimal patient care. These individual attributes that are necessary to provide the care described in EPAs have been further outlined through the delineation of competencies, sub-competencies, and developmental milestones, described in more detail below.

A CBME system also requires that curricula are designed in a way that sequences progression (core component 2) with both learning (core component 3) and teaching (core component 4), all designed to achieve the desired outcomes defined by EPAs as described above (core com-

K. Nowicki
University of Colorado School of Medicine, Aurora, CO, USA

D. A. Turner (✉)
American Board of Pediatrics, Chapel Hill, NC, USA
e-mail: DTurner@abpeds.org

H. McPhillips et al. (eds.), *Graduate Medical Education in Pediatrics*, Excellence in Medical Education 3, https://doi.org/10.1007/978-3-032-12952-9_21

ponent 1). These components of a CBME system create a learner-centeredness that promotes the development of an individual trainee so that each individual can reach their maximum potential. Programmatic assessment (core component 5) and the use of data from multiple sources to create a comprehensive and holistic view of an individual's performance, coupled with a curriculum based on defined outcomes, should exist to support and document the developmental acquisition of the knowledge, skills, and attitudes necessary for practice. A key element of a competency-based system is regular, frequent, and longitudinal assessment that allows programs to provide the feedback and coaching that is necessary to enable adjustments to learning plans and behavior changes [13, 14, 18, 23].

While assessment is an essential part of CBME and the focus of this chapter, it cannot be considered in isolation from the other components of a competency-based system. Consequently, we will discuss the topic of assessment in the context of the five core components of CBME and note that the additional non-assessment elements that are essential to successful implementation of a competency-based philosophy are largely covered in other chapters in this text.

Such an approach shifts the emphasis from assessment *of* learning to assessment *for* learning, which is a critical distinction in an authentic CBME system. This shift is important because assessment "conveys what we value as important and acts as the most cogent motivator of student learning" [33]. We will also discuss assessment within the context of a genuine CBME pediatric medical education system. We will begin with a discussion of expected outcomes and standards for assessment and follow that with a discussion about data collection and interpretation. We will then transition to discussing the critical task of providing feedback to trainees and address the importance of creating a learning environment that is conducive to growth and authentic competency-based learning. Finally, we will conclude the chapter with an overview of a programmatic assessment and its importance for a successful approach to CBME.

Desired Outcomes for Assessment

When designing a competency-based approach to assessment, it should begin "with the end in mind" and focus on the first core component of CBME—the outcomes competency framework defined based on the needs of patients. In pediatrics, our outcomes framework was defined by our community over a decade ago using the Entrustable Professional Activities (EPAs) [2]. EPAs are observable, routine activities that a pediatrician or pediatric subspecialist should be able to perform safely and effectively to meet the needs of their patients, and these EPAs should serve as the foundation for a competency-based approach to assessment. EPAs are tasks or responsibilities that a competent pediatrician should be entrusted to perform without supervision [37] and have been colloquially referred to by many in our specialty as "Everyday Pediatrician Activities." These EPAs serve as the foundation for the standards currently in place for GME training in our specialty in the US. The "Definition of Specialty" section of the ACGME Pediatric program requirements (effective July 2025) includes the content of the EPAs that have been defined for our specialty, examples of which include providing comprehensive care for children, managing acute, common diagnoses, and managing children with behavioral and mental health problems, to name a few [1]. These foundational activities should be the drivers of assessment and curriculum such that each program has a system in place to prepare each individual trainee to be ready to execute these EPAs without supervision when they transition to practice.

While EPAs represent the activities expected of pediatricians and thus, the expected outcomes of training, EPAs are only one part of a comprehensive competency-based approach to assessment. As an example, considering the EPA, "Assess and Manage Patients with Behavioral and Mental Health Problems," there are numerous competencies that must be integrated for an individual trainee to be able to execute this activity. The necessary competencies likely include all 6 of the core competency domains, which include patient care (PC), medical knowledge

(MK), professionalism (PROF), interpersonal and communication skills (ICS), practice-based learning and improvement (PBLI), and systems-based practice (SBP) [1]. These six core competencies were defined by the ACGME in partnership with the American Board of Medical Specialties in 1999. These competencies have been further broken down by each specialty into a number of different sub-competencies, and each sub-competency has a developmental trajectory, or set of milestones, based on Dreyfus' model of skill acquisition [11]. Milestones are "brief, narrative developmentally based statements that describe the skills, knowledge, and behavior" for each sub-competency [17], and reporting of milestones to the ACGME has been the standard for many years as part of the GME program accreditation process. EPAs provide a holistic view of a trainee's ability to execute a specific activity or core task that a pediatrician needs to be able to perform while competencies and milestones represent a more zoomed-in view of the demonstrable skills and behaviors that are required to execute a given EPA. In thinking about assessment from a practical perspective, there are times when it is necessary to use different lenses in different circumstances, as demonstrated in Fig. 21.1.

The current approach to assessment in pediatric GME is primarily milestone-based, largely driven by the requirement for twice-annual reporting of these data to the ACGME. However, data demonstrate that the current approach to assessment in pediatric GME often leaves gaps, with large percentages of graduating residents and fellows not being ready for practice when using the EPA outcomes framework [30, 38, 43]. These gaps are one reason that assessment in a CBME system needs to include not only determination of individual behaviors for specific sub-competencies (i.e., milestones), but also an assessment of how well these behaviors are integrated to execute a specific set of activities required of us by our patients (i.e., EPAs).

As a concrete example, many Clinical Competency Committees (CCCs) have become increasingly facile with milestones and their usefulness in understanding the developmental trajectory of a trainee (i.e., milestone level) for a given behavior or sub-competency, but the actual practice of assigning a milestone level to an individual trainee is often a challenge. Consider the

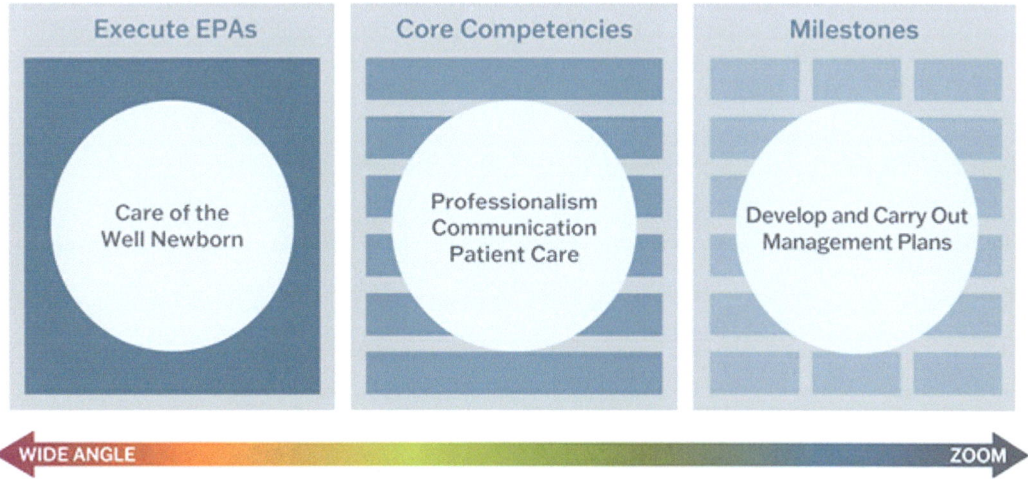

Fig. 21.1 Example of the relationship between Milestones, Competencies, and the ability to execute EPAs

general pediatrics Patient Care competency and its sub-competency, History (Fig. 21.2). As one assesses a trainee, it is often exceptionally challenging for faculty to determine which of the milestone levels most accurately reflects a given trainee's performance without clinical context. For example, when caring for a newborn in the nursery, a resident might be at Level 4: "*Filters, prioritizes, and synthesizes the history to develop a differential diagnosis in real time for complicated or atypical presentations*," while in the context of managing an adolescent with abdominal pain, the trainee might be at Level 2: "*Adapts template to filter and prioritize pertinent positives and negatives based on broad diagnostic categories or possible diagnoses.*" This difference in ability based on the clinical scenario can make assigning a milestone rating confusing and even frustrating for faculty and clinical competency committees. This scenario is typically encountered when the milestones are used as an assessment tool at the conclusion of a rotation or other experience rather than being applied in a specific context, which is not how milestones were intended to be used. If the focus of assessment is exclusively on the behaviors of the individual (i.e., milestones and sub-competencies), the ultimate outcome in a CBME framework—the needs of the patients—is lost, as is the ability to meaningfully and defensibly determine an individual's readiness to care for patients. In contrast, if the overall frame for assessment integrates the needs of the patients with a shift towards an EPA-based lens—for example, "How much supervision is required to care for an adolescent with abdominal pain"—faculty and trainees can discuss this determination and how ready a given trainee is for a specific situation and use this information to outline what behaviors (i.e., competencies, sub-competencies, and milestones) they need to focus on for improvement. Using the same example, it might be that a trainee caring for this adolescent excels at history taking but has a deficit in medical knowledge. To that end, assessment based on EPAs can be used to develop an individual competency/milestone profile of a trainee that is specific and can then be used for individualized learning plans, coaching, reports to the ACGME, and a variety of other purposes.

As this example demonstrates, an approach to assessment in a competency-based system must include holistic elements to determine readiness for patient-centered activities (i.e., EPAs) while integrating elements that describe specific behaviors (i.e., milestones) that can be used to help trainees develop. Too often an "either-or" perspective is taken when the various aspects of our CBME outcomes framework are considered. Instead, these elements, namely EPAs, sub-competencies, competencies, and milestones, should be considered complementary and important parts of a comprehensive approach to assessment and tracking of the developmental trajectory of a trainee in their progression toward reaching their full potential and readiness for practice.

To that end, expectations in program requirements and future requirements for individual certification include all of these elements of the

Patient Care 1: History

Level 1	Level 2	Level 3	Level 4	Level 5
Gathers information strictly following a template	Adapts template to filter and prioritize pertinent positives and negatives based on broad diagnostic categories or possible diagnoses	Filters, prioritizes, and synthesizes the history to develop a differential diagnosis in real-time for uncomplicated or typical presentations	Filters, prioritizes, and synthesizes the history to develop a differential diagnosis in real time for complicated or atypical presentations	Recognizes and probes subtle clues from patients and families; distinguishes nuances among diagnoses to efficiently drive further information gathering

Comments:

Not Yet Completed Level 1 ☐
Not Yet Assessable ☐

Fig. 21.2 Pediatrics Patient Care 1: History. (Used with permission from the ACGME)

CBME outcomes framework. As noted above, milestones are required by the ACGME as part of program accreditation but cannot be considered in isolation. While EPAs are not yet a part of the standards included by the ABP for individual physician certification, they will be in the coming years, and the EPAs already serve as the foundation for the development of the content outlines used for the general pediatrics and pediatric subspecialty initial certification examinations.

As programs work to develop an authentic approach to CBME to prepare their trainees for practice, it is critical that efforts to build *both* curricula and assessments designed to achieve these outcomes be prioritized. The remainder of this chapter continues to focus on the assessment side of the CBME equation, but the other key elements of a competency-based system, including the nuances and specifics of curriculum development and teaching/learning focused on the outcomes framework, are covered elsewhere in this text.

Collecting Data for Assessment

With the educational standards of an outcomes-based training program in mind, data needs to be collected to provide evidence regarding each individual trainee's knowledge, skills, and behaviors. Determining the appropriate approach by which to gather this information can be a daunting task, but when selecting instruments and approaches to assessment, categorization can help programs organize their strategy. An example of one way to categorize assessments might include: (1) written assessments, (2) clinical/practical assessments, (3) observation, (4) portfolios, and (5) peer and self-assessment [32]. Table 21.1 provides a list of potential GME examples from each category. Each of these different categories of assessment has their own advantages and disadvantages, but in an ideal state, programs should utilize multiple elements of assessment from each of these different categories. For example, a program might use the In-Training Exam as an assessment of overall knowledge, hold a simulation-based session to evaluate competency in procedures, and then gather data from peer assessments to evaluate a trainee's ability to hand over patients to other colleagues.

While the benefits of different types of assessments vary, the spirit of a competency-based approach to assessment is integrating a wide range of sources of data to develop the most complete picture of a trainee. This approach, termed programmatic assessment, is often described as each source of data adding additional pixels to an image so one can move from a fuzzy outline of a picture that has only limited pixels to a sharp and easily recognizable image that integrates many pixels.

One important source of data to be collected in the GME environment involves assessments from the frontline assessors involved in caring for patients with trainees. In the CBME literature, the approach to assessment of trainees by frontline faculty is described as workplace-based assessment (WBA). WBA is an approach to assessment that strives to authentically determine a trainee's knowledge, skills, and attitudes through observation of what they do with patients, families, and colleagues in a real-world context. In pediatric GME, authentic WBA is often missing, with the vast majority of assessment happening at the conclusion of a rotation or clinical

Table 21.1 Categories and examples of assessments relevant for GME

GME assessment examples	
Category	Examples
Written assessments	Multiple choice questions Clinical note review Clinical case reviews
Clinical/practical assessments	Observed structured clinical examination (OSCE) Oral examinations Virtual/Augmented Reality Online Assessments Simulation-based assessments
Observation	Workplace-based assessments 360-degree multi-rater assessments Patient/family assessments
Portfolios	Case or procedure logs
Peer and self-assessment	Narrative assessments Milestone behavioral ratings

experience, which may be weeks or even months after a given clinical encounter. This separation in time between a clinical encounter and the assessment is a substantial barrier to gathering the information necessary for successful trainee development and for program decision-making.

The spirit of WBA is to integrate the assessment into the clinical workflow and temporally connect the assessment as closely as possible to the clinical encounter. A key component of effective WBA is the inclusion of both quantitative (e.g., checklists or ratings) and qualitative data (e.g., narrative comments). Narrative comments are particularly important and can amplify low or high quantitative measures and provide explanations for trainees and CCCs about strengths and opportunities for improvement. Furthermore, narrative comments frequently address aspects of a trainee's performance not directly included in the quantitative portion [46]. Quantitative aspects of WBA instruments can establish a shared mental model of what competence looks like. The results of ratings also provide discrete data points that can be trended over time. However, the risk of an overemphasis on quantitative aspects of WBA assessment tools is that form completion is prioritized over providing meaningful verbal feedback or constructive written comments [5]. This problem can be mitigated by thoughtful WBA tool design, iterative change, and faculty development. As programs consider WBAs and their overall approach to data collection, critical elements of consideration are feasibility, impact on the learner, equity, reliability, validity, and acceptability—as described in more detail below.

To be sustainable, assessment in a busy GME program must be *feasible*. Assessment instruments need to be carefully crafted in an iterative, user-centered process with attention to efficiency and ease of use in the environment in which they will be utilized. To achieve these goals, educators may need to develop new assessment tools specific to their program's needs and local context, but in many cases, particularly in pediatric GME where collaboration is frequent and highly valued, it is possible to adapt existing tools. One increasingly popular and feasible approach is completing WBA with the use of a smartphone-based application (app). WBAs can be conveniently integrated into the clinical workflow with a well-designed app that includes thoughtful instrument design and a user-friendly interface. From a practical perspective, developing a system in which faculty can assess trainees in "real-time" as part of their daily work with residents and fellows can be a challenge, but if assessment forms are created to be patient-oriented (i.e., based on the EPA framework), short, and simple, the burden of assessment for trainees and faculty can be decreased—despite the increased volume of assessments being created. This approach also can greatly increase the perceived value of assessment by faculty and trainees. There are many examples across a wide range of specialties, including pediatrics and the pediatric subspecialties, in which an app-based approach to assessment using the EPA framework has been demonstrated as both a feasible and effective approach to creating a growth mindset and an authentic competency-based assessment program. Using EPAs as the frame for assessment allows for faculty and trainees to focus on activities that are essential for their future practice. While cost may be a potential barrier to implementation of an app-based approach to WBA, most existing resident management systems used in pediatric GME programs in the US have an app for assessment that can be used without adding additional cost to programs. Given the importance of this aspect of CBME, investment in a good assessment system is also an investment in teaching and learning and may improve satisfaction with the assessment process [39].

The *impact of assessment on the trainee* is another critical aspect of assessment to consider. Assessment, particularly in the CBME context, should have both educational and catalytic effects. Educational effects refer to the effects on behavior that occur before the assessment, that is, to the extent of which anticipation of the assessment prompts the trainee to engage in preparatory activities that are valuable and worth the time [46]. If an assessment instead prompts the trainee to cram knowledge or take another undesirable action, then changes in the assessment need to be made [32]. Assessment may also have a catalytic effect, which refers to effects that follow the assessment. For example, specific feedback on areas of needed improvement might encourage the trainee to put more effort into learning certain material moving forward. Ideally, assessments in pediatric GME motivate trainees to engage in high-yield activities before and after assessments [46]. Research to date has shown mixed results with respect to the impact of CBME-based assessment on trainees. In one national survey study of Canadian residents, trainees in CBME programs reported greater self-reflection and being more proactive in their learning (i.e., positive catalytic effects) but also described some undesirable behaviors (i.e., educational effects), including seeking out patient encounters that meet assessment requirements "rather than those that are interesting" or challenging [6]. These findings highlight the importance of creating a shared responsibility for assessment between programs, faculty, and trainees, while proactively evaluating the impact of assessment strategies on trainees to continuously improve.

Ensuring assessment is *equitable* relates closely to the impact of assessment on trainees and is also a critical priority. As described by Lucey et al., "equity in assessment is present when all [trainees] have fair and impartial opportunities to learn, be evaluated, coached, graded, advanced, graduated, and selected for subsequent opportunities based on their demonstration of achievements that predict future success in the field of medicine, and that neither learning experiences nor assessments are negatively influenced by structural or interpersonal bias related to personal or social characteristics of learners or assessors" [25]. Unfortunately, many studies show inequities in assessment across medical education based on race, ethnicity, gender, and more [3, 4, 22, 28, 29, 44]. Furthermore, studies have demonstrated that even minor differences in assessment outcomes can have a large impact on future opportunities [4, 34].

Traditionally, assessment has often focused on identifying "struggling" trainees, a label that continues to be disproportionately applied to trainees from underrepresented in medicine (URiM) groups. In addition, data still demonstrate bias in milestone-based assessments against US-born Black residents, which suggests that more needs to be done to improve equity in assessment [16]. In contrast to the focus on "struggling" trainees, the CBME perspective is that all trainees are on a developmental continuum and are continuously learning and growing, such that every trainee should have an individualized learning plan (ILP) plan, regardless of where they are on the spectrum of competency [25]. In addition to this helpful shift in mindset, Holmboe et al. in their 2023 paper, outline multiple strategies to improve assessment equitability. The five strategies described are stereotype replacement, perspective taking, individuation, counter-stereotypic imaging, and increased opportunities for contact. Each of these are practical strategies that can be readily employed by faculty [19]. When done in an authentic way, with proper attention to the core components, CBME has been described as well designed to create a more equitable system for assessment within GME [8, 15].

Reliability and validity are also important concepts when establishing an approach to assessment. A detailed discussion of these concepts is beyond the scope of this chapter, but the general principles are important considerations for programs. "Validity refers to whether an instrument actually does measure what it is purported to," and "reliability refers to the reproducibility of the scores obtained from an assessment" and is impacted by sources of variance including bias [40]. Importantly, no one assessment "method is inherently unreliable, and any method can be sufficiently reliable, provided sampling is appropriate across conditions of measurement" [40]. This point highlights that adopting an authentic, competency-based assessment approach (i.e., programmatic assessment) that includes diversity of data sources inherently addresses both reliability and validity [41].

Acceptability is the final factor to consider when determining the appropriateness of a data collection strategy for assessment. Acceptability describes the degree to which stakeholders such as trainees, faculty, CCCs, and external observers like regulatory agencies and the public agree that the assessment approach is credible [46]. If care is taken to select feasible assessment instruments that positively impact the trainee, have validity and reliability evidence, and are designed and administered equitably, then acceptability should follow.

While considering the various elements of an approach to assessment has the potential to be overwhelming, from a practical perspective, there are many opportunities to partner and share assessment techniques and instruments. If programs work to develop a comprehensive approach to CBME that integrates multiple data points from as many sources as possible, many of the challenges of an effective assessment approach are naturally solved.

Interpreting Data for Assessment

After data is collected, it must be interpreted. Ideally, the quantitative and qualitative data collected over time is collated into a portfolio or dashboard, which can inform formative feedback provided by coaches and program directors as well as summative decisions made by CCCs. As required by the ACGME, all pediatric GME programs have CCCs involved in the analysis and interpretation of assessment data, which is described in more detail elsewhere in this text.

However, it is important to note that there is often a substantial lack of data available for CCC decision-making in the current state of assessment in GME. As described by Lucey et al., "absent well-rounded data from multiple sources, group members may default to making decisions based on impressions or limited data, a process that again introduces risk for bias" [25]. The existence of this problem was further confirmed in a recent study in pediatrics in which the "default" approach to decision-making by CCCs was described as the most common pathway [31]. This issue is best mitigated by proactively creating a well-rounded assessment program that is focused on outcomes (i.e., EPAs) and establishes a broad set of instruments that gather data designed to inform decisions about progression, advancement, and ultimate readiness to practice.

An important priority when gaps in data are identified is to determine a process for adding additional information into the assessment portfolio. Drawing upon multiple sources and relying on committees rather than individuals to make assessment determinations, particularly high-stakes ones, is critical to promoting equity, as this approach considers the wisdom of the group and diversity of opinion [25].

Another important aspect of data interpretation that is often not explicitly discussed or considered is referencing, which may be done in either a criterion-referenced or a norm-referenced manner. Criterion-referencing measures performance against a fixed standard, such that all trainees being assessed could meet or not meet the standard—regardless of the performance of other individuals. Norm-referencing ranks performance against a group of individuals so that a trainee's performance is always relative to others being assessed. CBME should exclusively involve criterion-referencing, which is focused on the achievement of a specific set of tasks (i.e., EPAs) that either can or cannot be performed. This perspective is in contrast to norm-referencing, which creates a relative ranking compared to the performance of other peers [12]. Unfortunately, many aspects of the educational system, and even GME training, encourage a norm-referenced frame in which many individuals feel obliged to compete to be the best in a group rather than focus on becoming the best possible pediatrician. Creating an atmosphere where the entirety of a program—trainees and faculty alike—are focused on a criterion-referenced approach to data analysis is consistent with CBME and encourages a growth-oriented mindset, described in more detail later. The focus of analysis in a competency-based education and assessment system must prioritize gleaning what the trainee can and cannot do so that they can be coached appropriately to develop to their maximum potential. This approach is critical because in the end, "our focus must be to design assessments to ensure every graduate exceeds the competency thresholds necessary to [provide] safe, high-quality patient care, rather than to identify the top 10% of a graduating class" [25].

Feedback for the Trainee and Program

With the goal of achieving or surpassing the expected outcomes in mind, timely and actionable feedback is an integral part of the developmental process for each trainee so that goals can be established and individualized learning plans can be developed to facilitate achievement of those goals. Most programs and trainees recognize the importance of feedback, but this area is a frequent area of frustration and dissatisfaction in GME across multiple specialties. Supervisors and trainees are often not trained in feedback best practices, and a shared mental model of the optimal approach to feedback is often not present. The working and learning environment also is often not conducive to feedback, particularly with respect to creating sufficient time for meaningful conversations [10, 26]. Another challenge is that the structure of many clinical experiences leads to frequently changing supervisory relationships, which do not allow for longitudinal relationships and strong educational alliances—increasing the risk that trainees will perceive feedback as less credible [35, 42]. Trainees sometimes adapt to these challenges by taking on a performance approach where they change their behavior to conform to what they perceive to be desired by a specific supervisor rather than authentically caring for the patient with a mindset focused on growth [24].

A qualitative study of a direct observation program in a psychiatry residency continuity clinic found that bundling strategies for successful feedback together can help mitigate challenges and shift the focus from judgment to growth. In this study they designed a structured feedback program that featured (1) protected time for repeated direct observation and feedback, (2) longitudinal supervisory relationships, (3) assessment tools with evidence of validity, (4) ongoing faculty and resident training on program goals, resident autonomy, structured observation, and bidirectional feedback, and (5) monitoring faculty and resident participation. Semi-structured interviews of participating residents and supervisors found that participants were aligned with respect to the goals of feedback and that educational alliances existed between supervisors and trainees characterized by trust and respect. Longitudinal relationships and repeated practice encouraged trainees to abandon the performance approach and more authentically interact with patients. Feedback was generally perceived as credible, although when residents did disagree with the feedback they received, they often internally discounted the feedback. Findings from this study suggest that an intentionally designed feedback program can yield positive results [45, 46].

There is often a substantial disconnect between faculty expectations regarding providing feedback and trainees receiving it. Trainees often are reluctant to request feedback for a variety of reasons, with one concern being that they do not want to burden the faculty. This issue of the burden of assessment is an important one to overcome when developing an assessment system, and a clear best practice is for the approach to be simple and built into the clinical workflow of the day for trainees and faculty as described above. Faculty often prioritize clinical duties over making time to provide feedback to trainees and may often be "placing the onus for observation on the resident [which] may represent an attempt by faculty to juggle competing demands, in essence deferring the burden of deciding between clinical and educational responsibilities until prompted" [10]. There are many approaches to address these challenges, including the creation of "direct observation shifts" where faculty observers have no clinical or administrative responsibilities and are instead focused on providing feedback [10]. Carving out dedicated, protected time in a shift or clinic schedule is another approach, but there is a risk that other tasks will slip into the time set aside for feedback. Both approaches require faculty resources that may not be available in many programs, reinforcing the importance of a simple mechanism for faculty to provide feedback integrated into their clinical workday.

Feedback also should be supplemented with observations and conversations with allied health professionals, more senior or junior trainees (i.e., peers), and patients and caregivers who are all uniquely poised to provide feedback [36]. None of these sources of feedback should be seen as a replacement for faculty-trainee interactions. An important consideration is that feedback from others in the learning environment may not be perceived as relevant or credible in some aspects of a trainee's performance, but this input is particularly useful with respect to the trainee's communication skills, bedside manner, and professionalism [7].

This feedback "in the moment" associated with observation and WBA should be thought of separately from coaching, which is an important, but different, element of trainee feedback and development. Conversations with a dedicated coach provide a mechanism for feedback and other discussions to be synthesized through the lens of an experienced faculty member who has a meaningful and longitudinal relationship with the trainee. A best practice for every program working to embrace a competency-based system of education and assessment is the assignment of a coach to each trainee and the creation of specific expectations around how the coach can support each trainee's growth and development. Examples of specific expectations for coaches include regular meetings with the trainee, interpretation of assessment data, and establishment of a specific and individualized learning plan. Ideally, coaches have longitudinal relationships with trainees and are not involved in summative decisions by the program. Coaches can also advocate for the trainee at the program level as they provide a unique holistic perspective on the trainee's performance [5]. Coaching provides benefits beyond delivery of feedback to trainees including impacts on both professional identify formation and well-being, which are described elsewhere in this text. Tips for developing a coaching program can be found elsewhere in this text and also in the paper, *Tips for developing a coaching program in medical education* [27].

Feedback and coaching are not only essential for trainees' development, but also the successful evolution of a CBME-oriented training program. Individual trainee assessments can be aggregated at the level of the program to conduct robust program evaluation to identify strengths and gaps in the training program. These results should be used to evaluate and revise both the assessment program and curriculum, with a particular eye toward how bias and inequity may be influencing the results and impacting the trainees [19]. In fact, as part of the accreditation process, the ACGME requires that programs elicit confidential, written feedback from residents and faculty at least annually. This feedback is then expected to be reviewed, and if deficiencies are identified, the program is tasked with creating a written action plan. The program is also expected to document formal, systematic evaluation of resident performance, faculty development, graduate performance (including performance of program graduates on the certification examination) and program quality [1]. Beyond the required program evaluation, programs may find it beneficial to gather feedback from trainees and faculty more frequently than once per year. Taking time at faculty meetings, gathering data from coaches, and regularly scheduling check-ins with individual trainees or groups of trainees can all facilitate eliciting feedback for the program which can drive iterative change. Alumni are another important source of feedback for the program, and their input might best be gathered via anonymous surveys.

Establishing a Learning Environment Conducive to CBME

Clinical learning environments (CLEs) are defined as places where learners are engaged in healthcare-related activities. Pediatric GME programs in the US exist in unique learning environments, and each context has a complex interplay of a variety of factors. In the literature, the four primary domains of a learning environment have been defined as physical, organizational, social, and personal [21]. Each of these components provides unique and important contributions to how conducive (or not) a given CLE might be for competency-based education and assessment. A detailed discussion of the complexities of the CLE and how to optimize the CLE for learning is beyond the scope of this chapter and covered elsewhere in this text, but as programs work to implement a competency-based approach to education and assessment, the impact of the CLE cannot be understated. Increasing demands of faculty and trainees, structures and processes that contribute to inequities and social and personal factors that hinder learning all degrade trust in the CLE, which is foundational to an authentic and genuine approach to competency-based education and assessment [8, 9, 20]. Trust is an essential component for competency-based assessment since the focus in a CBME environment is on growth, to help equip each individual to not only meet the standards as described above but to achieve their maximum potential.

A focus on growth in the CLE, commonly referred to in the literature as a "growth mindset," as alluded to earlier in this chapter, is an essential component of a competency-based approach to assessment. Growth mindset can be defined as an individual's (and in this case, a program's) perspective that an individual trainee can develop talents and skills by working to integrate feedback in a continuous cycle of improvement. This growth mindset is often contrasted to a "fixed" mindset, in which one believes that an individual has an innate set of skills or talents. While many involved in medical education conceptually support the notion of a growth mindset, it is often woefully deficient in practice. One way this challenge is frequently manifested in GME is through the structures and processes set up for assessment. As briefly noted above, many programs' approaches to assessment are designed so that faculty formally assess trainees exclusively at the conclusion of a specific rotation or clinical experience [1]. While this approach is consistent with published requirements for evaluation, it does not lend itself to a growth-oriented approach to assessment and learning. In this scenario, faculty and trainees are often days, to sometimes weeks, removed from clinical encounters that contribute to assessments, which leads to limited and often generic information being included in assessments. In the eyes of trainees, and sometimes faculty, this approach also feels like a high-stakes "grade" that is being provided to document a trainee's performance—a clear depiction of assessment *of* learning.

In contrast, a more optimal approach to assessment in a competency-based system involves "real time" assessment and feedback as described earlier in this chapter, which happens as close to the time of a clinical encounter as possible and is part of the daily workflow for faculty and trainees. These assessments may be prompted by trainees or faculty, with a focus on growth and improvement. Frequent formative assessment that is low-stakes, individualized, and focused on helping each trainee reach their full potential should be the goal and is how competency-based assessment should be implemented—commonly referred to as assessment *for* learning. These frequent assessments take the pressure off both faculty and trainees since each individual assessment and conversation then becomes a very small piece of a large portfolio of assessments, allowing for authentic conversations focused on development and improvement.

Another important aspect of assessment that can be improved upon through frequent, formative assessment for learning is equity. As noted above, there is substantial evidence that many of our GME assessment systems are inequitable [25], and a competency-based approach focused on assessment for learning in this way can make the system more equitable [8, 15]. Clearly, this approach requires vulnerability on the part of the trainee and substantial trust in the system by both the trainee and faculty, which reinforces the importance of prioritizing diversity among faculty and putting structures and processes in place to optimize the CLE.

It is very likely that all aspects of the learning environment may not be in the control of GME programs, or even departmental leaders associated with a given program. However, there are ways to create structure and processes in training programs related to assessment that facilitate frequent and formative assessment, focus on growth, and are designed to allow for each resident or fellow to reach their full potential, and these approaches can go a long way in improving the environment for learning in a program and moving toward an authentic approach to

CBME. Competency-based education and assessment also sets the stage for early identification of trainees with differing trajectories and allows for individualized learning plans to be developed by programs, in partnership with trainees. This individualized learning is often discussed in the context of the development of remediation plans for a "struggling" trainee, but a competency-based system should be designed in a way that *all trainees* have an individualized plan to reach their maximum potential, whether it is achieving the minimum standard necessary for safe and effective care of patients, or mastering a certain area in which they excel.

Programmatic Assessment

The final of the five core components is programmatic assessment, simply defined as using multiple sources of data to contribute to a portfolio for decision-making about the progression of a trainee. While most pediatric GME programs have some structures in place to gather multi-source data regarding trainee development and progression, the full potential of programmatic assessment is often unrealized. As noted above, the current state of trainee assessment in pediatric GME is often limited to end of rotation evaluations, leading to an overall small number of total assessments available for programs and CCCs to consider for high-stakes decision-making. As mentioned above, in a recent qualitative study analyzing the data available and decision-making by CCCs in pediatrics, it was demonstrated that decisions are often being made with inadequate information [31]. In this study, the authors describe the most common pathway for progression and advancement decisions as one of "default" in which a trainee is advanced simply by the nature of time passed in the program unless concerns or "red flags" are reported in assessments [31]. These findings were further reinforced in a follow-up investigation revealing that there is a lack of intentionality and deliberateness in decision-making by CCCs, likely related to a paucity of data, in making high-stakes summative decisions about trainee progression and advancement [31].

Ensuring that the necessary data is available in a competency-based system and fully implementing this fifth core component of CBME requires intentionality in developing a comprehensive approach to assessment of trainees that integrates a wide range of formative and summative data points. An important element of programmatic assessment is described above and involves programs developing a robust system for "real-time" frontline assessments by faculty, peers, the interprofessional team, patients, and families. Termed workplace-based assessments in the literature and described in more detail above, these largely formative assessments are an essential element of programmatic assessment. These data can be triangulated with a wide range of other data points, including written knowledge assessments (e.g., multiple-choice exams), simulation-based assessments, oral exams, OSCEs, mini-CExs, and others, to paint a comprehensive picture of each individual trainee's progress that can be used for both longitudinal growth and development and summative decision-making.

Conclusions

In summary, competency-based assessment is a critically important component of CBME, but it cannot be considered in isolation. Without robust implementation of the five core components of CBME, competency-based assessment alone will likely not succeed in achieving our collective goal of preparing trainees to become the best possible pediatricians and pediatric subspecialists. Competency-based assessment starts and ends with the needs of patients—it should involve a focus on developing a comprehensive system of assessment that integrates data into specific and individualized learning plans designed to help each trainee achieve their fullest potential based on those patient needs. A competency-based approach to assessment also ensures that programs have the data necessary to make criterion-referenced, summative, high-stakes decisions about trainee promotion, advancement, and graduation.

References

1. Accreditation Council for Graduate Medical Education. Common Program Requirements. 2023. https://www.acgme.org/globalassets/pfassets/programrequirements/cprresidency_2023.pdf. Accessed 31 Aug 2024.
2. American Board of Pediatrics. 2024. https://www.abp.org/content/entrustable-professional-activities-general-pediatrics. Accessed 31 Aug 2024.
3. Anderson JE, Zern NK, Calhoun KE, et al. Assessment of potential gender bias in general surgery resident milestone evaluations. JAMA Surg. 2022;157:1164. https://doi.org/10.1001/jamasurg.2022.3929.
4. Boatright D, Ross D, O'Connor P, et al. Racial disparities in medical student membership in the alpha omega alpha honor society. JAMA Intern Med. 2017;177:659. https://doi.org/10.1001/jamainternmed.2016.9623.
5. Branfield Day L, Colbourne T, Ng A, et al. A qualitative study of Canadian resident experiences with competency-based medical education. Can Med Educ J. 2022; https://doi.org/10.36834/cmej.72765.
6. Braund H, Patel V, Dalgarno N, Mann S. Exploring residents' perceptions of competency-based medical education across Canada: a national survey study. MedEdPublish. 2024;14:2. https://doi.org/10.12688/mep.19247.1.
7. Brinkman WB, Geraghty SR, Lanphear BP, et al. Effect of multisource feedback on resident communication skills and professionalism. Arch Pediatr Adolesc Med. 2007;161:44. https://doi.org/10.1001/archpedi.161.1.44.
8. Busari JO, Diffey L, Hauer KE, et al. Advancing anti-oppression and social justice in healthcare through competency-based medical education (CBME). Med Teach. 2024;46:1167–74. https://doi.org/10.1080/0142159X.2023.2298763.
9. Caretta-Weyer HA, Smirnova A, Barone MA, et al. The next era of assessment: building a trustworthy assessment system. Perspect Med Educ. 2024;13:12–23. https://doi.org/10.5334/pme.1110.
10. Cheung WJ, Patey AM, Frank JR, et al. Barriers and enablers to direct observation of trainees' clinical performance: a qualitative study using the theoretical domains framework. Acad Med. 2019;94:101–14. https://pubmed.ncbi.nlm.nih.gov/30095454/.
11. Dreyfus SE, Dreyfus HL. A five-stage model of mental activities involved in directed skill acquisition. 1980. https://www.researchgate.net/publication/235125013_A_Five-Stage_Model_of_the_Mental_Activities_Involved_in_Directed_Skill_Acquisition
12. Elshama S. How to use and apply assessment tools in medical education? Iberoam J Med. 2020;2(4):351–9. https://doi.org/10.5281/zenodo.3978444.
13. Englander R, Frank JR, Carraccio C, et al. Toward a shared language for competency-based medical education. Med Teach. 2017;39:582–7. https://doi.org/10.1080/0142159X.2017.1315066.
14. Ferguson PC, Caverzagie KJ, Nousiainen MT, Snell L. Changing the culture of medical training: an important step toward the implementation of competency-based medical education. Med Teach. 2017;39:599–602. https://doi.org/10.1080/0142159X.2017.1315079.
15. Gilliam CA, Lurie B, Winn AS, et al. The role of competency based medical education in addressing health inequities and cultivating inclusive learning environments. Curr Probl Pediatr Adolesc Health Care. 2024:101641. https://doi.org/10.1016/j.cppeds.2024.101641.
16. Gray BM, Lipner RS, Roswell RO, et al. Adoption of internal medicine milestone ratings and changes in bias against Black, Latino, and Asian internal medicine residents. Ann Intern Med. 2024;177:70–82. https://doi.org/10.7326/M23-1588.
17. Hamstra SJ, Yamazaki K. A validity framework for effective analysis and interpretation of milestones data. J Grad Med Educ. 2021;13(2 Suppl):75–80. https://doi.org/10.4300/JGME-D-20-01039.1. Epub 2021 Apr 23. PMID: 33936537; PMCID: PMC8078069.
18. Holmboe ES, Sherbino J, Long DM, et al. The role of assessment in competency-based medical education. Med Teach. 2010;32:676–82. https://doi.org/10.3109/0142159X.2010.500704.
19. Holmboe ES, Osman NY, Murphy CM, Kogan JR. The urgency of now: rethinking and improving assessment practices in medical education programs. Acad Med. 2023;98:S37–49. https://pubmed.ncbi.nlm.nih.gov/37071705/.
20. Hsu D, Rassbach C, Leaming-Van Zandt K, et al. Competency based medical education and trust in the learning environment. Curr Probl Pediatr Adolesc Health Care. 2024:101640. https://doi.org/10.1016/j.cppeds.2024.101640.
21. Irby DM. Improving environments for learning in health professionals professions. Josiah Macy Jr Foundation; 2018. https://macyfoundation.org/assets/reports/publications/macy_monograph_2018_webfile.pdf. Accessed 31 Aug 2024.
22. King JT, Angoff NR, Forrest JN, Justice AC. Gender disparities in medical student research awards: a 13-year study from the Yale School of Medicine. Acad Med. 2018;93:911–9. https://doi.org/10.1097/ACM.0000000000002052.
23. Kogan JR, Holmboe ES. Realizing the promise and importance of performance-based assessment. Teach Learn Med. 2013;25 https://doi.org/10.1080/10401334.2013.842912.

24. LaDonna KA, Hatala R, Lingard L, et al. Staging a performance: learners' perceptions about direct observation during residency. Med Educ. 2017;51:498–510. https://pubmed.ncbi.nlm.nih.gov/28247495/.
25. Lucey CR, Hauer KE, Boatright D, Fernandez A. Medical education's wicked problem: achieving equity in assessment for medical learners. Acad Med. 2020;95:S98–S108. https://doi.org/10.1097/ACM.0000000000003717.
26. Massie J, Ali JM. Workplace-based assessment: a review of user perceptions and strategies to address the identified shortcomings. Adv Health Sci Educ. 2015;21:455–73. https://doi.org/10.1007/s10459-015-9614-0.
27. Miller-Kuhlmann R, Sasnal M, Gold CA, et al. Tips for developing a coaching program in medical education. Med Educ Online. 2023;29 https://doi.org/10.1080/10872981.2023.2289262.
28. Mueller AS, Jenkins TM, Osborne M, et al. Gender differences in attending physicians' feedback to residents: a qualitative analysis. J Grad Med Educ. 2017;9:577–85. https://doi.org/10.4300/JGME-D-17-00126.1.
29. Rojek AE, Khanna R, Yim JWL, et al. Differences in narrative language in evaluations of medical students by gender and under-represented minority status. J Gen Intern Med. 2019;34:684–91. https://doi.org/10.1007/s11606-019-04889-9.
30. Schumacher DJ, Schumacher DJ, West DC, et al. Longitudinal assessment of resident performance using entrustable professional activities. 2020;3:19316. https://doi.org/10.1001/JAMANETWORKOPEN.2019.19316.
31. Schumacher DJ, Michelson C, Winn AS, et al. A realist synthesis of prospective entrustment decision making by entrustment or clinical competency committees. Med Educ. 2023;58:812–24. https://doi.org/10.1111/medu.15296.
32. Shumway JM, Harden RM. AMEE Guide No. 25: The assessment of learning outcomes for the competent and reflective physician. Med Teach. 2003;25:569–84. https://doi.org/10.1080/0142159032000151907.
33. Tabish SA. Assessment methods in medical education. Int J Health Sci. 2008;2:3–7.
34. Teherani A, Hauer KE, Fernandez A, et al. How small differences in assessed clinical performance amplify to large differences in grades and awards: a cascade with serious consequences for students underrepresented in medicine. Acad Med. 2018;93:1286–92. https://doi.org/10.1097/ACM.0000000000002323.
35. Telio S, Regehr G, Ajjawi R. Feedback and the educational alliance: examining credibility judgements and their consequences. Med Educ. 2016;50:933–42. https://doi.org/10.1111/medu.13063.
36. ten Cate O, Sargeant J. Multisource feedback for residents: how high must the stakes be? J Grad Med Educ. 2011;3:453–5. https://doi.org/10.4300/JGME-D-11-00220.1.
37. ten Cate O. How can Entrustable Professional Activities serve the quality of health care provision through licensing and certification? Can Med Educ J. 2022;13:8–14. https://doi.org/10.36834/cmej.73974.
38. Turner DA, Schwartz A, Carraccio C, et al. Continued supervision for the common pediatric subspecialty entrustable professional activities may be needed following fellowship graduation. Acad Med. 2021;96 https://doi.org/10.1097/ACM.0000000000004091.
39. van der Vleuten CPM. The assessment of professional competence: developments, research and practical implications. Adv Health Sci Educ. 1996;1:41–67. https://doi.org/10.1007/BF00596229.
40. van der Vleuten CPM, Schuwirth LWT. Assessing professional competence: from methods to programmes. Med Educ. 2005;39:309–17. https://doi.org/10.1111/J.1365-2929.2005.02094.X.
41. Van Melle E, Frank JR, Holmboe ES, et al. A core components framework for evaluating implementation of competency-based medical education programs. Acad Med. 2019;94:1002–9. https://doi.org/10.1097/ACM.0000000000002743.
42. Watling C, Driessen E, van der Vleuten CPM, Lingard L. Learning from clinical work: the roles of learning cues and credibility judgements. Med Educ. 2012;46:192–200. https://pubmed.ncbi.nlm.nih.gov/22239333/.
43. Weiss PG, Schwartz A, Carraccio CL, et al. Achieving entrustable professional activities during fellowship. Pediatrics. 2021;148 https://doi.org/10.1542/peds.2021-050196.
44. Woolf K, Viney R, Rich A, et al. Organisational perspectives on addressing differential attainment in postgraduate medical education: a qualitative study in the UK. BMJ Open. 2018;8:e021314. https://doi.org/10.1136/bmjopen-2017-021314.
45. Young JQ, Sugarman R, Schwartz J, O'Sullivan PS. Overcoming the challenges of direct observation and feedback programs: a qualitative exploration of resident and faculty experiences. Teach Learn Med. 2020;32:541–51. https://doi.org/10.1080/10401334.2020.1767107.
46. Young JQ, Frank JR, Holmboe ES. Advancing workplace-based assessment in psychiatric education. Psychiatr Clin N Am. 2021;44:317–32. https://doi.org/10.1016/j.psc.2021.03.005.

Clinical Competency Committees 22

Su-Ting T. Li

Introduction

The purpose of a Clinical Competency Committee is to review and synthesize information on resident performance in order to advise the Program Director on each resident's performance and progression toward autonomous practice [1–5]. Residents and fellows will be referred to as residents throughout this chapter unless referring only to fellows.

At a minimum, CCCs must (1) review all resident evaluations at least twice a year prior to the residents' semiannual evaluations to (2) determine each resident's progress on achievement of specialty-specific Milestones and (3) advise the PD on each resident's progress. If an Accreditation Council for Graduate Medical Education (ACGME)-accredited pediatric fellowship program accepts an "exceptionally qualified" international applicant who did not complete an ACGME-accredited, ACGME-International Advance Specialty-accredited, American Osteopathic Association-approved, Royal College of Physicians and Surgeons of Canada-accredited, or College of Family Physicians of Canada-accredited residency program, the CCC must additionally evaluate their performance within the first 12 weeks of starting fellowship [4].

The PD is the ultimate arbiter and has final responsibility for resident assessment, promotion decisions, and decisions on whether a resident is ready to practice independently without supervision. With input from the CCC, the PD or designee must: (1) meet with each resident to review their semiannual evaluation of performance, including progress along specialty-specific Milestones, and (2) help residents develop individualized learning plans to "capitalize on strengths and identify areas for growth" [4, 5]. For residents who are failing to progress, this includes developing plans for improvement following institutional policies and procedures. A 2022 study of family medicine program directors evaluating features of effective CCCs found that programs with formal faculty development for CCC members, written policies for synthesizing data, written policies describing a standardized way for residents to receive feedback, use of multiple sources of assessment data, and sufficient time for CCC members to discuss residents were more likely to report effectively identifying residents who performed below expectations [6].

CCC Membership

The CCC is appointed by the PD and must include a minimum of 3 faculty members,

S.-T. T. Li (✉)
University of California Davis, Davis, CA, USA
e-mail: sutli@health.ucdavis.edu

H. McPhillips et al. (eds.), *Graduate Medical Education in Pediatrics*, Excellence in Medical Education 3, https://doi.org/10.1007/978-3-032-12952-9_22

including at least one core faculty member [4, 5, 7]. Core faculty members are American Board of Pediatrics (ABP)-certified or American Osteopathic Board of Pediatrics (AOBP)-certified faculty with a significant role in the education and supervision of residents and must devote a significant portion of their entire effort to resident education and/or administration. They must teach, evaluate, and provide formative feedback to residents. The PD may choose as additional CCC members faculty from the same program, faculty outside the division/department, or other health professionals with extensive contact and experience with the program's residents, such as nurses, or faculty who only interact with residents in one aspect, such as scholarship [8]. Current residents are not allowed to serve as members of the CCC. Chief residents who have already completed their core residency and are eligible for board certification in their specialty may serve as an observer or member of the CCC. As near-peers, chief residents may offer valuable insight, particularly in the areas of professionalism or interpersonal and communication skills. However, some chief residents may find it challenging to engage in these high-stakes evaluations of residents who they view as friends. The PD may decide to instate term limits for CCC members (e.g., 5 years with the opportunity to serve for a second term). If the PD decides that CCC members should have term limits, the PD should consider having CCC members with staggered appointments so that not all members of the CCC rotate off at the same time. Ideal size of the CCC may be dependent on the size of the program. Larger programs may consider having multiple CCC subgroups to discuss subsets of residents or subsets of Milestones, with each CCC subgroup potentially consisting of 5–10 members, which is considered the ideal group size for each member to contribute substantively, be large enough to allow for diverse viewpoints, and small enough to avoid side conversations [9]. Table 22.1 describes CCC membership.

When constructing a CCC and determining CCC processes, the PD should consider how to ensure equitable assessment of residents [10]. This includes ensuring diverse CCC membership to bring different perspectives into CCC deliberations [11]. Diverse groups can make more accurate decisions than individuals when engaging in discussion using a structured process to arrive at a group decision [9, 11]. Diverse groups bring diverse perspectives, focus more on facts, make fewer factual errors, encourage greater scrutiny of each member's decisions, and may process information more carefully [12–14]. PDs should consider composition of CCCs that include considerations of diversity in race, ethnicity, gender, academic rank, program role, specialty, and clinical sites among other factors. CCC members with different lived experiences can offer insight into performance through differing perspectives, which allow the CCC to "consider multiple decision options and avoid premature closure" [11]. In addition, PDs should consider requiring CCC members to receive formal training on implicit bias [11]. It may be helpful to have a bias disruptor in the CCC, whether that is a member of the CCC whose additional role is to call out any potential bias or to empower all CCC members to call out any perceived potential bias. Once potential bias is recognized, this allows the CCC to slow down and reexamine their processes and decision making to ensure that bias is mitigated. All CCC discussions must be kept strictly confidential, and some programs have CCC members sign a confidentiality agreement. In small programs, if all faculty are members of the CCC, it may be challenging to ensure confidentiality for residents discussed.

The PD may choose their level of involvement in the CCC, from not being involved in CCC meetings, being an observer in the CCC meetings, being a member of the CCC meetings, or being the Chair of the CCC meetings [1, 15]. A PD may choose to be involved in CCC meetings to be able to provide additional information about concerns raised by other faculty [16]. A PD may choose not to be a member of the CCC meetings so that the CCC functions independently of the PD without undue influence from the PD, as the CCC is giving recommendations to the PD. The PD may choose, due to the PD's additional roles as resident advocate, advisor, mentor, and confidante, not to be involved with CCC meetings.

Table 22.1 Clinical Competency Committee (CCC) membership

Minimum requirement for CCC members[a]	Optional CCC members	Notes
1. Core faculty[b]	Program director may be chair, member, observer, or not involved in CCC meetings	Program director may be the core faculty member
2. Additional faculty	Additional members of CCC must be faculty from the same program or other programs, or other health professionals with extensive contact and experience with the residents	Consider including faculty from diverse backgrounds to encourage diverse perspectives
	Non-voting members of CCC may be part of the CCC or invited to participate in a discussion on a particular resident. Non-voting members of the CCC may observe or contribute to the discussion of residents but may not contribute to the final decision on resident performance	In smaller programs, all program faculty may be CCC members
	In some instances, a program coordinator/manager may be a voting member of the CCC and may contribute to the final decision on resident performance. In other programs, a program coordinator/manager observes the CCC meeting to document minutes but does not contribute to the discussion on residents.	Chief residents who have completed their residency program and are eligible for board certification in their specialty may serve as members of the CCC. Non-voting members may include chief residents, faculty mentors/advisors, other health care providers, and medical education specialists. Faculty advisors or coaches may be asked to attend a portion of a CCC meeting where their resident advisee is being discussed. Residents may be asked to attend a portion of a CCC meeting when they are discussed Program coordinator / manager often attends the CCC meeting as a nonvoting member to take notes on the decision process, including the final agreed-upon milestone score for residents discussed

[a]CCC members are responsible for discussing resident performance data, determining resident progress on Milestone achievement, and advising the PD on each resident's progress. If the CCC utilizes voting to determine a resident's performance, only voting members of the CCC are eligible to vote

[b]Core faculty are American Board of Pediatrics certified or American Osteopathic Board of Pediatrics certified and must have a significant role in the education and supervision of residents. They must devote a significant portion of their time to resident education and/or administration and teach, evaluate, and provide feedback to residents. The CCC must include at least 1 core faculty member

The presence of the PD, whether or not the PD is Chair of the CCC, may hamper other CCC members from freely expressing their opinions [16]. If the PD is present during the CCC meeting, they should be cognizant of their potential effect on the discussion and endeavor to encourage open discussion and elicit everyone's viewpoints.

The Chair of the CCC should be familiar with assessment and Milestones and effective at creating a psychologically safe environment for CCC members to have open discussion about resident progress in their Milestone path toward unsupervised practice [11, 15]. If the PD chooses not to be Chair of the CCC, the PD should consider who might be best qualified to facilitate open discussion about residents to enable an equitable Milestone score based on available data. The PD might find that the best person to serve as CCC Chair may be an Associate Program Director, another faculty member, be elected by CCC members, or rotated among CCC members.

Depending on the number of residents in the program, how the CCC is constructed, prework needed by CCC members, and the frequency and duration of CCC meetings, faculty on CCCs may need to devote a significant amount of their time to this work. It may be challenging to recruit busy faculty to serve as CCC members, especially if there is no mechanism to account for their time. Some programs provide compensation for CCC members in the form of monetary compensation, protected time for CCC membership as part of their funded educational role in the department, and/or credit toward merit or promotion. Often, if CCC members are compensated, their role is expanded beyond just serving as a CCC member and may include serving as a faculty coach, advisor, and/or on the recruitment committee. PDs should be intentional in their decision to either include or exclude coaches or advisors on the CCC, particularly when discussing their specific advisee. Some PDs may intentionally invite the resident's coach and/or advisor to the CCC when their advisee is discussed, even when the coach/advisor is not a member of the CCC, to provide additional insight into the resident's performance and serve as the resident advocate. Other PDs may intentionally exclude a resident's coach and/or advisor from CCC meetings when discussing their specific advisee to allow the coach/advisor to be a safe faculty member not involved with assessment of the resident. The new Accreditation Council for Graduate Medical Education (ACGME) program requirements for graduate medical education in categorical pediatrics, effective July 1, 2025, require at least 1 core faculty member for every 5 approved resident positions in the program [17]. In addition, since required core faculty members, in aggregate, excluding program leadership, are required to be provided with support equal to an "average dedicated minimum of 0.1 FTE for educational and administrative responsibilities for the program that do not involve direct patient care," [17] it is possible that some PDs may be able to provide CCC members who are core faculty with some FTE support for their time.

In order for CCC members to effectively assess residents, they need a shared mental model of the subcompetencies, each Milestone level, and how each resident has progressed on the subcompetencies [11, 18]. In addition, in conjunction with their education team, PDs may want to consider how and if CCCs will play a role in determining level of entrustment for all graduating residents based on the American Board of Pediatrics Entrustable Professional Activities (EPAs) [19]. With the requirement to report EPAs to the ABP for initial certification decision making by 2028 [20], developing a shared mental model will require CCC member development [1, 16]. PDs, in conjunction with the CCC chair, needs to develop an onboarding process for new CCC members. There will need to be a recalibration of the shared mental model to ensure equity in CCC assessment of residents. Faculty development for CCC members may occur before, during, or after CCC meetings, or faculty may be encouraged to participate in institutional faculty development programs [16]. The ACGME's Clinical Competency Committees: A Guidebook for Programs, 3rd edition, includes resources for faculty development, including a quiz about CCCs and vignettes about challenging CCC cases [1]. A 2022 Canadian study of 8 residency programs identified challenges in CCC decision making, including different mental models of entrustment interpretation and performance standards, challenges with workplace-based assessment, including having residents directly observed, timely completion of assessments, and receiving high-quality written comments, and challenges with CCC resident performance review and competency decision making [21]. Suggestions included revising assessment tools, faculty development to ensure both assessors and CCC members have a single shared mental model, and adding resident representatives to the CCC. As stated above, the ACGME does not allow current residents to serve as members of the CCC, though chief residents who have already completed their residency program and are eligible for board certification are allowed to serve as members of the CCC. Others have suggested allowing the resident to attend the portion of a CCC meeting where they are being discussed to defend their portfolio [10]. If resident data reviewed ahead of the CCC meeting indicates concerns, inviting the resident's advisor, coach, or the resident themselves to that portion of the CCC meeting may provide additional insight and allow for a more equitable CCC decision. As the Program Evaluation Committee (PEC) does have resident members, the PEC could review the processes of the CCC to help ensure equitable CCC processes.

CCC Processes

CCC processes may be categorized into: pre-CCC meeting preparation, during-CCC meeting group process and decision making, and post-CCC meeting feedback, documentation, and follow-up. Table 22.2 shows the roles of CCC participants before, during, and after CCC meetings. There are a variety of ways to set up a CCC [1]. Programs with few residents may decide to schedule CCC meetings twice a year with ad hoc CCC meetings as concerns arise about residents. Programs with many residents may recognize that they will be unable to discuss all their residents in a single CCC meeting twice a year. Instead, they may decide to (1) meet more frequently (e.g., monthly) to discuss a subset of residents at each meeting, (2) have separate CCC subgroups for smaller subsets of residents, such as separate CCC subgroups for each post-graduate-year (PGY) cohort, (3) separate CCC subgroups by activity (e.g., separate CCC subgroups for quality improvement, research, inpatient rotations, outpatient rotations, procedures, etc.) or by subcompetency or EPA. For example, a CCC subgroup focused on quality improvement Milestone could review all information on quality improvement for each resident to make a Milestone determination on each resident. For programs who decide to have separate CCC subgroups for each PGY cohort, they may decide that the CCC subgroup follows the same cohort throughout their training at the program or stays with the same PGY year of training. Some programs may assign CCC members a subset of resident data to review prior to the CCC meeting to better identify and discuss residents with concerns. Other programs may present resident data to the entire CCC during the CCC meeting to make decisions on the resident. Programs with more than one CCC must ensure that all CCCs have a shared understanding of criteria for decision making to ensure fairness.

Pre-CCC Meeting Preparation

CCC members will need to receive, evaluate, and synthesize raw data from frontline assessments [22, 23] and other data [24–27] to determine individual resident performance, improvement toward unsupervised practice, and assign Milestone scores to each resident. It is important that members of the CCC clearly understand their role and how it fits into the role of the other members of the CCC. CCC members may be assigned residents from the same PGY cohort, assigned residents from all years of the program, assigned to review a type of assessment or rotation, or assigned a single subcompetency or activity to review across residents. If CCC members are assigned a group of residents to review, they may be assigned to follow the progress of those residents longitudinally through their residency. Table 22.3 shows examples of data which can be collected for CCC members to review. Program coordinators play a critical role in collating the necessary data ahead of time. Data management systems (e.g., MedHub, New Innovations) and Excel may be used to create dashboards to help synthesize the enormous quantity of data and make it digestible. Resident dashboards [28] could contain comparison data to help assess the resident in context—prior Milestone assessments, Milestone minimum expected by level of training, mean Milestone scores of peers within the program, and national Milestone scores of peers available on the ACGME website [29]. Both quantitative and qualitative data from multiple assessors (e.g., faculty, peers, patient/family, self, other health professional staff) are important [30]. Reliance on just quantitative assessments (e.g., mean scores) may not accurately represent resident performance as outlier assessments may inappropriately skew results out of context, or concerning outlier results may be missed. Asking CCC members to review resident Milestone aver-

Table 22.2 Clinical Competency Committee (CCC) processes

Role	Prior to CCC meeting	During CCC meeting	After CCC meeting
Program coordinator	Collects and collates resident data for CCC member review	Takes notes on CCC discussion and decisions, including agreed-upon milestone scores	Gives notes and milestone scores to PD
	Generates dashboard of resident data (e.g., milestone spider graph with prior milestone scores, minimum milestone expectations by level of training, mean milestone scores, and mean peer milestone scores for level of training)	Observes CCC meeting dynamics to provide feedback to CCC chair on how to improve group dynamics	Enters milestones scores to ACGME ADS site
	Distributes resident data / dashboards to CCC members		Coordinates meetings between PD or designee and resident to discuss milestone scores
	Invites CCC members and any non-CCC members determined by CCC chair (e.g., faculty advisor, faculty coach, resident) to CCC meeting		
CCC chair	In collaboration with CCC members and program director, determines agenda, including which residents discussed and in which order, faculty development planned during CCC meeting, and how to improve CCC processes	Facilitates discussion of residents to reach a consensus of milestone levels recommended for each resident and recommendations for promotion, remediation, suspension, non-renewal, non-promotion, or dismissal.	Relays discussion to PD
	Decides if / which non-CCC members are invited to CCC meeting (e.g., resident advisor; resident)	For residents who are not progressing as expected, with CCC members, develop a remediation plan (performance improvement plan)	
	In collaboration with the PD, schedules ad hoc CCC meetings when needed in response to concerning resident assessments, follow up on the progress of residents on remediation plans (performance improvement plans), plans CCC faculty development, or discusses ways to improve CCC processes	For advanced residents, discuss innovative educational opportunities to further enhance their development	
		Facilitates discussion of how to improve CCC processes (including additional sources of data if needed) to provide equitable assessment of residents.	
		Facilitates discussion to identify areas for improvement in the program (e.g., areas of weakness or gaps in assessment shared by multiple residents)	

CCC member	Reviews resident data for assigned residents if distributed prior to meeting Synthesizes assessments to arrive at a potential milestone level for each subcompetency for assigned residents Alerts program coordinator / CCC chair if any assigned residents require additional discussion at CCC meeting	Presents synthesized data of resident to support milestone levels they are recommending, including recommendations for promotion, remediation, suspension, non-renewal, non-promotion, or dismissal of a resident Participates in discussion of milestone levels, promotion, remediation, suspension, non-renewal, non-promotion, and dismissal of residents. Participates in discussion of remediation planning (performance improvement plan) for residents who are not progressing as expected. Discusses how to improve CCC processes (including additional sources of data if needed) to provide equitable assessment of residents	May be involved in remediation of residents not progressing as expected
Program director	Varies depending on whether PD is not a member of the CCC, an observer in the CCC, member of the CCC, or chair of CCC Ensures specialty-specific milestones, and when applicable, specialty-specific case logs will be used to assess resident progress.	Varies depending on whether PD is not a member of the CCC, an observer in the CCC, member of the CCC, or chair of CCC	Reviews and finalizes milestone scores for each resident Reviews, finalizes, and submits ACGME ADS milestone scores for each resident PD or their designee discusses milestone scores with each resident Ensures each resident receives annual summative and final summative evaluations. At least annually, the summative evaluation must include whether the resident is ready to progress to the next year of the program. The final summative evaluation must verify the resident has the knowledge, skills, and behaviors needed to practice autonomously after completing the program. In collaboration with CCC chair, develops a remediation plan (performance improvement plan) for residents who are failing to progress Collaborates with program evaluation committee (PEC) to ensure each resident receives sufficient performance data for CCC to make performance decisions on each resident
Resident	May utilize self-assessment to reflect on strengths and areas for improvement for individualized learning plan (ILP)	Residents may not serve as members of the CCC May be invited to participate in CCC meeting when they are discussed. Chief residents who have completed their core residency program and eligible for certification in their specialty may serve as observers or members of CCC	Meet with PD or their designee to discuss milestone scores, including areas of strengths and areas for growth

Table 22.3 Potential sources of data for Clinical Competency Committees to review to determine resident Milestone scores by competency

Patient care	Medical knowledge	Interpersonal and communication skills	Professionalism	Practice-based learning and improvement	Systems-based practice
Work-place based assessments	In-training exam scores	Multi-source assessments (e.g., self, peer, patient/ family, healthcare professional , faculty)	Conference attendance	Journal club presentation	Incident reports
End-of-rotation assessments	Multiple-choice questions (during residency, post-rotation, etc.)		Timely completion of administrative tasks (e.g., program evaluation, faculty assessments, online modules)	Grand rounds presentation	Electronic health record (notes, benchmarks)
Multi-source assessments (e.g., self, peer, patient/ family, healthcare professional)	Faculty assessments of medical knowledge		Multi-source assessments (e.g., self, peer, patient/ family, healthcare professional, faculty)	Scholarly project	Quality improvement and patient safety data
Electronic communication (e.g., email)	Chart stimulated recall		Professionalism in electronic communication	Self-assessment	Participation in quality improvement projects
Verbal communication				Learner assessment of teaching skills	Electronic health record (medical record audits, benchmarks)
Objective structured clinical exam (OSCE)				Evidence-based practice logs	Root cause analysis
Procedure logs				Development of individualized learning plan	
Simulated procedures					
Electronic health record (medical record audits, benchmarks)					
Resident-sensitive quality measures					
Videotaped performance					
Virtual reality					

age scores prior to the CCC meeting shortened the amount of time needed to discuss each resident during the CCC meeting [31]. CCC members found written comments were key to identifying residents who were not meeting expectations [32, 33]. Some programs only collect narrative evaluations and receive no numeric Milestone data, requiring CCC members to utilize the narrative comments to assign all Milestone scores. To comply with ACGME requirements, at a minimum, residents should be assessed after completion of every rotation and at least every 3 months for longitudinal experiences such as continuity clinic. At a minimum, residents should be assessed by faculty and one additional source. It is not the responsibility of the CCC to ensure that residents receive the minimum number of assessments. However, if CCC members note that a paucity of assessments interferes with their ability to assign Milestone scores, this should be discussed with the PD. The PD, in conjunction with the PEC, could then discuss a program improvement plan to collect additional assessments on residents.

Assessment tools utilizing a competency-based medical education framework, such as tools assessing Entrustable Professional Activities (EPAs) using an entrustment scale, can inform mapping of trainees to specialty-specific Milestones. This work will be enhanced by specific mapping of EPAs to subcompetencies, as many EPAs map to more than one of the subcompetencies and Milestones. It is essential that assessments be structured to mitigate implicit bias. Studies in internal medicine [34], emergency medicine [35], and surgery have shown gender, racial, and ethnic inequities in Milestone assessments of residents, including differences in qualitative comments on residents. Lack of high-quality written feedback, including lack of actionable corrective feedback in written assessments, makes it challenging for CCCs to make informed Milestone decisions [36]. Development of all front-line assessors (faculty, peers, other health care professionals) to ensure a shared mental model of each Milestone level, as well as how to support that assessment with written comments containing both reinforcing and corrective feedback, is important and will make it easier for CCC members to synthesize assessments. Utilizing learning analytics and natural language processing may help CCCs synthesize data from disparate sources to make data-informed decisions on residents [37–40]. The use of artificial intelligence to summarize narrative data should be used with caution, as it has the potential to amplify bias [41] and carries privacy concerns if a public source such as ChatGPT is utilized. Studies of the use of natural language processing in surgery [38], anesthesia [39], and dermatology [40] to synthesize narrative data for use in Milestone scoring is promising. A multicenter anesthesia study trained a natural language processing model to categorize feedback subcompetencies using data from 3 sites to evaluate the performance at a fourth site, which showed good model performance for competency domains of professionalism, interpersonal and communication skills, and practice-based learning and improvement (area under the receiver operating characteristic curve (AUC) 0.75–0.79), fair performance for medical care and patient care competencies (AUC 0.63–0.88), and poor performance for systems-based practice competency (AUC 0.59) [39].

CCC Meeting

In order to ensure equitable resident assessment, the CCC Chair should ensure all CCC members understand decision options, criteria for decision-making, and consequences of each decision [11, 42, 43]. In addition to Milestone level determinations and perhaps EPA level determinations (in preparation for the ABP requiring EPAs in 2028), CCC members will need to determine if the resident is progressing sufficiently in order to recommend promotion, remediation, suspension, non-renewal, non-promotion, or dismissal. All CCC members should have a shared understanding of the Milestones, assessment data, how to make decisions based on the data, and how to assess whether additional data is needed prior to deciding. The designation of one CCC member as a bias disruptor, whose role it is to call out the potential for bias in an individual assessment or committee decision either in a positive or negative direction, can help facilitate robust discussion and reduce bias. A structured process transparent to all members of the CCC may help ensure that all voices are heard [1, 11]. For example, the CCC Chair may first invite the CCC member who was responsible for reviewing the resident's data in advance of the CCC meeting to present the resident. Then, the CCC Chair may open the discussion to all CCC members, asking the most junior member of the CCC to comment first. To encourage open discussion, the CCC Chair should state their opinion last. In addition, if present, the PD should consider observing the discussion to provide clarifying information and refrain from offering their opinion, or wait to offer their opinion until all other voices have been heard.

Making data available for all CCC members in advance of the CCC meeting, or at least during the CCC meeting, will allow all CCC members the opportunity to make initial independent decisions based on the data before discussion and final decisions are made. Ideally, CCC meetings should be long enough to allow elicitation of diverse perspectives and ample time for discussion to reach consensus [9, 11]. The ACGME CCC Guidebook recommends that residents are discussed until a consensus is reached rather than calling for a vote on the resident, as "calling for a vote may lead to a situation in which the CCC may appear 'divided' and set up a situation in which its recommendation may be considered uncertain, leaving the program more vulnerable to a future challenge." [1]. While many CCCs focus primarily on residents who are not progressing as expected, [44] many recommend that the CCC take a developmental approach to help all residents optimize their education and progress in attaining competency [45]. For residents who are not progressing as expected, CCCs should also discuss recommendations for remediation plans (performance improvement plans) to help the resident based on areas of deficiency in one or more of the 6 competency domains. CCCs then recommend an action to the PD; PDs make the final decision on Milestone scores, promotion, remediation, or any adverse actions. Including the CCC is important so that it does not appear that the PD is making these high-stakes decisions independently. By including the CCC in resident assessment, including high-stakes decision making helps ensure the resident is assessed equitably and helps support the PD's decision.

CCC meetings are not only for accomplishing the goal of review and recommendations for each resident, but also an opportunity for CCC members to develop a shared understanding of assessment, Milestones, and group processes. CCC meetings are an opportunity to improve internal processes, identify program gaps, and offer suggestions to improve the program's curricula or assessment. The CCC may identify subcompetencies where most residents do not have sufficient data to assign a Milestone score as areas where the program may need to identify alternative assessment data. Additionally, the CCC may identify subcompetencies where most residents are not meeting expectations as an area where the program needs to improve its curricula and share that information with the Program Evaluation Committee. The CCC may also identify feedback that may be useful to faculty, including potentially identifying faculty who may benefit from additional faculty development and faculty who are role models in the way they provide specific reinforcing and corrective actionable feedback in their evaluations. These faculty role models might be recognized for merit and promotion committees or may make excellent faculty coaches. In an effort to ensure equitable assessment of residents, PDs with their educational leadership team should examine the program's own data for evidence of systematic group differences in performance, which could demonstrate bias, such as differences based on gender or race/ethnicity, and share this information with the CCCs.

Post-CCC Meeting

Post-CCC meeting, the CCC Chair needs to communicate the CCC discussion and recommendations for decisions to the PD. The PD is the final arbiter of resident Milestone scores and decisions and may disagree with CCC recommendations [46]. The program coordinator documents CCC discussions and decisions for each resident. Milestone scores are then entered into the ACGME Accreditation Data System (ADS), often by the program coordinator, and verified and submitted by the PD. The PD or their designee needs to communicate Milestone scores and decisions to each resident twice a year. At least annually, the PD needs to ensure each resident receives a summative evaluation describing their readiness to progress to the next year of training. At the completion of training, a final summative evaluation must attest that the resident has "demonstrated the knowledge, skills and behaviors necessary to enter autonomous practice" [47]. Residents who are not progressing as expected must receive a remediation plan (performance improvement plan) documenting specifically where they are not meeting expectations and a plan to support the resident to improve. Each institution or Designated Institutional Official (DIO) may have policies and procedures in place on how to communicate and document performance improvement expectations to residents. Oftentimes the DIO, human resources, Chair, and sometimes the institutional lawyer are involved with developing and approving, or at least made aware of, adverse actions including a performance improvement plan. CCCs may play different roles in these performance improvement plans, including whether or not they help develop, implement, and/or oversee the performance improvement plan.

Observers may be invited to contribute to the discussion of single or multiple residents, but may not contribute to the final decision of the resident's performance.

References

1. Andolsek K PJ, Hauer KE, Ekpenyong A, Edgar L, Holmboe E. Clinical Competency Committees. A Guidebook for Programs, 3rd Edition. 2020. https://www.acgme.org/globalassets/ACGMEClinicalCompetencyCommitteeGuidebook.pdf#:~:text=guidebook%20will%20briefly%20review%20of%20the. Accessed 24 Sept 2024.
2. Andolsek KM, Jones MD Jr, Ibrahim H, Edgar L. Introduction to the milestones 2.0: assessment, implementation, and clinical competency committees supplement. J Grad Med Educ. 2021;13(2 Suppl):1–4.
3. Ekpenyong A, Padmore JS, Hauer KE. The purpose, structure, and process of clinical competency committees: guidance for members and program directors. J Grad Med Educ. 2021;13(2 Suppl):45–50.
4. Accreditation Council for Graduate Medical Education. ACGME Common Program Requirements (Fellowship), effective July 1, 2023. https://www.acgme.org/globalassets/pfassets/programrequirements/cprfellowship_2023.pdf. Accessed 2 Oct 2024.
5. Accreditation Council for Graduate Medical Education. ACGME Common Program Requirements (Residency), effective July 1, 2023. https://www.acgme.org/globalassets/pfassets/programrequirements/cprresidency_2023.pdf. Accessed 2 Oct 2024.
6. Rowland K, Edberg D, Anderson L, Wright K. Features of effective clinical competency committees. J Grad Med Educ. 2023;15(4):463–8.
7. Accreditation Council for Graduate Medical Education. ACGME Program Requirements for Graduate Medical Education in Pediatrics, effective July 1, 2007. https://dconnect.acgme.org/acWebsite/downloads/RRC_progReq/320_pediatrics_07012007.pdf. Accessed 11 Feb 2014.
8. Langhan ML, Stafford DEJ, Myers AL, et al. Clinical competency committee perceptions of entrustable professional activities and their value in assessing fellows: a qualitative study of pediatric subspecialty program directors. Med Teach. 2023;45(6):650–7.
9. Hauer KE, Cate OT, Boscardin CK, et al. Ensuring resident competence: a narrative review of the literature on group decision making to inform the work of clinical competency committees. J Grad Med Educ. 2016;8(2):156–64.
10. Al-Bualy R, Ekpenyong A, Holmboe E. Effective clinical competency committee meeting practices: before, during, and after. Acad Med. 2023;98(11):1340.
11. Hauer KE, Edgar L, Hogan SO, Kinnear B, Warm E. The science of effective group process: lessons for clinical competency committees. J Grad Med Educ. 2021;13(2 Suppl):59–64.
12. Sommers SR. On racial diversity and group decision making: identifying multiple effects of racial composition on jury deliberations. J Pers Soc Psychol. 2006;90(4):597–612.
13. Phillips KW, Liljenquist KA, Neale MA. Is the pain worth the gain? The advantages and liabilities of agreeing with socially distinct newcomers. Personal Soc Psychol Bull. 2009;35(3):336–50.
14. Levine SS, Apfelbaum EP, Bernard M, Bartelt VL, Zajac EJ, Stark D. Ethnic diversity deflates price bubbles. Proc Natl Acad Sci USA. 2014;111(52):18524–9.
15. Blau JA, Atia AN, Powers DB. Clinical competency committees in plastic surgery residency. Plast Reconstr Surg Glob Open. 2021;9(9):e3833.
16. Ekpenyong A, Edgar L, Wilkerson L, Holmboe ES. A multispecialty ethnographic study of clinical competency committees (CCCs). Med Teach. 2022;44(11):1228–36.
17. Accreditation Council for Graduate Medical Education. ACGME Program Requirements for Graduate Medical Education in Pediatrics, effective July 1, 2025. https://www.acgme.org/globalassets/pfassets/programrequirements/2025-prs/320_pediatrics_2025.pdf. Accessed 3 Oct 2024.
18. Edgar L, Jones MD Jr, Harsy B, Passiment M, Hauer KE. Better decision-making: shared mental models and the clinical competency committee. J Grad Med Educ. 2021;13(2 Suppl):51–8.
19. American Board of Pediatrics. Entrustable Professional Activities (EPAS). https://www.abp.org/content/entrustable-professional-activities-epas. Accessed 3 Oct 2024.

20. American Board of Pediatrics. Next Steps for Training Programs. https://www.abp.org/content/next-steps-training-programs. Accessed 3 Oct 2024.
21. Szulewski A, Braund H, Dagnone DJ, et al. The assessment burden in competency-based medical education: how programs are adapting. Acad Med. 2023;98(11):1261–7.
22. Carney PA, Palmer RT, Fuqua Miller M, et al. Tools to assess behavioral and social science competencies in medical education: a systematic review. Acad Med. 2016;91(5):730–42.
23. Choe JH, Knight CL, Stiling R, Corning K, Lock K, Steinberg KP. Shortening the miles to the milestones: connecting EPA-based evaluations to ACGME milestone reports for internal medicine residency programs. Acad Med. 2016;91(7):943–50.
24. Kimbrough MK, Thrush CR, Barrett E, Bentley FR, Sexton KW. Are surgical milestone assessments predictive of in-training examination scores? J Surg Educ. 2018;75(1):29–32.
25. Martin SK, Farnan JM, McConville JF, Arora VM. Piloting a structured practice audit to assess ACGME milestones in written handoff communication in internal medicine. J Grad Med Educ. 2015;7(2):238–41.
26. O'Sullivan P, Greene C. Portfolios: possibilities for addressing emergency medicine resident competencies. Acad Emerg Med. 2002;9(11):1305–9.
27. Schumacher DJ, Martini A, Sobolewski B, et al. Use of resident-sensitive quality measure data in entrustment decision making: a qualitative study of clinical competency committee members at one pediatric residency. Acad Med. 2020;95(11):1726–35.
28. Friedman KA, Raimo J, Spielmann K, Chaudhry S. Resident dashboards: helping your clinical competency committee visualize trainees' key performance indicators. Med Educ Online. 2016;21:29838.
29. Sangha S KS, Shah H, Yamazaki K, Lekdee A, Edgar L, Hogan SO. Pediatrics Milestones Report 2024. 2024. https://www.acgme.org/globalassets/pdfs/milestones/specialty-specific/pediatrics-2024-milestones-national-report.pdf. Accessed 22 Mar 2025.
30. Ginsburg S, Watling CJ, Schumacher DJ, Gingerich A, Hatala R. Numbers encapsulate, words elaborate: toward the best use of comments for assessment and feedback on entrustment ratings. Acad Med. 2021;96(7s):S81–s86.
31. Nabors C, Forman L, Peterson SJ, et al. Milestones: a rapid assessment method for the clinical competency committee. Arch Med Sci. 2017;13(1):201–9.
32. Schumacher DJ, Michelson C, Poynter S, et al. Thresholds and interpretations: how clinical competency committees identify pediatric residents with performance concerns. Med Teach. 2018;40(1):70–9.
33. Ekpenyong A, Baker E, Harris I, et al. How do clinical competency committees use different sources of data to assess residents' performance on the internal medicine milestones? A mixed methods pilot study. Med Teach. 2017;39(10):1074–83.
34. Boatright D, Anderson N, Kim JG, et al. Racial and ethnic differences in internal medicine residency assessments. JAMA Netw Open. 2022;5(12):e2247649.
35. Mamtani M, Shofer F, Scott K, et al. Gender differences in emergency medicine attending physician comments to residents: a qualitative analysis. JAMA Netw Open. 2022;5(11):e2243134.
36. Anderson LM, Rowland K, Edberg D, Wright KM, Park YS, Tekian A. An analysis of written and numeric scores in end-of-rotation forms from three residency programs. Perspect Med Educ. 2023;12(1):497–506.
37. Carney PA, Sebok-Syer SS, Pusic MV, Gillespie CC, Westervelt M, Goldhamer MEJ. Using learning analytics in clinical competency committees: increasing the impact of competency-based medical education. Med Educ Online. 2023;28(1):2178913.
38. Abbott KL, George BC, Sandhu G, et al. Natural language processing to estimate clinical competency committee ratings. J Surg Educ. 2021;78(6):2046–51.
39. Booth GJ, Ross B, Cronin WA, et al. Competency-based assessments: leveraging artificial intelligence to predict subcompetency content. Acad Med. 2023;98(4):497–504.
40. Ramachandran V, Jairath N, Cheraghlou S, Pahalyants V. Revolutionizing dermatology residency: artificial intelligence for knowledge and clinical milestones assessment. Clin Exp Dermatol. 2024;49(7):732–3.
41. Glickman M, Sharot T. How human-AI feedback loops alter human perceptual, emotional and social judgements. Nat Hum Behav. 2025;9(2):345–59.
42. Schumacher DJ, King B, Barnes MM, et al. Influence of clinical competency committee review process on summative resident assessment decisions. J Grad Med Educ. 2018;10(4):429–37.
43. Schumacher DJ, Bartlett KW, Elliott SP, et al. Milestone ratings and supervisory role categorizations swim together, but is the water muddy? Acad Pediatr. 2019;19(2):144–51.
44. Hauer KE, Chesluk B, Iobst W, et al. Reviewing residents' competence: a qualitative study of the role of clinical competency committees in performance assessment. Acad Med. 2015;90(8):1084–92.
45. Goldhamer MEJ, Martinez-Lage M, Black-Schaffer WS, et al. Reimagining the clinical competency committee to enhance education and prepare for competency-based time-variable advancement. J Gen Intern Med. 2022;37(9):2280–90.
46. Schumacher DJ, Poynter S, Burman N, et al. Justifications for discrepancies between competency committee and program director recommended resident supervisory roles. Acad Pediatr. 2019;19(5):561–5.
47. Accreditation Council for Graduate Medical Education. Reformatted ACGME Common Program Requirements (Residency), effective July 1, 2025. https://www.acgme.org/globalassets/pfassets/programrequirements/2025-reformatted-requirements/cprresidency_2025_reformatted.pdf. Accessed 23 Mar 2025.

23 Resident Performance Challenges and Remediation

Katherine Mason and Christine Barron

Introduction

Medical education requires a consistent commitment to being a lifelong learner and to embracing the continuous improvement needed to incorporate emerging therapies and evolving knowledge. During residency and fellowship training, progressive independent practice is largely cultivated through ongoing supervision, assessment, and feedback. Trainees are observed, supported, and assessed, and receive both encouragement and constructive critique frequently to promote iterative skill acquisition and career expertise.

One successful outcome of pediatric residency is to confidently ascertain that the trainee consistently demonstrates the requisite knowledge, skills, and professional behaviors to care for well and sick children without direct supervision [1]. Inevitably, many medical learners will be identified as underperforming in one or more areas of competency during their graduate medical education training programs. These identified areas for improvement will require clear communication, correction and remediation. These areas for improvement may include one or more elements of the six core competencies. In the field of remediation, these have been expanded to the ACGME Competencies "Plus," which includes Medical Knowledge, Patient Care (Clinical Skills, Clinical Reasoning and Judgement), Time Management and Organization, Interpersonal Skills, Communication, Professionalism, Practice-Based Learning and Improvement, Systems-Based Practice, and Mental Well-Being [2].

Despite the universal understanding that residents will need to learn new ideas and skills, demonstrate professional growth, and improve their competencies over the course of their training, the process of remediation is often hampered by anxiety, uncertainty, stress, and even avoidance. This poses a tension between the inevitable need to improve knowledge, skills, behaviors, and mindset during residency and a hesitancy to provide clear, equitable, and compassionate remediation systems and processes that empower our learners and other stakeholders in medical education to support the development of an optimally trained pediatric workforce.

The barriers to fully embracing a culture of supportive remediation are numerous. From the learner perspective, residents are generally incredible academic and personal performers who are unfamiliar and uncomfortable with being told that their performance is suboptimal. This can lead them to feel defensive and to believe that the constructive feedback offered is unfair, discriminatory, or outright wrong. These common reactions to critique should be explored and considered, as it is entirely possible that bias and

K. Mason (✉) · C. Barron
Warren Alpert Medical School of Brown University, Providence, RI, USA
e-mail: katherine_mason1@brown.edu

H. McPhillips et al. (eds.), *Graduate Medical Education in Pediatrics*, Excellence in Medical Education 3, https://doi.org/10.1007/978-3-032-12952-9_23

inequity in the provision of constructive criticism can occur in even the best-designed and well-intentioned programs. The learner and remediation team should also explore the alternate perspective that constructive critique is being offered as a means to promote growth and excellence. From the program leadership perspective, remediation can be demoralizing for the program, requires extensive labor and time, is emotionally taxing for the remediation team, and can seem to conflict with the desire to provide a supportive environment for the learners [3]. Faculty may be concerned that they are not adequately trained to provide actionable remediation, that they lack sufficient time, expertise, or power to lead impactful remediation efforts. However, ensuring that residency graduates consistently demonstrate clinical competency, professionalism, and social responsibility is fundamental to the program's social contract to the community, and to the patients and families who will ultimately entrust graduates with the care of their children. Providing course correction and remediation for struggling learners is an ACGME requirement for sponsoring institutions and an expectation of the public and the communities we serve in health care. Tailored improvement interventions ranging from the supervision of taking a clinical history to the completion of disciplinary measures are required to support the learner in their professional identity formation and personal growth and to honor our contract with society to ensure our graduates meet high academic and professional standards. As pediatric faculty, we provide individually tailored clinical care that is developmentally appropriate, conscientious, sensitive, and unequivocally strives for the best outcomes for our patients and families. We can absolutely do the same for our learners, who are our legacy to the communities we serve.

Considerations Specific to Pediatric Training Programs

Pediatricians and pediatric training programs have specialty-specific areas of emphasis, expertise, and group norms that contribute to the framework of remediation of trainees. Pediatricians and their training programs are characterized by an embedded culture of discerning developmental patterns and understanding the continuity of skill development. The emphasis on family-centered care in pediatrics can translate into a view of remediation which includes a diversity of key stakeholders and a more holistic approach to learner assessment and the development of learning plans. The pediatric emphasis on preventative care aligns nicely with the development of systems to preemptively ensure the best outcomes for learners, as well as processes for the early identification of residents in need of more support and oversight. Finally, there are important parallels between understanding the benefits of early intervention for pediatric patients and the benefits of early intervention for struggling learners.

Pediatric trainees are most commonly identified as needing remediation for deficits in Medical Knowledge and Patient Care [4]. This differs from the earlier report by Guerrasio, in which residents from multiple disciplines who were referred to an institution-wide remediation program most commonly had difficulties with Practice-Based Learning and Improvement and Professionalism [5]. Importantly, more than one area of deficit is generally present in trainees requiring remediation, necessitating the ability to prioritize the most impactful areas for learner improvement within a holistic framework for supporting best performance in all areas.

It is also worth noting that, in general, educational budgets vary greatly between specialties and even between individual programs. The impact of providing resources to assist in remediation, such as coaching, protected and funded faculty time, consultation with educational and psychological experts, engaging with paid systems and programs for the assessment of potential learning deficits and neurodiverse challenges, board prep programs, and countless others, cannot be overstated in the discussion of optimizing learner remediation.

Remediation in the Pediatric GME context thus has unique cultural, environmental, and learner characteristics that inform and can enrich or detract from optimal outcomes.

Strategies to Mitigate Performance Challenges in Residency

While remediation interventions and programs are often constructed for individual trainees, a robust system-wide approach to cultivating excellent learner outcomes clearly offers great value. The process of remediation is time- and labor-intensive for the remediation team, the training program members and the learner. One recent study cited that remediation faculty required between 25 and 75 h per learner for an effective remediation process [6]. Residents involved in remediation often describe the process as stressful, painful, destabilizing, and even a threat to their personal and professional identities [7, 8]. Investing in some preventative care and anticipatory guidance to minimize and mitigate the need for formalized remediation is as consistent with good practice in medical education as it is in clinical care. The creation of a strong educational culture that is both supportive of learners and grounded in the responsibility to train excellent physicians is an achievable task.

Some general best practices in building a culture of educational excellence in pediatric residency to minimize performance challenges are described below. Setting clear expectations for the residents, faculty, and other team members regarding roles and responsibilities is foundational to trainee success. These may focus on professionalism, performance, knowledge, specific rotation goals and objectives, timeliness, communication, or others. As an example, a resident in an outpatient clinic may have specific learning goals around age-appropriate anticipatory guidance that they will discuss with the families, review with their preceptors, and then accurately document in the medical record in a timely fashion. They may be expected to ask for feedback from their preceptor, communicate clearly with the medical assistant, use official interpreter services when there is a language barrier, and finish their charting by 6 p.m. on clinic days. The preceptor may have clear expectations to provide verbal feedback to the learners daily, written feedback once per block, provide a 5-minute talk on a relevant teaching, clinical, research, or career development topic at lunch time, and review rotation objectives and resources periodically to ensure they are up to date and relevant. The clinic nurse may be expected to give verbal feedback to the trainees and/or the preceptor about the trainees in a meeting once per week and may be expected to direct medical questions to the patient's primary resident or to a senior resident covering urgent questions. Working to define these expectations, having them available for reference and revision, and communicating them clearly and often to all involved in the educational mission is an important part of establishing a culture of educational excellence for trainees.

1. Establish *core values of embracing a growth mindset* and in giving, receiving, and acting upon constructive feedback at all levels of medical training and practice as a means for iterative improvement, professional development, and practice-based learning. Normalize the expectation that all learners and faculty can benefit from reflection, compassionate critique of performance, and a consistent commitment to learning and improvement. Provide models and examples of senior learners and faculty receiving and acting upon feedback in an open, transparent manner that emphasizes iterative growth as clinicians and teachers.
2. Create a program culture of achieving one's best through *high expectations* coupled with support for learner and team performance. Emphasize a firm belief in the ability of the learners to do difficult and impactful things within safe learning spaces, through eliciting feedback, practicing reflection and self-awareness, deliberate practice, and exhibiting respect and positive regard for everyone. In this culture, the program will support trainees with respect and compassion while believing in their capacity for excellence in patient care that is evidence based, family centered, inclusive and equitable, and incorporates team-based practices.
3. Emphasize *learner ownership* of showing up as their best self when on duty and participating in program activities and events. While

recognizing that learners have conflicting demands and need to invest in their personal relationships, fiscal stability, personally fulfilling activities, and sound mental health; it is helpful to set the expectation early and often that they are responsible for their engagement with the required activities and duties of residency. Learners should demonstrate self-directed learning and actively seek feedback, demonstrate a drive to practice evidence-based medical practice by consulting and integrating up-to-date medical literature into their care for patients. Program leadership and faculty should demonstrate support for learner-led processes of obtaining feedback and acting on it as a core value of the training program. Residents can be expected to create skill development and cognitive goals that are specific, measurable, achievable, relevant, and time-bound (S.M.A.R.T.) goals that can be reviewed with rotation directors and advisors periodically.

4. Encourage very *early identification and action* on areas for growth with medical learners. This is a joint responsibility of the learners, faculty, and program leaders. For the learners, the identification of areas for growth can be manifested as goal setting for each rotation, periodic reviews with their advisors, working with coaches, practice examinations for medical-knowledge assessment, and written reflection exercises. For faculty, this would include timely and actionable feedback to the learner, a focus on competency-based assessments, providing direct observation and feedback to the learner that considers all six core competencies, as well as other elements such as making use of opportunities for advocacy, scholarship, and the preservation of well-being. For program leadership, early identification and action on areas of growth for the learners may be manifested by the development and maintenance of processes for collecting supervisor feedback, the development of QR code-linked feedback collection to improve immediacy of written feedback, the development and delivery of faculty development on the importance of early identification of nascent areas for improvement, and ensuring a culture of empathic expectations of excellence.
5. Use *competency-based medical education* (CBME) as the foundational framework for curriculum development, assessment, and feedback [9]. CBME is dependent upon work-based assessments of the learner, necessitating synthesis of the observations and judgments of clinical faculty, staff, and senior trainees. Both residents and faculty have described an increased burden of assessment as the CBME framework is incorporated into residency programs, necessitating innovation in assessments, enhancement of data platforms for assessment, and increasing resident representation in assessment and feedback planning, design, and implementation.
6. Ensure high-quality *faculty development* resources and programming to share best practices in feedback, encourage success-oriented coaching, and ensure that all teaching faculty have a clear understanding of the need for high-quality evaluations and the early identification of learners at risk for sub-optimal performance. Longitudinal, multi-modal faculty development, which creates a shared mental model of CBME-based assessment and rotation objectives, is a good investment to provide accurate assessments and actionable feedback, which should aid in the early identification of learners with performance challenges. There are several known barriers to faculty engagement in remediation: time; self-doubt regarding faculty expertise, authority, or the impact of their efforts; a perception of lack of cultural support for efforts, lack of organizational infrastructure and resources; and fear of repercussions for honest critical feedback [10].
7. Highlight examples of how *leadership demonstrates commitment to and value for the educational mission* of the training program. Ensure that faculty, staff, and trainees are aware of educational-related promotion

criteria, awards, professional development opportunities, and venues for educational scholarship. Develop and advertise recognition of those who advocate for and participate in the educational mission. This can be residency, departmental, or institutional teaching awards; Education-scholarship-focused Individual Learning Plans (ILP); allocation of funds for educational conference attendance and certificate or master's-level programs; contributions to blogs or newsletters highlighting educational accomplishments and opportunities; among others.

8. *Celebrate successes*, large and small, to avoid a culture of deficit-based recognition and action. In the busy world of residency training and clinical care, it is tempting to focus on problem-solving and prevention rather than a holistic view that includes consideration of positive performance. Including feedback and communication on things well done reinforces positive behaviors, engenders a sense of belonging and appreciation, and improves perceptions of the overall learning environment. Educational leaders will find that encouraging positive feedback, as well as collecting negative feedback, can assist in normalizing ongoing reflection and feedback and possibly improve the quality of assessments and perceptions of the learning environment.

Frameworks for Diagnosis of Learners in Need of Remediation

In addition to creating a programmatic culture of normalizing focused learner improvement, effective remediation requires several important components:

1. Timely, detailed, and accurate evaluations.
2. Early identification of deficiencies and areas to focus improvement.
3. Investment and commitment of Clinical Competency Committee (CCC) members and frontline teaching faculty.
4. The consistent application of a universal process to minimize bias and ensure equity, while also allowing flexibility to implement different means of intervention based on the specific situation.
5. Institutional and Program policies addressing evaluation, advancement, and due process.

Timely, detailed, and actionable evaluations are essential to identify and assist an underperforming learner. Narrative evaluations are particularly helpful, as they often contain most of the necessary information to correctly identify areas for improvement and inform which level of intervention is most appropriate to implement and monitor for successful and sustained improvement.

Remediation can require different levels of intervention. Underperforming learners may have minor areas for improvement, which require only minimal intervention to prompt self-awareness and improvement, such as immediately addressing an observed lapse in behavior or performance and providing real-time feedback directly to the learner. Other situations will require a more carefully documented and structured individualized plan, for example, a Focused Individualized Learning Plan (FILP). This variation of an individualized learning plan can be implemented and monitored, is often more acceptable to trainees, and is not considered to meet the reporting requirement for disclosure that formal remediation plans require. In cases where the learner's underperformance is more persistent or consequential, initiation of a formalized remediation or even termination may be appropriate levels of intervention.

Regardless of the level of remediation intervention decided upon, it is often discovered that there have been several missed opportunities for earlier intervention for the learner. A pervasively common missed opportunity occurs when supervisors and ancillary providers ascribe observed deficits to the learner being early in their career or just starting a specific rotation. While the expectation is that the learner will improve with more time and experience, they are more likely to be successful if they are provided with clear and specific feedback and goals to tailor changes. It is most constructive to provide the learner with the opportunity to demonstrate improvements within the rotation through multipoint observation, assessment, and documentation by the same faculty. The provision of vague or only positive feedback is a significant barrier to learners achieving success in acquiring knowledge and skills in all aspects of their roles. Establishing an expectation within your program that clinical and non-clinical activities require the provision and receipt of actionable, constructive feedback allows for any observed learner deficits to be addressed in a timely fashion with the learner, and encourages learner engagement focused on improvement with the opportunity to demonstrate improvement and progress, and may mitigate the need for informal or formal remediation later in their training.

High-quality, timely assessments allow for the early identification of underperforming medical learners by CCCs. The CCCs are composed of Core Faculty and other individuals who are appointed by the Program Director and review evaluations to make recommendations to the PD regarding resident progress, the need for acquiring more information about a learner's performance, any concerns that remediation or disciplinary action is required, and the resident's suitability for promotion and graduation. As such, they are deeply invested in the educational mission, and many should have ACGME-mandated protected time for their contributions to the educational enterprise. Therefore, the CCC members are well suited to play an important role in remediation. CCC members can review available assessments and feedback to provide input on the level of intervention that would be appropriate to implement for that particular situation. The investment and commitment of Clinical Competency Committee (CCC) members is a cornerstone for successful programs.

Once a learner is identified as underperforming, the next important step is to clarify the specific area(s) of deficits on which to focus improvement efforts. Often this can be approached in a manner similar to the process of formulating a differential diagnosis, which is familiar and aligns with the faculty member's experiences. While several frameworks have been used, one recognizable framework is SOAP (Subjective, Objective, Assessment, and Plan).

Subjective: Reviewing feedback and eliciting additional feedback from multiple sources, including the learner's perspective.

Objective: The documentation of specific instances of demonstrable difficulties with achieving a competency or milestone, with dates, with a focus on the learner's observed behaviors or communication.

Assessment: Based upon both the subjective and objective findings, in conjunction with input from others such as CCC members, preceptors, supervising attendings, and nursing colleagues, to accurately diagnose the area(s) of concern. Importantly, this cannot be done accurately and equitably without eliciting information from the learner directly.

Plan: Delineate the specific ways that the program and learner will be expected to partner to address the areas of concern. Define who is involved in monitoring the remediation process, the frequency of meetings with the learner, and expected outcomes from each meeting. Clearly define specific outcomes that are expected and the frame within which they are to occur. Consider the provision of additional resources depending on the assessment and outcomes desired, such as counselling, coaching, additional knowledge testing programs, and experiences tailored to the learner's needs. What is the length of time during which this remediation program will take place? Review the program's policies for assessment, disciplinary action, promotion, and dismissal.

We have found that this clinically analogous framework is readily understood by all involved in remediation, is flexible and adaptable enough to serve well for a variety of remediation concerns, and is effective; but it is only one of many excellent frameworks for the diagnosis of learners in need of remediation. A discussion of all published frameworks for remediation is beyond the scope of this chapter, but the literature is replete with examples [10–14].

Correctly identifying the specific deficit(s) of any learner requires a comprehensive review of all available information. Often, additional information is necessary to accurately diagnose the problem. There are several ways to obtain additional information. Sometimes, this may simply require requesting faculty to complete outstanding evaluations; often, it will require more thought and planning. Frequently, CCCs may only receive verbal reports of concerns despite the necessity of written feedback to create an intervention plan. When your CCC or program leadership receives a verbal report of concerns, encourage the person providing the information to complete a written evaluation. If they are reluctant to do this, then ask that they send details of the incident in writing by email to the program director, or a CCC member, so this important information can be documented and included in the learner's evaluation portfolio.

Once the CCC has received and reviewed all relevant information, it is helpful to use readily available resources such as Milestones 2.0 and Entrustable Professional Activities (EPAs) to accurately determine the learner's deficits within each specific competency. If only one area is identified, that will be the focus of the intervention. However, it is more frequent that careful inquiry will reveal deficiencies in more than one area of the ACGME-plus competencies: Medical Knowledge, Patient Care (Clinical Skills, Clinical Reasoning and Judgement), Time Management and Organization, Interpersonal Skills, Communication, Professionalism, Practice-Based Learning and Improvement, Systems-Based Practice, and Mental Well-Being [2]. The CCC and program leadership will have to prioritize which are the top two to three competencies to focus on, while clearly communicating to the learner that there are concerns in each area.

While assessing for potential bias throughout each step in the process is imperative, it's just as important not to create bias. For example, if additional information is needed from the learner's continuity clinic, it would be prudent to avoid asking for an evaluation for only that one learner and instead ask the supervising faculty to provide written evaluations for the 3–6 residents that they supervise in a particular clinic that includes this specific learner. This will mitigate potential bias when faculty members are providing requested evaluations. It is well documented in the literature that written feedback is often biased by gender and race [15, 16], which requires ongoing faculty development to address implicit bias as essential to optimizing the learning culture of any program [17–19].

Codified, transparent, and readily available documentation of the institution's and program's policy specifically addressing evaluation, promotion, disciplinary action, and graduation that describes the ways that learner performance is assessed and aggregated, the review process for promotion and retention within the program, the process for the initiation of a remediation plan or Focused Individualized Learning Plan, and the appeals process for learners is essential.

Refining a Remediation Strategy (Focused Individualized Learning Plan (FILP) vs. Formal Remediation)

Remediation can often be perceived as a negative, punitive action, but should rather be identified as a process of learner-focused, team-facilitated improvement for correction of a performance deficit. The goal of remediation is for a learner to demonstrate sustainable improvements to meet at least the minimal threshold of competency. Therefore, it is imperative to provide faculty development specifically on remediation to create a learning environment that normalizes and destigmatizes the process of iterative, focused improvement and learning, instead of punitive interventions at times of failure.

Circumstances that include concerns for patient safety, or if a learner is identified to be unfit for duty, or if a crime has been committed, mandate immediate reporting to the Designated Institutional Officer (DIO) and following the Graduate Medical Education (GME) Due Process Policy. This may result in formal remediation, probation, suspension, or termination as determined by the GME office in conjunction with the

PD. However, there are many situations in which another form of intervention can be implemented to identify and address concerns, which allows the learner to demonstrate improvement and the attainment of competency while avoiding having to embark on a high-stakes formalized remediation or disciplinary plan. The majority of situations requiring some degree of attention to the improvement of learner performance are opportunities to implement a Focused Individualized Learning Plan (FILP), which provides a structure and documentation that contains clear, fair, comprehensive, and precise identification of the deficit(s), expectations, monitoring, and next steps for all involved.

When implementing a FILP, it is important to assemble a team of 2–3 providers, rather than assigning a solitary remediator. The team should first review all available information on performance and any concerns, meet together, discuss the information and known context of the learner's underperformance, identify any need for further information gathering, such as ensuring the learner's perspective has been included, prepare a draft of the FILP, and then schedule a meeting with the learner. We have found it helpful if the Program Director meets with the remediation team at the preparatory meeting and again during the initial meeting with the learner, but otherwise does not have to participate in each subsequent meeting and instead can be provided updates from team members.

Preparing for the meeting with the learner is a critical component. All team members should maintain a supportive, growth-oriented mindset throughout the entire process. One suggested framework is borrowed from the field of psychology and the process of appreciative inquiry, and the work of Carl Rogers on maintaining "unconditional positive regard" in relationships with clients. Anticipate that the learner may not agree with the team's assessment and often will initially respond defensively and/or externalize blame. It is possible to support the learner's emotions while also keeping focused on the knowledge, skills, and behaviors that need to be addressed. The learner may need some time and space after this meeting to complete some self-reflection and return to discuss additional questions and obtain some clarification from the team.

For interventions to be effective, it is important to engage learners throughout the entire process with a shared goal of improving their performance within a supportive team approach. It may prove useful to help them focus on the behaviors they demonstrate and how those are perceived, rather than their internal intentions. As stated above, at the onset of this intervention, it is helpful to assess the learners' understanding and engagement. This can be accomplished by having the learner provide the team with an email communication summarizing their understanding of the first meeting. This exercise can help assess the learner's insight and self-motivation to be fully engaged in this process. Additionally, after reviewing the areas requiring focused improvements, it is helpful to request that the learner create draft SMART (specific, Measurable, Attainable, Relevant, and Time-bound) goals that will become part of the documented FILP. Anticipate that the team members will need to work with the learner to edit these goals, ensuring that there is a clear plan for measuring improvement, and the FILP should include a time frame by which this must occur. The FILP is a process and will require ongoing assessments to demonstrate sustainable improvements in competencies. In some circumstances, processes for the collection of information from evaluations and direct observations that already exist will be sufficient to capture the necessary updated feedback to determine if a learner is improving. However, there will be other circumstances where the team may need to create additional evaluation forms, opportunities for mentored practice, reviews of documentation, or implement a plan where the learner requests specific feedback from faculty members during identified rotations that would provide the necessary updated feedback to assess improvement and inform changes to the plan.

Throughout the FILP process, the team members will schedule regular meetings with the learner. At a minimum, the identified team members should meet with the learner monthly, but generally more frequent meetings with the learner are more effective. Depending on the area of concern, weekly or even more frequent meetings may be necessary. For example, when Interpersonal and Communication is an area of focus, it is helpful to meet weekly or more often and review actual communication completed by the learner in verbal and electronic forms to provide mentorship and role modeling to improve communication across all team members.

The Focused Individualized Learning Plan serves as a standardized process that provides clear expectations, transparent and detailed documentation, and helps to mitigate bias. See the appendix at the end of the chapter for an example of a templated FILP.

If the situation requires immediate formal remediation, or an informal remediation plan is unsuccessful resulting in a progression to formal remediation, then the DIO must be involved, and the PD will follow their institutional policy on formal remediation. Formal remediation can have long-standing consequences, as this will become part of the learner's permanent portfolio with mandatory reporting to credentialing organizations, included in reference letters, and must be acknowledged by the learner for all future applications for positions, medical staff privileges, and licensures.

Outcomes in Remediation

A FILP should be implemented for a clearly defined time, such as 3 months.

Remediation interventions can be successful for deficits in any of the competencies. However, not every remediation intervention is successful. Success is limited, if not impossible, when a learner declines to participate in the remediation process, demonstrates poor insight that minimizes their engagement in this process, or when the training program lacks resources or a remediation infrastructure. There are four possible outcomes for learners, which should be documented within the FILP. They include:

1. *Completion of the Focused Individualized Learning Plan:* When the learner has satisfactorily demonstrated improvement and there is no additional need for corrective action or any other intervention. The FILP is deemed successfully completed, and the remediation group and learner sign as successfully completed.
2. *Continuation of the Focused Individualized Learning Plan:* When the learner has performed satisfactorily on a significant portion of the plan but it is determined that the learner would benefit from continuing the remediation intervention to successfully complete all areas defined within the original plan. In this option, revising the FILP to note which elements of the original plan have been completed and no longer warrant ongoing action, as well as a revised SMART goal approach to the assessment of other elements of competency still evolving, is necessary. If new problems have been identified in the interim which were not addressed in the initial FILP, the program can opt to create a separate FILP or append the continuation of the original with the new elements.
3. *Implement Formal Remediation, Imposition of a Term of Probation:* When the learner has not performed satisfactorily and there is a continued need for remediation. This is utilized when the learner's continuation in the program does not constitute a serious threat to the welfare or safety of patients, employees, or other staff members or to the integrity of the program.
4. *Other Appropriate Action:* When the learner has not performed satisfactorily, the GME will determine based upon the institution's Due Process Policy, if probation, suspension, or termination is deemed appropriate.

Legal Considerations for Remediation in Residency

When embarking on decisions to implement any level of intervention for a learner, there needs to be consideration for potential legal involvement. Understanding your institution's Due Process Policy is very important. Program directors, CCC members, and any remediation team members should have clear knowledge of this policy, which is available from the office of the DIO. Learners are also able to review the Due Process Policy at any time. Program directors should meet and review this policy and the different levels of intervention that are acceptable and approved by your institution's DIO.

Documentation is essential in these situations. Included in the documentation is the CCC's review of all information, including any additional information that was obtained during the process of generating the FILP or any other remediation plan. Ensure documentation of all relevant information, including personnel involved, the dates of the primary review and any subsequent meetings, the specific findings of deficiencies, the date the learner was notified, the date the learner submitted draft SMART goals, the start and anticipated end date of the remediation intervention, and the specific plan for continued reassessment throughout this intervention. In the first formal letter to start a remediation intervention, include the four potential outcomes of the plan described above.

Historically, courts have not reversed an academic decision if there was a review of the entire learner's record. The documentation is important to demonstrate not only compliance with the Due Process policy but also the reasoned academic decision. Learners cannot sue for libel, as courts have already determined that negative evaluations are not defamatory. It is the burden of the learner to prove that the decision was irrational and unreasonable [20].

While it is important to consider possible legal consequences, this is rare and is usually mitigated by creating and implementing a uniform and equitable process and ensuring that remediation actions are in compliance with your institutional policies and are consistently and clearly documented [21].

Tips and Perspectives from Leaders and Learners

Normalize an educational culture of evaluating strengths and opportunities for improvement as an iterative part of lifelong learning. Work to shift the academic culture away from a focus on punitive interventions. Instead, normalize and destigmatize the process of iterative focused improvement and learning that is embraced across the continuum from students to leaders. Provide balanced and timely feedback to learners and help them to develop skills of goal setting for personal improvement.

Provide faculty development on writing high-quality assessments, mentoring, implicit bias, and Competency-Based Medical Education principles on an ongoing basis.

Ensure the documentation, availability, and use of a consistent and equitable due process for all remediation initiatives. Share program policies for assessment, promotion, disciplinary action, and graduation where they are readily accessible for all learners and leaders.

Encourage early communication, preferably in writing, regarding concerns about deficiencies and opportunities for improvement, and share these with the learner using a growth-oriented framework of lifelong learning.

Meticulously document all communications regarding the remediation process from initial concerns leading through investigation and diagnosis, stakeholder and any consultant's reports, communications with the learner, SMART goals, learner reflections, subsequent evaluations, reassessments and outcomes of interventions.

Initiate the process with the learner in a manner that conveys appreciative inquiry, compassionate curiosity, respect, and unconditional positive regard [22].

Expect and plan to address more than one deficit per learner.

Have the learner document minutes of meetings with the remediation team and revisions incorporated by the team leaders to ensure closed-loop communication.

Assess the learner's insight and desire to improve, anticipating that this may evolve and shift over time.

Recognize and reward faculty that provide high-quality feedback and contribute to the success of the educational mission.

Tips for creating a culture of educational excellence

1. Set clear expectations and communicate them clearly and often
2. Emphasize competency-based learning and assessment and a growth mindset
3. Embrace high expectations for learners, leaders, and the learning environment
4. Encourage learner ownership for bringing their best to educational endeavors
5. Include learner-led processes for obtaining feedback
6. Practice respect, curiosity, and compassion when working with a learner who is struggling. Emphasize a culture of unconditional positive regard for learners, while emphasizing the duty to society for ensuring reliable clinical competency
7. Employ systems and processes for the early identification of learners needing help
8. Provide high-quality faculty development resources and programs
9. Engage senior leadership in demonstrating commitment to and the value of the educational mission
10. Celebrate successes

Summary

Remediation in Pediatric Graduate Medical Education is an integral part of the training program continuum that ensures learners achieve competency. Pediatric faculty and providers are well suited to participate in learner remediation by nature of their training in preventative care, early intervention, and the holistic assessments of complex determinants of well-being. A key foundation is the creation of a learning environment that embraces high expectations while providing the necessary support to facilitate success. Clear communication about expectations, policies, and processes for the determination of competency, the decision to promote or remediate, and graduation requirements should be readily accessible and reviewed periodically with faculty and trainees. Other key elements for successful remediation in Pediatric GME training include ongoing faculty development about assessment and remediation and the support of departmental and institutional leadership for work being done as part of the educational mission. Early identification of learners who are facing challenges and are demonstrating suboptimal performance is extremely helpful in correcting the trajectory back towards the attainment of competence and excellence. The importance of written documentation and adherence with institutional policies for Due Process cannot be overstated. Egregious or persistent poor performance in knowledge, skills, or behaviors will require a formalized remediation plan created in partnership with the Designated Institutional Official and the GME office. For less severe lapses, a Focused Individualized Learning Plan (FILP) is a structured, outcomes-based format for remediation of performance with oversight from a remediation team and active engagement of the learner in the process, ensuring clarity and learner engagement.

Appendix: Sample Focused Individualized Learning Plan (FILP) Document

Date
Trainee Name e.g. Willie Flourish, MD
PGY-level

Initiation of Focused Individualized Learning Plan
Dear Dr. Flourish:
Our recent Residency Program Clinical Competency Committee (CCC) on *DATE* highlighted the following strengths:

1.
2.
3.

In addition, the CCC raised the following concerns about your performance as a pediatric resident. It was the assessment of the CCC that you had not yet achieved the expected milestones for your level of training in relation to several ACGME competencies. Progress towards independence in some EPAs requires focused attention. These EPA's competencies and sub-competencies were:

- EPA 4: Manage patients with acute, common diagnoses in an ambulatory, emergency, or inpatient setting
- EPA 15: Lead an interprofessional health care team
- **Interpersonal and Communication Skills**
  - ICS-2: Interprofessional and Team Communication
- **Systems Based Practice**
  - SBP3: Work in interprofessional teams
- **Professionalism**
  - PROF 1: Professional Behavior
  - PROF 3: Accountability/Conscientiousness
- **Wellness**
  - PROF4: Well-Being

After careful discussion, it was the recommendation of the CCC that you embark on a **focused individualized learning plan** (**FILP**) with special attention paid to the areas noted above
On *DATE* these concerns were discussed in a meeting attended by yourself, *NAME OF ALL ATTENDEES AND ROLES.*
During this meeting you were informed that you would be enrolled in a FILP which would consist of several SMART goals designed by you based on your summative evaluations and the feedback from the CCC. You were asked at the conclusion of the meeting to provide *Remediation team members* a summary of our discussion, an ACGME competency-based self-assessment and 3–4 SMART goals which could be linked back to the specific sub-competencies and EPAs listed above. After receiving your summary, self-assessment, and your revised SMART goals on *DATE*, after careful review, editing, and approval, your Focused Individualized Learning Plan was finalized on *DATE*.
Your FILP will begin *DATE* and extend for approximately 3 months until *DATE*. During this time, you will be expected to obtain 360-degree just-in-time feedback; this includes feedback from your peers and from members of the interdisciplinary care team as well as your faculty preceptors. Your clinical settings will be the following:
DATES AND ASSIGNED ROTATIONS
Each week/2 weeks/month you will meet with members of your FILP team. At each meeting, your FILP and performance will be reviewed, and strategies developed to keep you on track with the plan. You will also be expected to meet with your advisor *NAME* for further guidance and additional support during this time.
A decision to undertake 1 of 4 courses of action will be made at the conclusion of the FILP based on the progress towards achievement of your smart goals and the 360-degree written and verbal feedback from your interdisciplinary team members and from your supervisors during this period:

1. *Termination of the focused individualized learning plan*, with a statement provided to you that the conditions of the plan were satisfactorily resolved and there is no present need for corrective action.
2. *Continuation of the focused individualized learning plan* for an additional specified period, provided that you have performed satisfactorily on a significant portion of the plan.
3. *Imposition of a term of probation,* provided that your continuation in the program does not constitute a serious threat to the welfare or safety of patients, employees, or other staff members or to the integrity of the program.
4. *Other appropriate action,* including Termination of your participation in the residency program.

I greatly appreciate your commitment to this program, your patients, and your desire to improve. We believe that you will successfully address the concerns raised and resolve the conditions of the FILP and continue in your progress towards board eligibility and emerge as the outstanding physician that we know you to be capable of becoming.
Sincerely,

_______________ _______________

NAME *DATE*
Residency Director

_______________ _______________

NAME OF FILP MEMBER *DATE*

_______________ _______________

NAME OF FILP MEMBER *DATE*

Recipient Attestation:
I have had an opportunity to read the above letter and understand the terms, conditions, and implications of the issues presented. I have had the opportunity to discuss these issues with
NAME and to ask relevant questions.

_______________ _______________

Trainee name Date:

References

1. American Board of Pediatrics. "Program Directors Training Verification". Accessed 15 Jan 2025. https://www.abp.org/content/program-directors-training-verification
2. Guerrasio J. Remediation of the struggling medical learner. Association for Hospital Medical Education; 2017.
3. Ziring D, Frankel RM, Danoff D, Isaacson JH, Lochnan H. Silent witnesses: faculty reluctance to report medical students' professionalism lapses. Acad Med. 2018;93(11):1700–6. https://doi.org/10.1097/ACM.0000000000002188.
4. Riebschleger MP, Haftel HM. Remediation in the context of the competencies: a survey of pediatrics residency program directors. J Grad Med Educ. 2013;5(1):60–3. https://doi.org/10.4300/JGME-D-12-00024.1.
5. Guerrasio J, Garrity MJ, Aagaard EM. Learner deficits and academic outcomes of medical students, residents, fellows, and attending physicians referred to a remediation program, 2006–2012. Acad Med. 2014;89(2):352–8. https://doi.org/10.1097/ACM.0000000000000122.
6. DeKosky AS, Sedrak MS, Goren E, Dine CJ, Warburton KM. Simple frameworks for daily work: innovative strategies to coach residents struggling with time management, organization, and efficiency. J Grad Med Educ. 2018;10(3):325–30. https://doi.org/10.4300/JGME-D-17-00756.1.
7. McLeod K, Woodward-Kron R, Rashid P, Archer J, Nestel D. "I'm on an Island": a qualitative study of underperforming surgical trainee perspectives on remediation. Am J Surg. 2024;234:11–6. https://doi.org/10.1016/j.amjsurg.2024.01.033.
8. Bourgeois-Law G, Regehr G, Teunissen PW, Varpio L. Strangers in a strange land: the experience of physicians undergoing remediation. Med Educ. 2022;56(6):670–9. https://doi.org/10.1111/medu.14736.
9. Keeley MG, Bray MJ, Bradley EB, Peterson CM, Waggoner-Fountain LA, Gusic ME. Fidelity to best practices in EPA implementation: outcomes supporting use of the core components framework from the University of Virginia Entrustable Professional Activity program. Acad Med. 2022;97(11):1637–42. https://doi.org/10.1097/ACM.0000000000004944.
10. Kalet A, Chou CL. Remediation in medical education: a mid-course correction. text. 2nd ed. Springer International Publishing: Imprint: Springer; 2023. p. 342.
11. Merriam SB, McNeil MA, Spagnoletti CL. A 5-step framework for the assessment and remediation of a struggling medical learner in the clinical environment. South Med J. 2019;112(3):135–6. https://doi.org/10.14423/SMJ.0000000000000939.
12. Warburton KM, Goren E, Dine CJ. Comprehensive assessment of struggling learners referred to a graduate medical education remediation program. J Grad Med Educ. 2017;9(6):763–7. https://doi.org/10.4300/JGME-D-17-00175.1.
13. Ridinger H, Cvengros J, Gunn J, et al. Struggling medical learners: a competency-based approach to improving performance. Mededportal. 2018;14:10739. https://doi.org/10.15766/mep_2374-8265.10739.
14. Lacasse M, Audetat MC, Boileau E, et al. Interventions for undergraduate and postgraduate medical learners with academic difficulties: a BEME systematic review: BEME guide no. 56. Med Teach. 2019;41(9):981–1001. https://doi.org/10.1080/0142159X.2019.1596239.

15. Gorth DJ, Magee RG, Rosenberg SE, Mingioni N. Gender disparity in evaluation of internal medicine clerkship performance. JAMA Netw Open. 2021;4(7):e2115661. https://doi.org/10.1001/jamanetworkopen.2021.15661.
16. Rojek AE, Khanna R, Yim JWL, et al. Differences in narrative language in evaluations of medical students by gender and under-represented minority status. J Gen Intern Med. 2019;34(5):684–91. https://doi.org/10.1007/s11606-019-04889-9.
17. Chapman EN, Kaatz A, Carnes M. Physicians and implicit bias: how doctors may unwittingly perpetuate health care disparities. J Gen Intern Med. 2013;28(11):1504–10. https://doi.org/10.1007/s11606-013-2441-1.
18. Champagne-Langabeer T, Hedges AL. Physician gender as a source of implicit bias affecting clinical decision-making processes: a scoping review. BMC Med Educ. 2021;21(1):171. https://doi.org/10.1186/s12909-021-02601-2.
19. Sabin JA. Tackling implicit bias in health care. N Engl J Med. 2022;387(2):105–7. https://doi.org/10.1056/NEJMp2201180.
20. Lefebvre C, Williamson K, Moffett P, et al. Legal considerations in the remediation and dismissal of graduate medical trainees. J Grad Med Educ. 2018;10(3):253–7. https://doi.org/10.4300/JGME-D-17-00813.1.
21. Irby DM, Milam S. The legal context for evaluating and dismissing medical students and residents. Acad Med. 1989;64(11):639–43. https://doi.org/10.1097/00001888-198911000-00001.
22. Kendrick SB, Simmons JM, Richards BF, Roberge LP. Residents' perceptions of their teachers: facilitative behaviour and the learning value of rotations. Med Educ. 1993;27(1):55–61. https://doi.org/10.1111/j.1365-2923.1993.tb00229.x.

24 Faculty Performance

Hayley Gans

Importance of Faculty Performance

Faculty create the environment in which future healthcare providers acquire the knowledge and attitudes necessary to deliver optimal care. The importance of teaching style on student achievement has long been appreciated outside the medical field. However, an evolving understanding of the impact of faculty-specific behaviors on medical trainee achievement highlights the importance of individual faculty members on the learning climate and the efficacy of the clinical learning environment [1]. Studies illustrate how a favorable learning climate is associated with greater trainee achievement [2], and a challenging environment predicts higher trainee burnout [3]. In addition, the learning climate is explicitly linked with faculty performance [2]. Specific behaviors that facilitate a positive learning climate include providing assessments, especially with a coaching lens; meeting learners at their level of competence; and teaching with learner involvement [1, 2]. Faculty behaviors and interactions that support a positive learning climate and the acquisition of trainee competency include positive reinforcement by supervisors through frequent interactions for feedback and fostering inquiry and trust, especially by utilizing "mistakes" as a tool for improvement [4].

In the complex team-based environments in which faculty teach and trainees learn, effective leadership is multidimensional. For faculty to prepare trainees to meet the needs of today's medicine, they must be content experts as well as serve as mentors, role models, and motivators [5–9]. Most importantly, effective faculty cultivate an atmosphere of inquiry, encouraging trainees to think critically and develop their clinical skills as lifelong learners, communicators, and educators. Ultimately, a positive learning environment translates to competent trainees with a positive professional identity and results in higher-quality patient interactions and health outcomes [5–7]. For instance, medical students trained by faculty known for their effective teaching competencies tend to demonstrate superior clinical skills and improved patient communication [8]. Well-functioning faculty lead to enhanced trainee engagement, better teaching outcomes, and improved patient care, which translates into higher-quality patient interactions and health outcomes [9].

H. Gans (✉)
Stanford University, Stanford, CA, USA
e-mail: drhayley@stanford.edu

H. McPhillips et al. (eds.), *Graduate Medical Education in Pediatrics*, Excellence in Medical Education 3, https://doi.org/10.1007/978-3-032-12952-9_24

Goals of Faculty Performance Assessment

The primary goal of faculty performance assessment is to provide feedback that enhances self-efficacy in teaching, team leadership, and creating a positive learning environment. Assessments are crucial for creating an environment that promotes psychological safety, where faculty members feel supported and motivated to innovate and learn. According to the Accreditation Council for Graduate Medical Education (ACGME), the continuous assessment and enhancement of teaching faculty must occur annually and provide assessments in teaching and areas of interpersonal skills [10].

Evaluation of faculty performance is critical in academic medicine, helping faculty identify areas of strength and opportunities for improvement in their educator skills [11]. Since specific behaviors, such as coaching methodology and learner-centered styles, are linked to creating a favorable learning climate and improved trainee performance, these provide a framework for evaluating faculty for improvement in these domains. The assessment process should not only focus on outcomes that are traditionally part of faculty performance, such as formal teaching sessions (i.e., morning report, noon conferences, medical school courses), rotations (i.e., clerkships, clinics, programs), mentoring (i.e., scholarship), program initiatives (i.e., curriculum, recruitment, advocacy and advancing diversity, equity, and inclusion), awards, publications, and local and national presentations, but to be effective must also incorporate self-reflection.

Reflective practice, although still in its infancy, is endorsed by the ACGME, which expects learners and practicing physicians to utilize reflection to enhance their practice [12]. Many benefits are associated with reflective practice, including preparation for the rapid changes found in the medical field, lifelong learning, learning from experiences, handling difficult and complex situations, and fostering a more meaningful learning environment [13]. While reflection is practiced throughout all levels of medicine, its implementation varies. Typically targeted at the learner, assessments of reflection include journaling and written reflections on performance, as well as questionnaires that focus on reflections on learning. A scoping review [14] highlighted several themes that emerged across tools designed to fulfill the goals of reflective practice (Table 24.1), while also acknowledging the limitations of these tools, including a lack of global validation and limited application in a single population. While journaling, descriptive writing, and scenario reflections are effective reflective tools, questionnaires are more easily administered and assessed and have been used successfully in medical practice [15]. Faculty assessments have not routinely incorporated reflective questions into annual reviews. However, sufficient evidence supports their value, and thus the evaluation process should include metrics on self-reflection, as well as those that foster practice in students and trainees, utilizing questions that align with the desired practice [14].

Peer evaluation is an important component of faculty assessment, and most academic centers employ some form of this tool. Peer evaluations are shown to be more reliable than trainee assessments [16] and thus have considerable potential as a valuable tool for improvement. However, few institutions have a process to provide peer feedback to the faculty being assessed. This is a missed opportunity to harness the expertise of peer physicians [17] and provide a mechanism for building a culture of psychological safety. Peer evaluations using ACGME competencies that are specific and reliable [18] could be incorporated into an evaluation metric. These domains would include clinical practice, teaching, and research metrics. Currently, most institutions utilize select groups of faculty to assess other faculty; however, this has the potential to introduce bias and limit engagement. A study evaluating peer faculty reviews, in which all faculty members reviewed each other, resulted in more robust and consistent peer evaluations, ultimately improving the annual review process for all faculty [18]. Furthermore, this study supports the inclusion of questions on division, departmental, and institutional contributions, providing an opportunity for career and professional

Table 24.1 Reflective practice domains, subdomains, and subscales

Reflection in action		Reflection on action					Reflection for action	
One's beliefs and biases	Patient's beliefs and biases	Multiple perspectives	Context	Past situations	One's limitations	Alternatives	New learnings	Plan for change
Check state of mind and whether one's beliefs influence decision-making	Understand if one is considering the beliefs and concerns of the patient	Learn how others approach a situation; be aware of things one did not consider	Understand the nuances of the circumstances and how this influenced one's decision-making; appreciate the climate for the interaction	Consider if past experiences are impacting the thought process; consider if anchoring	Think and apply strengths, and understand what strategies one uses; consider where one was challenged	Develop new perspectives: What other strategies could be employed; what new techniques can be applied	How can one improve: Approach the situation differently	Open to change and learning: Apply new approaches; strive for more knowledge

Adapted from Refs. [14, 15]

development discussions. It may also serve to educate faculty on each other's contributions and to raise awareness of such opportunities [18].

Additionally, there is a growing awareness that the most effective feedback tool utilizes a coaching methodology, which has been increasingly used in residency programs but should also be incorporated into faculty feedback and assessment (see Chap. 30). Coaching can be applied broadly but is effective in guiding improvements in clinical, communication, and leadership skills [19]. By creating a culture of continuous improvement, institutions empower faculty to enhance their teaching methodologies and cultivate critical thinking and inquiry among trainees. Using peers to act as reliable and safe evaluators and coaches fosters an environment that includes all participants and supports a persistent and stable culture.

An essential goal of faculty assessment is to foster effective mentorship skills in both the clinical and scholarship realms [20]. While the importance of mentorship relationships is well established, studies measuring what constitutes an effective mentor are limited. A significant hurdle is inherent in the mentoring role, as successful mentoring should be measured by the mentee's success, which can be challenging to capture. However, several frameworks have been proposed, reflecting evidence that mentoring skills can be taught [21], with specific known knowledge and skills that affect positive outcomes, and thus these can be measured. Therefore, evaluations should incorporate mentorship metrics and provide clear standards for mentorship roles [22]. This scoping review summarizes the key areas that lead to effective mentoring, including efficacy in developing competence (either clinical or scholarly), which can be measured through the acquisition of knowledge and technical skills in the mentee. Interpersonal skills vital to academic success can also be determined by assessing attention to task and communication skills in the mentee. Professional identity is vital for mentee success and should therefore be included in the evaluation process through the affirmation of the mentee's view of themselves as a clinician and scientist. Team building is foundational to physician success and must include advancing cultural awareness and responsiveness in the mentee. Lastly, but vitally important, is the role of the mentor as a sponsor, who actively promotes and creates opportunities for the mentee [22].

Faculty as role models is crucial to the development of competent physicians who have a positive professional identity [6]. Yet, standards are elusive and, until more recently, developing and defining effective role models was undervalued and left to vague assumptions that physicians will "naturally" role model. Role models are distinct from mentors (who may also act as role models) as they teach more by example and demonstrate specific aspects of professional behavior, such as values and attitudes, that contribute to a professional identity through experience. Trainees learn better in environments where their professional roles can be observed and practiced. Effective role models should be fostered through faculty development, institutional recognition of this skill, and creating environments that promote reflection and improvement. Currently, there are no specific metrics for assessing faculty as role models; however, these can be embedded in trainee evaluations, similar to reflection.

Role of Faculty Performance in Academic Advancement

Most academic centers use faculty teaching evaluations as part of the advancement process. Teaching and contributions to medical education are more difficult to assess than other academic metrics, such as publications. However, there is a growing appreciation for the need to develop tools such as educator portfolios to increase visibility and value in teaching and scholarship in the medical education field. Recognizing that these portfolios complement traditional curriculum vitae and are a powerful tool for career advancement, especially when professional effort includes medical education, the ACGME has developed guidelines [23]. In addition, many institutions include templates and guidance for educators' portfolios, and the Academic

Pediatrics Association (APA) published a template that can be adapted [24]. The intention is to document educational activities in terms of quantity, quality, scope, and impact. Portfolios promote an understanding of the academic currency in medical education, such as peer-reviewed workshops, which are not typically included in traditional academic metrics, such as abstracts. An educational portfolio should include educational contributions in teaching, learner assessment, curriculum development, mentoring and advising, educational leadership, and administration. However, until this is routinely recognized, faculty assessments by learners remain one of the primary measures of a faculty member's teaching skills and can significantly impact their professional advancement. Data on how these assessments are used for promotion is lacking, which puts a burden on programs, given the ACGME requirement to have faculty assessments, to provide an assessment tool that promotes faculty excellence and a positive pathway to promotion. In addition, there is evidence that trainee evaluations tend to be biased, often providing high scores and exhibiting poor internal consistency [16, 25]. In addition, the one-size-fits-all strategies commonly employed lack the nuance to provide valid feedback to faculty members in their varied professional roles [25].

Frameworks and Models for Faculty Performance Assessment

General Considerations A variety of frameworks exist to evaluate faculty performance systematically. Given the complexity of the learning climates and the diverse faculty skills needed to foster a positive learning climate, multiple assessment tools are likely required. Commonly employed models include peer review systems and student and trainee evaluations. As mentioned, peer evaluations allow faculty members to provide insight into each other's teaching styles and, if used correctly, can facilitate constructive feedback cycles. Peer assessment can be incorporated into 360 feedback, providing a more comprehensive reflection of faculty performance in the multiple domains in which they practice and roles they participate in [18].

The criteria for evaluating faculty performance must align closely with institutional goals and accreditation standards. Institutions should establish criteria encompassing teaching, scholarship, and service to education, ensuring that expectations are clear and measurable. Currently, data indicate that many faculty members experience misalignment, lack of transparency, and inconsistency, along with hierarchical structural issues and barriers to effective feedback systems; thus, change is warranted [26]. Additionally, faculty feel their teaching efforts and scholarship in the field are undervalued and under-supported. Efforts to restructure the evaluation system and criteria for promotion include the incorporation of the Educator's Portfolio (see section "Role of faculty performance in academic advancement") and Education Value Unit (EVU) into the process. The current system utilizes work relative value units (wRVUs) for physician compensation, which does not recognize non-clinical efforts. As a result, there is a growing adoption of an EVU system to complement compensation, using a points system to assess and reward faculty for their educational efforts. While published data show variable metrics measured under EVU systems, the general themes include lectures, courses, advising, mentoring, workshops, publications, presentations (regional and national), teaching awards, program leadership, rotation directions, conference attendance, committee membership (regional and national), among other activities [27]. In a recent scoping review [28], the authors note that "EVU systems increase the number of faculty who meet baseline educational requirements, promote educational productivity, redistribute educational burden and funding among faculty members, and shift physician priorities towards education." While the study found only 40 US academic medical centers use an EVU system, the clear benefits support increased adaptation. Importantly, the studies showed that the "monetary reward associated with EVU systems is unlikely to be a significant factor contributing to these changes; instead, intrinsic motivation and a sense of academic responsibility play a larger role." In developing assessment tools, it is crucial to collaborate with accrediting bodies to ensure that performance assessments align with broader educational goals, thereby creating a shared vision of excellence among faculty members.

Specific Considerations

Student and Trainee Evaluations Validated tools are needed, given the importance of trainee evaluations for faculty promotion and excellence. The Stanford Faculty Development Program (SFDP) framework is a widely disseminated framework, which includes many of the essential domains: a) learning climate, (b) control of the teaching session, (c) communication of goals, (d) promoting understanding and retention, (e) evaluation, (f) feedback, and (g) promoting self-directed learning [29]. The advantages of the tool include validity in both inpatient and outpatient settings, excellent internal consistency when applied to students and residents, and targeted skills that are linked with student and trainee success. Initially, the tool included twenty-five items; however, the feasibility of student and trainee completion was low in some settings. Consequently, attempts have been made to iterate and validate shorter versions [30], which have met with some success. The model has given rise to other frameworks, with a recent trend toward a milestones-based approach. Given the introduction of milestones in 2013 by the ACGME for resident assessments and the general acceptance of this method, application to faculty assessments has been investigated. The advantage of this method is that it improves the accuracy of evaluations, given the use of specific skill- and behavior-language in place of the typical Likert-based assessments, and it provides more standardization. Success using milestone evaluation of surgical faculty has shown improved quality of trainee feedback, positive impact on faculty who improved in areas with lower milestone scores, and overall improvement of faculty satisfaction with resident feedback [31]. Others have successfully adapted and validated tools in a large academic center. In the latter system, a learner tool was coupled with a faculty self-evaluation, and both were perceived as helpful and reflective of essential domains, with faculty adjusting their teaching based on the feedback [11]. The ACGME has proposed milestones for clinician educators [32], developed through a rigorous and collaborative process, that identify key skills defining competence and expertise in medical educators and provide a pathway for assessing clinician educators (CE). These milestones can be integrated into learner, peer, and self-evaluation [33], and while 20 subcompetencies have been identified, each represents a unique skill and can be used independently. The CE milestones project identified five competency areas, Universal pillars, which assess commitment to lifelong learning, personal growth, well-being, bias mitigation, and professional responsibilities [32]. These are meant to be part of a reflective practice of self, with the remaining subcompetencies applying to the learning environment and learner outcomes [33]. These include the application of educational theory to clinical practice to facilitate respectful, unbiased communication and problem-solving, promote evidence-based decisions and scientific learning, foster effective feedback, and support learner lifelong learning. Additional subcompetencies relate to curriculum development, scholarship, leadership, and administrative skills [32]. Overall, this framework provides a comprehensive and granular roadmap with developmental milestones detailing the knowledge, skills, and attitudes needed to master each of the subcompetencies, and thus represents a powerful tool for faculty assessment and improvement.

Measuring the Mentorship Relationship As mentioned, faculty are mentors, and success in this domain is linked to the clinical and scholarly success of trainees. It also provides an avenue for faculty academic advancement and increased faculty satisfaction. Assessments in this area are rarely used. However, frameworks exist that could be utilized by programs and institutions to support faculty as scholarship mentors (see section "Goals of faculty performance assessment"). Programs can use current infrastructure within graduate medical education (GME), such as scholarly concentrations and scholarship oversight committees (SOC), as a source to assess scholarly mentors. For scholarship success, recognized mentoring skills that have been shown to be effective and should be incorporated into assessment tools include the ability to individualize trainee projects and skills, role-modeling ethical and inclusive scholarly conduct, continuous assessment and improvement of trainees, sponsoring trainee professional development, and empowering and motivating trainees [22]. Mentorship in the clinical arena is equally necessary and should thus be assessed and incorporated into the required faculty assessment by students and trainees. These assessment tools should ask about leading a team, a competency that can be extrapolated through the ACGME milestones.

Role of Program Leadership in Faculty Performance

Program leadership is crucial in enhancing faculty performance, and the ACGME requires program leaders to establish structured processes for providing timely and constructive faculty feedback [10]. The information outlined above provides the content for assessment development. In addition to designing assessment tools, regular performance reviews must occur and should be designed as developmental conversations that foster growth and improvement rather than punitive evaluations. Program leadership can also establish a mechanism to value teaching excellence by publicly honoring faculty deemed exceptional teachers by trainees. Evaluations serve as one metric that can be used in algorithms to identify excellence, and by sharing the criteria with faculty, leadership establishes a framework for them to work toward this goal. This recognition can also increase the importance of teaching throughout an institution, which may have additional impacts at the institutional level.

Program leadership can also provide or facilitate faculty coaching. As few as five coaching sessions coupled with other feedback tools have provided enhanced support for faculty and can be tailored to specific domains, such as leadership [19], skills that must be developed rather than passively acquired. Additionally, institutions may provide coaches to faculty once a deficit is identified. Program leadership, thus, should be using assessment tools to identify potential areas for improvement among faculty and facilitate coaching in this area, which creates a positive rather than punitive approach.

Building an educator culture by implementing a community of practice is a powerful tool that has been shown to provide skills, professional identity as an educator, psychological safety, peer support, and role modeling. These communities have been used successfully in medical environments [34] and have shown value in sharing best practices, skill building, fostering innovation, and improving faculty retention [35].

Conclusion

Faculty are the foundation of medical education, having the most direct impact on learners. Thus, their skill in developing competent physicians is critical and a prized resource. The ever-changing and increasingly complex skills faculty need to be effective teachers in the current medical environments require a culture that promotes continual reflection, open and positive skill assessment, and motivation to improve. Advancements in knowledge related to assessment strategies highlight the roles of innovative tools such as coaching integration into feedback, development of reflective practice, skill and behavior-based assessment tools, and attention to value alignment and psychological safety. Additionally, multiple tools are likely the only effective strategy for comprehensively evaluating faculty competence. Importantly, institutions have an evolving appreciation of the value of medical education and medical education scholarship as the bedrock of the academic mission and thus may serve as resources for programs to implement innovative assessment tools. While this increased value on educational metrics is essential, more work is needed to harmonize the value of medical education with historical academic metrics. Program leadership is well poised to create dynamic and positive learning climates where faculty are supported and there is a culture of feedback, learning, and improvement, leading to better and competent clinicians and improved healthcare outcomes.

References

1. Lucas CA, Benedek D, Pangaro L. Learning climate and students' achievement in a medicine clerkship. Acad Med. 1993;68(10):811–2.
2. Lombarts KM, Heineman MJ, Scherpbier AJ, Arah OA. Effect of the learning climate of residency programs on faculty's teaching performance as evaluated by residents. PLoS One. 2014;9(1):e86512.
3. Dyrbye LN, Thomas MR, Harper W, et al. The learning environment and medical student burnout: a multicentre study. Med Educ. 2009;43(3):274–82.
4. Hoff TJ, Pohl H, Bartfield J. Creating a learning environment to produce competent residents: the roles of culture and context. Acad Med. 2004;79(6):532–9.
5. Cruess SR, Cruess RL, Steinert Y. Supporting the development of a professional identity: general principles. Med Teach. 2019;41(6):641–9.
6. Kenny NP, Mann KV, MacLeod H. Role modeling in physicians' professional formation: reconsidering an essential but untapped educational strategy. Acad Med. 2003;78(12):1203–10.
7. Leape LL, Shore MF, Dienstag JL, et al. Perspective: a culture of respect, part 2: creating a culture of respect. Acad Med. 2012;87(7):853–8.
8. Schmidt HG, Vermeulen L, van der Molen HT. Longterm effects of problem-based learning: a comparison of competencies acquired by graduates of a problem-based and a conventional medical school. Med Educ. 2006;40(6):562–7.
9. Torralba KD, Jose D, Byrne J. Psychological safety, the hidden curriculum, and ambiguity in medicine. Clin Rheumatol. 2020;39(3):667–71.
10. https://www.acgme.org/globalassets/pfassets/programrequirements/cprresidency_2023.pdf. Published 2023. Accessed.
11. Kassis K, Wallihan R, Hurtubise L, Goode S, Chase M, Mahan JD. Milestone-based tool for learner evaluation of faculty clinical teaching. MedEdPORTAL. 2017;13:10626.
12. Colleges AoAM. Core entrustable professional activities for entering residency: curriculum developers' guide. Published. 2014. Accessed 9/29/24.
13. Mann K, Gordon J, MacLeod A. Reflection and reflective practice in health professions education: a systematic review. Adv Health Sci Educ Theory Pract. 2009;14(4):595–621.
14. Prefontaine C, Gaboury I, Corriveau H, Beauchamp J, Lemire C, April MJ. Assessment tools for reflection in healthcare learners: a scoping review. Med Teach. 2022;44(4):394–400.
15. Rogers SL, Priddis LE, Michels N, et al. Applications of the reflective practice questionnaire in medical education. BMC Med Educ. 2019;19:47.
16. Beckman TJ, Lee MC, Mandrekar JN. A comparison of clinical teaching evaluations by resident and peer physicians. Med Teach. 2004;26(4):321–5.
17. Ramsey PG, Wenrich MD, Carline JD, Inui TS, Larson EB, LoGerfo JP. Use of peer ratings to evaluate physician performance. JAMA. 1993;269(13):1655–60.
18. Rosenbaum ME, Ferguson KJ, Kreiter CD, Johnson CA. Using a peer evaluation system to assess faculty performance and competence. Fam Med. 2005;37(6):429–33.
19. Schwartz R, Weimer-Elder B, Wilkins E, et al. Developing a feedback-rich culture in academic medicine: the effect of coaching and 360-feedback on physician leadership. BMC Med Educ. 2022;22(1):733.
20. Sambunjak D, Straus SE, Marusic A. Mentoring in academic medicine: a systematic review. JAMA. 2006;296(9):1103–15.
21. Pfund C, House SC, Asquith P, Fleming MF, Buhr KA, Burnham EL, Eichenberger Gilmore JM, Huskins WC, McGee R, Schurr K, Shapiro ED, Spencer KC, Sorkness CA. Training mentors of clinical and translational research scholars: a randomized controlled trial. Acad Med. 2014;89(5):774–82.
22. Pfund C, Byars-Winston A, Branchaw J, Hurtado S, Eagan K. Defining attributes and metrics of effective research mentoring relationships. AIDS Behav. 2016;20(Suppl 2):238–48.
23. Baldwin CD, Gusic M, Chandran L. The educator portfolio: a tool for career development, https://www.aamc.org/professional-development/affinity-groups/gfa/faculty-vitae/educator-portfolio-tool. Accessed 28 June 2025.
24. Gusic M, Chandran L, Balmer D, D'Alessandro D, Baldwin C. Educator portfolio template of the academic pediatric association's educational scholars program. MedEdPORTAL. 2007;3:626.
25. Beckman TJ, Ghosh AK, Cook DA, Erwin PJ, Mandrekar JN. How reliable are assessments of clinical teaching? A review of the published instruments. J Gen Intern Med. 2004;19(9):971–7.
26. Jones RF, Froom JD. Faculty and administration views of problems in faculty evaluation. Acad Med. 1994;69(6):476–83.
27. Beck Dallaghan GL, Wright ST, Plant J, Butani L, Morgenstern BZ. Educational relative value units as a measure of academic productivity: a systematic review. Cureus. 2023;15(4):e36995.

28. Husain A, Chen DA, Lelli GJ. A review on the use of the educational value unit (EVU) among teaching hospitals. Healthcare. 2023;11(1):136.
29. Litzelman DK, Stratos GA, Marriott DJ, Skeff KM. Factorial validation of a widely disseminated educational framework for evaluating clinical teachers. Acad Med. 1998;73(6):688–95.
30. Mintz M, Southern DA, Ghali WA, Ma IW. Validation of the 25-item Stanford faculty development program tool on clinical teaching effectiveness. Teach Learn Med. 2015;27(2):174–81.
31. Schoen J, Birch A, Adolph V, et al. Four-year analysis of a novel milestone-based assessment of faculty by general surgical residents. J Surg Educ. 2018;75(6):e126–33.
32. https://www.acgme.org/education-and-resources/faculty-development/clinician-educator-milestones/. Accessed 28 June 25.
33. Mahan JD, Kaczmarczyk JM, Miller Juve AK, et al. Clinician educator milestones: assessing and improving educators' skills. Acad Med. 2024;99(6):592–8.
34. Chen HC, Wamsley MA, Azzam A, Julian K, Irby DM, O'Sullivan PS. The health professions education pathway: preparing students, residents, and fellows to become future educators. Teach Learn Med. 2017;29(2):216–27.
35. de Carvalho-Filho MA, Tio RA, Steinert Y. Twelve tips for implementing a community of practice for faculty development. Med Teach. 2020;42(2):143–9.

Part VI

Resident Development and Support

Advising, Mentoring, and Coaching

25

Caroline E. Rassbach and Kim Hoang

Why Residents Need Advising, Mentoring, and Coaching

Graduate medical education has become increasingly complex in recent years. During the 3 years of residency training, programs must find the right combination of direction, guidance, and oversight to ensure that each resident is equipped with the appropriate clinical competency to practice in a variety of complex medical systems when they graduate. In addition, residents have individualized professional needs that the program must support and develop during training, including well-being, career exploration, and skills in research, teaching, communication, and leadership. Programs can support all of these professional needs by developing a system for residents to receive advising, mentoring, and/or coaching from their faculty members. All three approaches, which we will discuss further below, can be used to support residents in any of these different professional areas, and residents can benefit from a tailored approach to their specific needs and goals.

C. E. Rassbach (✉) · K. Hoang
Stanford School of Medicine, Stanford, CA, USA
e-mail: crassbac@stanford.edu

Defining Advising, Mentoring, and Coaching

Advising, mentoring, and coaching occur on a continuum and can be distinguished by (1) the amount of time the faculty member spends asking questions, giving advice, and making connections; (2) the types of questions the faculty member asks; (3) the goals of the relationship; and (4) the individual learners' needs [1, 2].

Advising Advisors typically focus on a specific event or issue with a resident and offer strategies and solutions based on their expertise [1–4]. These faculty are typically the ones leading the conversation, speaking approximately 75% of the time, and directly giving their advice and/or answers that the residents may choose to follow or not. The relationship between the advisor and resident is typically more episodic and centered around a session based on what the resident needs to know or asks, compared with mentoring and coaching. Advising can be useful for early learners who need more assistance with their educational needs and for specific needs such as test-taking preparation, preparing for a specific educational experience, or developing study habits.

Residents need advising during residency training to ensure that they achieve their ACGME milestones through assessment and feedback,

H. McPhillips et al. (eds.), *Graduate Medical Education in Pediatrics*, Excellence in Medical Education 3, https://doi.org/10.1007/978-3-032-12952-9_25

meet their graduation requirements, maintain their administrative responsibilities, and achieve their academic and career goals [4, 5]. Faculty advisors understand the workings of the program and are liaisons to the program director, gathering knowledge to advise residents during training.

Mentoring Mentoring relationships are often formed serendipitously between a more senior faculty and a resident mentee with similar career or professional interests [2, 6]. In contrast to advising, this relationship is more personal, bidirectional, longitudinal, and focused on a resident's longer-term professional and career development. Mentors, similar to advisors, will often direct the conversation with their expertise, but often balance their own speaking with eliciting ideas from the resident so that each party is speaking approximately half of the time. Mentors often provide their expertise by sharing their own experiences with the resident to help guide the resident in their career. Mentors may introduce the resident to their own professional network to elevate the resident into their field of interest, and may provide opportunities for shadowing, research, or other academic development. There can also be a mutual benefit to the mentoring relationship, as the resident may assist in the mentor's scholarly projects.

The importance and benefits of mentoring in academic medicine have been well established and are recognized as a key components of facilitating career choice and success, personal development, and academic productivity [6]. ACGME requires residency programs to support core faculty who will mentor their residents during training to maximize their fullest potential [7]. In particular, the ACGME guidelines highlight that, in order to advance residents' knowledge and practices of a scholarly approach to evidence-based patient care, there must be faculty mentoring them through their scholarly activities [7].

Coaching Coaching is a newer approach in GME that seeks to guide learners through asking deep questions and often complements advising and mentoring in meeting residents' overall professional needs [8, 9]. Unlike advisors and mentors, coaches do not require subject expertise. A coach's approach is inquiry-based, framing questions that lead the residents to their own conclusions and solutions. Coaches spend more time probing and listening than telling and answering, often speaking 25% of the time or less [1]. The goals of the conversation are typically directed by the residents, who have a challenge or skill that they want to focus on, and the coaches help guide the residents to find strategies by asking clarifying questions, listening deeply, reflecting, and assisting in identifying potential strategies, action items, and future goals [1]. Coaching can also be broken down into four archetypes: academic, skills, developmental, and at risk [10].

The Coalition of Physician Accountability assembled the UME-GME Review Committee to improve the UME-to-GME transition and calls for programs to support targeted coaching of resident physicians, especially in the transition to residency [11]. The organization highlighted that this major transition from medical school to residency comes with many challenges, and each resident has their own unique strengths and potential gaps. Coaching allows residents to move from a performance to a growth mindset for effective lifelong learning as they transition from medical school to being physicians.

There are instances where the same faculty member can serve as an advisor, mentor, and coach, especially in programs that are smaller in size with fewer core faculty. The key for success here is that the faculty members understand the circumstances in which they should utilize advising, mentoring, and coaching and apply the different techniques in the different circumstances. It is best to have a shared mental model of the resident's needs by asking them explicitly what guidance they are seeking so the faculty can align their approach. Marcdante et al. created a table that compares and contrasts the different approaches of advising, mentoring, and coaching and is a good reference to remember the specific focus and strategy that each role entails ([2], Table 25.1).

Table 25.1 Marcdante et al's comparing and contrasting advisor, mentor, and coach [2]

Comparing and contrasting four forms of guidance				
Item	Advisor	Coach	Coach with wisdom	Mentor
Focus	Specific event	Task/skill	Task/skill with long-term view in the field	Career; focus on character development, socialization into field
Expert	In target area	Global/not specific	In specific performance target	In same field, "been there" and shares
Control	Advisor directed	Learner directed	Mostly learner directed	Mentor directed with repeated interchanges
Strategy	Give advice or answer	Help learner find a strategy through asking clarifying questions	Combines coaching and mentoring on specific topic; when mentor, explicitly states he/she is doing so	After discussion with learner, mentor transmits information intentionally based on his/her own experience and expertise; networks learner with others in field
Benefits	None for advisor	No direct benefit for coach	No direct benefit for coach	Mutual benefit with mentor often involved in learner products
Time	Single session	Time limited, current	Time limited, current	Long-term, future oriented

Frameworks for Advising, Mentoring, and Coaching

The next thing to consider is what frameworks to use when considering advising, mentoring, and coaching conversations. Frameworks are useful tools for faculty in these roles to have as a guide when they meet with their residents. All of these frameworks can be adapted for use in an advising, mentoring, or coaching relationship.

An advising framework that may be useful to guide the relationship between the advisor and the learner is a framework for Fostering Learner Agency in academic advising [12]. In this framework, the advisor considers three elements: voice, choice, and collaboration, in promoting agency for the learner. Voice includes the learner's values, beliefs and perspectives; choice includes ensuring the learner understands the choices available to them, and collaboration refers to the partnership between the learner and advisor.

The Master Adaptive Learner (MAL) framework is particularly relevant in residency education because it provides strategies for the development of skills necessary for learning [13]. The MAL framework's four phases (planning, learning, assessing, adjusting) allow learners to identify learning needs, identify resources for learning, engage with learning, assess what they learned, and then incorporate this learning into their practice. As MAL is an iterative framework, residents can then plan again based on their new level of knowledge to identify their next learning goal. The MAL framework is based in part on the Plan-Do-Study-Act framework used in quality improvement, which is also very useful in medical education [14]. In MAL, the advisor, mentor, or coach supports the resident by asking questions to identify learning needs, resources, and strategies for learning. The faculty also help the resident prioritize and set goals, actively listen to and reflect with them about their self-assessment, review performance data, and provides encouragement and accountability in the learning process.

A third framework, the R2C2 (Relationship, Reaction, Content, Coaching) model, is particularly useful when reviewing performance data or secondhand feedback with a resident. This can be done by an advisor, mentor, or coach, but is particularly helpful in a coaching relationship. This model includes four elements: (1) rapport and relationship building, (2) exploring reactions to feedback, (3) exploring feedback content, and (4) coaching for change. The R2C2 model is an evidence-based method for coaching conversations toward performance improvement [15].

A fourth framework, the Stanford Coaching Framework [16], is particularly useful as a guide for workplace-based coaching. The coaching begins when a resident identifies a learning or performance goal. The coach then observes the resident in real time performing a clinical task, or alternatively can discuss performance data [17] or resident self-assessment related to the learning goal outside of direct observations. The coach asks for the resident's reflection and self-assessment, provides their own feedback, and works with the resident to identify subsequent learning goals. The Stanford Coaching Framework is an iterative cycle, such that the resident incorporates what they learned from coaching into their future practice and creates further learning goals as part of ongoing learning and in the setting of a longitudinal coaching relationship.

Finally, the GROW (Goal, Reality, Options, Will) and WOOP (Wish, Outcome, Obstacle, Plan) frameworks can be used for career and leadership development coaching conversations [18, 19]. These frameworks allow learners to identify a goal they are hoping to achieve, identify challenges to achieving that goal, and select strategies to make progress toward that goal.

In addition to using a framework, faculty should understand that their role is multifaceted and often includes role modeling, providing psychosocial and emotional support, extending career guidance, facilitating skill development, and providing sponsorship [20]. An expert educator can adapt to the real-time needs of a resident to determine which roles to focus on during a given conversation and whether to take an advising, mentoring, or coaching approach. A number of effective behaviors have been established for advisors, mentors, and coaches, including building rapport and trust, sharing strengths and limitations, aligning expectations, and identifying with and authentically engaging with the learner. In addition, faculty in these roles may need to address diversity and equity factors with the learner, navigate power differentials, affirm the learner's sense of belonging and physician identity, maintain open communication, and facilitate learner agency [20].

Structures for Advising, Mentoring, and Coaching in Residency

A resident's needs around advising, mentoring, and coaching can change over time and require shared responsibility between the resident and faculty member. Programs also have a duty to provide a structure and expectations around advising, mentoring, and coaching, and each program has the opportunity to build on its unique strengths in defining its approach to advising, mentoring, and coaching. All residents need faculty guidance around clinical skills development, including medical knowledge, clinical reasoning, patient care, procedural skills, communication skills, and professionalism. In addition, all residents will need faculty guidance around career development, board preparation, leadership, and scholarship. Structured meetings between a resident and their advisor, mentor, or coach are needed to allow for discussion of these topics over time. Programs should set expectations about the frequency of these scheduled meetings. In addition, a resident may request additional meetings with their advisor, mentor, or coach, for example, to discuss pros and cons of various career options, to discuss scholarship, or to process an experience or feedback the resident experienced. Programs should encourage resident-initiated meetings, as they signal agency, engagement in learning, and leadership.

Feedback, which is an important part of advising, mentoring, and coaching for all residents, must be provided in a timely, constructive, and individualized manner [21]. Depending on the specific context being discussed and the developmental stage of the learner, faculty may choose to take an advising, mentorship, or coaching approach. The R2C2 model, discussed above, is a particularly useful framework for reviewing feedback with a learner to foster growth [14]. Another commonly used framework for feedback is the ADAPT (Ask-Discuss-Ask-Plan Together) framework [22].

In addition to regularly scheduled advising, mentoring, or coaching meetings, some residents will need more targeted support as part of a remediation plan if they are not progressing at the expected rate. Residency programs may provide additional advising, mentorship, or coaching around time management, test- taking skills, clinical skills, professionalism, or other topics.

Advising, mentoring, and coaching are also essential for supporting residents' well-being and professional identity, especially for residents with unique challenges, identities, or struggles during residency [23, 24]. Residents may need multiple levels of support, including from professional counselors or psychiatrists as well as from their advisor, mentor, or coach. Coaching, in particular, has been shown to help residents develop their professional identity, which includes how they "think, act, and feel like a physician" [25]. In addition, serving as a coach for residents has been shown to help build the professional identity of the faculty member [26].

A number of structures have been utilized for advising, mentoring, and coaching during residency. For example, in our Stanford program, the Advising Associate Program Director serves as an advisor for each resident in a class and holds semiannual meetings with each resident in that class. These meetings entail reviewing the resident's well-being and experiences to date during residency, review of performance data, discussion of career and academic goals, discussion of elective plans, boards preparation, scholarly development, and other topics. Our residents receive mentorship from Scholarly Concentration and research mentors and Chief Residents. In addition, each resident has a Coach who is assigned to work with a smaller number of residents and meets with each resident to discuss their strengths, weaknesses, and learning goals and also performs clinical coaching. Clinical coaching occurs in the setting of a resident's clinical or leadership experiences, and the role of the coach is to directly observe the resident in action, and then later to prompt their reflection, provide feedback based on their observations, and encourage ongoing goal development toward clinical competence.

Other programs utilize faculty as academic or career advisors to support residents in their clinical skills and career development. Others have described trainee-led mentorship selection [27]. An increasing number of pediatric residency programs, including our own, have dedicated coaching programs for their residents [16, 28]. For programs seeking to develop scholarship skills for residents, consider creating a mentorship program focused on scholarship skills and experiences. Various research mentorship models have been described, including dyadic [29], multiple, apprenticeship, peer, and team mentorship models [30].

Program Development

As you build your program's advising, mentorship, and coaching goals, consider utilizing frameworks such as curriculum development or logic model frameworks. In addition, a prior publication specifically outlined steps in developing a coaching program in medical education, including the following 12 steps: (1) Identify "the why" or reasons a coaching program is needed, (2) Learn from established programs and prior literature, (3) Conduct a needs assessment of key stakeholders, (4) Identify and obtain resources needed, (5) Outline program goals and objectives, (6) Design programmatic approach, (7) Gather, adapt, or design tools for coaching, (8) Recruit coaches, (9) Design and implement faculty development for coaches, (10) Create and implement an orientation for learners, (11) Gather feedback on the program to assess feasibility and acceptability and to guide program development, and (12) Collect program outcome data to demonstrate programmatic impact [31].

Faculty and Learner Development of Advisors, Mentors, and Coaches

Faculty and learners need orientation and training around the expectations and structure of advising, mentoring, and coaching during residency. In particular, each group needs to understand their roles and expectations, as well as any specific frameworks or structures used in the program. Both groups should also be encouraged to utilize techniques that foster mutual trust, investment, co-creation, and psychological safety, and mitigate unconscious biases.

References

1. Deiorio NM, Foster KW, Santen SA. Coaching a learner in medical education. Acad Med. 2021;96(12):1758. https://doi.org/10.1097/ACM.0000000000004168.
2. Marcdante K, Simpson D. Choosing when to advise, coach, or mentor. J Grad Med Educ. 2018;10(2):227–8. https://doi.org/10.4300/JGME-D-18-00111.1.
3. Kuhn TL. Historical foundations of academic advising. In: Gordon VN, Habley WR, Grites TJ, editors. Academic advising: a comprehensive handbook. San Francisco: JosseyBass; 2008. p. 3–16.
4. Woods S, Burgess L, Heflin M. Resident advising toolkit. MedEdPORTAL. 2010;6:7800. https://doi-org.laneproxy.stanford.edu/10.15766/mep_2374-8265.7800.
5. Woods SK, Burgess L, Kaminetzky C, McNeill D, Pinheiro S, Heflin MT. Defining the roles of advisors and mentors in postgraduate medical education: faculty perceptions, roles, responsibilities, and resource needs. J Grad Med Educ. 2010;2(2):195–200. https://doi.org/10.4300/JGME-D-09-00089.1.
6. Sambunjak D, Straus SE, Marušić A. Mentoring in academic medicine. JAMA. 2006;296(9):1103.
7. 2024 Accreditation Council for Graduate Medical Education (ACGME). Guide to the Common Program Requirements (Residency). Version 4.1; updated March 2024. https://www.acgme.org/globalassets/pdfs/guide-to-the-common-program-requirements-residency.pdf.
8. Deiorio NM, Carney PA, Kahl LE, Bonura EM, Juve AM. Coaching: a new model for academic and career achievement. Med Educ Online. 2016;21(1):33480. https://doi.org/10.3402/meo.v21.33480.
9. Beyond Advising and Mentoring: Competencies for Coaching in Medical Education. https://www.tandfonline.com/doi/epdf/10.1080/0142159X.2021.1947479?needAccess=true&role=button. Accessed 12 Jan 2023.
10. Love LM, Simonsen KA, Bowler C, Beck Dallaghan GL. Archetypes of coaching across the medical education continuum. Acad Med. 2021;96(12):1757. https://doi.org/10.1097/ACM.0000000000004169.
11. American Medical Association. 2 huge steps to ease transition from medical school to residency. June 21, 2024. https://www.ama-assn.org/medical-students/preparing-residency/2-huge-steps-ease-transition-medical-school-residency.
12. A framework for fostering student agency in academic advising. https://nacada.ksu.edu/Resources/Academic-Advising-Today/View-Articles/A--Framework-for-Fostering-Student-Agency-in-Academic-Advising.aspx. Accessed 23 Feb 2025.
13. Cutrer WB, Miller B, Pusic MV, Mejicano G, Mangrulkar RS, Gruppen LD, Hawkins RE, Skochelak SE, Moore DE Jr. Fostering the development of master adaptive learners: a conceptual model to guide skill acquisition in medical education. Acad Med. 2017;92(1):70–5. https://doi.org/10.1097/ACM.0000000000001323.
14. Frankel A, Haraden C, Federico F, Lenoci-Edwards J. A framework for safe, reliable, and effective care, White Paper. Cambridge, MA: Institute for Healthcare Improvement and Safe & Reliable Healthcare; 2017.
15. Sargeant J, Mann K, Manos S, et al. R2C2 in action: testing an evidence-based model to facilitate feedback and coaching in residency. J Grad Med Educ. 2017;9(2):165–70. https://doi.org/10.4300/JGME-D-16-00398.
16. Rassbach CE, Blankenburg R. A novel pediatric residency coaching program: outcomes after one year. Acad Med. 2018;93(3):430. https://doi.org/10.1097/ACM.0000000000001825.
17. Mourad R, Archana P, Miller JA. Chapter 6: applications of coaching. In: Hammoud MM, Deiorio NM, Moore M, Wolff M, editors. Coaching in medical education. Elsevier – Health Sciences Division; 2022. p. 58.
18. Saddawi-Konefka D, Baker K, Guarino A, et al. Changing resident physician studying behaviors: a randomized, comparative effectiveness trial of goal setting versus use of WOOP. J Grad Med Educ. 2017;9(4):451–7. https://doi.org/10.4300/JGME-D-16-00703.1.
19. Kang: Nursing students' experience of online peer tutoring based on the grow model: a qualitative study
20. National Academies of Sciences E, Affairs P and G, Workforce B on HE and, Stemm C on EM in, Dahlberg ML, Byars-Winston A. The science of mentoring relationships: what is mentorship? In: The science of effective mentorship in STEMM. National Academies Press (US); 2019. https://www.ncbi.nlm.nih.gov/books/NBK552775/. Accessed 13 Sept 2023.
21. Lefroy J, Watling C, Teunissen PW, Brand P. Guidelines: the do's, don'ts and don't knows of feedback for clinical education. Perspect Med Educ. 2015;4(6):284–99. https://doi.org/10.1007/S40037-015-0231-7.
22. Padmore J, Hauer KE, Ekpenyong A, Edgar L, Holmboe E. Kathryn Andolsek Duke University. n.d.. https://www.acgme.org/globalassets/ACGMEClinicalCompetencyCommitteeGuidebook.pdf
23. Deb L, Desai S, McGinley K, et al. Mentorship in postgraduate medical education. In: Contemporary topics in graduate medical education – volume 2. IntechOpen; 2022. https://doi.org/10.5772/intechopen.98612.
24. International Medical Graduates (IMG) toolkit: Mentorship. American Medical Association. Published July 8, 2024. https://www.ama-assn.org/education/international-medical-education/

international-medical-graduates-img-toolkit-mentorship. Accessed 22 July 2024.
25. Hoang K, Grow HM, Rooholamini SN, McPhillips H, Selling SK, Rassbach CE, Blankenburg R. Impact of longitudinal coaching on pediatric residents' professional identity formation: a multi-institution qualitative study. Acad Pediatr. 2024;24(5):866–74. https://doi.org/10.1016/j.acap.2024.04.012.
26. Selling SK, Rooholamini SN, Mollie Grow H, McPhillips H, Hoang K, Blankenburg R, Rassbach C. The effects of coaching pediatric residents on faculty coaches' relationships, learning, and professional identity formation. Acad Med. 2023;98(3):376–83. https://doi.org/10.1097/ACM.0000000000005011.
27. Caruso TJ, Steinberg DH, Piro N, et al. A strategic approach to implementation of medical mentorship programs. J Grad Med Educ. 2016;8(1):68–73. https://doi.org/10.4300/JGME-D-15-00335.1.
28. Thomas MW, Hill TA, Walz A, Rassbach CE, Naifeh MM, Blankenburg R. The landscape of pediatric residency coaching programs in the United States. Acad Pediatr. 2025;
29. Kashiwagi DT, Varkey P, Cook DA. Mentoring programs for physicians in academic medicine: a systematic review. Acad Med. 2013;88(7):1029–37, Cited 266 times.
30. Henry-Noel N, Bishop M, Gwede CK, Petkova E, Szumacher E. Mentorship in medicine and other health professions. J Cancer Educ. 2019;34(4):629–37. https://doi.org/10.1007/s13187-018-1360-6.
31. Miller-Kuhlmann R, Sasnal M, Gold CA, Nassar AK, Korndorffer JR, Van Schaik S, Marmor A, Williams S, Blankenburg R, Rassbach CE. Tips for developing a coaching program in medical education. Med Educ Online. 2024;29(1):2289262. https://doi.org/10.1080/10872981.2023.2289262.

26 Well-Being in GME: Finding Meaning in Medicine

Jennifer G. Duncan and Elizabeth L. Seashore

An Introduction to Well-being: Finding Meaning in Medicine

Pediatric residency is an incredibly formative experience, one in which trainees move through the rigor of the academic learning environment as they translate their evolving medical knowledge to clinical practice. Sleep can be sparse, emotions high, learning curves steep, and the risk of burnout ever-present. Well-being efforts in residency programs have historically focused on mitigating the negative effects of these challenges; reducing work hours, providing opportunities to engage in wellness activities, and ensuring access to emotional support services are all necessary components of a well-being program and will be expanded on in this chapter. It is also critical to recognize that physician well-being depends on a sense of purpose in the work. A study by Shanafelt et al. examined the impact of meaning-making interventions on trainees physicians. The authors found that structured interventions aimed at helping trainees find meaning in their work can significantly improve their sense of professional fulfillment and reduce burnout [1]. Meaning-centered practice can help trainees stay connected to their initial motivations for pursuing pediatrics as a specialty and sustain their passions throughout their training and careers. Furthermore, great meaning often comes from moments of challenge and growth. In her book *Untamed*, author and queer activist Glennon Doyle offers "we can do hard things" and expounds on the value of leaning into struggle with a deep knowing of one's own resilience [2]. This concept can be applied to the clinical learning environment.

Rather than sheltering trainees from the difficult aspects of their medical training and the career that follows, programs can instead prepare them by setting expectations at the start of their training about the challenges they are likely to encounter in residency and in practice. This involves giving intention to curriculum on how to do hard things, helping trainees to process and cope after challenging events, and guiding them to translate these formative experiences into passion and meaning so they can continue this important work throughout their training and beyond.

J. G. Duncan (✉)
Washington University in St. Louis School of Medicine, St. Louis, MO, USA
e-mail: duncan_j@wustl.edu

E. L. Seashore
University of California, San Francisco School of Medicine, San Francisco, CA, USA

Starting the Conversation

A key aspect of finding meaning in medicine is the development of a strong professional identity by integrating personal values with the

H. McPhillips et al. (eds.), *Graduate Medical Education in Pediatrics*, Excellence in Medical Education 3, https://doi.org/10.1007/978-3-032-12952-9_26

professional roles and responsibilities of being a physician. Professional identity formation is a dynamic process influenced by various factors, including mentorship, clinical experiences, and reflective practices [3]. It helps trainees understand who they are as doctors and how they fit into the broader medical community. However, the framework for professional identity formation has not always been inclusive. Research by Wyatt et al. highlights that traditional models often fail to consider the unique experiences of trainees who are underrepresented in medicine (UIM) [4]. These models can inadvertently perpetuate feelings of isolation and identity threat among these individuals. Wyatt et al. call for an approach that recognizes and values diverse identities within the medical profession, ensuring that all trainees feel a sense of belonging and are equitably supported in their professional growth. Further supporting this, Trevino et al. emphasize the distinct challenges faced by UIM learners, such as identity fusion, stereotype threat, and lack of mentorship. They advocate for tailored strategies to support the professional identity formation of UIM trainees, including institutional support, building communities of practice, and fostering an inclusive environment [5].

The language used to discuss well-being for medical trainees can be likewise problematic and requires intention. The word 'resilience,' for example, has fallen out of favor with many graduate medical education learners for the ways in which some feel it has been weaponized to place the burden of achieving well-being on the individual learner. Resilience has been used to denote a characteristic that each trainees does or does not demonstrate within their training program and does not always honor the remarkable circumstances in which that trainees has lived and achieved to get to this moment in their medical journey. In reclaiming this word in the well-being literature, resilience should be more clearly defined as a shared goal between trainees and educators, one that harnesses the strengths of the trainees and the support of their program to foster humanism through completion of training and as part of an ongoing well-being practice. A study by Pu et al. expands upon this concept, highlighting humanistic values such as empathy, compassion, and patient-centered care as central to their professional identity formation. It goes on to offer a modification to Cruess' professional identity framework to reflect humanism in identity formation during pediatrics residency [6]. Another framework that can be utilized to move beyond 'resilience' is the concept of human flourishing. Flourishing incorporates a broad range of states or outcomes, including mental and physical health, happiness and life satisfaction, meaning and purpose, character and virtue, and social relationships.

Barriers and Opportunities

Several barriers can impede the cultivation of meaning in pediatric residency. Generational and cultural differences significantly influence what defines well-being, leading to varying expectations and experiences among trainees. For instance, younger generations may prioritize work-life integration and mental health more than older generations, who might have different views on professional dedication and resilience. Additionally, cultural backgrounds can shape how trainees perceive and manage stress, impacting their overall well-being. The principles of diversity, equity, and inclusion (DEI) and well-being are deeply connected and cannot be addressed independently. Each trainee enters training with a unique background and set of lived experiences. For many trainees, the burdens of systemic and institutionalized racism and bigotry can compound high-intensity clinical events and interpersonal interactions, leading to feelings of isolation and burnout. By integrating a DEI-centered lens into well-being initiatives, residency programs can provide wraparound support in fostering a sense of belonging so that all trainees feel valued in their academic community [7].

Another critical barrier is the scarcity mindset prevalent in academic medicine. The mindset is defined by a constant sense of competition for limited resources (funding, opportunities, recognition), which can exacerbate stress and hinder collaboration. This often leads to a focus on short-term achievements and survival, rather than long-term growth and well-being. Naming and re-evaluating systems that contribute to the scarcity mindset can demystify its existence and disempower its influence for trainees and faculty alike. Finally, the imposter phenomenon, also known as imposter syndrome, can pose a significant barrier to cultivating meaning in medicine. It is characterized by persistent self-doubt and a fear of being exposed as a fraud despite evident success and is common among high-achieving individuals, including medical trainees. Learners experiencing imposter syndrome may attribute their successes to luck rather than their abilities, leading to increased anxiety and decreased self-esteem. This presents a unique opportunity for well-being programming that centers on helping trainees to develop confidence in addition to competence [8].

Prevalence of Burnout in Pediatric Residency

Improving well-being in pediatric residency requires an understanding of burnout. Importantly, burnout is a World Health Organization-designated condition and is considered a workplace phenomenon, not a result of individual factors such as personal resiliency or vulnerability [9]. Burnout is characterized by emotional exhaustion, depersonalization, and a reduced sense of personal accomplishment. Over 50% of pediatric trainees experience burnout at some point during their training [10]. A study by Koressel et al. followed a cohort of pediatric trainees over three years and found that burnout, stress, and fatigue significantly increased within the first six months of residency and persisted throughout the training period [11]. Emotional exhaustion and moderate stress were prevalent in over 65% of trainees at every time point measured. The increase in burnout over time in training has been shown in multiple subspecialties and is a strong indicator that factors within our medical training systems, rather than individual deficits in coping or resilience, are the primary drivers of burnout [12].

Drivers of Well-being vs. Burnout

Shanafelt et al. have extensively studied the drivers of burnout and engagement in physicians [13]. Key factors affecting burnout include excessive workload, inefficient work processes, lack of control and flexibility, insufficient reward, breakdown of community, absence of fairness, and conflicting values (Fig. 26.1). Conversely, drivers of engagement and well-being include meaning-

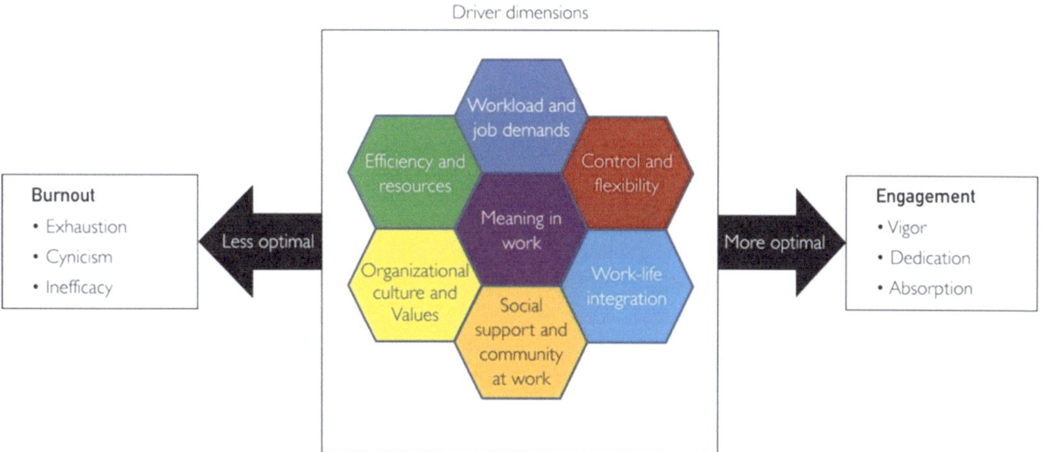

Fig. 26.1 Factors contributing to physician burnout and engagement. (Reprinted with permission from Shanafelt TD, Noseworthy JH) [13]

ful work, a supportive work environment, effective leadership, and opportunities for professional growth, with meaning in work being the most critical factor in driving engagement.

The drivers of well-being and burnout can also be understood through the Job Demands-Resources framework [14]. This model posits that job constraints (e.g., high workload, time pressure, emotional demands) can lead to burnout, especially when job resources (e.g., support, autonomy, opportunities for professional development) are insufficient.

What Is at Stake

The consequences of burnout are well-documented and include impaired professional behavior, reduced quality of patient care, and increased risk of medical errors [15]. Burnout can also lead to mental health issues such as depression, anxiety, and increased risk for substance use disorder, which in turn can contribute to suicidal ideation [16, 17]. Among pediatric trainees specifically, studies show trainees with evidence of burnout are more likely to report suboptimal patient care behaviors, including earlier discharge, making treatment or medication errors, or spending less time answering questions [18]. Additionally, Staples et al. showed that trainees with burnout scored lower on all pediatric milestones, suggesting an association with decreased overall performance [19]. Three years of data from the Pediatric Trainees Burnout-Resilience Study Consortium confirms many of the smaller studies, demonstrating that trainees who meet criteria for burnout have worse mental health, more sleepiness, and greater stress. They also had lower self-compassion and mindfulness scores, lower quality of life, and less satisfaction with work-life balance as well as career choice [10]. Thus, addressing the factors that contribute to burnout is critical for maintaining both high-quality patient care and for ensuring the health and sustained engagement of our pediatric workforce.

ACGME Requirements for Trainee Well-being

The Accreditation Council for Graduate Medical Education (ACGME) has established requirements to ensure the well-being of trainees. Historically, these requirements have focused on duty hours, supervision, and the learning environment. However, recognizing the growing concerns about trainees burnout, the ACGME has introduced new requirements that emphasize a more holistic approach to trainee health. In 2017, the ACGME began mandating that residency programs implement comprehensive well-being initiatives, and these requirements remain in effect in the newest common program requirements [20]. Requirements include access to mental health self-assessment tools and counseling services, structured wellness curricula, and arttention to work intensity, workplace safety, and fatigue mitigation. Programs are also required to provide resources for stress management and resilience training and to create a supportive environment that encourages trainees to seek help without fear of stigma. These requirements offer a challenge and an opportunity for pediatric training programs to re-evaluate and reimagine their systems of support for trainees. In the remainder of this chapter, we outline key characteristics of successful well-being programs, offering residency programs suggestions for meeting the ACGME requirements and beyond.

Characteristics of Successful Well-being Programs

Well-being means different things to different people; therefore, successful well-being programs need to have a multi-faceted approach. Given the multiple drivers of physician distress and burnout, addressing individual needs and system-level challenges and ensuring a culture within the learning environment that supports well-being and professional growth are all important (Table 26.1).

Table 26.1 Characteristics of successful well-being programs

Individual well-being support		
	Well-being curricula	
		Moral distress and injury, grief and loss, imposter phenomenon, burnout, depression, suicide, substance use, and fatigue
	Coping skill development	
		Self-care: Sleep, exercise, nutrition, health care
		Psychological skill building: Mindfulness, self-compassion, positive psychology
		Creative expression
		Relational practices
		Debriefings
	Peer support and coaching	
Mental health resources		
	Awareness building, stigma reduction	
	Screening tools for well-being and mental health	
	Confidential and affordable mental health care	
	Crisis response plans	
Community and culture		
	Establish inclusive community	
	Develop psychological safety	
	System interventions	
		Address workload, workflow and efficiency
		Establish clear expectations and policies in the learning environment
		Address mistreatment, microaggressions and bias
	Tools for monitoring well-being	

Supporting Well-being at the Individual Level

Teaching Towards Meaning-Making

With fostering meaning in medicine as the north star, pediatric training programs can design well-being curricula that offer a variety of options to reach the individualized needs of each trainees. Work by Shanafelt discusses approaches to meaning-centered education in residency, including reflective writing and practice, narrative medicine, and facilitated group discussions, all of which help trainees connect with a deeper purpose in their work and foster a sense of community among peers [1]. Recently, Vermette and colleagues described a flourishing-focused advising strategy that incorporates self-assessment, guided reflections, and discussion with an advisor to generate a strengths-based approach to optimizing well-being that also holds promise for helping trainees focus on meaning in work [21].

Essential Components of a Well-being Curriculum

Targeted Didactic Topics

Moral Distress and Moral Injury

Moral distress occurs when individuals feel compelled to act against their beliefs due to external constraints, leading to feelings of powerlessness and frustration [22]. The AMA Journal of Ethics discusses the different types of moral distress experienced by medical students and trainees physicians [23]. It examines how moral distress arises from conflicts between deeply held values and the demands of clinical practice and how this can lead to burnout and other negative outcomes. The article also discusses strategies for addressing and mitigating moral distress, including ethics education and ethics rounds, facilitated discussions and debriefings, and organizational support in the creation of policies and support systems. Moral injury, on the other hand, involves a deeper violation of one's moral or ethical code, often resulting from witnessing or participating in actions that contradict deeply held values. Rosen et al. discusses the continuum between moral distress, moral injury, and burnout among healthcare professionals, particularly in the context of the COVID-19 pandemic [24]. Both moral distress and moral injury are prevalent in medical training and can significantly impact trainees' mental health and professional satisfaction. Addressing these issues through education and support can help mitigate their effects.

Grief and Loss

Pediatric trainees education on death and bereavement is foundational to supporting well-being and cultivating meaning for trainees. Trainees should receive didactics proactively on how to care for a dying patient, from recognizing signs of imminent death to providing comfort at the end of life to both the child and their loved ones. Following patient loss, trainees should be offered support utilizing an interdisciplinary team of facilitators with experience and skill in processing such events. The AAP Resilience in the Face of Grief and Loss Curriculum, developed by Serwint et al., addresses the need for structured education on grief and loss for pediatric healthcare providers [25]. This curriculum includes modules on understanding grief, high-stakes communication, managing emotions after high-intensity clinical experiences, and provisions for personal wellness. It also provides guidance on implementing such a curriculum and offers opportunities for faculty development. The curriculum emphasizes the importance of equipping healthcare providers with the skills and support needed to handle the emotional challenges of pediatric care.

Imposter Phenomenon

As previously discussed, imposter phenomenon can be a significant barrier to trainees well-being and meaning making. Supporting trainees through this involves creating a culture of open communication, providing mentorship, and offering workshops that address self-doubt and build confidence. Work by Ogunyemi and colleagues on a longitudinal GME-led assessment of burnout and learning environments incorporated one such workshop on imposter syndrome as part of a larger resiliency training program, with reported improvements in levels of burnout and clinical learning environment measures [26].

Required Education: Burnout, Mental Health, Substance Use and Fatigue

The ACGME does require education of trainees and faculty on specific topics, including burnout, depression and substance use disorders, suicidal ideation or potential for violence, and how to assist individuals with these concerns [20]. Additionally, programs are required to educate faculty and trainees on signs of fatigue and fatigue mitigation strategies. Addressing all these topics in a manner that keeps trainees engaged can be challenging, and lectures on these topics are often met with frustration. We encourage programs to partner with local experts in psychiatry, psychology, and sleep medicine to develop compelling approaches to these discussions. Additionally, programs can consider the use of online educational modules that serve to satisfy these requirements.

Promoting Coping Strategies

Meaningful Self-Care

Actively encouraging self-care activities, including things like identifying a primary care physician and other health providers, attending to good nutrition, and getting adequate sleep and exercise when possible, is an important foundational approach. However, given that lack of time is the leading reason for poor self-care by physicians, limiting the definition of self-care only to strategies that generally must occur outside of work hours can be problematic. Considering a holistic approach to self-care that incorporates dimensions of well-being beyond only physical health may allow incorporation of sustaining practices during the workday. Recently, Hussain, Yaden, and Tomescu outlined "strategic self-care" that highlights physical, psychological, and relational/spiritual domains of self-care [27]. Faculty and program leadership can help trainees learn to incorporate components of each of these domains into their workdays, such as breathing exercises to calm the nervous system or attending to nutrition and hydration while at work. Intentionally helping trainees to foster meaningful relationships, or to address moments of perfectionism with cognitive reframing can also support well-being while at work. Faculty modeling of these self-care activities is a critical component of establishing a culture that supports well-being. Establishing a culture that supports individual health also includes setting clear expectations related to physical illness and transparency around illness and leave policies, as well as ensuring trainees have awareness of a variety of resources to meet individual needs. Another essential aspect of self-care is boundary-setting, which involves establishing clear limitations to protect one's time, energy, and emotional resources. Boundary-setting requires recognizing one's limitations, communicating them effectively, and adhering to them consistently. In the context of medical training, boundary-setting can help trainees manage their workload, avoid over-commitment, and ensure they have time for rest and personal activities.

Sleep

Despite duty hour regulations, sleep deprivation is still a major challenge in medical training and is associated with poor cognitive performance, perceived medical errors, depression, and burnout [28]. Trainees appreciate leaders that acknowledge the difficulties of training rather than simply telling them to sleep more. Commonly, physicians do not recognize our own symptoms of fatigue; thus an important approach to addressing fatigue is ensuring trainees and faculty recognize signs of fatigue and are able to have supportive conversations with trainees. It is most beneficial to focus on strategies for mitigating fatigue, including strategic napping, circadian shift strategies related to light exposure, strategic use of caffeine and melatonin, and even nutritional strategies to improve sleep [29–31]. Facilitated discussions are one approach to optimize personal recognition of sleep deprivation tolerance. For some trainees, sleep issues are not simply a result of their clinical schedules, and so ensuring awareness of resources to address sleep difficulties, including sleep specialists and internet-based insomnia applications [32], is important. Finally, programs must ensure trainees have options for safe transportation home when too fatigued to drive [20].

Exercise

Exercise has many physical and emotional health benefits. Individuals with established exercise routines are less likely to experience burnout [33]. However, maintaining physical activity is often difficult during residency. Multiple strategies have been studied to facilitate regular exercise for trainees, including team-based competitions, activity trackers, and easier access to fitness equipment/facilities with positive results [34–36]. While challenging, a programmatic approach to promote and incentivize the physical activity domain may be a worthwhile investment.

Health Care

Many GME trainees do not attend to routine healthcare needs [37]. Mental health resources are even more significantly underutilized [38]. Program- and institution-level interventions to ensure easy access to healthcare and to reduce stigma associated with taking the time needed to address physical and mental health needs are critical. Simple strategies to improve access to care, such as providing lists of recommended physicians accepting new patients, offering flexible days off, on-site clinics dedicated to trainees or hospital/school of medicine employees, and opt-out scheduling of mental health visits, are all strategies that have been deployed [39, 40]. Programs should be transparent about how trainees can attend to health care needs during the regular workweek, as is required by the ACGME.

Nutrition

Maintaining healthy eating habits is also challenging for medical trainees [29, 41]. Lack of time, cost of healthy food, and limited food choices in the hospital setting are all contributors to poor eating habits for trainees. Additionally, food insecurity among trainees is likely under-recognized. Providing access to regular healthy snacks, on-site resources for healthier food alternatives, and program-level attention to food insecurity are all considerations for supporting good nutrition.

Psychological Skill-Building

Skill-building that strengthens our ability to face adversity and grow is essential throughout training and our future careers. Incorporating practices that promote healthy emotional processing into didactic curricula can be beneficial in building resilience. This can include introductions to strategies for recognizing negative self-talk and using cognitive restructuring to reframe thinking in the moment, as well as promoting self-compassion, psychological flexibility, creative expression, and relational connections.

Fostering Psychological Flexibility

The concept of psychological flexibility refers to the ability to remain open to experiences, including challenging thoughts and emotions, while also taking actions that align with one's values. Values are freely chosen guiding principles that hold personal meaning and shape our everyday decisions across different life domains, including how we care for patients, pursue career growth, and engage in relationships [42]. For pediatric trainees, these values at work might include providing compassionate care, personal growth in knowledge, or being a supportive team member. Unlike specific goals, such as completing a certain number of procedures, values cannot be fully achieved or checked off a list [43]. Value-based actions are behaviors that align with these personal values, even in times of distress. For a trainee, this might mean focusing on supporting and teaching the interns during a particularly difficult rotation, because it aligns with their value of teaching others. These principles are the basis of a form of cognitive behavioral therapy called acceptance and commitment therapy. In recent years these principles have formed the basis of workplace interventions, including in healthcare settings [44], with improvement in psychological distress. While these interventions involved structured, longitudinal workshops that may not be feasible to fit into a training program curriculum, program leadership and mentors can support trainees in utilizing this framework by teaching about the concepts of psychological flexibility and values, providing opportunities for personal reflection, and guiding trainees to consider their values when faced with challenges during training. By focusing on values rather than just goals, pediatric trainees can find deeper meaning and satisfaction in their work, even amidst the challenges of residency.

Mindfulness Techniques

Mindfulness techniques, including meditation, have been increasingly studied as effective coping strategies for trainees physicians. Mindfulness involves maintaining a moment-by-moment awareness of thoughts, feelings, bodily sensations, and the surrounding environment, typically through a gentle, nurturing lens. Studies have shown that mindfulness-based interventions can significantly reduce stress, anxiety, and depression among trainees physicians [45]. These practices help trainees manage the emotional demands of patient care, particularly at the bedside with patients and their families, by promoting a calm and focused presence. Benefits of mindfulness extend beyond immediate stress relief, contributing to long-term self-care practices that support sustained mental health and professional satisfaction. For instance, an 8-week mindfulness program developed by Fendel et al. and tailored for trainees physicians demonstrated medium-to-large improvements in perceived stress, mental health, self-attributed mindfulness, and self-compassion. Additionally, small-to-medium improvements were observed in job strain, effort-reward imbalance, work-related burnout, thriving at work, and physician empathy [46]. Another study by Minichiello and colleagues developed a mindfulness training program for family medicine trainees, resulting in significant decreases in perceived stress and increases in mindful awareness. Trainees reported personal and professional benefits, including improved relationships with patients and reduced burnout [47]. While not all programs are able to develop longitudinal mindfulness interventions, mindfulness strategies can also be incorporated into daily work. Teaching trainees to consider brief (micro) moments of mindfulness throughout the day, such as just before eating a meal, while washing hands prior to a procedure, or before starting a difficult conversation can help reduce stress [48].

Self-Compassion

Self-compassion is a specific type of mindfulness practice that involves treating oneself with the same kindness, concern, and support that one would offer to others experiencing a difficult situation. Groundbreaking work by psychologist Kristin Neff describes self-compassion, including its three main elements: self-kindness—being warm and understanding toward oneself when encountering pain and personal shortcomings, rather than ignoring them or being self-critical; common humanity—recognizing that suffering and personal inadequacy are part of the shared human experience—something that everyone goes through rather than being something that happens to "me" alone; and mindfulness—holding one's painful thoughts and feelings in balanced awareness rather than over-identifying with them. Medical trainees can use self-compassion practices to navigate the challenges of their training, maintain their mental health, and foster a more supportive and compassionate approach to themselves and their patients. Neff and Germer's study on the Mindful Self-Compassion (MSC) program found that self-compassion training can significantly reduce stress, anxiety, and depression while increasing well-being and resilience among participants, and this has been adapted to the healthcare environment [49, 50]. Additionally, in a randomized clinical trial, Fainstad et al. demonstrated the effectiveness of self-compassion training through group coaching in reducing burnout in female trainees physicians specifically [51]. The study found significant improvements in emotional exhaustion, depersonalization, personal accomplishment, and self-compassion scores among participants. Work by Liu et al. found that well-being factors such as greater mindfulness, self-compassion, and empathetic concern are associated with increased confidence in providing calm, compassionate care among pediatric trainees [52]. These factors contribute to trainees' ability to manage the emotional demands of patient care and maintain a compassionate presence at the bedside. Programs can incorporate these principles into their well-being curriculum as part of their strategy to support overall well-being.

Positive Psychology

The concept of positive psychology and the benefits of specific practices, such as gratitude and strengths-based reflections, can be introduced as part of a curriculum and then reinforced in daily work. For example, team leaders might encourage members of the team to share something they are grateful for or reflect on who they helped today as a means of encouraging those positive connections. Sexton and colleagues have developed multiple "bite-size" well-being strategies that are publicly available [53] and have been shown, when used regularly, to have a positive impact on work-life integration, happiness, depressive symptoms, and emotional thriving and recovery [54].

Creative Expression

Creative expression, including reflective writing and art-based interventions, can be promoted either individually or as group-based activities. Art-based interventions with GME trainees are associated with increased empathy for patients and positive impact on awareness, time for reflection, and normalization of experiences through their time with peers [55, 56]. Many GME programs have integrated forms of narrative medicine into their regular curricula, allowing trainees an opportunity to share experiences and vulnerability with others, reducing isolation, and promoting connection and meaning making [57, 58]. In recent years, several programs have extended their narrative medicine curricula to include storytelling events, which has further extended community-building among trainees [59, 60].

Relational Practices

A sense of belonging is critical to one's well-being [61]. The recent COVID-19 pandemic provided important insights into the negative impact of isolation on mental health. Programs should proactively work to promote connections between trainees and optimize opportunities for connection outside of the program [62]. This maybe particularly important for individuals that identify as part of minoritized communities (UIM, LGBTQIA+, and international graduates, as some examples) [63]. For some trainees, religious and spiritual practices can also be a key coping mechanism [64]. Programs can provide information and resources to help connect trainees to preferred spiritual communities.

Connecting with values to find meaning in work is another important self-care strategy. Studies in practicing physicians indicate a positive association between a sense of greater meaning and domains of greater well-being [65]. The

Healer's Art program, implemented at medical schools around the world, introduces reflective practices to medical students with a focus on specific themes, including finding a sense of awe in clinical practice [66, 67]. The benefits of this curriculum have been sustained [68]. Lader et al. reported that an adaptation of this curriculum for pediatric trainees resulted in a greater sense of belonging and renewed commitment to patient-centered care [69].

Pediatric programs now also have a unique opportunity to connect with an already developed curriculum that promotes many of the above strategies. The Pediatric Trainees Burnout-Resilience Study Consortium (PRB-RSC), in collaboration with the American Foundation for Suicide Prevention, developed a novel curriculum—Sustaining and Training for Resilience, Engagement, and Meaning [STREAM]—that includes five modules related to promoting mental health, engagement, resilience, and positive emotions and enhancing the joy and meaning of our work [70]. While there is no published data yet, it is our understanding that the early experiences with the curriculum have been positive (personal communication).

Debriefing After High-Intensity Clinical Events

Debriefing sessions provide an opportunity for trainees to reflect on and process their experiences, an approach that is essential for emotional and psychological recovery. Providing protected time and a safe space to reflect can help trainees express their emotions, share their experiences, and receive validation and support from their peers and facilitators. This process can mitigate the risk of developing post-traumatic stress disorder (PTSD) and other stress-related conditions. Studies have shown that structured debriefings improve team performance, enhance learning, and provide critical emotional support. Additionally, participation in debriefing and reflective sessions also helps facilitators process their own grief, which in turn creates a culture of shared support and meaning [71]. A number of toolkits exist to help educators, physicians, and interdisciplinary staff facilitate peer-led debriefs, including publications by the Quality Palliative Care in Long Term Care Alliance [72].

Peer Support and Coaching

Systems of support, such as peer support programs, coaching, and group discussions, can provide a formal well-being structure that enhances the overall culture of well-being within programs. Support from peers can be in the form of sibling-type pairings, with more senior trainees paired with junior trainees to help optimize the transition into residency and offer guidance for various challenges, or in structured peer group discussions [73]. Many programs have created peer support initiatives that address trainee needs after adverse events, interprofessional conflicts, or other challenges faced in the workplace [74, 75]. Peer supporters are trained in active listening and psychological first aid [76] and provide a space to process these events. Evidence shows that in these circumstances many physicians would prefer to talk to a physician colleague to process the event. Some peer support programs are structured such that colleagues from a different department or division provide confidential support, but more recently, training programs have trained and embedded GME peer supporters within their programs that fulfill a similar role [77].

Coaching programs offer personalized guidance and support, helping trainees develop strategies for self-reflection, improvement, and personal and professional success. These programs have been implemented in several residency programs and are associated with improved coping skills and lower levels of emotional exhaustion [78, 79]. Recently, Fainstad et al. and Mann et al. have published on a group coaching intervention that utilizes virtual group coaching sessions, self-study materials, recorded videos, and a small number of 1:1 coaching sessions. This particular group coaching approach demonstrated improvements in burnout, moral injury, impostor phenomenon, and self-compassion [51, 80]. A study by Redman et al. on a GME "success coaching" program found that coaching helped trainees address various areas of need, including medical knowledge, clinical skills, efficiency, interpersonal skills, communication, professionalism, and mental health and well-being [81].

Discussion groups that offer an opportunity for reflective practices and processing are also beneficial. Some programs have offered faculty-facilitated discussion groups or Balint groups that allow participants to process training challenges or events from the clinical setting with the help of a trained facilitator [82, 83]. In our own programs, palliative care faculty have been willing to facilitate these debriefs, allowing trainees to process emotionally challenging experiences that occur during high-intensity rotations. Recently, support groups facilitated by a therapist were shown to improve surgery trainees' perceptions of their own competency and increase the likelihood of shared problem-solving with peers [84].

Establishing Resources

Beyond structured well-being curricular offerings, there are several additional resource considerations.

Mental Health Programming and Resources

Mental health support is a critical component of well-being programming for individuals. Trainees and fellows have higher levels of mental health diagnoses compared to other professions [16, 17, 38, 85]. The COVID-19 pandemic further highlighted these concerns. Importantly, mental health diagnoses are distinct from burnout, though potentially related. Thus, recognition of changes in a trainee's behavior should result in broad considerations for the cause. Addressing stress in a proactive manner can help prevent the development of more serious mental health concerns. Openly discussing physician distress and mental health needs is a foundational approach to reducing stigma and promoting help-seeking [86]. Providing education to faculty and trainees about signs and symptoms of burnout, depression, and suicidal ideation are ACGME requirements [20]. This knowledge is key to building awareness and ideally helps arm individuals with resource information for referrals if needed. One systematic approach is psychological first-aid training [76].

Beyond education, promoting regular well-being and mental health screening also promotes a culture where help-seeking is encouraged. Multiple anonymous screening tools focus on overall well-being (see section on Well-being Assessment). These tools, coupled with resource awareness, can help identify individuals prior to the development of serious mental health concerns. Additionally, the American Foundation of Suicide Prevention developed a tool (Interactive Screening Program) [87] that allows individuals to anonymously submit stress and depression questionnaires and receive responses from a licensed mental health professional at the individual's institution. The platform aims to identify at-risk individuals and connect them more rapidly with therapy services. This is an approach that some institutions are taking to ensure trainees in need are accessing mental health care [88].

The ACGME requires that programs provide access to confidential and affordable mental health counseling and treatment. There are multiple potential approaches to providing access to counseling and psychiatric care, with the specific approach dependent on institutional structure and feasibility. Some institutions have internal resources for care, while others have used employee assistance programs, contracts with local providers, or tele-mental health platforms. A few institutions have published on the establishment of GME-specific mental health programs noting program structure and costs [89, 90]. Regardless of approach taken, it is also essential for programs to ensure trainees have the ability to attend appointments, even during working hours, as required by the ACGME. Tracking de-identified utilization data is important for programs to understand whether efforts to reduce stigma and promote awareness are effective. In well-established programs, utilization rates for mental health services are now greater than 30%. Clear program policies are needed to facilitate accessing appointments, including reducing the stigma associated with asking for the time needed. A strategy many programs have taken to reduce barriers to seeking help is "opt-out" therapy or wellness check-in appointments, where the program schedules trainees for a one-time appointment and they have the option to cancel. This approach has resulted in a large percentage (>50%) of trainees keeping appointments and high satisfaction ratings, as well as increased self-reporting of willingness to engage in mental health services [91, 92]. In one study, 39% of trainees self-initiated additional appointments, compared to only 6% prior to implementation of the opt-out strategy [91]. Another study found that in addition to increased utilization of mental health services, the opt-out strategy was associated with fewer reports of professionalism issues [93].

Regardless of services offered, programs should consider plans for responding to crises. The ACGME and American Foundation for Suicide Prevention have published an excellent toolkit for crisis planning [94]. This guide provides direction for proactive planning, including communication strategies and resource needs in the event of any unexpected death of a trainee. Programs should also consider how they would approach wellness checks in the event that a trainee does not show up for work. Finally, clear processes should be in place for responding in the event of a serious mental illness that presents itself during working hours, including the specific location for referral for emergency services in a manner that optimizes confidentiality for the trainee.

Creating Culture and Systems That Support Meaning in Medicine

The well-being interventions discussed thus far are primarily aimed at the individual. Importantly, pediatric programs also need to address the systems-level challenges that contribute to burnout and inhibit thriving. Medical students who enter training begin with high resilience and low burnout, but this worsens over time in training [85], providing a strong argument that the system of training itself must be examined rather than focusing solely on the individual. Additionally, when interventions that specifically target trainees have been assessed, systems-level interventions have been more effective in reducing burnout [95]. Systems-level interventions are those that impact workload, workflow, and culture, and generally include structural support or policies that address challenges faced by individuals in the program. While some of these interventions can occur at the program level, others may require broader institutional change. Program leaders may not always have the authority to address system issues, but they can serve as advocates for change and engage with appropriate stakeholders.

Team Culture

The culture within the clinical learning environment is a critical factor in overall well-being. The importance of "teaming" is highlighted by the ACGME identifying it as a core component of the Clinical Learning Environment Review [96]. Team structure, interprofessional relationships and collaboration, and communication can be both sources of support and difficulty for pediatric trainees [97]. Additionally, the workload carried by members of the team can impede collaboration, and the manner in which disagreements are resolved can contribute to ongoing conflict [98]. Frequently changing teams adds an additional challenge in academic medicine, so effective culture work needs to reach beyond the individual team to engage broadly across an organization. An intervention focused on workplace civility, where individuals had the opportunity to express gratitude with electronic dissemination across teams and specialties, resulted in an improvement in team attitudes [99]. Highlighting accomplishments and showing appreciation are important components of ensuring that individuals feel valued within a program and organization.

Psychological safety within teams is one of the most important components of team culture; this concept describes a sense that people can take interpersonal risks, admit mistakes, and seek help without fear of retribution [100]. Higher levels of psychological safety are associated with more trust. Interventions that aim to enhance team structure can have a significant impact on overall well-being. One pediatric residency program described the use of an interprofessional simulation curriculum to address team culture, which, while helpful, was not sufficient to address all culture issues [98]. Pierce et al. describe a multi-pronged intervention that focused on leadership and team development, shared problem solving to address workflow challenges, and cultivating positive emotions [101]. This longitudinal program had a positive impact on burnout measures and satisfaction with the workplace. The multi-faceted approach underscores that addressing team culture requires attention to more than one aspect of team dynamics. Nevertheless, beginning to address culture with even small changes is beneficial.

Hierarchy within teams is another aspect of team dynamics that should be considered. Supervisor support has been identified as an important contributor to trainee burnout [102]. Educators that are open to discussing opinions and who empower trainees to ask questions are more likely to establish mutual respect within teams. Faculty development in communication and feedback helps to promote positive teamwork dynamics. Additionally, the balance of supervision and autonomy for pediatric trainees is linked to their well-being. Self-determination theory defines our basic psychological needs of relatedness, competency, and autonomy [103]. These basic needs are linked with intrinsic motivation and overall satisfaction. Faculty and senior trainees behaviors that foster competence (a sense of mastery and effectiveness) and autonomy (feeling one has a choice in aspects of their work) can positively influence pediatric trainees well-being. Ensuring trainees are using their highest level of skills, focusing predominantly on physician-specific tasks, is one way to help foster a sense of competence. Offering choices, where possible, in how a trainees manages a particular condition or responds to a diagnostic challenge can help foster autonomy. Promoting these behaviors through faculty and senior trainees professional development is one approach programs can take, in addition to ensuring opportunities for observation and feedback to individuals leading trainees teams. An additional approach to supporting these basic psychological needs is through mentorship and coaching programs (see above for coaching). Both faculty and peer mentoring programs can be effective in providing support for professional growth and protection from burnout [104, 105].

A critical component of culture within any program is bias within the learning environment. Microaggressions and implicit bias impact every aspect of well-being [106]. Learners can feel invalidated, resulting in a lack of focus and ability to learn for the impacted individual, as well as reduced trust and teamwork within the group. Repeated microaggressions and incivility have a cumulative effect leading to worsening stress, impaired coping, increased burnout, and an overall decreased sense of well-being. Programs should partner with champions in diversity, equity, and inclusion to address these issues in the learning environment.

A final note on team culture: it is also notable that there is a social contagion effect associated with burnout, such that a portion of individual burnout can be attributed to burnout of team members [107]. Thus, attention to all of these components of team culture—relational practices, team dynamics, psychological safety, and inclusion—are critical for every member of the healthcare team.

Mistreatment and Well-being

Several studies have linked experiences of unprofessional behavior and mistreatment with burnout in physicians [108–110]. Importantly, female physicians and physicians from ethnic and racial minority groups are more likely to experience mistreatment. Among pediatric trainees in one study, nearly 20% reported experiencing bullying or discrimination. Trainees who have experienced mistreatment are more likely to experience burnout [109, 110]; in pediatric trainees there was nearly a

2-fold increased likelihood of reporting burnout symptoms with exposure to mistreatment [110]. There are multiple sources for the mistreatment behavior, with patients, families, and clinical staff making up the largest group in the pediatric study. Proactive work to address civility within organizations is critical for reducing harmful behaviors in the clinical learning environment. This can occur through education and group discussions that promote listening to all perspectives, reducing power imbalances, and training individuals to be "upstanders" when they witness unprofessional behaviors [111]. It is important to have clear systems in place for reporting and addressing mistreatment that occurs in the workplace. Hickson et al. described their graduated intervention approach to addressing disruptive behaviors, including informal feedback conversations, non-punitive "awareness" interventions when patterns of behavior are detected, leader-developed action plans for persistent patterns, and ultimately disciplinary processes [112]. While individual residency programs may not have the ability to develop such a robust system, a mechanism for collecting concerns, tracking them, and partnering with appropriate leaders and human resource staff to address behaviors systematically can help promote an improved culture and help trainees feel supported. Addressing patient-derived mistreatment also requires clear organizational policies regarding expected behavior as well as education of trainees and faculty in how to address the behaviors when they occur. Empowering trainees to respond to these behaviors is important for ensuring their self-efficacy and confidence, which may protect them from the negative consequences of stress and burnout. The Macy Foundation funded several GME Catalyst Awards that include structured approaches to addressing mistreatment such as practical skills training using a variety of strategies, for example, observed structured clinical exams (OSCEs) and simulation [113–118]. An important component of education for patient-derived mistreatment is ensuring faculty understand strategies for supporting trainees and fellows, including offering an opportunity for trainees to have a voice in the response.

Creating a Learning Environment Structure That Supports Meaning Making

Program leaders can attend to specific structural supports that serve to enhance well-being and therefore optimize meaning making for pediatric trainees. These include attention to leadership communication strategies, schedules, policies, and monitoring of workload and workflows. Finally, we will address leadership behaviors that support well-being.

Communication, Transparency, and Setting Expectations

Clear communication and transparency are foundational for a supportive learning environment. Program directors and faculty must articulate program goals, policies, expectations, and evaluation criteria with clarity and consistency. Regular feedback sessions, with faculty from rotations and with program leadership, should be established, providing trainees with insights into their progress and areas for improvement. Equally important is the creation of channels for trainees to voice their concerns and contribute to program development. This bidirectional feedback fosters a sense of ownership and engagement among trainees and fellows. The COVID-19 pandemic highlighted the importance of communication in reducing stress and anxiety among healthcare workers [119]. Some of the routines established during the crisis have been maintained, such as regular town halls and structured emails or newsletters. Transparency in decision-making processes that affect trainees is also crucial. When modifications to rotations, schedules, or program structures are necessary, involving trainees in the discussion or at least providing clear explanations for these changes can significantly reduce anxiety and resistance. By setting clear expectations and maintaining open lines of communication, programs can create an atmosphere of trust and mutual respect, essential for trainee well-being and professional growth.

Fostering Competence

The development of clinical competence and professional confidence involves a delicate balance between providing autonomy and ensuring appropriate supervision. We have already touched on the importance of autonomy and competence as basic psychological needs. Programs can establish clear expectations and guidance around graduated responsibility and ensure both faculty development and trainee awareness of these general goals. This approach should be coupled with clear guidelines on when to seek supervision or assistance, creating a safety net that allows trainees to push their boundaries without compromising patient care. Additionally, ensuring protected time for education and reflection is important in developing their competence and professional identity. Building reflective activities into the regular curriculum can help foster this learning mindset. Debriefing after challenging cases is another opportunity to foster reflection and professional growth, as well as a culture in which discussing tough issues is normalized. Encouraging reflective practice through journaling, guided reflection, and storytelling can help trainees process their experiences and extract meaningful lessons from their daily work [59].

Schedules and Attention to Workload

The design of trainees schedules plays a role in preventing burnout and promoting well-being. Balancing high-intensity rotations with less-demanding ones allows for recovery periods and helps maintain sustainable work patterns. A study evaluating the association between burnout and signals of workload from electronic health record (EHR) data logs in pediatric, internal medicine, and anesthesia trainees demonstrated fluctuations in burnout over the course of the year and found that variations in burnout were associated with higher clinical load in the preceding month [120]. Importantly, this study showed that clinicians have periods of recovery from burnout, and those time periods can be relatively short, so strategic scheduling to allow for intervals of reduced workload is beneficial. This may be accomplished by adding outpatient or elective rotations following rotations with high clinical workloads or scheduling periods of non-clinical time [121]. The newer X + Y scheduling model, where blocks without continuity clinic (X) are interspersed with blocks of continuity clinic (Y), may emerge as a strategy that helps to address recovery from burnout. Initial data of X + Y scheduling in pediatric training programs indicates improvement in inpatient workflow and time for teaching [122]; improving workflow is another well-being improvement strategy.

Attention to Workload and Work Efficiency

Understanding and managing workload is a key factor in addressing trainee well-being. The health care system is a complex environment, and trainees have the added cognitive burden of learning while also providing clinical care. In 2018, Harry et al. described the relationship between cognitive load and burnout and developed a framework for the physician task load (PTL) index. The PTL index incorporates multiple domains, including effort, mental and physical demands, and time demands [123] (Fig. 26.2). Their study found a dose-response relationship between the quintile of the PTL and risk of burnout. This multidimensional approach to workload assessment can help programs identify specific areas of strain and target interventions accordingly.

The Job Demands-Resource Model, proposed by Demerouti et al., offers a complementary framework for understanding the interplay between job demands (such as workload and time pressure) and job resources (including discharge assistants, faculty feedback) [14]. Strategies to address the balance between demands and resources are an important component of any well-being program.

Program leaders should also consider the connection between meaningful work and workload. Most pediatric trainees and fellows enter training with a strong calling to their field of medicine and connection to meaning in work reduces burn-

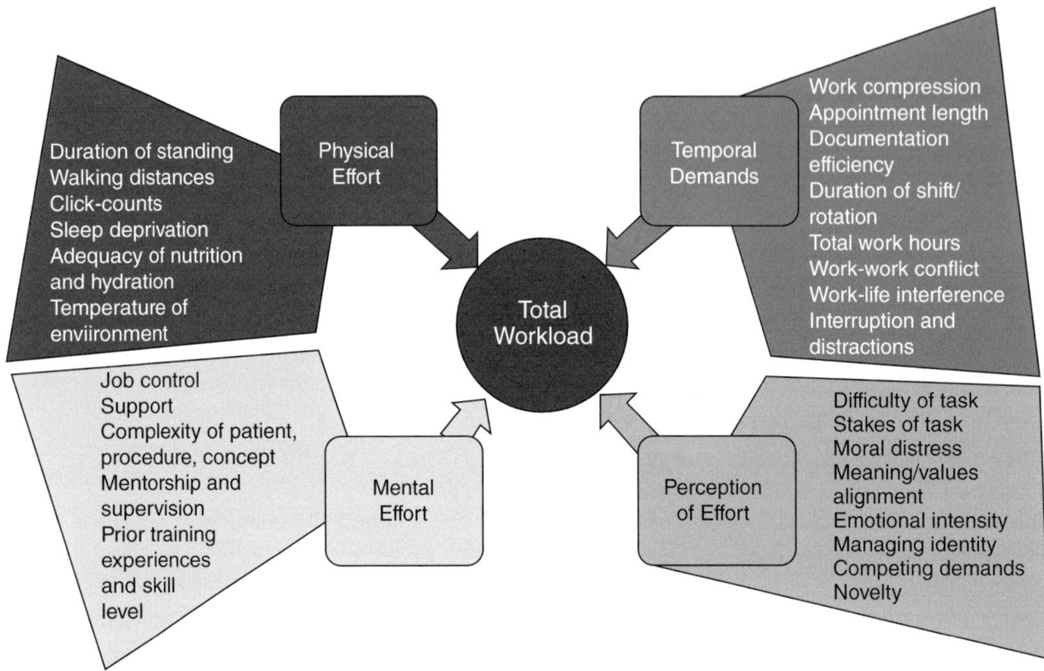

Fig. 26.2 Physician task load index domains that contribute to total workload. (Reprinted with permission from Caring for Caregivers to Be) [124]

out [125]. However, there are many work activities for trainees that may not be associated with a strong connection to meaning in work. Strategies that promote all healthcare workers functioning at the "top of their license" such that the primary activities they are doing are those that use the full extent of their knowledge and skills are beneficial to all team members. Attention to addressing non-physician task loads and demands associated with the EHR is an important strategy for reducing burnout. Structures that promote more team-based care and improve interprofessional collaboration can also help to reduce burnout [126]. Example interventions include adding medical assistants to clinics and increasing in-room support [127], using pharmacy staff to assist with medication histories [128], and interprofessional team rounding innovations [129]. Engaging trainees, faculty, and staff to identify areas for improvement and target interventions is critical for success.

Monitoring Well-being and Assessing Outcomes

A key component of any improvement program is data collection and monitoring. Additionally, we know that physicians in general are poor judges of their own objective well-being, so utilization of self-assessment tools can be beneficial in recognizing signs of distress and considering steps for improvement. The National Academy of Medicine (NAM) has developed an action plan for health workforce well-being, which includes several key actions to measure and assess burnout and well-being among health workers and learners and sharing the de-identified data with organizational leaders to assist in identifying interventions [130].

Given that well-being is a broad term, any assessment needs to consider which domains are important well-being targets. In the context of the clinical learning environment, some key domains include stress, fatigue, quality of life, engage-

Table 26.2 Common tools for assessing and monitoring well-being

Assessment tool	Domains measured
Mini-Z	Multiple
Mayo well-being Index	Multiple
Stanford Professional Fulfillment Index	Multiple
Maslach burnout inventory	Burnout
Copenhagen burnout inventory	Burnout
Oldenburg burnout inventory	Burnout
Physician Job Satisfaction Scale	Job satisfaction
The Flourish Index	Flourishing
Professional quality of life scale (PROQOL)	Quality of life
Perceived Stress Scale	Stress

ment, burnout, joy in work, and professional fulfillment. There are numerous instruments available to measure each of these domains, as well as several tools that aim to measure multiple domains (Table 26.2). Awareness of these tools is beneficial for programs that are designing specific wellness interventions with a desire to measure outcomes pre- and post-intervention. Separate from improvement efforts or research, programs are required by the ACGME to provide access to self-assessment tools. Importantly, any self-assessment tool should be anonymous and confidential so that trainees can answer honestly without fear of program leader awareness of their scores. This can be accomplished by providing links to appropriate online assessment tools that provide real-time feedback, for example, Mental Health America offers screening tools for a variety of different problems, such as stress, depression, anxiety, and addiction [131]. Some programs have customized assessment tools that provide immediate results and feedback. For a fee, the Mayo Well-being Index [132] and the Professional Well-being Academic Consortium (using the Stanford Professional Fulfillment Index [133]) offer options for programs to access aggregate data from their trainees' assessments with comparisons to trainees nationally. Recently, the American Medical Association began offering institutions the opportunity to partner with them at no cost to conduct an organizational assessment [134] using a customized survey that includes the Mini-Z [135], as well as additional questions that assess organizational culture, leadership, workplace efficiency, and intention to leave. Another approach is to utilize the already available ACGME Well-being Survey data that is required for trainees and faculty annually. By comparing program means to the national mean and establishing a metric for concern (e.g., greater a certain amount from the national mean), overall well-being can be tracked over time. Coupled with direct conversations with trainees, this type of monitoring can help guide improvement efforts to target areas of greatest need.

For pediatrics specifically, the Association of Pediatric Program Directors (APPD) Longitudinal Educational Assessment Research Network (LEARN) conducts the Pediatric Trainees Burnout-Resilience Study Consortium (PRB-RSC) [136]. This study involves over 40 residency programs in the US and aims to understand the epidemiology, natural history, and impact of interventions designed to address burnout and resilience in pediatric trainees. The PRB-RSC collects data on burnout, stress, and resilience, providing insights into the effectiveness of wellness interventions. Programs can register for the consortium via the PRB-RSC website.

Well-being Centered Leadership

Program leaders play an important role in fostering well-being for pediatric trainees. Beyond the attention to developing systems and culture that promote well-being, leadership structure and leadership skills are critical factors. Leadership structures that ensure strong collaborations between the clinical/unit leadership, human resources, and leaders in the belonging and inclusion space are important so that program directors can effectively advocate on behalf of their trainees. Leaders' attention to their own well-being also has an important impact on their team. Leaders with lower levels of burnout and higher self-valuation and professional fulfillment have team members with lower burnout scores [137]. Additionally, higher leadership scores, as rated by members of a team, are associated with lower individual burnout scores of team members [138]. Also, in work areas where leaders demonstrate positive psychology principles (e.g., asking what is going well, recognizing achievements), there are improved work-life integration norms and safety culture [139]. Shanafelt et al. described a framework for well-being-centered leadership that incorporates leadership philosophies with a focus on relationship building [140]. We encourage attention to this framework that starts with a foundation of caring for people (including self), builds to cultivating relationships between individuals, and ultimately evolves into fostering team relationships. They propose that only after strong relationships and trust are in place are leaders able to inspire change. Importantly, there are many levels of leaders within our learning environments, from Chairs, Division Chiefs, and Program Directors to Chief Trainees, individual faculty who lead trainees teams, and senior trainees supervising interns. Encouraging all trainees to consider themselves leaders in some respect and teaching leadership skills will serve them and the rest of the team well. Program and departmental attention to leadership training with relational skills in mind will help to further the culture of well-being within all training programs.

Conclusion

Well-being has multiple dimensions; therefore, it is imperative for training programs to have broad approaches in the design of their well-being programs. Attention to personal factors as well as workplace factors is critical in supporting all individuals in a program. Addressing only individual factors without attending to problems in the learning environment, including culture, workflow inefficiencies, and workload, risks creating more frustration among pediatric trainees. Offering multiple resources and curricular approaches to address coping strategies is important to meet the diverse needs of pediatric trainees and fellows. Additionally, addressing as many factors as possible related to workplace systems and culture is critical. Finally, attention to leadership skill development is a key component of fostering the culture of well-being within a program; where there is well-being, there is meaning in medicine.

References

1. Shanafelt TD. Enhancing meaning in work: a prescription for preventing physician burnout and promoting patient-centered care. JAMA. 2009;302(12):1338–40. https://doi.org/10.1001/jama.2009.1385.
2. Doyle G. Untamed. 1st edn. The Dial Press; 2020:xvi, 333 pages
3. Toubassi D, Schenker C, Roberts M, Forte M. Professional identity formation: linking meaning to Well-being. Adv Health Sci Educ Theory Pract. 2023;28(1):305–18. https://doi.org/10.1007/s10459-022-10146-2.
4. Wyatt TR, Balmer D, Rockich-Winston N, Chow CJ, Richards J, Zaidi Z. 'Whispers and shadows': a critical review of the professional identity literature with respect to minority physicians. Med Educ. 2021;55(2):148–58. https://doi.org/10.1111/medu.14295.
5. Trevino R, Poitevien P. Professional identity formation for underrepresented in medicine learners. Curr Probl Pediatr Adolesc Health Care. 2021;51(10):101091. https://doi.org/10.1016/j.cppeds.2021.101091.
6. Pu H, Bachrach LK, Blankenburg R. Finding meaning in medicine: pediatric trainees' perspectives on humanism. Acad Pediatr. 2022;22(4):680–8. https://doi.org/10.1016/j.acap.2021.12.007.
7. Association of American Medical Colleges (AAMC). Cultivating Excellence in Medical Education. Accessed 10 June 2025, https://www.aamc.org/about-us/excellence-academic-medicine/cultivating-excellence-medical-education
8. Gottlieb M, Chung A, Battaglioli N, Sebok-Syer SS, Kalantari A. Impostor syndrome among physicians and physicians in training: a scoping review. Med Educ. 2020;54(2):116–24. https://doi.org/10.1111/medu.13956.
9. World Health Organization. ICD-11 for Mortality and Morbidity Statistics. QD85 Burn-out. 2024; https://icd.who.int/browse/2024-01/mms/en#129180281
10. Kemper KJ, Schwartz A, Wilson PM, et al. Burnout in pediatric trainees: three years of National Survey Data. Pediatrics. 2020;145(1) https://doi.org/10.1542/peds.2019-1030.
11. Koressel LR, Groothuis E, Tanz RR, Palac HL, Sanguino SM. Natural history of burnout, stress, and

fatigue in a pediatric trainees cohort over three years. Med Educ Online. 2020;25(1):1815386. https://doi.org/10.1080/10872981.2020.1815386.

12. Grow HM, McPhillips HA, Batra M. Understanding physician burnout. Curr Probl Pediatr Adolesc Health Care. 2019;49(11):100656. https://doi.org/10.1016/j.cppeds.2019.100656.
13. Shanafelt TD, Noseworthy JH. Executive leadership and physician well-being: nine organizational strategies to promote engagement and reduce burnout. Mayo Clin Proc. 2017;92(1):129–46. https://doi.org/10.1016/j.mayocp.2016.10.004.
14. Demerouti E. The job demands–resources model: challenges for future research. IEEE Electr Insul Magazine. 2011;37 https://doi.org/10.4102/sajip.v37i2.974.
15. Rathert C, Williams ES, Linhart H. Evidence for the quadruple aim: a systematic review of the literature on physician burnout and patient outcomes. Med Care. 2018;56(12):976–84. https://doi.org/10.1097/MLR.0000000000000999.
16. Mousa OY, Dhamoon MS, Lander S, Dhamoon AS. The MD blues: under-recognized depression and anxiety in medical trainees. PLoS One. 2016;11(6):e0156554. https://doi.org/10.1371/journal.pone.0156554.
17. Mata DA, Ramos MA, Bansal N, et al. Prevalence of depression and depressive symptoms among trainees physicians: a systematic review and meta-analysis. JAMA. 2015;314(22):2373–83. https://doi.org/10.1001/jama.2015.15845.
18. Baer TE, Feraco AM, Tuysuzoglu Sagalowsky S, Williams D, Litman HJ, Vinci RJ. Pediatric trainees burnout and attitudes toward patients. Pediatrics. 2017;139(3) https://doi.org/10.1542/peds.2016-2163.
19. Staples BB, Burke AE, Batra M, et al. Burnout and association with trainees performance as assessed by pediatric milestones: an exploratory study. Acad Pediatr. 2021;21(2):358–65. https://doi.org/10.1016/j.acap.2020.08.006.
20. Accreditation Council for Graduate Medical Education (ACGME). ACGME Program Requirements for Graduate Medical Education in Pediatrics. Accessed 18 Oct 2024, https://www.acgme.org/globalassets/pfassets/programrequirements/2025-prs/320_pediatrics_2025.pdf
21. Vermette D, Doolittle B, Gielissen KA. Assessing well-being in milestones 2.0: a case for flourishing-focused advising. J Grad Med Educ. 2022;14(4):390–3. https://doi.org/10.4300/JGME-D-21-00970.1.
22. Morley G, Ives J, Bradbury-Jones C, Irvine F. What is 'moral distress'? A narrative synthesis of the literature. Nurs Ethics. 2019;26(3):646–62. https://doi.org/10.1177/0969733017724354.
23. Moral Distress and Medicine. AMA J Thics. 2017;19(6):515–634.
24. Rosen A, Cahill JM, Dugdale LS. Moral injury in health care: identification and repair in the COVID-19 era. J Gen Intern Med. 2022;37(14):3739–43. https://doi.org/10.1007/s11606-022-07761-5.
25. Serwint JR, Bostwick S, Burke AE, et al. The AAP resilience in the face of grief and loss curriculum. Pediatrics. 2016;138(5) https://doi.org/10.1542/peds.2016-0791.
26. Ogunyemi D, Darwish AG, Young G, et al. Graduate medical education-led continuous assessment of burnout and learning environments to improve trainees' wellbeing. BMC Med Educ. 2022;22(1):292. https://doi.org/10.1186/s12909-022-03366-y.
27. Hussain FNYM, Tomescu O. Individually focused well-being interventions. In: Ripp J, Thomas L, editors. Caring for caregivers to be. Oxford University Press; 2023. p. 132–67. chap 7.
28. Trockel MT, Menon NK, Rowe SG, et al. Assessment of physician sleep and wellness, burnout, and clinically significant medical errors. JAMA Netw Open. 2020;3(12):e2028111. https://doi.org/10.1001/jamanetworkopen.2020.28111.
29. Hamidi MS, Boggild MK, Cheung AM. Running on empty: a review of nutrition and physicians' Well-being. Postgrad Med J. 2016;92(1090):478–81. https://doi.org/10.1136/postgradmedj-2016-134131.
30. Makowski MS, Shanafelt TD, Hausel A, Bohman BD, Roberts R, Trockel MT. Associations between dietary patterns and sleep-related impairment in a cohort of community physicians: a cross-sectional study. Am J Lifestyle Med. 2021;15(6):644–52. https://doi.org/10.1177/1559827619871923.
31. Makowski MS, Trockel MT, Menon NK, Wang H, Katznelson L, Shanafelt TD. Performance nutrition for physician trainees working overnight shifts: a randomized controlled trial. Acad Med. 2022;97(3):426–35. https://doi.org/10.1097/ACM.0000000000004509.
32. Ito-Masui A, Sakamoto R, Matsuo E, et al. Effect of an internet-delivered cognitive behavioral therapy-based sleep improvement app for shift Workers at High Risk of sleep disorder: single-arm, Nonrandomized Trial. J Med Internet Res. 2023;25:e45834. https://doi.org/10.2196/45834.
33. Taylor CE, Scott EJ, Owen K. Physical activity, burnout and quality of life in medical students: a systematic review. Clin Teach. 2022;19(6):e13525. https://doi.org/10.1111/tct.13525.
34. Nutting R, Grant JT, Ofei-Dodoo S, Runde MS, Staab KA, Richard BR. Increasing trainees physician well-being through a motivational fitness curriculum: a pilot study. Kans J Med. 2020;13:228–34.
35. Weight CJ, Sellon JL, Lessard-Anderson CR, Shanafelt TD, Olsen KD, Laskowski ER. Physical activity, quality of life, and burnout among physician trainees: the effect of a team-based, incentivized exercise program. Mayo Clin Proc. 2013;88(12):1435–42. https://doi.org/10.1016/j.mayocp.2013.09.010.
36. Thorndike AN, Mills S, Sonnenberg L, et al. Activity monitor intervention to promote physical activity

of physicians-in-training: randomized controlled trial. PLoS One. 2014;9(6):e100251. https://doi.org/10.1371/journal.pone.0100251.
37. Rangel EL, Castillo-Angeles M, Kisat M, Kamine TH, Askari R. Lack of routine healthcare among trainees physicians in New England. J Am Coll Surg. 2020;230(6):885–92. https://doi.org/10.1016/j.jamcollsurg.2019.11.005.
38. Guille C, Speller H, Laff R, Epperson CN, Sen S. Utilization and barriers to mental health services among depressed medical interns: a prospective multisite study. J Grad Med Educ. 2010;2(2):210–4. https://doi.org/10.4300/JGME-D-09-00086.1.
39. Caldwell KE, Kushner BS, Donald C, Wise PE. Implementation of flexible days off improves surgical trainees attendance of personal health appointments, perceived wellbeing, and sense of control. J Surg Educ. 2024;81(11):1522–8. https://doi.org/10.1016/j.jsurg.2024.07.024.
40. Major A, Williams JG, McGuire WC, Floyd E, Chacko K. Removing barriers: a confidential opt-out mental health pilot program for internal medicine interns. Acad Med. 2021;96(5):686–9. https://doi.org/10.1097/ACM.0000000000003965.
41. Wee CE, Petrosky J, Mientkiewicz L, Liu X, Patel KK, Rothberg MB. Changes in health and well-being during trainees' training. South Med J. 2020;113(2):70–3. https://doi.org/10.14423/SMJ.0000000000001061.
42. Lundgren T, Luoma JB, Dahl J, Strosahl K, Melin L. The bull's-eye values survey: a psychometric evaluation. Cogn Behav Pract. 2012;19(4):518–26.
43. Finkelstein-Fox L, Pavlacic JM, Buchanan EM, Schulenberg SE, Park CL. Valued living in daily experience: relations with mindfulness, meaning, psychological flexibility, and stressors. Cogn Ther Res. 2020;44:300–10.
44. Prudenzi A, Graham CD, Flaxman PE, Wilding S, Day F, O'Connor DB. A workplace acceptance and commitment therapy (ACT) intervention for improving healthcare staff psychological distress: a randomised controlled trial. PLoS One. 2022;17(4):e0266357. https://doi.org/10.1371/journal.pone.0266357.
45. Ameli R, Sinaii N, West CP, et al. Effect of a brief mindfulness-based program on stress in health care professionals at a US biomedical research hospital: a randomized clinical trial. JAMA Netw Open. 2020;3(8):e2013424. https://doi.org/10.1001/jamanetworkopen.2020.13424.
46. Fendel JC, Aeschbach VM, Schmidt S, Goritz AS. The impact of a tailored mindfulness-based program for trainees physicians on distress and the quality of care: a randomised controlled trial. J Intern Med. 2021;290(6):1233–48. https://doi.org/10.1111/joim.13374.
47. Minichiello V, Webber S. Trainees physician perspectives on mindfulness education in residency: a multispecialty qualitative assessment of clinical care impact. J Grad Med Educ. 2023;15(3):356–64. https://doi.org/10.4300/jgme-d-22-00492.1.
48. Heppner WL, Shirk SD. Mindful moments: a review of brief, low-intensity mindfulness meditation and induced mindful states. Soc Personal Psychol Compass. 2018;12(12):e12424. https://doi.org/10.1111/spc3.12424.
49. Neff KD, Germer CK. A pilot study and randomized controlled trial of the mindful self-compassion program. J Clin Psychol. 2013;69(1):28–44. https://doi.org/10.1002/jclp.21923.
50. Neff KD, Knox MC, Long P, Gregory K. Caring for others without losing yourself: an adaptation of the mindful self-compassion program for healthcare communities. J Clin Psychol. 2020;76(9):1543–62. https://doi.org/10.1002/jclp.23007.
51. Fainstad T, Mann A, Suresh K, et al. Effect of a novel online group-coaching program to reduce burnout in female trainees physicians: a randomized clinical trial. JAMA Netw Open. 2022;5(5):e2210752. https://doi.org/10.1001/jamanetworkopen.2022.10752.
52. Liu A, Ben-Zion S, Schwartz A, Mahan JD, Reed S. Well-being factors associated with confidence in providing calm, compassionate care in pediatric trainees. Patient Educ Couns. 2023;115:107906. https://doi.org/10.1016/j.pec.2023.107906.
53. Duke Center for Healthare Safety and Quality. Well-being Tools. Accessed 18 Oct 2024, https://hsq.dukehealth.org/tools/
54. Sexton JB, Adair KC, Cui X, Tawfik DS, Profit J. Effectiveness of a bite-sized web-based intervention to improve healthcare worker wellbeing: a randomized clinical trial of WISER. Front Public Health. 2022;10:1016407. https://doi.org/10.3389/fpubh.2022.1016407.
55. Orr AR, Moghbeli N, Swain A, et al. The fostering resilience through art in medical education (FRAME) workshop: a partnership with the Philadelphia Museum of Art. Adv Med Educ Pract. 2019;10:361–9. https://doi.org/10.2147/amep.S194575.
56. Quinn MA, Fletcher KE, Floden SL, Zelenski AB. A visual arts activity to support trainees as they care for "difficult patients". J Grad Med Educ. 2025;17(1):89–95. https://doi.org/10.4300/JGME-D-24-00469.1.
57. Bajaj N, Phelan J, McConnell EE, Reed SM. A narrative medicine intervention in pediatric trainees led to sustained improvements in trainees well-being. Ann Med. 2023;55(1):849–59. https://doi.org/10.1080/07853890.2023.2185674.
58. Sinha A, Slater CS, Lee A, Sridhar H, Gowda D. "The forest and the trees": a narrative medicine curriculum by trainees for trainees. Pediatr Res. 2024;96(2):313–8. https://doi.org/10.1038/s41390-024-03142-2.
59. Olson ME, Trappey BE. Making space for stories: promoting physician and medical student well-being through successful medical education storytelling

events. BMC Med Educ. 2024;24(1):1172. https://doi.org/10.1186/s12909-024-06130-6.
60. Washington University School of Medicine. In Our Words: A Storytelling Series. Accessed 18 Oct 2019, https://inourwords.wustl.edu/
61. Allen K-A. The psychology of belonging. 1st ed. ed. Routledge; 2020.
62. McKenna KM, Hashimoto DA, Maguire MS, Bynum WE. The missing link: connection is the key to resilience in medical education. Acad Med. 2016;91(9):1197–9. https://doi.org/10.1097/acm.0000000000001311.
63. Leep Hunderfund AN, Saberzadeh Ardestani B, Laughlin-Tommaso SK, et al. Sense of belonging among medical students, trainees, and fellows: associations with burnout, recruitment retention, and learning environment. Acad Med. 2024; https://doi.org/10.1097/acm.0000000000005892.
64. Doolittle BR, Windish DM, Seelig CB. Burnout, coping, and spirituality among internal medicine trainees physicians. J Grad Med Educ. 2013;5(2):257–61. https://doi.org/10.4300/JGME-D-12-00136.1.
65. Yoon JD, Daley BM, Curlin FA. The association between a sense of calling and physician Well-being: a National Study of Primary Care Physicians and Psychiatrists. Acad Psychiatry. 2017;41(2):167–73. https://doi.org/10.1007/s40596-016-0487-1.
66. Remen RN, O'Donnell JF, Rabow MW. The healer's art: education in meaning and service. J Cancer Educ. 2008;23(1):65–7. https://doi.org/10.1080/08858190701821394.
67. Rabow MW, Wrubel J, Remen RN. Authentic community as an educational strategy for advancing professionalism: a national evaluation of the Healer's Art course. J Gen Intern Med. 2007;22(10):1422–8. https://doi.org/10.1007/s11606-007-0274-5.
68. Jaiswal C, Anderson K, Haesler E. A self-report of the Healer's art by junior doctors: does the course have a lasting influence on personal experience of humanism, self-nurturing skills and medical counterculture? BMC Med Educ. 2019;19(1):443. https://doi.org/10.1186/s12909-019-1877-3.
69. Lader M, Burke AE, Stolfi A, Andarsio E, Hanson C, Boreman C. A Program's Experience with Healer's Art: fostering compassionate healing and human connection. Acad Pediatr. 2018;18(5):e33. https://doi.org/10.1016/j.acap.2018.04.091.
70. Sustaining and Training for Resilience, Engagement and Meaning [STREAM]. Accessed 18 Oct 2024,
71. Eng J, Schulman E, Jhanwar SM, Shah MK. Patient death debriefing sessions to support trainees' emotional reactions to patient deaths. J Grad Med Educ. 2015;7(3):430–6. https://doi.org/10.4300/jgme-d-14-00544.1.
72. Quality Palliative Care in Long Term Care Alliance. Peer Led Debriefing Toolkit: Guidelines for Promoting Effective Grief Support Among Front Line Staf. Accessed 19 Oct 2024, https://www.palliativealliance.ca/assets/files/Alliance_Reources/Org_Change/Peer_Led_Debriefing-_Final.pdf
73. Abrams MP. Improving trainees well-being and burnout: the role of peer support. J Grad Med Educ. 2017;9(2):264. https://doi.org/10.4300/jgme-d-16-00805.1.
74. Hu YY, Fix ML, Hevelone ND, et al. Physicians' needs in coping with emotional stressors: the case for peer support. Arch Surg. 2012;147(3):212–7. https://doi.org/10.1001/archsurg.2011.312.
75. Shapiro J, Galowitz P. Peer support for clinicians: a programmatic approach. Acad Med. 2016;91(9):1200–4. https://doi.org/10.1097/ACM.0000000000001297.
76. Everly GS. Psychological first aid to support healthcare professionals. J Patient Safety Risk Manag. 2020;25(4):159–62. https://doi.org/10.1177/2516043520944637.
77. Moore KA, Ureste P, Davis DL, Boscardin C, Thomas LR. Peer support ambassadors: a program to advance a supportive and inclusive clinical learning environment. Acad Med. 2024;99:S62.
78. Palamara K, Kauffman C, Chang Y, et al. Professional development coaching for trainees: results of a 3-year positive psychology coaching intervention. J Gen Intern Med. 2018;33(11):1842–4. https://doi.org/10.1007/s11606-018-4589-1.
79. Huang EY, Saberi RA, Palamara K, Katz D, Chen H, Neville HL. Coaching program to address burnout, well-being, and professional development in pediatric surgery trainees: a randomized controlled trial. Ann Surg. 2024; https://doi.org/10.1097/SLA.0000000000006257.
80. Mann A, Shah AN, Thibodeau PS, et al. Online well-being group coaching program for women physician trainees: a randomized clinical trial. JAMA Netw Open. 2023;6(10):e2335541–51. https://doi.org/10.1001/jamanetworkopen.2023.35541.
81. Redman C, Chung CG, McFarlane D, Meara A, Ejaz A. Graduate medical education success coaching for trainees and fellows: a single-institution real-world experience. Med Educ Online. 2024;29(1):2342102. https://doi.org/10.1080/10872981.2024.2342102.
82. Slavin S, Shoss M, Broom MA. A program to prevent burnout, depression, and anxiety in first-year pediatric trainees. Acad Pediatr. 2017;17(4):456–8. https://doi.org/10.1016/j.acap.2016.12.016.
83. Player M, Freedy JR, Diaz V, et al. The role of Balint group training in the professional and personal development of family medicine trainees. Int J Psychiatry Med. 2018;53(1–2):24–38. https://doi.org/10.1177/0091217417745289.
84. Zárate Rodriguez JG, Naaseh A, Caldwell KE, et al. Promoting surgical trainees well-being through therapist-facilitated discussion groups: a quantitative and qualitative analysis. J Surg Educ. 2024;81(11):1798–806. https://doi.org/10.1016/j.jsurg.2024.08.014.
85. Dyrbye LN, West CP, Satele D, et al. Burnout among U.S. medical students, trainees, and early career physicians relative to the general U.S. population. Acad

Med. 2014;89(3):443–51. https://doi.org/10.1097/ACM.0000000000000134.
86. Bannatyne AJ, Jones C, Craig BM, Jones D, Forrest K. A systematic review of mental health interventions to reduce self-stigma in medical students and doctors. Front Med (Lausanne). 2023;10:1204274. https://doi.org/10.3389/fmed.2023.1204274.
87. American Foundation of Suicide Prevention. Interactive Screening Program. Accessed 19 Oct 2024, https://afsp.org/interactive-screening-program/
88. Mortali M, Moutier C. Facilitating help-seeking behavior among medical trainees and physicians using the interactive screening program. J Med Regul. 2018;104(2):27–36.
89. Ey S, Moffit M, Kinzie JM, Brunett PH. Feasibility of a comprehensive wellness and suicide prevention program: a decade of caring for physicians in training and practice. J Grad Med Educ. 2016;8(5):747–53. https://doi.org/10.4300/JGME-D-16-00034.1.
90. Hasan S, Pozdol SL, Nichelson BK, Cunningham SJ, Lasek DG, Dankoski ME. The development of a comprehensive mental health service for medical trainees. Acad Med. 2022;97(11):1610–5. https://doi.org/10.1097/ACM.0000000000004789.
91. Guldner G, Siegel JT, Broadbent C, et al. Use of an opt-out vs opt-in strategy increases use of residency mental health services. J Grad Med Educ. 2024;16(2):195–201. https://doi.org/10.4300/JGME-D-23-00460.1.
92. Kevern T, Davies DR, Stiel K, Raaum S. Impact of opt-out therapy appointments on trainees physicians' mental health, Well-being, stigma, and willingness to engage. J Grad Med Educ. 2023;15(6):734–7. https://doi.org/10.4300/JGME-D-22-00898.1.
93. Sofka S, Lerfald N, Reece J, Davisson L, Howsare J, Thompson J. Universal well-being assessment associated with increased trainees utilization of mental health resources and decrease in professionalism breaches. J Grad Med Educ. 2021;13(1):83–8. https://doi.org/10.4300/JGME-D-20-00352.1.
94. Accreditation Council for Graduate Medical Education. After a Suicide: A Toolkit for Physician Residency/Fellowship Programs. ACGME Updated 2018. Accessed 18 Oct 2024, https://www.acgme.org/Portals/0/PDFs/13287_AFSP_After_Suicide_Clinician_Toolkit_Final_2.pdf
95. Busireddy KR, Miller JA, Ellison K, Ren V, Qayyum R, Panda M. Efficacy of interventions to reduce trainees physician burnout: a systematic review. J Grad Med Educ. 2017;9(3):294–301. https://doi.org/10.4300/jgme-d-16-00372.1.
96. Accreditation Council for Graduate Medical Education. Accreditation Council for Graduate Medical Education. CLER pathways to excellence: Expectations for an optimal clinical learning environment to achieve safe and high-quality patient care, version 3.0. Accessed 18 Oct 2024, https://www.acgme.org/globalassets/pdfs/cler/acgme-cler-2024-pte3.pdf
97. Leiter M, Maslach C. The impact of interpersonal environment on burnout and organizational commitment. J Organ Behav. 1988;9:297–308.
98. Haviland C, Green J, Dzara K, et al. Psychological safety between pediatric trainees and nurses and the impact of an interdisciplinary simulation curriculum. BMC Med Educ. 2022;22(1):649. https://doi.org/10.1186/s12909-022-03709-9.
99. Lee KC, Oppenheim IM, Do D, Lin TC, Rosin R, Merchant RM. Making workplace civility go viral. NEJM Catalyst. 2020;1(1) https://doi.org/10.1056/CAT.19.1088.
100. Edmondson A. Psychological safety and learning behavior in work teams. Adm Sci Q. 1999;44(2):350–83. https://doi.org/10.2307/2666999.
101. Pierce RG, Maples WJ, Krippner J, et al. Results from the National Taskforce for humanity in healthcare's integrated, organizational pilot program to improve Well-being. Jt Comm J Qual Patient Saf. 2021;47(9):581–90. https://doi.org/10.1016/j.jcjq.2021.05.010.
102. Prins JT, Hoekstra-Weebers JE, Gazendam-Donofrio SM, et al. The role of social support in burnout among Dutch medical trainees. Psychol Health Med. 2007;12(1):1–6. https://doi.org/10.1080/13548500600782214.
103. Deci EL, Ryan RM. Intrinsic motivation and self-determination in human behavior. Plenum Press; 1985.
104. Pethrick H, Nowell L, Paolucci EO, et al. Peer mentoring in medical residency education: a systematic review. Can Med Educ J. 2020;11(6):e128–37. https://doi.org/10.36834/cmej.68751.
105. Gaeta ED, Gilbert M, Johns A, Jurkovich GJ, Wieck MM. Effects of mentorship on surgery trainees' burnout and Well-being: a scoping review. J Surg Educ. 2024;81(11):1592–601. https://doi.org/10.1016/j.jsurg.2024.08.001.
106. Gilliam C, Russell CJ. Impact of racial microaggressions in the clinical learning environment and review of best practices to support learners. Curr Probl Pediatr Adolesc Health Care. 2021;51(10):101090. https://doi.org/10.1016/j.cppeds.2021.101090.
107. Sexton JB, Adair KC, Proulx J, et al. Emotional exhaustion among US health care workers before and during the COVID-19 pandemic, 2019–2021. JAMA Netw Open. 2022;5(9):e2232748. https://doi.org/10.1001/jamanetworkopen.2022.32748.
108. Dyrbye LN, West CP, Sinsky CA, et al. Physicians' experiences with mistreatment and discrimination by patients, families, and visitors and association with burnout. JAMA Netw Open. 2022;5(5):e2213080. https://doi.org/10.1001/jamanetworkopen.2022.13080.
109. Hu YY, Ellis RJ, Hewitt DB, et al. Discrimination, abuse, harassment, and burnout in surgical residency training. N Engl J Med. 2019;381(18):1741–52. https://doi.org/10.1056/NEJMsa1903759.

110. Kemper KJ, Schwartz A. Pediatric Trainees Burnout-Resilience Study C. Bullying, discrimination, sexual harassment, and physical violence: common and associated with burnout in pediatric trainees. Acad Pediatr. 2020;20(7):991–7. https://doi.org/10.1016/j.acap.2020.02.023.
111. Mundo W, Vaughn J, Odetunde A, et al. A national pilot study on simulation-based upstander training for emergency medicine clinicians. AEM Educ Train. 2024;8(3):e10990. https://doi.org/10.1002/aet2.10990.
112. Hickson GB, Pichert JW, Webb LE, Gabbe SG. A complementary approach to promoting professionalism: identifying, measuring, and addressing unprofessional behaviors. Acad Med. 2007;82(11):1040–8. https://doi.org/10.1097/ACM.0b013e31815761ee.
113. Dunne D, Asnes A, Berg D, et al. Developing CLOUT: A Longitudinal, Cross-Program Chief Trainees Curriculum to Increase Psychological Safety in the Clinical Learning Environment. Acad Med 9900
114. Shofer SL, Gagliardi JP, Bryant S, et al. Championing Civility in the Clinical Learning Environment: Evaluation of a Novel Training Program. Acad Med 9900
115. Srinivasan S, Evaristo CE, Ali H, et al. Simulation Training to Interrupt Microaggressions. Acad Med 9900;
116. Fraley L, Sheffield V, Houchens N. Enhancing an Experience-Based Patient-Initiated Mistreatment Training. Acad Med 9900;
117. Fernandez D, Gorgens S, McCann-Pineo M, Sperandeo M, Cassara M, Moadel T. Simulation vs RISE UP: A Comparative Study of Approaches for Teaching Emergency Medicine Trainees How to Manage Microaggressions. Acad Med 9900;
118. Torres C, Morales D, Whitley A, Porter B, Greene R, Zabar S. Diversity and Inclusion Through Collaboration: Co-Producing a Simulation Curriculum to Address Discrimination Against Trainees. Acad Med 9900;
119. Ripp J, Peccoralo L, Charney D. Attending to the emotional well-being of the health care workforce in a New York City health system during the COVID-19 pandemic. Acad Med. 2020;95(8):1136–9. https://doi.org/10.1097/acm.0000000000003414.
120. Lou SS, Lew D, Harford DR, et al. Temporal associations between EHR-derived workload, burnout, and errors: a prospective cohort study. J Gen Intern Med. 2022;37(9):2165–72. https://doi.org/10.1007/s11606-022-07620-3.
121. Stevens K, Davey C, Lassig AA. Association of weekly protected nonclinical time with trainees physician burnout and well-being. JAMA Otolaryngol Head Neck Surg. 2020;146(2):168–75. https://doi.org/10.1001/jamaoto.2019.3654.
122. Myers RE, Thoreson L, Howell HB, et al. Impact of X+Y scheduling on pediatric trainees and faculty perceptions of education and patient care. Acad Pediatr. 2021;21(7):1273–80. https://doi.org/10.1016/j.acap.2021.02.018.
123. Harry E, Sinsky C, Dyrbye LN, et al. Physician task load and the risk of burnout among US physicians in a National Survey. Jt Comm J Qual Patient Saf. 2021;47(2):76–85. https://doi.org/10.1016/j.jcjq.2020.09.011.
124. Quinn MABL, McFadden K, McGrath KP. System-level interventions. In: Ripp J, Thomas L, editors. Caring for caregivers to be. Oxford University Press; 2023. p. 170. chap 8.
125. Shanafelt TD, West CP, Sloan JA, et al. Career fit and burnout among academic faculty. Arch Intern Med. 2009;169(10):990–5. https://doi.org/10.1001/archinternmed.2009.70.
126. DeChant PF, Acs A, Rhee KB, et al. Effect of organization-directed workplace interventions on physician burnout: a systematic review. Mayo Clin Proc Innov Qual Outcomes. 2019;3(4):384–408. https://doi.org/10.1016/j.mayocpiqo.2019.07.006.
127. Sinsky CA, Bodenheimer T. Powering-up primary care teams: advanced team care with in-room support. Ann Fam Med. 2019;17(4):367–71. https://doi.org/10.1370/afm.2422.
128. Hillmann W, Hayes BD, Marshall J, et al. Improving burnout through reducing administrative burden: a pilot of pharmacy-driven medication histories on a hospital medicine service. J Gen Intern Med. 2021;36(8):2511–3. https://doi.org/10.1007/s11606-020-06066-9.
129. Li J, Talari P, Kelly A, et al. Interprofessional teamwork innovation model (ITIM) to promote communication and patient-centered, coordinated care. BMJ Qual Saf. 2018;27(9):700–9. https://doi.org/10.1136/bmjqs-2017-007369.
130. National Academy of Medicine. National Plan for Health Workforce Well-Being. 2024.
131. Mental Health America. Take a Mental Health Test. Accessed 15 Oct 2024, https://screening.mhanational.org/screening-tools/
132. Dyrbye LN, Satele D, Sloan J, Shanafelt TD. Ability of the physician well-being index to identify trainees in distress. J Grad Med Educ. 2014;6(1):78–84. https://doi.org/10.4300/JGME-D-13-00117.1.
133. Trockel M, Bohman B, Lesure E, et al. A brief instrument to assess both burnout and professional fulfillment in physicians: reliability and validity, including correlation with self-reported medical errors, in a sample of trainees and practicing physicians. Acad Psychiatry. 2018;42(1):11–24. https://doi.org/10.1007/s40596-017-0849-3.
134. American Medical Association. Organizational Well-being Assessment. Accessed 15 Oct 2024, https://www.ama-assn.org/system/files/org-well-being-assessment.pdf
135. Linzer M, McLoughlin C, Poplau S, Goelz E, Brown R, Sinsky C. The mini Z worklife and burnout reduction instrument: psychometrics and clinical implications. J Gen Intern Med.

2022;37(11):2876–8. https://doi.org/10.1007/s11606-021-07278-3.
136. Association of Pediatric Program Directors. Pediatric Trainees Burnout-Resilience Consortium Study. Accessed 18 Oct 2024, Pediatric Trainees Burnout-Resilience Consortium Study.
137. Shanafelt TD, Makowski MS, Wang H, et al. Association of Burnout, professional fulfillment, and self-care practices of physician leaders with their independently rated leadership effectiveness. JAMA Netw Open. 2020;3(6):e207961. https://doi.org/10.1001/jamanetworkopen.2020.7961.
138. Dyrbye LN, Major-Elechi B, Hays JT, Fraser CH, Buskirk SJ, West CP. Physicians' ratings of their supervisor's leadership behaviors and their subsequent burnout and satisfaction: a longitudinal study. Mayo Clin Proc. 2021;96(10):2598–605. https://doi.org/10.1016/j.mayocp.2021.01.035.
139. Sexton JB, Adair KC, Profit J, et al. Safety culture and workforce well-being associations with positive leadership WalkRounds. Jt Comm J Qual Patient Saf. 2021;47(7):403–11. https://doi.org/10.1016/j.jcjq.2021.04.001.
140. Shanafelt T, Trockel M, Rodriguez A, Logan D. Wellness-centered leadership: equipping health care leaders to cultivate physician well-being and professional fulfillment. Acad Med. 2021;96(5):641–51. https://doi.org/10.1097/ACM.0000000000003907.

Supporting Residents with or Planning Families

27

Ann E. Burke and Sabrina Ben-Zion

Historical Perspective: Residents as Parents

Over the last five decades, the percentage of women entering medical school has risen from 6.9% in 1966 to 47% in 2005 to 55% in 2024 [1]. About one-quarter of pediatric graduates are parents of children by the time they graduate residency [2]. Perspectives and practices around women having children have changed over time due in part to women being a greater majority of medical school graduates. In 2000, the Future of Pediatric Education (FOPE) II published a notable report in the *Journal of Pediatrics* titled "Organizing Pediatric Education to Meet the Needs of Infants, Children, Adolescents, and Young Adults in the 21st Century." [3] This report covered a wide range of issues around pediatric workforce and education, including concern over the low number of women progressing in academia and entering fellowships. To address that concern, a "Women in Medicine Task Force" was created to consider the issues [4]. The FOPE II report resulted in recommendations that actively encouraged fair parental leave policies, access to quality childcare, flexibility in timing of advancement in academic rank, and coordinated scheduling [5]. In a study from 2006 that surveyed pediatric chairs and program directors, 74% of programs reported lactation facilities, although only 57% provided access to breast pumps [6]. At that time, 90% of programs reported maternity leave policies, but only 27% offered any part-time re-entry into the training program. In 2015, a study of members of the AAP Section on Medical Students, Residents, and Fellowship Trainees (SOMSRFT) were surveyed about parental leave policies at their institutions. Thirty percent of the over 900 respondents did not know if their program had a written policy for parental leave [7]. In another study, only 8 of 15 had written family leave policies for residents, while all had leave policies for faculty [8]. The Accreditation Council for Graduate Medical Education (ACGME) now mandates that programs have a parental leave policy, and starting July 1, 2022, put new institutional requirements into effect to have leave policies that include a minimum of six paid weeks off for medical, parental, and caregiver leave. Additionally, institutions must provide at least one additional week of paid time off. However, variability remains in regard to funding and payers. A systematic review in 2024 found that in 11 studies the presence of a written leave policy was associated with lower anxiety levels among trainees and stronger feelings/perceptions of support [9]. While a stan-

A. E. Burke (✉)
Dayton Children's Hospital/Wright State University Boonshoft School of Medicine, Dayton, OH, USA
e-mail: ann.burke@wright.edu

S. Ben-Zion
Akron Children's Hospital, Akron, OH, USA

H. McPhillips et al. (eds.), *Graduate Medical Education in Pediatrics*, Excellence in Medical Education 3, https://doi.org/10.1007/978-3-032-12952-9_27

dardized leave policy across all pediatric programs is desired, challenges remain not only in the aforementioned differences in funding and payers, but in length of leave based on program size, program assessment to verify competence, and individual trainee preferences. We posit that it is best practice to have a written, well-advertised, and flexible family leave policy that aligns with program culture.

Pregnancy and Delivery Considerations

Graduate medical training is a stressful time of physical demands and rapid experiential learning. There are concerns that this stress may lead to health consequences in the perinatal time for mothers and their babies. Becoming a parent is a life-changing decision and can weigh heavily on a trainee. Literature has shown downstream effects of the demands of residency on outcomes of health. While many studies were performed prior to work-duty–hour restrictions, obstetrical complications such as placental abruption, hypertension, intrauterine growth restriction, and miscarriage rates were higher in trainees than in a control group with an obstetrical complication rate of 34% [10]. In a larger study done at Stanford in 2018, many women expressed concern about the potential negative impact of the physical demands of their jobs on pregnancy [11]. But, in addition to concerns about their health and safety during pregnancy and the perinatal period, women had particular concerns about the negative impact that taking maternity leave may have on their professional reputation and career. Compared to men, a higher proportion of women worried that having a child during training would lead to negative professional perceptions of them [11]. Open communication with the trainee is of utmost importance to be able to effectively and supportively plan for absences due to foreseen and unforeseen circumstances and more must be done to ensure women physicians who choose to have children are offered the same opportunities as their male counterparts.

Parental Leave

Planning for Leave

Many programs develop a process regarding planning for parental leave and review this with trainees at orientation. Typically, program leadership appreciates knowing about parenting news and plans sooner rather than later. Each resident has different goals, health needs, and interests. For instance, are they planning on pursuing a fellowship, do they foresee any prebirth restrictions or complications, have they planned childcare for after they return to work, do they have thoughts about their pre-delivery rotations, and are they considering a restricted schedule or rotation changes when they return to work? Meeting with each trainee, understanding their goals, and demonstrating flexibility within the program can reduce anxiety and worry. Using a worksheet to keep track of leave, plan for time off, and develop contingency plans is helpful for record-keeping and clarity. Conveying honest and deep happiness about the learner and the good news of a new baby is of course also important to reinforce programmatic support.

Leave Duration

The length of time that residents take for parental leave varies widely. A study from 2015 reported that the average allowed parental leave time was 8.5 weeks, but almost 30% of participants said they took less than 6 weeks off [7]. In 2016, the median length of resident maternity leave was 5–8 weeks, while paternity leave was 1 week or less [12]. Four years later, in 2019, maternal leave was still short among resident trainees with a median leave time of 7 weeks, with most mothers taking less than 6 weeks of leave [13]. As recent as 2021, a large study of 845 pediatric trainees at 13 programs that was powered by the Association of Pediatric Program Directors research network called the Longitudinal Educational Assessment Research Network (LEARN) [14] showed that almost half of the respondents had parental leaves of less than or equal to 6 weeks, with a mean leave time of 8 weeks [15]. In that study, 64% of partner leaves were less than 2 weeks in duration. Additionally, this study demonstrated that there was less burnout with longer parental leave in pediatric residents. The predicted probability of burnout was 56%, 36%, and 20% when the mean leave duration was 4 weeks, 8 weeks, and 12 weeks, respectively. This suggests that longer parental leave is important for trainee health and well-being and should be encouraged.

The Impact of Leave on Well-Being Leave Time and Wellness

There have been a number of studies that have explored the relationship of factors related to parental leave and well-being.

In a rather large pediatric fellowship study, the authors found that greater than 40% of fellows indicated they received greater than 5 weeks of *paid* parental leave, with most indicating they used vacation, sick leave time, and unpaid leave to lengthen their leave as they preferred more time off for their wellness [16]. They also found 45% of fellows indicated their program's leave policy increased the stress of having a child, though it was unclear why. A major theme that emerged from the qualitative part of that study was that equity in parental leave between parent fellows and co-fellows, and fostering a more supportive program culture were most important to them [16]. Lack of support for return-to-work considerations and breastfeeding support are strongly associated with negative emotions in residents and students [17].

In a systematic review of several studies [9], the relationship of various factors around parental leave and well-being has been explored. Presence of a written policy, extended leave duration over 6 weeks, and perceived support from the program correlate with higher levels of well-being in trainees. Conversely, dissatisfaction was perceived by trainees around topics that were inadequately addressed by programs such as breastfeeding support and time, stigma and bias associated with parental leave, and return-to-work considerations [9].

Leave Policies

Program directors and institutions must follow US federal laws regarding parental leave. By the Amendment of Title VII of the 1964 Civil Rights Act (Civil Rights Act of 1964. Public Law 88-352, 78. Stat. 241. 1964), [18] it is unlawful to discriminate against women affected by pregnancy and conditions related to that. The American with Disabilities Act disallows discrimination against anyone with a disability. Women who may be unable to perform their duties at a job due to medical conditions related to pregnancy or the birth of the child are treated, under the law, like any person with disabilities [18]. Furthermore, any educational program that receives funds from the federal government, which includes most GME training programs, calls for protection for trainees from gender discrimination under Title IX [19].

A milestone in federal law in support of rights of employees and job security for family leave was enacted in 1993 as the Family Medical Leave Act (FMLA) [20]. This affords employees the opportunity to take unpaid leave for a variety of family and medical issues for up to 12 weeks in a 12-month period. One caveat is that an employee must have been employed for 12 months prior to using this leave. A hotly debated issue was whether residents and fellows in GME programs are students vs. employees, and this was ruled upon by the Supreme Court in 2011. The court ruled that residents are indeed employees such that they do qualify for FMLA. While FMLA is a law that ensures job security after leave, it does not require employers to compensate workers for their time off.

The American Board of Pediatrics (ABP) current "absences from training policy" allows trainees 1 month of absence each year, which includes vacation, sick, or family leave. For example, if a residency program has 3 weeks of vacation and one study week per academic year, those residents have 1 month of absence per year and do not need to make up time. Additional paternal leave, however, would need to be "made up." There are some caveats to this policy that are important. Since July 2021, the ABP allows for up to a total of 8 weeks of additional parental, medical, or caregiver leave (one time) over a training period [21]. However, the trainee must be deemed competent by the PD and the Clinical Competency Committee (CCC) for this time to be waived. Additionally, the resident must have met all mandatory (nonelective) training requirements. In previous years, a written waiver would need to be submitted to the ABP but that is no longer required. As the ABP has been a pioneer among specialties in competency-based medical education, the community of program directors looks forward to the future where flexibility with individual trainees is based on data driven evidence of competence more so than time in training.

Parental leave for residents and pediatric training programs is a significant topic for the American Academy of Pediatrics (AAP) [22]. The AAP is the membership organization for pediatricians, and over the years they have contributed to the various FOPE convenings, as well as publishing policies and guidance on this topic. The most recent policy statement was published in 2022 [23]. This policy statement had input from residents, fellows, and liaisons from other organizations who are baby and family oriented. The general summary of the eight recommendations is as follows:

1. Each program must have a written policy that is more inclusive of all types of parenting situations (fostering, adoption, gender neutral leave) with a minimum of 12 weeks guaranteed.
2. Pediatric organizations should work with the American Board of Pediatrics to expand competency-based residency completion. Further, there should be options for flexible examination dates to accommodate off-cycle trainees.
3. Pediatric training programs should have a culture that embraces parenting residents.
4. Serious consideration should be given to 24-hour on-site childcare centers and sick childcare arrangements.
5. Programs should have lactation sites and equipment available to all residents. This includes the concept of time for pumping that is protected.
6. Creative training opportunities that may be less vigorous should be explored, such as remote learning and parenting electives.
7. Parental leave should be paid for each individual trainee. This may take some collaboration with the Centers for Medicare and Medicaid Services and other organizations to accomplish all programs.
8. Residency directors should build a culture of early sharing of information about planned leave.

Given the above rules, requirements, and laws, trainees in pediatrics most commonly work directly with their program leadership to determine an agreed-upon parental leave plan. Many residents have accrued sick time and forgo vacation to extend their parental leave and remain being paid. This "banking" of time is discouraged as having sick and vacation time available after return to work is important for trainees' health and well-being. Some programs, such as those in military training programs, allow residents to take up to 12 weeks or more for leave and receive pay during that time. The Department of Defense (DoD) mandates 12-week paid leave, for example. Some pediatric programs within larger adult systems may be constrained by GME funding via the Center for Medicare and Medicaid for extending a resident's training. Some programs, especially those with funding from the Children's Hospital Graduate Medical Education (CHGME) through the Health Resources and Funding Administration (HRSA), may have more flexible funding to allow for extending an individual resident's training. Emphasis should be on working with the trainee and finding a timeline that follows the rules but most importantly supports the trainee's needs.

The guiding principle of support and communication with the resident is similar regarding rotation requirements. It is good to remember that the ACGME accredits programs, and the ABP certifies pediatricians. If a resident misses an ACGME-required rotation, they may or may not have to make that up. With the flexibility and individualized curriculum requirements with the 2025 ACGME program requirements, program leaders have even more flexibility in tailoring a trainee's experiences to align with their future plans and career goals [24].

Return to Work

Family-friendly considerations include not only parental leave but also on-site childcare availability, sick-care for children, part-time residency positions, lactation support, flexibility with schedules, and paid leave. In one study, not surprisingly, residents with children (both men and women) were more likely than residents without children to rate these family-friendly considerations as very important when they were choosing a residency [2]. Details about program flexibility in scheduling and handling unforeseen needs, along with benefits such as longer leave options, paid leave, and paternity leave, may go into decisions regarding choosing training programs as well as satisfaction retrospectively with training [2, 6, 25].

Parenting Electives

The use of parenting electives can provide learning opportunities consistent with training requirements that afford trainees paid time at home while nurturing a child. There is much to be experienced from the hands-on learning of taking care of a baby. Factors that influence a resident's leave length include financial considerations, as well as the desire to graduate "on-time." [26] Extending training may delay fellowship start and have other consequences with subsequent employment. The idea of parenting electives diminishes the need to prolong residency and may increase paid time to care for a child. One study examined the characteristics of paternal leave pre- and post-implementation of 2- to 4-week neonatal at-home elective with pay. Notable changes occurred post-implementation, including those taking greater than 7 weeks of leave increased, mothers using unpaid FMLA time decreased, and partners' leave duration increased [27].

Another study aimed at describing the prevalence and structure of parenting electives in pediatric residency programs gathered data from 36 programs [28]. Eighty-one percent of the programs queried offered specific parenting and/or individualized electives that can be tailored to trainees wanting to spend more time at home. Some specific activities shared by most included self-reflective exercises, reading parenting books or articles, and exploring available community resources. Another activity many programs include is a teaching component by the new parent to their peers, which is a benefit to all. It is important to note that during parenting electives most programs require some clinical time, such as continuity clinic days or attendance at didactics.

Program directors can and should be flexible and creative when discussing and arranging parenting electives. The use of goal-setting and learning plans can assist in making sure the trainee has direction and aim while experiencing this type of elective. It is important to communicate expectations for parenting electives. When used, parenting electives can both teach and help new parents alleviate the stress of returning to work too soon, while also learning and benefiting from paid time at home.

Part-Time and Flexible Time

Part-time residencies were implemented in several specialties in the 1970s [29, 30]. Flexible and part-time pediatric residency options were more prevalent 20 years ago, and today very few are advertised and/or offered [31]. In a part–time model, this could mean a resident would complete the required months of training over 4–6 years, taking interval month or block rotations off. A flexible training option may be two residents who "job-share" a residency position with both working half-time for some or all their rotations. In 2005, around 12% of residency programs reported offering a part-time training option; however, only about 1% of residents reported working part time [6, 32]. In a survey of pediatric residents by the American Academy of Pediatrics in 2010, 2% of the respondents held part-time residency slots; however, 23% expressed interest in this option [25]. Offering part-time training requires multiple considerations, including the American Board of Pediatrics certification requirements, programmatic details of how it may work from a scheduling standpoint, awareness of the concept in the first place, and benefits to the resident [29]. However, given that a strong driving factor to decreasing paternal leave time is the goal of finishing residency on time, training time is prolonged significantly with a part-time program. Multiple other sources highlight the point that working reduced hours as a resident can still feel like working full time (e.g., 40 h/week vs 80 h/week); thus, why not simply have a regular schedule and not spend 6 years in residency? Despite this, in reflecting on participating in part-time residency training 15–25 years later, almost all participants in a qualitative study reported that it was beneficial for their mental health and well-being as a professional [33]. Reduced hour training and part-time schedules remain the desired options for some residents [29, 32]. Given the waning interest in pediatrics by US medical graduates, this option may be something to consider in making a residency program more family friendly.

Lactation Considerations

Many organizations, including the AAP, the American Academy of Family Physicians (AAFP), the American College of Obstetricians and Gynecologists (ACOG), the World Health Organization (WHO), and others, recommend infants be exclusively breastfed for the first 6 months of life, with continued breastfeeding for at least the first year and beyond [34]. It has been shown that longer maternity leaves promote higher breastfeeding rates as well as longer duration of breastfeeding. Unfortunately, breastfeeding rates in the United States fall short of national and global recommendations, and the demand of medical training often causes trainees to stop breastfeeding before their desired goal [35].

Recognizing this and with a focus on promoting wellness, in 2019, the ACGME added a new common program requirement to "… provide for clean and private facilities for lactation that have refrigeration capabilities, with proximity appropriate for safe patient care." [36]

Most institutions and hospitals have their own lactation policies that extend to all employees, but these often do not ensure lactation spaces are close to clinical areas where trainees work, nor do they ensure refrigeration capabilities. In fact, most policies state that human milk may not be stored in patient refrigerators, thereby requiring separate spaces to store milk pumped during the workday. Trainees are often left having to cart coolers or chilling canisters to and from their worksites. In addition, hospital lactation spaces often need to be shared by patients and staff, so they may not be available when a trainee needs them. Reviewing and visiting available lactation spaces at all training sites is an important first step in identifying the gaps and advocating for additional spaces or refrigeration if necessary.

Recognizing the need for GME-specific policies around lactation, in 2019, Johnson and Walsh published a template for institutions to craft an ACGME-compliant lactation policy for trainees [37]. The policy template focuses on the delineation of responsibilities of administrators, trainees, and supervisors and includes minimum requirements for lactation rooms, specifies necessary time for lactation, and emphasizes the importance of a supportive workplace culture. The AAP also has a step-by-step guide to help institutions create or revise policies to best support medical trainees to breastfeed [38].

Childcare Considerations

In addition to the stress of returning to training for parents, the paucity of affordable and effective childcare can have large repercussions on well-being and happiness. Pediatrics as a specialty has advocated for on-site childcare for trainees, as well as sick childcare in the fourth recommendation from the parental leave guidelines from the AAP cited above. There are no recent data about on-site childcare for trainees; however, in a small study asking pediatric program directors about the implementation of clinical learning environment components, one of the least implemented was on-site childcare, with only 11 of 35 program directors reporting that exists [39]. One qualitative study looking at the perspectives of pediatric residents who were parents during the Covid-19 pandemic revealed that one of the major themes identified was the difficulty of work obligations vs. childcare "challenges." [40] When talking with trainees about maternity leave in that qualitative study, one of the five major themes was the tensions and conflicts around "balance of work obligations versus childcare challenges." In the surgical literature, one study with 347 female surgery residents as participants found that only 18% had institutional support for childcare [41].

In an ideal future state, childcare centers would be readily available to all in the pediatric workforce. Many tools for advocacy exist to raise awareness, including Children's Hospital Association (CHA) and family-friendly checklists through the American Academy of Pediatrics.

Competency-Based Medical Education

Competency-based medical education (CBME) is built on the concept that the competencies of learners should ensure they are ready to meet the ever-changing healthcare needs of patients [42]. Education outcomes in a CBME system are defined based on the needs of patients, and in healthy CBME systems, there is a dramatic paradigm shift from a focus on process and time on rotations to outcomes of learners [43, 44]. CBME promotes progressive development of expertise toward mastery of a defined set of outcomes, which our community has defined using Entrustable Professional Activities (EPAs) [42, 45]. In 2028, the American Board of Pediatrics will be asking programs to verify clinical competence in the EPA language [46]. This change in framework from time-based to outcome-based programs allows trainees who take parental leave to potentially not have to make up time they may have missed by being on parental leave. In the future, the idea that making up time may be a moot point as training in a true CBME system will not be time-based, nor time-defined. In 2024, our pediatric community and training programs are not structured to allow and support this in several areas. Those details include licensing that is bound by time in training, no workable system to "graduate" trainees early and release them to a job or fellowship, and no system to fill service needs if residents leave programs at variable times. However, it is good to recognize the flexibility of time-based training in the future [47].

Conclusions

Faced with the well-described benefits of longer duration of leave after having a child and the importance of paid leave, pediatric education leaders should be advocating for generous parental leave, generous paid time off, availability of daycare and sick childcare options, as well as modification of work schedules to support optimal breastfeeding practices. The move to more individualized curricular time within pediatric residency training that can support the expansion of parenting electives and the move to CBME are both promising changes. As pediatricians, we are uniquely suited to lead the way in promoting a family-friendly work environment. Our resident parents and their children deserve the best possible outcomes for their families.

References

1. Magrane D, Lang J, Alexander H. Women in US academic medicine and medical school benchmarking 2004–2005. AAMC. www.aamc.org/members/wim/statistcis/stats05/start.htm
2. Berkowitz CD, Frintner MP, Cull WL. Pediatric resident perceptions of family-friendly benefits. Acad Pediatr. 2010;10(5):360–6. https://doi.org/10.1016/j.acap.2010.06.013. Epub 2010 Aug 7. PMID: 20692217.
3. The Future of Pediatric Education II. Organizing pediatric education to meet the needs of infants, children, adolescents, and young adults in the 21st century. A collaborative project of the pediatric community. Task Force on the Future of Pediatric Education. Pediatrics. 2000;105(1 Pt 2):157–212.
4. Alexander D, Boat T, Britto M, Burke A, Homes A, Sectish T, Stanton B, Stevenson D. Federation of Pediatric Organizations Task Force on Women in Pediatrics: considerations for part-time training and employment for research-intensive fellows and faculty. J Pediatr. 2009;154(1):1–3.e2. https://doi.org/10.1016/j.jpeds.2008.08.010.
5. Britto MT, Fuentes-Afflick E, Sectish TC, Stanton B. Federation of Pediatric Organizations Task Force on Women in Pediatrics II: survey of active members of the Society for Pediatric Research regarding part-time and flexible work. J Pediatr. 2009;155(4):459–460.e1. https://doi.org/10.1016/j.jpeds.2009.06.051.
6. McPhillips HA, Burke AE, Sheppard K, Pallant A, Stapleton FB, Stanton B. Toward creating family-friendly work environments in pediatrics: baseline data from pediatric department chairs and pediatric program directors. Pediatrics. 2007;119(3):e596–602. https://doi.org/10.1542/peds.2006-2397. Epub 2007 Feb 5.
7. Dixit A, Feldman-Winter L, Szucs KA. Parental leave policies and pediatric trainees in the United States. J Hum Lact. 2015;31(3):434–9. https://doi.org/10.1177/0890334415585309. Epub 2015 May 6.
8. Magudia K, Bick A, Cohen J, et al. Child-bearing and family leave policies for resident physicians at top training institutions. JAMA. 2018;320(22):2372–4.
9. Corbisiero MF, Stellern JJ, Kyllo HM, Burnet G, DeSanto K, Christian N, Acker SN. Formal Parental leave policies and trainee well-being in US graduate medical education: a systematic review. J Grad Med Educ. 2024;16(5):532–44. https://doi.org/10.4300/JGME-D-24-00018.1. Epub 2024 Oct 15. PMID: 39416406; PMCID: PMC11475440.
10. Behbehani S, Tulandi T. Obstetrical complications in pregnant medical and surgical residents. J Obstet Gynaecol Can. 2015;37(1):25–31. https://doi.org/10.1016/S1701-2163(15)30359-5. PMID: 25764033.
11. Kin C, Yang R, Desai P, Mueller C, Girod S. Female trainees believe that having children will negatively impact their careers: results of a quantitative survey of trainees at an academic medical center. BMC Med Educ. 2018;18(1):260. https://doi.org/10.1186/s12909-018-1373-1. PMID: 30424762; PMCID: PMC6234638.
12. Blair JE, Mayer AP, Caubet SL, Norby SM, et al. Pregnancy and parental leave during graduate medical education. Acad Med. 2016;91(7):972–8.
13. Stack SW, Jagsi R, Biermann JS, Lundberg GP, Law KL, Milne CK, Williams SG, Burton TC, Larison CL, Best JA. Maternity leave in residency: a multicenter study of determinants and wellness outcomes. Acad Med. 2019;94(11):1738–45. https://doi.org/10.1097/ACM.0000000000002780.
14. Schwartz A, Young R, Hicks PJ, APPD Learn. Medical education practice-based research networks: Facilitating collaborative research. Med Teach. 2016;38(1):64–74. https://doi.org/10.3109/0142159X.2014.970991. Epub 2014 Oct 16. PMID: 25319404; PMCID: PMC4776698.
15. Dundon KM, Powell WT, Wilder JL, et al. Parenthood and parental leave decisions in pediatric residency. Pediatrics. 2021;148(4):e2021050107. https://doi.org/10.1542/peds.2021-050107.
16. Dyess NF, Weikel BW, Barker JM, Garrington TP, Parker TA. Parental leave during pediatric fellowship training: a national survey. PLoS One. 2022;17(12):e0279447. https://doi.org/10.1371/journal.pone.0279447. PMID: 36548290; PMCID: PMC9779013.
17. Dixit A, Feldman-Winter L, Szucs KA. "Frustrated," "depressed," and "devastated" pediatric trainees: US academic medical centers fail to provide adequate workplace breastfeeding support. J Hum Lact. 2015;31(2):240–8. https://doi.org/10.1177/0890334414568119. Epub 2015 Jan 14. PMID: 25588382.
18. The Pregnancy Discrimination Act of 1978. Public Law 95-555. 92 Stat. 2076. 1978. https://www.law.cornell.edu/cfr/text/29/appendix-to_part_1604#:~:text=On%20October%2031%2C%201978%2C%20President,on%20the%20basis%20of%20sex.
19. United States Department of Justice. Overview of Title IX of the Education Amendments of 1972, 20 USC. https://www.justice.gov/crt/title-ix-education-amendments-1972.
20. United States Department of Labor. Family Medical Leave Act of 1993. Pub L 103-3, 29 USC. https://www.dol.gov/agencies/whd/laws-and-regulations/laws/fmla.
21. American Board of Medical Specialties Policy on Parental, Caregiver, and Medical Leave During Training. Effective July 1, 2021 https://www.abms.org/policies/parental-leave/.
22. American Academy of Pediatrics (aap.org).
23. https://publications.aap.org/pediatrics/article/154/5/e2024068958/199722/Paid-Family-and-Medical-Leave-Policy-Statement?autologincheck=redirected.

24. https://www.acgme.org/specialties/pediatrics/program-requirements-and-faqs-and-applications/.
25. Sectish TC, Rosenberg AR, Pageler NM, Chamberlain LJ, Burgos A, Stuart E. Making pediatrics residency programs family friendly: views along the professional educational continuum. J Pediatr. 2006;149(1):1–2.
26. Stack SW, McKinney CM, Spiekerman C, Best JA. Childbearing and maternity leave in residency: determinants and well-being outcomes. Postgrad Med J. 2018;94(1118):694–9. https://doi.org/10.1136/postgradmedj-2018-135960. Epub 2018 Dec 15. PMID: 30554173; PMCID: PMC7466823.
27. Cree-Green M, Cree J, Urban K, Bunik M, Sass AE, Rosenberg A. A structured neonatal parenting elective: an approach for parenting leave during residency. Acad Pediatr. 2020;20(5):595–9. https://doi.org/10.1016/j.acap.2020.02.008. Epub 2020 Feb 8.
28. Ben-Zion S, Lehmann A, Price L, Burnett HQ, Michelson CD. The use of parenting electives in pediatric residency [published online ahead of print, 2021 Dec 2]. Acad Pediatr. 2021:S1876-2859(21)00613-6. https://doi.org/10.1016/j.acap.2021.11.017.
29. Gordon MB, McGuinness GA, Stanton BF, Brooks S, Chiang VW, Vinci R, Sectish TC. Part-time training in pediatric residency programs: principles and practices. Pediatrics. 2008;122(4):e938–44. https://doi.org/10.1542/peds.2008-0719. Epub 2008 Sep 22.
30. Kamei RK, Chen HC, Loeser H. Residency is not a race: our ten-year experience with a flexible schedule residency training option. Acad Med. 2004;79(5):447–52.
31. Cull WL, Frintner MP, O'Connor KG, Olson LM. Pediatricians working part-time has plateaued. J Pediatr. 2016;171:294–9. https://doi.org/10.1016/j.jpeds.2015.12.062. Epub 2016 Feb 1. PMID: 26795679.
32. Holmes AV, Cull WL, Socolar RR. Part-time residency in pediatrics: description of current practice. Pediatrics. 2005;116(1):32–7. https://doi.org/10.1542/peds.2005-0127.
33. Alexander SM, Byerley JS, Page CP, Holmes AV, Beck Dallaghan GL. Reflections on part-time residency training, 15-25 years later: a qualitative study on wellness and career impact. Teach Learn Med. 2023;35(3):315–22. https://doi.org/10.1080/10401334.2022.2050241. Epub 2022 Apr 17.
34. Breastfeeding Support. https://www.healthychildren.org/English/ages-stages/baby/breastfeeding/Pages/Where-We-Stand-Breastfeeding.aspx.
35. Peters GW, Kuczmarska-Haas A, Holliday EB, et al. Lactation challenges of resident physicians- results of a national survey. BMC Pregnancy Childbirth. 2020;20:762. https://doi.org/10.1186/s12884-020-03436-3.
36. Common Program Requirements. ACGME. Common Program Requirements – Residency (acgme.org). Last accessed 21 May 2025.
37. Johnson HM, Walsh DS. Crafting an evidence-based, accreditation Council of Graduate Medical Education-Compliant Lactation Policy for residents and fellows. Breastfeed Med. 2020;15(1):49–55. https://doi.org/10.1089/bfm.2019.0201. Epub 2019 Dec 17.
38. https://www.aap.org/en/patient-care/breastfeeding/policies-on-breastfeeding. Last accessed on 19 May 2025.
39. Zwemer E, Serwint JR, Sieplinga K, Wilson PM, Webber S, Lien ER, Babal JC, Donnelly KM, Nichols MH, Batra M, Schwartz A, Reese JW. Implementation and maturity of clinical learning environment components across pediatric residency programs. Acad Pediatr. 2023;23(7):1301–6. https://doi.org/10.1016/j.acap.2023.04.008. Epub 2023 Apr 23. PMID: 37094643.
40. Wilder JL, Hark CM, Marcus CH, Rabinowitz EC, Michelson CD, Winn AS, Pingree EW. Pediatric trainees as parents: perspectives from a pandemic. Acad Pediatr. 2021;21(6):927–33. https://doi.org/10.1016/j.acap.2021.04.006. Epub 2021 Apr 16.
41. Rangel EL, Smink DS, Castillo-Angeles M, Kwakye G, Changala M, Haider AH, Doherty GM. Pregnancy and motherhood during surgical training. JAMA Surg. 2018;153(7):644–52. https://doi.org/10.1001/jamasurg.2018.0153. PMID: 29562068; PMCID: PMC5875346.
42. Carraccio C, Burke AE. Beyond competencies and milestones: adding meaning through context. J Grad Med Ed. 2010;2(3):419–22.
43. Carraccio C, Wolfsthal SD, Englander R, Ferentz K, Martin C. Shifting paradigms: from Flexner to competencies. Acad Med. 2002;77:361–7.
44. Powell DE, Carraccio C. Toward competency-based medical education. N Engl J Med. 2018;378(1):3–5.
45. ten Cate O. Entrustability of professional activities and competency-based training. Med Educ. 2005;39:1176–7.
46. https://www.abp.org/content/entrustable-professional-activities-general-pediatrics.
47. Schumacher DJ, Caretta-Weyer H, Busari J, Carraccio C, Damodaran A, Gruppen LD, Hall AK, Kinnear B, Warm E, Ten Cate O, ICBME Collaborators. Competency-based time-variable training internationally: ensuring practical next steps in the wake of the COVID-19 pandemic. Med Teach. 2021;43(7):810–6. https://doi.org/10.1080/0142159X.2021.1925098. Epub 2021 May 26. PMID: 34038645.

Developing an Inclusive and Safe Learning Environment

28

Courtney A. Gilliam and Deawodi Ladzekpo

Historically, the design and operational norms of CLEs have predominantly reflected the values and experiences of the dominant cultural and professional groups in medicine [1]. This often leaves trainees who are underrepresented in medicine (URiM) facing unique challenges that can affect their learning outcomes and overall training experience. Many institutions and programs aim to cultivate inclusive environments, yet the paradigm of inclusion assumes the subjugation of identities to adapt to a static medical culture designed by individuals with historical privilege and power. URiM trainees describe being perceived as "other" in CLEs and must downplay core elements of their authentic selves to survive [2]. Daily instances of micro- and macroaggressions, discrimination, bias, and racism negatively affect trainees' learning, ability to provide high-quality patient care, and well-being. Intentionally cultivating a safe and inclusive learning environment in which everyone's authentic selves are valued, respected, and celebrated is imperative to ensure trainee success.

C. A. Gilliam (✉)
Department of Pediatrics, University of Cincinnati College of Medicine, Cincinnati, OH, USA
e-mail: Courtney.Gilliam@cchmc.org

D. Ladzekpo
Cincinnati Children's Hospital Medical Center, Cincinnati, OH, USA

Setting the Culture of Inclusion in CLE

Mission and Vision Integration Developing a culture that genuinely integrates DEI within a CLE begins with the explicit incorporation of these values into all mission and vision statements of medical education institutions. This foundational step signals the program's commitment to these principles and sets the stage for more detailed strategic actions. Setting a tone of inclusion and safety spans efforts across the residency training program and hospital, and it requires early, diverse, consistent, and intentional approaches. Starting with the residency training program leadership team, expectations of constant learning, commitment and action, and humble grace when inevitable mistakes are made to guide trainees in their growth [3]. It is critical that program leadership individually and collectively work to understand DEI and antiracism through reading, activism, and their lived experiences, such as identity, privilege, race, ethnicity, age, or positionality, and those of their trainees. The expectation should be made early that program leaders will hold one another accountable, as well as push and support each other through mistakes and uncomfortable moments. This framework helps ensure that values of inclusion and safety are reflected in daily operations and decision-making processes at all levels.

H. McPhillips et al. (eds.), *Graduate Medical Education in Pediatrics*, Excellence in Medical Education 3, https://doi.org/10.1007/978-3-032-12952-9_28

Setting Expectations for Engagement It is crucial for programs to set clear expectations for ongoing reflection, conversation, and education to foster support in the clinical learning environment. This involves regular training sessions, facilitated discussions, and the incorporation of DEI goals into the performance evaluation criteria of both trainees and faculty.

Intentional Recruitment and Retention Strategy While diverse recruitment is essential, it must be accompanied by a culture strategy that prevents burnout, attrition, and resignation among trainees. This means creating an environment where diverse trainees feel genuinely included and supported throughout their educational journey.

The Impact of Medical Education, Teaching, and Feedback on the Clinical Learning Environment

Over the last several years, the Accreditation Council for Graduate Medical Education (ACGME) and the American Academy of Pediatrics (AAP) have called for changes to curricular components related to DEI. Residency training programs continue to build DEI-focused didactics for trainees to gain understanding on healthcare inequities and ongoing solutions. In one study of a curriculum addressing racism, pediatric residents reported improvement in the development of skills and named strategies to combat racism and improve patient care [4]. While specific lecture series and specific equity curricula are important, there is a need for standard incorporation of DEI into all competency-focused education. This allows for intentional application of all content through an inclusion lens.

Formal Education on Racism and Discrimination

For learners and educators to be effective advocates for DEI, they must receive formal education on racism, discrimination, and structural inequities. This education must go beyond individual biases, encompassing the interpersonal, institutional, and systemic dimensions of discrimination. By understanding the history of racism in the United States and its impact on healthcare, trainees can develop a critical awareness of how these inequities manifest in patient care and medical practice.
Educational initiatives aimed at recognizing and responding to implicit and explicit bias are instrumental. They provide a shared language for discussing difficult issues such as microaggressions, health inequities, and mistreatment in the clinical learning environment (CLE). These initiatives must also address the skills needed to intervene when witnessing bias or discrimination. For pediatric trainees, communication skills that enable active engagement and the ability to shift conversations away from biased perspectives are particularly vital. When educators are equipped to handle these situations, they can create an environment where all trainees, regardless of background, feel supported and respected.

Multimodal Education for Competency Progression

Medical education should emphasize experiential learning and the application of knowledge, rather than focusing solely on knowledge acquisition. Multimodal educational approaches can be used to help learners develop a variety of skills, yet these approaches are often underutilized when it comes to addressing disparities in the CLE [5]. Integrating diverse educational strategies ensures that learners engage with content in ways that enhance their ability to recognize and address inequities.

1. *Case-Based Learning*: Case-based learning encourages the application of medical knowledge to real-world scenarios. This method facilitates inquiry-based learning and teamwork, offering a collaborative approach to solving complex healthcare problems. For example, Boston Medical Center's longitudi-

nal curriculum, Health Equity Rounds, uses case-based learning to discuss the impact of racism in healthcare. Interdisciplinary teams analyze the effects of implicit bias and systemic racism on clinical outcomes, providing evidence-based tools for learners to recognize and mitigate bias in clinical settings.

2. *Simulation-Based Learning*: Simulations replicate real-world experiences in a controlled environment, promoting learning without exposing patients to unnecessary risks. While simulation-based learning is an invaluable tool in medical education, it remains underutilized in teaching competencies related to health inequities. Simulation can, however, be highly effective in developing skills such as culturally effective care for LGBTQ+ patients or recognizing disparities in pain management for Black children. Moreover, debriefing after simulations can highlight the importance of interprofessional teamwork in addressing healthcare disparities and mitigating bias.
3. *Experiential Learning Across Rotations*: Community pediatrics and advocacy rotations provide trainees with opportunities to understand their role as a collaborative leader, community needs and assets, and the upstream factors that impact health and well-being via experiences inside and outside of the healthcare system. Experiences engaging with local schools and community-based organizations are examples of opportunities learners can partake in while on these rotations. However, training programs rely heavily on community pediatrics and advocacy rotations as the primary vehicles to educate trainees on health inequities—even though these inequities exist across all phases of care and impact youth with various acute and chronic diseases. Training programs should consider ways to integrate experiential learning opportunities within other required and elective rotations. Practical ways to accomplish this goal include revising and incorporating learning objectives for each rotation that reflect competencies associated with identifying and mitigating health inequities. Additionally, programs can create elective and/or longitudinal experiences tied to specific competencies. Some residency programs have developed longitudinal advocacy and community tracks or pathways that incorporate didactics and immersive learning experiences to promote health equity. Mullett et al. describe a longitudinal DEI curriculum, developed in 2018, which offers residents innovative interdisciplinary training in delivering equitable, effective, and safe care and fostering inclusive working and learning climates. Every residency program has unique needs, challenges, and resources, and for that reason the residency program conducted a comprehensive needs assessment to inform the curriculum. Currently, the curriculum consists of 28 h of content yearly on a broad range of topics, including racism in medicine, LGBTQ2+ health, social determinants of health, and trauma-informed care. Residents learn DEI definitions, explore cultural humility, and practice responding to microaggressions [6].

Ensuring Equitable Feedback, Assessment, and Evaluation

Faculty Feedback for Continued Dialogue

Educators are crucial in modeling and teaching principles that promote an inclusive learning environment. Programs must advocate for robust faculty development and training across the healthcare system to promote shared language and dialogue. So, often the onus of advocating and educating on inclusive efforts falls on trainees. Education is necessary for everyone (supervising physicians, ancillary staff, etc.) in the clinical learning environment to shift this burden. Establishing a feedback-rich environment where faculty educators receive constructive critiques from their peers, superiors, and trainees can lead to continuous improvement in how DEI is integrated into teaching. A 360-degree feedback mechanism allows educators to understand their effectiveness from multiple perspectives, fostering a culture of openness and continuous learning.

Programmatic Assessment

Several tools and resources are available to help training programs achieve high-quality assessment of program performance in cultivating an inclusive learning environment. Tools such as the antiracism program scorecard can be a valuable way for programs to self-assess their performance using a validated tool to allow future targeting of gaps and areas needing improvement. The ABP's EPA-14 [7] also functions well for both individual trainee assessment and by providing insight into important areas to be included in training program curricula. Additionally, the original 52 pediatrics milestones (version 1.0) contain a Cultural Humility Milestone that can inform tools for trainee assessment [5].

Faculty Development

As medical institutions increasingly prioritize DEI, the need for comprehensive faculty development becomes clear. Faculty members play a critical role in modeling inclusive behavior and guiding trainees through the complexities of patient care in diverse settings. However, for faculty to effectively teach DEI principles, they must first develop their own understanding of these issues. Institutions must invest in faculty development programs that equip educators with the knowledge and tools necessary to foster safe and inclusive learning environments.

Institutional Example: Children's National Hospital

In June 2020, Children's National Hospital (CNH) expanded its Diversity, Equity, Inclusion, and Justice (DEIJ) initiative by developing the Racial Health Equity Curriculum (RHEC). This curriculum was designed to address the specific challenges of racism in healthcare, providing faculty with the tools they need to recognize and combat these issues. Delivered through four interactive virtual sessions, RHEC focused on the history of racism, its impact on healthcare, and strategies for addressing systemic inequities. Faculty who participated in the program reported significant increases in self-awareness, understanding of systemic racism, and a greater ability to address bias in clinical practice [8].

The success of the RHEC highlights the importance of structured faculty development. CNH's national needs assessment, conducted as part of its DEIJ initiative, provided valuable data that informed the development of a health equity curriculum for pediatric faculty across the United States. This curriculum was designed to be generalizable, allowing other institutions to replicate CNH's success in addressing faculty development needs related to health equity.

National Examples: AAP, APA, and APPD Resources

National organizations, such as the American Academy of Pediatrics (AAP), the Academic Pediatric Association (APA), and the Association of Pediatric Program Directors (APPD), have also taken significant steps to promote DEI in medical education. These organizations have created a wealth of accessible resources, including publications, policy statements, toolkits, and virtual presentations, to support both passive and active learning on DEI topics.

One notable resource is the APA's Antiracism and Equity Toolkit [9], which divides information into three categories: tools for learning, tools for action, and a comprehensive resource list. This toolkit is designed for individual learners, institutions, and organizations at various stages of their DEI education journey. It includes journal articles, books, podcasts, toolkits, videos, and workshops, allowing users to engage with the content at their own pace.

APPD has also made strides in promoting DEI through its Confronting Racism Virtual Café, a series of webinars that began in 2020 [10]. These virtual sessions explore the intersection of DEI and medical education, offering trainees and educators alike the opportunity to engage in meaningful discussions about allyship, bias, microaggressions, and systemic racism. These seminars are valuable not only for their content but also for the opportunities they provide to foster dialogue and reflection in real time.

Mentorship

Mentorship is one of the most crucial components of building a safe and inclusive learning environment. It provides trainees with guidance, support, and role models that shape their personal and professional development. Effective mentorship is not just about academic and career advancement; it also fosters a sense of belonging, addresses the specific challenges that URiM learners face, and offers critical emotional support [11].

In traditional models, mentorship often involves senior faculty members guiding trainees. While this approach remains valuable, more modern frameworks—such as *mentorship families*—have proven to be even more effective in supporting today's diverse group of trainees. These families consist of multiple mentors at different career stages, including peers, junior faculty, and senior leaders, who together provide a more holistic support system. This structure allows for a range of perspectives and fosters a well-rounded mentoring experience that meets the diverse needs of trainees.

Classic and Peer Mentorship Models

In the classical mentorship model, senior faculty members serve as mentors who guide trainees through academic and professional challenges. While this model provides invaluable insight from established professionals, the significant power differential between senior mentors and trainees can sometimes inhibit open dialogue, especially regarding sensitive issues like racism, sexism, and discrimination. Trainees may hesitate to fully express themselves for fear of being misunderstood or facing negative consequences, particularly in environments where the "hidden curriculum" of medical training still includes systemic inequities like racism, colorism, sexism, homophobia, and ableism [12].

To address these challenges, institutions have increasingly recognized the importance of *peer mentorship*, where mentorship occurs between individuals at the same or near-same career stage. Peer mentorship offers a safe space for trainees to discuss shared experiences, providing support from those who have recently navigated similar challenges. Examples of peer mentoring models include both formal national programs and informal social media-enabled networks. Peer mentors from minoritized communities can play a unique role in identifying and normalizing experiences of imposter syndrome, providing antiracist mentorship, and creating brave spaces for trainees to share their struggles [13].

Mentoring Across Differences and Affinity Matching

Effective mentorship also involves *mentoring across differences*, where mentors and mentees may not share the same lived experiences. This type of mentorship is essential in nurturing humility, openness, and cross-cultural competency in trainees. Mentors with different backgrounds provide opportunities for trainees to learn how to engage with diverse patients and colleagues, broadening their perspectives and enhancing their ability to work in multicultural environments. Programs that focus on *mentoring across differences* often include educational initiatives that address assumptions, generational sensitivities, bias, and cultural nuances within mentoring relationships. These initiatives, as described by Osman et al., aim to build capacity for both mentors and mentees, ensuring that the relationship is grounded in understanding, respect, and mutual learning [14]. *Affinity matching*, on the other hand, groups mentors and mentees based on shared experiences, whether related to race, culture, gender, sexual orientation, or other identities. Affinity-based mentorship builds strong personal relationships and fosters social capital that is instrumental in helping trainees navigate professional environments. It also reinforces a sense of belonging, as trainees see mentors who share their identities succeed in the field.

Resident Well-Being and Inclusion

Promoting resident well-being is a cornerstone of building safe and inclusive learning environments, especially considering the high levels of stress, workload, and burnout that many trainees face. URiM trainees often experience an additional layer of stress as they navigate a medical system that was not originally designed with their experiences in mind [15]. The intersection of race, ethnicity, and well-being becomes even more complex when these trainees are subjected to microaggressions, bias, and systemic discrimination within the clinical learning environment.

Osseo-Asare and colleagues describe three major themes from the underrepresented in medicine (UiM) trainee experience in the workplace: a daily barrage of microaggressions and bias, UiM residents tasked as race/ethnicity ambassadors, and challenges with negotiating professional and personal identity while seen as "other" [2]. These challenges continue beyond training and affect attending physicians too, who describe discrimination, unsupportive climates, and limited promotion opportunities [16] [17]. Because of fundamental differences in lived experiences, when creating initiatives addressing well-being, understanding the breadth of diversity among trainees is crucial.

Creating a Supportive Environment for URiM Trainees

To foster well-being among all residents, institutions must adopt an equitable approach that ensures each trainee's voice is heard and represented. One successful strategy is the use of *affinity groups* or *caucusing*, where residents are grouped based on their racial or ethnic identity for discussions and debriefs. This allows trainees from marginalized groups to share their experiences in a safe space, free from the burden of educating their peers. Such sessions, like those described by Gilliam et al., are rich in educational value, offering an opportunity for mutual support, healing, and reflection [3]. When initiating this practice, it was critical to frame caucusing as a vital educational component that shifts away from centering the majority in education initiatives and allows URiM trainees protected time and space for sharing without the pressure of having to educate their peers. Caucused sessions can be held for educational sessions, that is, after a microaggressions training for residents to further explore the impact and trauma of microaggressions [18]. They can also be used for debriefs during acute events regarding injustice, inequity, and racism.

Caucusing has been especially valuable during discussions about racial injustice, such as after the high-profile killings of Breonna Taylor, Ahmaud Arbery, George Floyd, and Tony McDade in 2020. These sessions provided URiM trainees with a protected space to process the emotional impact of these events while offering white peers the opportunity to reflect on their roles as allies without placing the emotional burden on their URiM colleagues.

Addressing Burnout in the Clinical Learning Environment

Burnout among residents is well-documented and is further exacerbated for URiM trainees. The constant exposure to discrimination, bias, and the expectation to perform as both medical professionals and representatives of their racial or ethnic groups takes a significant toll on mental health. For these trainees, relying on traditional support systems may not be enough to mitigate the unique challenges they face.

To effectively address burnout, institutions must create robust support networks that include not only faculty and peers but also mental health services that are attuned to the specific needs of URiM trainees. Furthermore, well-being initiatives must be tailored to reflect the diversity of experiences within the residency cohort, recognizing that one-size-fits-all approaches are insufficient.

Promoting Professional Identity Formation by Ensuring Safety in the Clinical Environment

Professional identity formation (PIF)—the process through which an individual comes to "think, act, and feel like a physician"—is profoundly influenced by the clinical learning environment. While mentorship, peer relationships, and institutional culture play important roles in shaping PIF, interactions with patients and families also leave lasting impressions on how residents view themselves as healthcare providers. Safety in the clinical environment extends beyond physical security to encompass psychological and emotional well-being. A 2020 study by the Pediatric Resident Burnout and Resilience Study Consortium found that one-third of pediatric residents experienced mistreatment during training, with patients' families cited as the second most common source [19]. Such mistreatment is often underreported and underaddressed, contributing to an environment where residents feel unsafe or unsupported [20, 21]. Mistreatment by patients and families has been linked to increased medical errors, adverse patient outcomes, and higher rates of burnout among trainees. For residents, such experiences can also negatively impact their professional identity formation (PIF) [22].

When mistreatment by patients and families goes unaddressed, it can erode residents' sense of competence and belonging. To counteract this, institutions must

1. Provide clear guidelines for handling mistreatment and offer debriefing sessions that allow residents to process these experiences in a supportive setting.
2. Explore the use of behavioral response teams and de-escalation training that can empower residents to set boundaries with patients and families, protecting their emotional well-being while maintaining patient care.
3. Residents should receive training on how to recognize and mitigate the emotional impact of mistreatment.

Programs that foster emotional resilience, self-compassion, and peer support can mitigate the harmful effects of mistreatment, helping residents continue their professional development without compromising their mental health.

Collecting Clinical Learning Environment Climate Data

Data collection is an essential part of assessing the effectiveness of DEI initiatives and ensuring that clinical learning environments are safe, inclusive, and responsive to the needs of all trainees. Annual surveys, real-time feedback mechanisms, and climate evaluations provide valuable insights into the experiences of residents and help institutions identify areas for improvement.

Climate surveys should go beyond general questions to explore specific topics such as experiences of overt racism, bias, and mistreatment. Additionally, discussions facilitated by external experts can provide a deeper understanding of how these issues manifest in the clinical setting and what can be done to address them. By involving trainees in the process of data collection and solution-building, institutions demonstrate a commitment to transparency and continuous improvement.

Timely dissemination of climate data is critical. Annual reports on DEI should include actionable findings and be made publicly available to enhance accountability. Creating forums where trainees can react to these findings fosters a culture of openness, allowing institutions to adapt their strategies in real time to meet the evolving needs of the learning environment.

Partnering for Institutional Change

Collaboration between institutions is essential for driving meaningful, systemic change in medical education, particularly when it comes to fostering diversity, equity, and inclusion (DEI). Institutions that partner with each other can share best practices, pool resources, and create more impactful DEI initiatives than they could in isolation. These partnerships also provide opportunities for continuous learning and growth, as institutions can learn from one another's successes and challenges and intentionally break down the silos in the medical education DEI space.

Beyond institutional collaborations, partnerships with local communities are equally important. Community engagement ensures that educational programs are tailored to meet the specific needs of diverse populations. By working closely with the communities they serve, medical institutions can ensure that DEI efforts are not only theoretical but are grounded in real-world needs and outcomes.

Institutional Policy Changes

Implementing inclusive programming without concurrently addressing institutional policies and structures can result in only superficial or short-term changes. Truly inclusive environments require a thorough examination of existing policies and practices to identify and address implicit biases that may disadvantage underrepresented in medicine (URiM) trainees.

While much of the existing literature on policy change in medical education focuses on *removing bias from the application process* (such as through mission-driven holistic candidate reviews), there is relatively little attention paid to the policies and structures that govern trainees' experiences once they are accepted into a program. It is imperative that institutions regularly assess their policies, processes, and organizational structures to ensure they do not perpetuate inequities.

Equity impact assessments are a valuable tool for this purpose. Used in sectors like government and public health, these assessments provide a stepwise process for identifying, understanding, and mitigating potential harms to historically marginalized groups when creating policies or making institutional decisions. Medical education programs can adapt this model to review their own policies and practices.

For example, Children's National Hospital's pediatric residency program created an equity impact assessment tool, designed specifically for graduate medical education (GME) programs, to evaluate their clinical competency committees and the decision-making processes that influence trainee evaluation and remediation. By using such tools, institutions can proactively address areas where implicit bias may be affecting trainee outcomes and take steps to create more equitable policies.

Creating a Culture of Accountability

To ensure that DEI initiatives lead to long-term, sustainable change, institutions must cultivate a *culture of accountability*. This includes setting clear goals and benchmarks for DEI initiatives, tracking progress over time, and holding leaders accountable for achieving these objectives. Transparent reporting is essential to maintaining trust and ensuring that DEI efforts remain a priority. *Anonymous reporting tools* can be used in the clinical learning environment to give trainees a safer space to report concerns without repercussions. It is necessary that anonymous reporting tools have a robust committee to review concerns and provide recommendations on escalation and feedback.

One way to promote accountability is through *periodic external program audits*, which provide unbiased feedback on an institution's DEI progress. These audits can identify gaps, highlight successes, and offer recommendations for future improvements. Creating action plans based on these findings—complete with accountability timelines, designated leaders, and measurable outcomes—ensures that DEI remains an ongoing priority, not a one-time project.

Conclusion

Building a safe and inclusive clinical learning environment (CLE) is a critical strategy for improving the quality of medical education and patient care. A truly inclusive CLE fosters a sense of belonging, ensures that all trainees feel valued and respected, and equips them with the tools they need to navigate the complex social dynamics of healthcare. It also empowers URiM trainees to thrive in environments that have historically excluded or marginalized them.

Throughout this chapter, we have explored the various components of a safe and inclusive CLE, including mentorship, faculty development, resident well-being, the impact of mistreatment, and the importance of data collection. Each of these areas plays a vital role in creating an environment where all trainees, regardless of background, can succeed.

However, achieving this vision requires sustained commitment and action at every level of medical education. Institutions must actively work to address the systemic inequities that have shaped medical education for centuries. This includes revising curricula to reflect the experiences and needs of diverse populations, training faculty to address and mitigate bias, and creating policies that support the retention and success of underrepresented trainees.

Ultimately, building a safe and inclusive CLE is about more than diversity—it is about fostering *equity and belonging*. It is about creating spaces where trainees can bring their authentic selves to their work, without fear of discrimination or bias. And it is about ensuring that the future of healthcare is built on a foundation of justice, compassion, and respect for all.

By following the strategies outlined in this chapter—integrating DEI into curricula, supporting faculty development, promoting mentorship, addressing well-being and burnout, ensuring clinical safety, and holding institutions accountable for their progress—medical education programs can take meaningful steps toward achieving this goal. These interventions will not only improve the educational experience for all trainees but will also lead to better healthcare outcomes for the patients and communities they serve.

Summary of Key Strategies

To recap, the following strategies are essential for creating a safe and inclusive clinical learning environment:

1. *Integrating DEI into medical curricula*: Ensure that diversity, equity, and inclusion are not standalone topics but are woven into every aspect of medical training. This includes addressing racism, implicit bias, and health inequities in both didactic and experiential learning.
2. *Supporting faculty development*: Faculty must be equipped with the skills and knowledge necessary to foster inclusive learning environments. Structured DEI training programs for faculty are critical to achieving this goal.
3. *Promoting mentorship and affinity groups*: Mentorship is a key factor in trainee success. Institutions should implement diverse mentorship models, including peer mentorship and affinity matching, to support underrepresented trainees.
4. *Addressing resident well-being*: Burnout is a serious issue in medical training, particularly for underrepresented in medicine (URiM) trainees. Institutions should provide robust support networks and mental health resources that are tailored to the unique needs of BIPOC and other marginalized trainees.
5. *Ensuring clinical safety*: Mistreatment from patients and families can significantly impact

residents' mental health and professional identity formation. Institutions must develop clear protocols for addressing mistreatment and provide residents with the tools and support they need to navigate these challenges.

6. *Collecting and acting on climate data*: Regularly collect data on the learning environment to identify areas where improvements are needed. Use this data to inform DEI strategies and ensure that progress is measured and reported transparently.
7. *Partnering for institutional change*: Collaborate with other institutions and local communities to share best practices and resources. Ensure that DEI initiatives are supported by policy changes and a culture of accountability.

By implementing these strategies, medical education programs can create learning environments that not only meet the needs of diverse trainees but also prepare future physicians to deliver equitable and compassionate care to the communities they serve.

References

1. Zaidi Z, Rockich-Winston N, Chow C, Martin PC, Onumah C, Wyatt T. Whiteness theory and the (in)visible hierarchy in medical education. Med Educ. 2023;57(10):903–9. https://doi.org/10.1111/medu.15124. Epub 2023 May 18. PMID: 37199083.
2. Osseo-Asare A, Balasuriya L, Huot SJ, et al. Minority resident physicians' views on the role of race/ethnicity in their training experiences in the workplace. JAMA Netw Open. 2018;1(5):e182723. https://doi.org/10.1001/jamanetworkopen.2018.2723.
3. Gilliam CA, Olszewski AE, McDade JE, Homer P, Grow HM, McPhillips HA, Rooholamini SN. Grounded in justice: an equity framework for chief residents. Acad Med. 2021;96(12):1638–42.
4. Jindal M, Thornton RL, McRae A, Unaka N, Johnson TJ, Mistry KB. Effects of a curriculum addressing racism on pediatric residents' racial biases and empathy. J Grad Med Educ. 2022;14(4):407–13.
5. Gilliam CA, Lurie B, Winn AS, Barber A, Jackson D, Weisgerber M, Unaka N. The role of competency based medical education in addressing health inequities and cultivating inclusive learning environments. Curr Probl Pediatr Adolesc Health Care. 2024;54:101641.
6. Mullett TA, Rooholamini SN, Gilliam C, McPhillips H, Grow HM. Description of a novel curriculum on equity, diversity, and inclusion for pediatric residents. J Natl Med Assoc. 2022;113(6):616–25.
7. Unaka NI, Winn A, Spinks-Franklin A, et al. An Entrustable professional activity addressing racism and pediatric health inequities. Pediatrics. 2022;149(2):e2021054604. https://doi.org/10.1542/peds.2021-054604.
8. Anum-Addo SY, Hippolyte J, Barber A. Shifting the paradigm in workforce diversity: prioritizing an inclusive environment in graduate medical education. Acad Med. 2023;10:1097.
9. Diversity, Equity, and Inclusion Collection. Association of American Medical Colleges. Diversity, Equity, and Inclusion Collection. Accessed 24 Aug 2024.
10. Curricula for Anti-Racism. Association of pediatric program directors. https://www.appd.org/about/curricula-for-anti-racism/. Accessed Aug 22 2024
11. Bonifacino E, Ufomata EO, Farkas AH, Turner R, Corbelli JA. Mentorship of underrepresented physicians and trainees in academic medicine: a systematic review. J Gen Intern Med. 2021;36:1023–34.
12. McClinton A, Laurencin CT. Just in TIME: trauma-informed medical education. J Racial Ethn Health Disparities. 2020;7(6):1046–52.
13. Fraiman YS, Montoya-Williams D, Ellis J, Fadel CW, Bonachea EM, Peña MM. Plugging the leaky pipeline: the role of peer mentorship for increasing diversity. Pediatrics. 2022;150(4):e2021055925.
14. Osman NY, Gottlieb B. Mentoring across differences. MedEdPORTAL. 2018;14:10743. https://doi.org/10.15766/mep_2374-8265.10743.
15. Anthym M, Tuitt F. When the levees break: the cost of vicarious trauma, microaggressions and emotional labor for black administrators and faculty engaging in race work at traditionally white institutions. In: Black liberation in higher education. Routledge; 2021. p. 6–27.
16. Cyrus K. Why I gave up my dream of leading diversity efforts in medicine. AAMC News. https://www.aamc.org/news-insights/why-i-gave-my-dream-leading-diversity-efforts-medicine. Published August 10, 2020. Accessed 20 Aug 2024.
17. Blackstock U. Why Black doctors like me are leaving faculty positions in academic medical centers. STAT News. https://www.statnews.com/2020/01/16/black-doctors-leaving-faculty-positions-academic-medical-centers. Published January 16, 2020. Accessed 20 Aug 2024.
18. Gilliam CA, Grow HM, Yeboah D, Seimears TL, Rooholamini SN. Building safe spaces through race-based affinity groups in microaggressions trainings. Acad Pediatr. 2023;23(8):1492–3.
19. Kemper KJ, Schwartz A. Bullying, discrimination, sexual harassment, and physical violence: common and associated with burnout in pediatric residents. Acad Pediatr. 2020;20(7):991–7. https://doi.org/10.1016/j.acap.2020.02.023.

20. Mamede S, Van Gog T, Schuit SCE, et al. Why patients' disruptive behaviours impair diagnostic reasoning: a randomised experiment. BMJ Qual Saf. 2017;26(1):13–8. https://doi.org/10.1136/bmjqs-2015-005065.
21. Alwan IA, Babiker A, Yousif SMA, Badri M, Haqwi AA. Risk of diagnostic errors when dealing with aggressive patients: experimental study. Saudi J Kidney Dis Transplant. 2019;30(6):1310. https://doi.org/10.4103/1319-2442.275475.
22. Trevino R, Poitevien P. Professional identity formation for underrepresented in medicine learners. Curr Probl Pediatr Adolesc Health Care. 2021;51(10):101091. https://doi.org/10.1016/j.cppeds.2021.101091. Epub 2021 Nov 4. PMID: 34742661.

Chief Residents

29

Jason (Jay) Homme and Kristin Sundy

What Is a Chief Resident?

The term chief resident refers to residents chosen by their program to serve in roles beyond the typical expectations of the program. These roles and responsibilities are generally administrative, educational, and clinical. Historically, the term chief resident indicated a resident in their final year of a structured training program, but it has evolved to include additional leadership roles and often takes place after training has been completed. The term *resident* implies that these individuals are still considered trainees, but in many programs, chiefs serve in a junior faculty role and are credentialed as such. A chief resident is still supervised and guided by the program director and other members of the program leadership team and, as such, should have expectations for personal and professional growth throughout the academic year before progressing to their next professional stage.

J. (Jay) Homme (✉)
Mayo Clinic, Rochester, MN, USA
e-mail: homme.jason@mayo.edu

K. Sundy
University of North Carolina, Chapel Hill, NC, USA

Types of Chief Residents

Most chief residents at pediatric residency programs are fourth-year chiefs, meaning they have completed their 3 years of pediatric residency training and have stayed on to complete an additional year as a chief resident. Fourth-year chiefs are usually independent clinical practitioners and balance their time between clinical roles and administrative duties for the residency program. At most programs, fourth-year chiefs are not completing a “postgraduate year” (PGY) as they are not enrolled in a training program. Typically, chiefs are considered clinical instructors or an institutional equivalent.

At some programs, as in surgical residencies, chief residents are often in their third or final year of residency and may be selected to be an administrative chief resident. Given that such chiefs are still completing training and have the workload of a resident, they may have fewer administrative responsibilities than fourth-year chief residents. Third-year chiefs tend to carry scheduling roles and are responsible for urgent staffing needs for the residency program but may not be responsible for resident recruitment or sit on hospital committees.

The number of chief residents a program employs commonly depends on the size of the program and the amount of time chiefs are expected to dedicate to administrative tasks. Programs with third-year chief residents may

H. McPhillips et al. (eds.), *Graduate Medical Education in Pediatrics*, Excellence in Medical Education 3, https://doi.org/10.1007/978-3-032-12952-9_29

have multiple per year even in a small program as these chiefs will need to balance the responsibilities of their residency schedule with administrative roles. Overall, the number of chiefs tends to range from one to five, exceeding five in rare cases, with most programs in the middle of this range between two and three. Programs with only one chief resident, or a "solo chief," are in a unique category. The chief role is broad and can be challenging, and sharing the responsibility with co-chiefs typically supports wellness. Solo chiefs may need additional support from residency faculty to allow for true time off.

Two other unique types of chief residents include medicine-pediatrics chiefs and those doing a chief year at a program other than where they did residency. The role of a medicine-pediatrics chief varies widely by institution. Some programs select a resident from the graduating medicine-pediatrics class to do a fifth year as chief, where chiefs will split their time between the two programs. Others may select one or multiple fourth-year medicine-pediatrics chiefs and allow graduating medicine-pediatrics residents to apply for a position as either a medicine or a pediatrics chief as an independent process. At institutions with a medicine-pediatrics program, there is great value in having representation among chiefs in both departments who understand the intricacies and uniquities of the medicine-pediatrics resident experience and schedule. Programs may choose to hire an external graduate to fill a chief resident position as an alternative route to filling the role if there is no internal resident interest in the position. This happens in a minority of cases as chief residents at their home programs bring with them 3 years of experience at the institution and familiarity with residency program norms.

Selecting Chief Residents

The selection of a cohesive group of chief residents is imperative to the cohort's success as chiefs work very closely with one another, sharing numerous responsibilities. In most residency programs, selection of chief residents happens in the fall or winter of the categorical residents' second year [6]. This timing allows interested residents to know the outcome of their application to be a chief before they must apply for fellowship or a job. The program director (PD) is primarily responsible for making this selection with input from associate program directors, current chief residents, and, occasionally, the pediatric department chair [6]. Each program has its own approach to the selection process. Residents may be nominated by peers, faculty, or themselves, often followed by an application process involving a statement of interest and/or an interview. In assessing a chief applicant, PDs should consider the applicant's clinical acumen, teaching ability, professionalism, and interpersonal skills. A chief resident will typically spend a portion of their time as an attending in a variety of clinical settings, making it important for chiefs to be ready to step into this role. As we discuss later in the chief resident job description, chiefs are often responsible for the facilitation and/or presentation of resident didactics and will spend a significant portion of their time negotiating programmatic changes with residents and delivering feedback to residents and faculty alike. Without strong interpersonal skills and a high level of professionalism, chiefs will struggle to perform these duties and represent the program well. Finally, PDs should consider the group as a whole as they build their chief cohort, allowing for different but complementary personalities. An ideal chief group is one that is stronger together than the sum of its parts, taking advantage of each chief's individual talents and interests to form a well-rounded cohort.

An important, yet often forgotten, piece to consider throughout this process is the diversity and representation among chief groups. Less than 20% of PDs report having a system for mitigating bias in chief resident selection [6]. As we strive toward better representation of groups underrepresented in medicine (UIM) in residency cohorts, we must consider this in the selection of our chief residents, too.

Chief Resident Job Description

The chief resident role varies widely across pediatric residency programs, and in most cases has evolved based on the needs present at a specific program rather than based on a standardized set of expectations. In fact, nearly half of the chief residents in all specialties report having no official job description at all [12]. In this section, we will describe common practices among pediatric residency programs based on anecdotal evidence, highlighting published trends when available. While it may be challenging to encompass the many roles of a chief resident in a job description, PDs should attempt to do so for the purpose of expectation setting and the well-being of their chiefs.

Scheduling

Chiefs have traditionally been responsible for scheduling resident rotations, clinics, and call schedules. This typically starts in the spring after match day and may be a significant portion of the chief handoff that occurs around the same time. First, chiefs schedule rotations either in block format or X + Y, a process that varies widely between programs. Following rotation scheduling, clinics and shift or call schedules are filled in according to program needs and resident requests. In recent years and as ACGME requirements become more specific, some residency programs have shifted toward having a full-time, nonclinical administrator complete the rotation schedule. Typically, such administrators have longer tenure with a program than chief residents and can carry forward knowledge from experience. Once schedules are in place, chiefs tend to share an "on-call" role for urgent resident staffing needs such as last-minute activation of back-up call.

Program Representation

As recent residents and members of the residency program leadership team, chiefs play the key role of communication liaison between residents and PDs. Often, chiefs are the most approachable of the leadership team to residents and will field questions and concerns about all aspects of the residency program. Similarly, chief residents represent the residency program to educators and leaders throughout a hospital system and must respond to questions and concerns from faculty and support staff unaffiliated with the program. Many chief groups choose to consolidate such questions and concerns into a shared email inbox monitored by the chiefs. Like sharing "on-call" responsibilities, chiefs share the responsibility of triaging and responding to emails from residents and faculty alike. With a shared inbox, chiefs can respond to emails with a united front.

As previously described, chief residents have the opportunity to take on an apprenticeship-type role in education and hospital administrative leadership during their tenure. Chiefs will interface regularly with residency program leadership but will often attend and participate in meetings with greater hospital leadership such as rotation directors, division and department chairs, nursing leadership, the designated institutional official, and possibly executive leadership of their institution. Through these experiences, chiefs learn how to prepare for and lead or participate in a meeting. In some scenarios, chiefs may be the only representative of the residency program in a meeting and must use this opportunity to further the interests of the residents and PDs as a program leader, rather than an individual. Examples of committees chiefs may participate in outside of the residency program include divisional education committees, quality improvement teams, medical student scheduling and/or assessment committees, and larger hospital committees focused on throughput and patient flow, hospital capacity, or faculty recruitment. Within their residency program, chiefs often have roles on committees dedicated to resident assessment (such as clinical competency committees and remediation teams), program assessment (such as a program evaluation committee), and curriculum development.

Residency Recruitment

In many programs, resident recruitment is a core responsibility of chief residents. Specific responsibilities vary based on the program and style of interview days—in-person or virtual. During in-person interview days, chiefs may lead hospital tours, host dinners for applicants and residents, and interview applicants as faculty representatives of the program. During virtual interview days, chiefs similarly may welcome applicants, perform interviews, and facilitate social events between applicants and residents. Chief residents typically participate in program leadership meetings debriefing interviews and applicants, and are privy to, if not participants in, the ranking process. Recruitment, in particular, is an opportunity for chiefs to reflect on and develop programmatic initiatives for diversity, equity, and inclusion and the recruitment of residents from racial and ethnic populations historically underrepresented in medicine [10, 13]. Chiefs, along with program faculty, should participate in implicit bias training and reflect on their own biases in preparation for interacting with residency applicants.

Intern Orientation

Given that there is significant overlap between the timeline for new intern onboarding and the chief transition process, rising chief residents tend to have a significant role during intern orientation leading tours, setting professionalism expectations, establishing plans for well-being, offering clinical tips, and more. Chief resident involvement in orientation opens lines of communication between chiefs and new residents and sets the stage for chiefs to be the primary contact in residency leadership. Having just completed training, new chief residents are familiar with the day-to-day tasks of residents and can speak to common pitfalls that inform orientation content. Since much of the clinical and administrative content will be learned *on the job* by interns, orientation is an ideal time to discuss wellness resources, normalize the challenges interns will face, and build community that will foster resilience going forward. Inevitably, chiefs will encounter topics throughout the year that would have been well-placed during orientation and should take note when this happens to pass on to future chief classes.

Education

In its origin, the role of the chief resident was largely clinical and educational. With the increasing number of residents and complexity of resident schedules, the role has shifted to a primarily administrative set of responsibilities. With the increasing number of residents and complexity of resident schedules, the role has shifted to a primarily administrative set of responsibilities, yet continues to offer robust opportunities for development as a clinician educator. Chief residents are often responsible for the scheduling of resident conferences and their speakers and typically facilitate these conferences. Residency programs differ by didactic structure, with either a daily morning report and noon conference or an academic half day. Chiefs will instruct and support residents as they present morning reports or didactics and facilitate the delivery. In some programs, chiefs, themselves, may be the presenters at many conference sessions and can build a repository of case-based didactics for future use. Chiefs can use resident conferences to practice delivering high-yield teaching points, designing curricula, and facilitating their own preparation for the pediatric board exam. Conference scheduling and delivery is often an area for chief classes to innovate from year to year, and even within the year, based on their goals as a group. Having recently been the audience of resident lectures, chiefs will be familiar with the strengths and areas for improvement in their program's didactic curriculum and can modify accordingly. As they consider designing or reworking educational curricula, chiefs should review best practices for curriculum development, including Kern's Six Steps for Curriculum Development [14].

As they work to schedule faculty speakers, chiefs should be aware of any financial incentives for education at their institution. Many academic practices include participation in resident education in the annual bonus structure, as well as promotion and tenure on a clinician educator track. Chiefs can use this to their advantage to incentivize faculty to speak at resident didactics. For promotion purposes, faculty will need to receive evaluations on their teaching, which is a good practice for chiefs to include in lectures in general. A brief, generic evaluation form can be used for each conference and results distributed to faculty as needed.

Finally, chiefs may be responsible for monitoring attendance at educational conferences for residency purposes. Some programs require attendance at conferences for receipt of enrichment or academic funds, or meal stipends. Alternative means of incentivizing resident attendance include offering lunch at midday conferences, granting residents "points" for attendance that contribute toward a prize or "house cup."

Resident Support

As the most "on the ground" members of the residency leadership team, chiefs are often the first to hear news about residents who are struggling in their personal or professional lives. Preceptors may share concerns with chiefs via a shared email inbox or directly. Some of these concerns are minor and clinical performance-related and thus can be handled either by encouraging preceptors to give feedback to residents directly or by chiefs doing some basic remedial work with the resident involved. When there are recurrent concerns about clinical performance such as knowledge gaps, time management skills, or communication with families, chiefs should discuss the situation with the PD to ensure that the resident received appropriate, structured, remediation with any necessary scheduling adjustments. A common challenge is concerns about residents regarding their interpersonal or professionalism skills, which typically require a different skillset to remediate. Minor professionalism concerns may involve instances of disrespectful communication with team members or patients and families, late arrival to shifts, or failure to communicate scheduling changes, and these should be discussed with the PD when recurrent, but a singular occurrence may be appropriately managed by chief residents. Any single major professionalism lapse such as prejudiced statements reflecting racism or sexism, sexual harassment or assault, needs to be shared with the PD promptly to allow for disciplinary action. Of their responsibilities, remediation is the one that chiefs tend to feel least prepared for. PDs should dedicate time early in the academic year to teach chief residents general principles of remediation and set expectations about what chiefs should handle and what should be escalated. Throughout the year, PDs should continue to coach chief residents through remediation scenarios and remain available for questions. Common concerns about residents that might be brought to chiefs include challenges with efficiency, difficulties interacting with patients and families, and professionalism issues.

A particularly important role of the chief resident is in the support of resident well-being. This plays out on the scheduling side with respect to requests for days off, vacations, and honoring the celebration of the residents' choice of holiday and important life events. We also see this in the day-to-day interactions with residents who bring concerns about their work life or personal life to the chiefs seeking advice and/or support. Chiefs should be aware of the wellness resources available to residents, including any employee assistance programs that offer counseling or therapy services. As managers of the call schedule, it is generally the chiefs' responsibility to make accommodations for necessary medical and mental health treatment, which should be done without judgment or penalty. While most wellness concerns can be addressed by chiefs, "red flags" such as self-harm, suicidal ideation, or inability to make contact with a resident who has not reported to a scheduled shift should be quickly escalated to the PD. Workplace scenarios chiefs will encounter often include conflict between residents or other members of the care team, challenging patient interactions, and microaggressions from any of the above. This is an important area of chief resident development and preparation as chiefs may not have been in a position to field such concerns before. PDs should set expectations for communication around specific types of concerns and when chiefs should escalate issues to more senior members of the leadership team such as in the case of microaggressions, particularly from other staff or faculty members.

The examples described above offer an opportunity for chief residents to hone their skills delivering bidirectional feedback. Chiefs will be responsible for giving feedback to residents when working together in the clinical setting and may also deliver feedback about overall clinical performance or professionalism concerns that arise. PDs should mentor and coach chief residents through such conversations and give chiefs feedback on their delivery. Over the course of the chief year, chiefs will become more independent as they discuss performance with residents. Concurrently, chiefs may have to coach clinical preceptors to give their own feedback to residents. Occasionally, concerns are brought to chiefs by faculty supervising residents prior to delivering that feedback to the resident themselves. It is appropriate in this situation for chiefs to take note of the concern but encourage faculty to speak with the residents about their firsthand observations.

Transition Planning and the Chief Resident Handoff

A unique feature of the chief year is its short duration of only one year. Often, chief residents have their successors selected prior to starting their own time as chiefs and must begin thinking about how they plan to hand off their responsibilities nearly from the start. Since much of the chief resident year is on the job training, a good transition plan can help hasten the learning curve, decrease anxiety associated with the new roles/responsibilities, and limit the amount of *reinventing the wheel* that tends to occur in the absence of a thoughtful handover process. Transitions are a time for innovations that, along with the continuation of existing projects/plans and deliberate transition planning, increases the likelihood for success. As chief residents start their new role, they are guiding others that find themselves in new positions (interns, senior residents) and chief residents that benefit from a thoughtful transition plan are better suited to help others succeed.

Aspects that contribute to a successful transition for graduating chiefs include reflecting on the year, seeking feedback, setting timelines, and discussing expectations. For rising chief residents, a successful transition includes opportunities to set goals (personal and professional), understand job descriptions and assigned, or chosen, roles, and ask questions. Programs may have different expectations as to when transitions occur but a high-level sample timeline may include basic orientations to the job in fall/early winter, division of roles and planning block schedules during winter and early spring, followed by some dedicated time for formal training as assumption of certain aspects by the rising chiefs (e.g., communication with incoming intern class), culminating in officially assuming the chief resident role with the change of academic year.

A chief handbook/guide is an enduring document that is program specific and is updated in an ongoing manner with new policies/procedures and other components critical to successfully fulfilling the chief resident role. Some sample sections include instructions related to handling of absences/leaves, specific chief duties (scheduling lectures, recruitment, chief projects, etc.), communication preferences, key ACGME and program-specific policies, templates for scheduling, and other notable resources for recurring tasks throughout the chief year.

For chief residents concluding their year, it is also important that they have plans to successfully transition to their next activity. The breadth of activities and opportunities of the chief resident year is largely unmatched anywhere else during a career, so there is a significant role contraction that occurs after the chief year. Each individual is formulating a new professional identity, with some going on to further training (fellowship), others staying on at the same institution as a faculty member (moving in), and some taking faculty positions at other institutions (moving on). Seeking out advice and mentoring from trusted faculty, especially if they have formerly served as a chief resident, can be a valuable component to transitioning from the chief resident year.

Clinical Responsibilities

Informal surveys show that clinical time for chief residents ranges from 0% to 50%, averaging around 30%. During this time, the majority of chiefs will be credentialed as attending-level providers and will practice independently as any faculty member. As with other aspects of the chief job description, this varies by institution. Often, chiefs will be assigned a specific clinical full-time equivalent (FTE), but the definition of 1.0 FTE tends to vary as well. Traditionally, chiefs would work as general pediatricians on inpatient teaching services and in resident clinics. This remains true at many institutions, but others have begun to expand the options available to chief residents for their clinical time. Some may do all their clinical time either inpatient or outpatient within their residency program's institution. Some chiefs might work in a community clinic or outreach site, and others still may work in a fellow or advanced practice provider role on subspecialty services within the hospital or the intensive care units. Ideally, a chief's clinical time should align with and further their clinical goals, while still allowing for professional development in the administrative, education, and leadership realms. Importantly, academic and administrative time should be protected, and chiefs should not be expected to flex into clinical coverage beyond their contracted FTE without appropriate compensation as would be provided for other attending-level physicians.

Division of Labor Among Chief Residents

Each residency program with multiple chief residents has a unique system for division of labor. Chief residents may be selected for a specific administrative role, such as scheduling, lectures, or for a satellite residency program location, or chiefs may be selected as a group and divide responsibilities later. Viewing chief residency as an opportunity for academic and leadership development, it is ideal for chiefs to have responsibility for a variety of roles rather than a single expertise. For example, a chief resident who is responsible for all the resident scheduling may not get the opportunity to present and facilitate resident didactics, missing important development as an educator. Similarly, a chief resident responsible for all didactic scheduling and facilitation may not develop the necessary skills to help residents process and respond to microaggressions or examples of injustice in the workplace. We have seen these roles divided between chiefs for the duration of the year, and we have seen chiefs rotate roles throughout the chief year to get exposure to each one. Each role comes with its own set of trials and challenges with potential for burnout, so sharing roles allows chiefs to divide and conquer to support each other.

Another important division of labor is that between chief residents and residency program administrators. In general, chiefs should take on roles that are resident-facing, need clinical context, or involve scholarly output. Administrative tasks that occur annually, require institutional memory, or involve coordination with larger administrative bodies within the institution may be best completed by program coordinators, managers, or administrators who spend more than one year with the residency program. Program administrators are often best positioned to facilitate leave time for new parents, prolonged illness, or other extended absences and otherwise ensure adherence to ACGME requirements that chiefs may not be as familiar with. Regardless of who performs the tasks, chiefs must be familiar with the processes, so they are able to answer questions from residents and troubleshoot time-sensitive resident needs. For example, program administrators may do the initial block or rotation scheduling for residents with chiefs completing the day-to-day or call schedules. Residents will come to chiefs with questions about schedule swaps or time-off requests, and chiefs will be best prepared to answer these questions and honor requests if they are familiar with the block scheduling process in addition to the call schedules.

Professional Development for Chief Residents

Training for the Chief Role

Chiefs undergo training for the role through local, regional, and/or national chief development programs. Most chiefs report receiving some training from their home institution, often described as a "bootcamp." This may be a direct handoff from their graduating chiefs, leadership training from residency program leadership, or hospital-wide training for institutional chief residents in a variety of specialties.

In addition to local training, there are several offerings on the national level for chief resident preparation. The Accreditation Council of Graduate Medical Education (ACGME) offers a Leadership Skills Training Program for Chief Residents available to all specialties that focuses on leadership skills and conflict resolution [1]. The Association of Pediatric Program Directors (APPD) offers a broad range of pediatric-specific chief development content, as well. At the annual APPD Spring Meeting, rising and graduating chief residents are invited to attend the Forum for Chief Residents that involves didactic teaching on presenting and facilitating resident lectures, responding to resident feedback, working with co-chiefs, and program development. Rising chiefs are also invited to a pre-conference session titled Leadership, Education, Growth and Advocacy in the Chief Year (LEGACY) that focuses on individual and group leadership skills, emotional intelligence, and negotiation. Chief residents are offered membership to APPD that comes with access to resources, leadership opportunities within APPD, and additional training via online seminars throughout the year [3].

Overall, chiefs find such national development programs to be important. However, chiefs often report a need for increased mentorship and development at their home institutions, particularly with regard to working with co-chiefs and receiving feedback about their leadership skills [10].

There are many professional societies and organizations that have resources available that can be helpful to chief residents and program leadership teams supporting chiefs. Some of the most active are included in Table 29.1.

These sites are frequently updated with new information and resources, and new sites may also become available.

Advancing Chief Residents' Goals

Chief residents tend to enter the year with big and bold hopes for what their time as chiefs might hold and the changes they can enact for their program. Program directors can help guide chief residents in developing thoughtful plans for their

Table 29.1 Professional societies and organizations that have chief resident resources available for program leadership, including chief residents

Organization	What it offers	Link
Association of Pediatric Program Directors (APPD)	Leadership development, chief-specific toolkits, networking	https://www.appd.org
Accreditation Council for Graduate Medical Education (ACGME)	Program requirements, policy updates, leadership skills training course for chief residents	https://www.acgme.org
American Board of Pediatrics (ABP)	Certification, assessment guidance, MOCA-Peds info	https://www.abp.org
American Osteopathic Board of Pediatrics (AOBP)	Osteopathic certification requirements and exams	https://www.acopeds.org/aobp/
American Academy of Pediatrics (AAP)	Clinical guidelines, advocacy, section memberships	https://www.aap.org

chief resident year by encouraging them to develop goals for various domains of the chief year, including personal goals (e.g., wellness/well being), programmatic goals (how they want to help advance the program), development as clinician, development as educators, scholarship opportunities, and planning for their next steps as several examples. Meeting in advance of the chief year to discuss these goals and establishing plans for follow-up can greatly increase the chances that the year will be productive well beyond the skill development of scheduling and other administrative tasks commonly associated with chief residency.

Advancing Chief Residents' Goals: Personal

Chiefs may be in their first administrative role that brings a new set of challenges for navigating work–life balance and integration. While residency hours are long, there is minimal work outside of the clinical duties and a clinical shift tends to end with the shift. Chief year often brings a lighter clinical schedule but a longer task list with many ongoing and long-term projects. Chiefs must learn to more intentionally set boundaries between work and home so that they are not continuously "on-call." Many new chiefs find this challenging, particularly since they tend to be high-performers and self-identified perfectionists. In programs with multiple chiefs, they can take turns being the primary contact for residents and faculty with urgent needs to maintain some protected time off outside of typical work hours. For daytime work, chiefs should come to an agreement together and with their program director regarding deadlines for recurring tasks so that they are clear on what must be done before leaving for the day and what can wait until tomorrow. Program directors should teach and encourage their chiefs to respect the boundaries they set with the role to minimize the risk of burnout, which is common among chief residents.

Advancing Chief Residents' Goals: Professional

Despite only lasting one year, the chief residency can have an enormous impact on a chief resident's future and can set chiefs up for success as leaders and scholars. Some key professional hurdles throughout the year include preparation for the pediatric board exam, applications to jobs or fellowship, and scholarly efforts both as a chief group and as individuals.

Preparing for the board certification exam is an important task throughout residency but intensifies during a chief resident year. Setting aside dedicated study time by blocking the calendar is an important strategy as the other demands of the chief year can easily push aside this priority. Since chief residents are commonly involved in the planning of educational conferences/activities, they can leverage this by choosing topics and/or speakers that concomitantly help fulfill their own study goals. Board review sessions can be structured such that they meet both personal needs and those of the junior residents in the program. There are a variety of board preparation courses and materials available, including question banks. Chiefs should set aside time to prepare in a simulated testing environment where blocks of questions are answered, but not reviewed immediately, to build up the testing *stamina* necessary on the day of the actual examination. Finally, blocking time for the test itself and delegation of duties to other members of the program leadership team in the days leading up to the exam can limit unnecessary stress.

When it comes to academics and scholarship, chiefs are exposed to a wide variety of quality improvement (QI) and medical education efforts. As discussed, chiefs tend to be heavily involved in residency didactic curricula but will also be asked to serve as representatives to the residency program on other education-related projects that may be rotation-specific. Many chief residents have a role in reviewing and/or debriefing safety events submitted by residents and may be sought out by QI scholars making changes to resident workflow. Chiefs can demonstrate the breadth of their involvement in these activities by keeping an updated curriculum vitae with descriptions of their role and responsibilities. It is worth documenting involvement in chief responsibilities such as clinical competency committees, program evaluation committees, and any hospital quality improvement teams. These are roles not often held by recent residency graduates that have not completed a chief year and thus offer unique discussion points in interviews and documentation of experience that can be built on in future roles.

Unlike residency, chief year offers the opportunity to dedicate a significant portion of time to scholarly efforts, allowing, hopefully, for completion of a project before the end of the year. Many chiefs present their work at national conferences such as the Association of Pediatric Program Directors Spring Meeting, Pediatric Academic Societies, and specialty-specific conferences. Without a plan and a timeline, chiefs might find that the year runs away from them with the many administrative demands, so it is important to set goals and share them with mentors so that chiefs can hold themselves accountable. Common chief projects include curriculum development, significant schedule or staffing changes, resident well-being initiatives, and work around remediation or struggling learners. Discussion with former chiefs from their home institution or current chiefs from other institutions can help chiefs decide on the feasibility of their proposed interventions. Chiefs greatly benefit from sharing ideas with chiefs at other programs as residency programs tend to grow and develop within the silo of their own institution. Chiefs may choose to enact changes that were successfully implemented within other programs and by working together they can do so with the wisdom earned by their fellow chiefs.

Advancing Programmatic Goals

Another important set of goals to consider are those of the residency program. A great residency program is constantly evolving to meet the expectations of residents, core faculty, and accrediting bodies and chief residents are well-positioned to both assist in and learn from these efforts. PDs can mentor their chiefs through enacting change, developing new curricula, and educating residents both on the wards and in the classroom.

Advancing Programmatic Goals: Change Management

Chiefs benefit from learning and implementing effective change management methodologies. One example is Kotter's eight steps to transforming an organization [8]. These individual steps can be applied to proposed changes during a chief year and include (1) establishing a sense of urgency, (2) forming a powerful guiding coalition, (3) creating a vision, (4) communicating the vision, (5) removing obstacles, (6) creating short-term wins, (7) consolidation of improvements, and (8) institutionalizing new approaches. Change takes time, and skipping important steps can create an illusion of speed but lead to unsatisfactory results. Some chief years will be defined by significant changes (e.g., implementing updated ACGME program requirements, switching from noon conference to academic half days) and others may have limited amounts of change (e.g., minor changes in curriculum or coverage schedules), but all chiefs will benefit from opportunities to build knowledge and skills related to effective change management. In addition to value during the chief year, having skills to implement change will benefit chief residents as future leaders in their chosen specialties.

Advancing Programmatic Goals: Curriculum Development

Most chief residents will have a role in curriculum development during their year. This may be via resident didactics and selection of speakers, creation of a simulation series, implementation of a diversity, equity, and inclusion curriculum, or any variety of other topics. While not all educational interventions must be published, chiefs deserve recognition for the work they do, and presentation (if not publication) of rigorous curriculum development is an achievable scholarly goal for a chief. It is best remembered that planning ahead for dissemination of scholarly work is a key step in making work presentable. Chiefs can refer to instructional journal articles on curriculum development or may go more in depth by reading Kern's six-step approach to curriculum development to ensure that their curriculum is well-thought out [9, 14]. One aspect to focus on is the value of a needs assessment, both general and targeted, to ensure that stakeholder opinions are considered and prevent prior work from being duplicated. As chiefs think ahead for their projects, developing a curricular change from a conceptual framework will increase the rigor of their scholarly output [11].

Chief Residents as Middle Management

The chief resident role is a classic example of middle management [4]. Chiefs help manage up working closely with other members of the program leadership team, including the program director, associate program directors, and program coordinators/administrators. Chiefs also commonly interact regularly with key faculty (e.g., department chair, vice-chair for education) and administrators. *Up work* can include understanding the needs of the program, program director, and the institution and may include implementation of new policies/procedures, changes to staffing models, or other institutional initiatives. Chiefs help manage downward through their interactions with residents currently in the program and prospective future residents. *Down work* is done on behalf of the program but done with residents and includes teaching/conferences, scheduling, and counseling/support. There is also *lateral* work when there are co-chiefs, clinical faculty, and committee work. Chiefs also engage in *internal* work related to reflection, dealing with stressors, and relationship building. This middle management role for chief residents can be both challenging and rewarding. Chiefs can be intentional about not sliding up or down too much, not losing contact with those they are serving, avoiding splitting or scapegoating behaviors, and can help look for system-level explanations and opportunities that can provide broad benefits and garner support/buy-in. As chief classes transition, residents and faculty may make requests to new chiefs that have been denied or deferred by prior chief classes, so it is important to have a prepared response that allows chiefs to touch base with each other or the program director before responding to such requests while they grow into the role. The guidance and support from the program director and other key supervisors can be instrumental in chiefs having success as middle managers.

Benefits and Outcomes of a Chief Resident Year

The chief resident year can be a highly beneficial and strategic portion of a career plan. The intensive interactions, multiple roles, and myriad novel opportunities can accelerate the trajectory of a chief resident's career planning by developing insight about areas of interest, strengths, and necessary growth. Working within multidisciplinary groups provides invaluable perspective that can further leadership capabilities. Chief residents are also commonly identified as skilled educators, and completion of a chief year is often viewed favorably for consideration for faculty positions at academic medical centers [7].

About half of the pediatric chief residents go on to complete a subspecialty fellowship versus general practice and more former chiefs report holding leadership positions and having academic time in their contracts than residency graduates who did not complete a chief year [2]. In another study, former chief residents were more likely to be described as "excellent role models" [15]. However, information is lacking on career paths of former pediatric chief residents. Anecdotally, former chief residents are overrepresented among pediatric residency leadership positions, and even undergraduate medical education leadership positions. For some chiefs, the chief resident year may be a deterrent to an academic career. In a survey of pediatric chief residents, about 25% of respondents would not agree to be a chief again in retrospect, and less than 20% planned to pursue an academic career directly out of the chief year [5]. Overall, though, completion of a chief resident year does seem to predict future leadership in academic medicine and medical education for those who are interested.

Compensation Models

As described, chief residents' appointments may vary considerably between institutions, and, as such, compensation models also vary widely. As employees, chief residents are provided with salary and benefits commensurate with their job posting. Third-year chiefs are commonly paid as a PYG-3, with some programs able to offer additional compensation in terms of a chief stipend/bonus or improved benefits (e.g., parking) to recognize the added roles/responsibilities to be completed concurrent with completion of the primary residency training program. PGY-4 chiefs may hold trainee status versus junior faculty status, and this can have a significant impact on compensation. Informal surveys of chief residents show that there is a wide range of strategies to compensate chief residents. A chief stipend/bonus and moonlighting opportunities are commonly used for chief residents who maintain a trainee designation within an institution. Chiefs that are appointed as junior faculty generally receive higher base salaries but may also be subject to similar structures as other faculty where at least a portion of pay is tied to distribution of clinical activities and ability to generate revenue for the institution. Careful consideration of compensation structures for programs/institutions to recognize the significant contributions of chief residents while recognizing the sacrifices (such as the additional year) can help facilitate strong interest in this critical role within residency training programs.

Summary

Individuals are chosen for and choose to pursue a chief residency year for a myriad of reasons. The chief year can be highly flexible, and career focused, offering roles and responsibilities to build knowledge, skills, and influence programs and trainees through a wide range of administrative, clinical, educational, and scholarly responsibilities. Program leaders can foster success in their chiefs through communicating clear expectations, facilitating adequate preparation, and providing mentorship throughout the year. This highly formative experience can serve as a springboard into long and satisfying careers, and it is often said: *Once a Chief, Always a Chief.*

References

1. ACGME. Leadership skills training program for chief residents. Accreditation Council for Graduate Medical Education; 2024. https://www.acgme.org/meetings-and-educational-activities/courses-and-workshops/leadership-skills-training-program-for-chief-residents/. Accessed 9 Aug 2024.
2. Alpert JJ, Levenson SM, Osman CJ, James S. Does being a chief resident predict leadership in pediatric careers? Pediatrics. 2000;105:984–8. https://doi.org/10.1542/peds.105.S3.984.
3. APPD. For Chief Residents. Association of Pediatric Program Directors; 2024. https://www.appd.org/resources-programs/program-resources/2555-2/. Accessed 9 Aug 2024.
4. Berg DN, Huot SJ. Middle manager role of the chief medical resident: an organizational psychologist's perspective. J Gen Intern Med. 2007;22:1771–4. https://doi.org/10.1007/s11606-007-0425-8.
5. Dabrow SM, Harris EJ, Maldonado LA, Gereige RS. Two perspectives on the educational and administrative roles of the pediatric chief resident. J Grad Med Educ. 2011;3:17–20. https://doi.org/10.4300/JGME-D-10-00039.1.
6. Gustafson S, Poitevien P, Acholonu R, et al. Opportunities for mitigating bias in the process and priorities for pediatric chief resident selection. Acad Pediatr. 2022;22:319–23. https://doi.org/10.1016/j.acap.2021.12.004.
7. Irby DM, Gillmore GM, Ramsey PG. Factors affecting ratings of clinical teachers by medical students and residents. J Med Educ. 1987;62:1–7. https://doi.org/10.1097/00001888-198701000-00001.
8. Kotter JP. Leading change, with a new preface by the author, 1R edition. Harvard Business Review Press; 2012.

9. Lai S, Buchheit BM, Kitamura K, et al. Five key articles on curriculum development for graduate medical educators. J Grad Med Educ. 2024;16:75–9. https://doi.org/10.4300/JGME-D-23-00208.1.
10. McDaniel LM, Molloy MJ, Blanck J, et al. The chief residency in U.S. and Canadian graduate medical education: a scoping review. Teach Learn Med. 2024:1–10. https://doi.org/10.1080/10401334.2023.2298870.
11. Mills DM, Teufel RJ II. Tools for medical education scholarship: from curricular development to educational research. Hosp Pediatr. 2020;10:452–7. https://doi.org/10.1542/hpeds.2019-0293.
12. Pettit JE. Coleadership among chief residents: exploration of experiences across specialties. J Grad Med Educ. 2015;7:203–7. https://doi.org/10.4300/JGME-D-14-00298.1.
13. Raphael JL, Giardino AP, Harris T, et al. Perceptions revisited: pediatric chief resident views on minority housestaff recruitment and retention in pediatric residency programs. J Natl Med Assoc. 2014;106:58–68. https://doi.org/10.1016/S0027-9684(15)30071-7.
14. Thomas PA, Kern DE, Hughes MT, et al. Curriculum development for medical education: a six-step approach. JHU Press; 2022.
15. Wright SM, Kern DE, Kolodner K, et al. Attributes of excellent attending-physician role models. N Engl J Med. 1998;339:1986–93. https://doi.org/10.1056/NEJM199812313392706.

Part VII

Faculty and Leadership Development

Faculty Development

30

H. Barrett Fromme and Nicola Orlov

Determining Your Needs

The Accreditation Council for Graduate Medical Education (ACGME) provides clear guidelines for faculty members in the common program requirements for residency and fellowship that faculty members must participate in faculty development "at least annually" [2, 3]. More specifically, the ACGME mandates faculty members who interact with residents and fellows must demonstrate professionalism and an interest in education; provide safe, cost-effective, and patient-centered care; and engage in annual faculty development around education, quality improvement, well-being, and the improvement of care delivery through practice-based learning and improvement [2, 3]. Additionally, annual faculty evaluations are required to include an assessment of faculty participation in the faculty development (FD) series [2], and the ACGME's program requirements instruct programs to use evaluations of faculty to guide the content introduced in FD sessions [2, 3].

Content that needs to go beyond that mandated by the ACGME should be determined and planned by systematically analyzing the needs of the faculty at the institution. Conducting this needs assessment can be done in a variety of ways. Internal data sources, including an internal annual program evaluation, rotation evaluations, and faculty evaluations, can provide insight into the areas of strength and opportunity for a faculty group. Additionally, the ACGME provides program directors with feedback from the annual core faculty and trainee surveys that not only delineates strengths and weaknesses in a program but also compares data from an individual program to other programs nationally [2]. Content needs for a faculty development curriculum can be driven by the ACGME survey and internal data collection systems. Further, engaging with faculty, understanding the culture of a department, and creating space to regularly meet and debrief with trainees and faculty about their experiences can help identify more subtle content needs or areas that are not explored on the ACGME survey. Program directors and faculty who oversee FD programming should also embrace these moments when faculty are together as an opportunity to share anticipated changes within the field, develop shared language about the department and program's mission, and foster a community of practice.

Traditionally, the organization of faculty development programs has occurred in an impromptu manner; however, emerging literature offers a more intentional and data-driven approach to faculty development, called competency-based faculty development (CBFD)

H. B. Fromme (✉) · N. Orlov
University of Chicago Pritzker School of Medicine, Chicago, IL, USA
e-mail: hfromme@bsd.uchicago.edu

H. McPhillips et al. (eds.), *Graduate Medical Education in Pediatrics*, Excellence in Medical Education 3, https://doi.org/10.1007/978-3-032-12952-9_30

[4]. CBFD proposes that rather than opportunistically offering faculty development sessions, frameworks should be used to ensure exposure to a wide breadth of necessary skills to all educators within a hospital system [4, 5]. The concept of developing a curriculum based on the needs of the faculty, department, program, and trainees aligns with the ACGME's suggestion that faculty evaluations be used to determine FD needs. Further, because the ACGME gives program directors the authority to determine which faculty should participate in supervision of residents and the responsibility of monitoring faculty performance in education, program directors should consider using existing CBFD frameworks as they determine the FD needs of their faculty body.

Knowing Your Audience

When developing any curriculum, it is important to know who your audience is and what their needs are. In faculty development, depending on the institution and site, there can be a broad range of the type of clinicians who teach learners. Faculty are defined by the ACGME as "the collective body of physicians who have individually received a formal assignment to teach resident/fellow physicians" [6]. This describes a highly varied group, with some employed by and working at the primary institution, and others recruited to teach at off-site locations. While, by definition, all designated faculty are expected to teach, there is another subset of physicians who identify as medical educators or clinician educators. These individuals have chosen to pursue a career where they develop skills beyond teaching, often in the areas of curriculum development, assessment, or evaluation [7]. Both groups, the clinical teachers and the clinician educators, have a tremendous impact on the clinical learning environment, and both need skills development. To provide the best support for both groups, it is essential to understand the two groups, and how even within those groups there is a large variation in experience, motivation, skills, and resource availability.

Clinical Teachers

While the ACGME defines who is considered a faculty member, the individuals who have been designated as such do not all have the same experience in, motivation for, or time to teach. Planning faculty development for the physicians who teach must consider these potentially different individuals.

The traditional faculty clinical teacher is one who is employed by the university or institution and has teaching as part of the expectation of their employment. These individuals often have protected time to engage with learners and develop their own skills. Despite that, faculty come in with varying degrees of training on teaching skills, and they have similarly varied interests in teaching. Examples of clinical teachers who work with residents can include (1) a pediatric intensivist who is 80% clinical, who has always loved teaching, completed a resident-as-teacher course in residency, and frequently attends teaching skills workshops within the department; (2) a senior hematologist/oncologist, with several leadership roles, who only has 4 weeks of service a year and one clinic a week, and who never attends teaching skills training due to other commitments; and (3) a pediatrician who owns and runs a robust clinical practice who has agreed to have residents rotate through the clinic during their ambulatory rotation. All offer unique opportunities for resident learning, but they also present challenges. Time is a challenge for all groups, as productivity demands for both clinical and nonclinical work are significant. In addition, lack of training, confidence in skills, and lack of best practices in training can be barriers [8]. Faculty development efforts will need to not only address key topics to build skills and confidence in teaching but will also need to be thoughtfully delivered to integrate easily into the other responsibilities of the teacher.

Medical Educators

As mentioned above, medical educators are faculty who have made the decision to pursue a career as a medical educator. While this includes having strong teaching skills, it also includes a focus on areas such as assessment, evaluation, curriculum, and, with all of those, scholarship. Within the language of the ACGME, this includes core faculty, defined as individuals who have a "significant role in the education of residents/fellows … evaluate the competency domains, work closely with and support the program director, assist in developing evaluation systems, and teach and advise" [2]. Implicit in this definition is that core faculty do more than teach, with the actual work of core faculty often going beyond evaluation. To be most prepared for their roles, these individuals will need additional training in areas beyond teaching skills, which can be provided within the residency or department, or it can be outsourced to institutional or national programs. Residency programs need to be able to offer at least foundational support in certain topic areas so that the core faculty, including the program director and associate program directors, have the skills they need to not only run the program, but to contribute to discovery within medical education.

Adult Learning

Regardless of the faculty role and aspiration, faculty development efforts need to be considered through the lens that the learners are adults. There is an abundance of adult learning theories and categories of theories, so it may be easiest to start with Malcolm Knowles, who coined the term "andragogy" [9]. Core to Knowles' theory was that adults are self-directed in their learning, they learn from experience, they are ready to learn when it is relevant to their work, and thus want it to be practical and applicable, and, finally, that there is internal motivation to learn [10]. In addition to Malcolm Knowles, David Kolb's Experiential Learning Cycle brings an additional framework to building learning experiences for adults by taking individuals through a cycle of having a concrete experience and reflecting on it, from there structuring new concepts, and then testing those new concepts. Learners, such as faculty in faculty development programs, benefit by being taught through relevant cases and problems, where they can build their own potential approaches and actively investigate their own theories [11]. Regardless of what format or framework one uses, it is essential to remember that faculty are adults who learn best when actively involved with content relevant to their own work. We will discuss specific methods for implementation with this in mind later in the chapter.

Key Content

While your needs assessment may identify areas that need more development than others for your clinical teachers and medical educators, there are core topics that will allow each group to perform their roles optimally. But what topics are most important for each group? Over the years, numerous organizations, in the United States and internationally, have recommended various skills in which teachers and educators need to be proficient. These have come from both subspecialty organizations, institutions, and larger organizations [12]. Most recently, the ACGME published the Clinician Educator Milestones, which are designed for "educators, educational scholars, and educational leaders," which were developed through a deliberate process [13]. While all these resources can serve as a guide for faculty development topics in response to a local needs assessment, we offer the following key topic areas for both clinical teachers and medical educators.

Clinical Teachers

Embedded with residents in the daily work of clinical care, clinical teachers are responsible for the immediate, day-to-day teaching of learners. Whether they encounter residents for a half day in a clinic or for 2 weeks on a service rotation, they need to have the skills to maximize the learning opportunities and further the growth of the learners. While it is important to recognize that the role of a clinical teacher is continually evolving, which will require continued development, there are core areas in which they need to be well versed. We will discuss each here [14]. This is not an exhaustive list, but it is an essential one.

Feedback

While there are many skills that clinical teachers need, perhaps one of the most important and the most challenging is the ability to provide effective formative feedback. Feedback is of paramount importance to guiding learners to improve their skills. While feedback in medical education existed before 1983, Jack Ende's classic article provides a phenomenal and succinct summary of the key features, emphasizing that "without feedback, mistakes go uncorrected, good performance is not reinforced, and clinical competence is achieved empirically or not at all" [15]. Feedback is a core element in competency-based education and depends on the relationships between those who are involved [16]. In the GME space, this includes clinical teachers providing formative feedback to residents and fellows. Formative (in contrast to summative feedback, or evaluations, which will be discussed later) allows learners to know where they currently are, where they need to go, and how to get there. It can be immediate (e.g., provided on the spot) or more formal (e.g., "Feedback Fridays" or at the end of clinic), and each is important for the growth of the learner. Most importantly, it should be an active, collaborative experience between teachers and learners, with both focused on the goals of the learner through discussion and reflection. Finally, it is important to create a culture of feedback that will "normalize feedback, promote trusting teacher-learner relationships, define clear performance goals, and ensure that the goals of the learners and teachers align" [17].

The challenge is that clinical teachers often feel unprepared or unwilling to provide honest and direct formative feedback. Challenges include those for the individuals, such as personal biases and fear of retaliation in teachers, as well as lack of trust in the teacher–learner dyad [18, 19]. The system can also present challenges by inadvertently connecting formative feedback to evaluations or prioritizing a culture of "niceness," which dissuades the provision of constructive feedback [20, 21]. By emphasizing feedback skill development in faculty development, one can address several of these issues. In fact, just by valuing and teaching feedback, the system culture can change [22].

There exist many resources to help with the process of delivering faculty development in feedback skills. There are numerous models that have literature to support them, including the ADAPT model [23], the R2C2 model [24], the Pendleton model [25], and Feedback Scripts [26]. While any of these can be used, it is important to be intentional when giving clinical teachers a framework to use when giving feedback. Of note, it is also important, though slightly outside the purview of faculty development, to enhance the feedback receiving skills of the learners, as they are a key part of this partnership.

Providing feedback training is an essential element in GME, and one must consider the balance of reaching the most faculty, while also allowing deeper exploration of the material. For this reason, the topic of feedback merits repetition and diversity in delivery. Large group virtual sessions allow for conveying foundational information to the largest group of faculty. While this is not ideal for small group work, especially role play, it does ensure that every faculty member has exposure to the material, and it can be repeated annually. It is then important to offer smaller sessions that allow for deeper discussion of real cases as well as role play, potentially utilizing Objective Structured Teaching Encounters with standardized learners if resources permit.

Establishing the Learning Climate Through Coaching

The learning climate, often described in teaching literature as "a safe learning environment," can include many elements, but the literature supports its impact on learner achievement, burnout, motivation, and success. The learning environment may include inpatient rotations, continuity clinic, community practices, morning reports, or noon conferences. In all of these settings, critical facilitators of learning include supervision, coaching and assessment, feedback, supportive behaviors from teachers, engagement, goal-focused teaching, motivation and stimulation of learning, and respect [27–29].

Coaching leverages many of these influencers and predictors of learning climate. Since Atul Gawande's 2011 article on coaching, there has been a renewed interest in this method in medicine. The application of a coaching framework to medical education was seen in 2014 in Watling's article comparing athletics and music careers to medicine [17], and there have been several articles and programs over the past decade focused on coaching programs in UME and GME [30, 31]. While formal coaching programs are valuable (and will be discussed later), the role of coaching in everyday clinical teaching should not be overlooked. Clinical teaching provides the ideal environment for a "coach" or clinical teacher to work with learners to set their goals, be observed, get feedback immediately, and improve their performance. Key to this is the recognition of the teacher that they are in a coaching role; attendings often think of themselves as teachers, not coaches, and reframing that expectation would be valuable. There are simple frameworks that can not only guide the process for individuals but also separate it from the role of mentorship and advising [32].

Introducing faculty to the learning climate and coaching can be done in larger groups for a varied audience. However, smaller group discussions can also be beneficial for clinical teachers who teach in the same context. Faculty in the same division (e.g., pediatric hospital medicine) may have much to gain from sharing experiences and successes in the same environment, while those in the pediatric emergency medicine may take a different approach or face different challenges. Having an opportunity for clinical teachers to analyze their own current environment and work through a case to see where they can improve their approaches is tremendously useful. Similarly, giving faculty time to work through a coaching framework through the lens of their own daily practice is more valuable than just providing the framework. These sessions can be done virtually as some of the work is introspective and personal and then group sharing can be utilized.

Goals, Expectations, and Growth Mindset

Within the role of the clinical coach are several unique skills besides feedback. They must work with learners to establish shared goals. Clinical teachers should be provided instruction on optimal ways to facilitate goal setting, both for learners and for themselves. While this should include a discussion of what a good clinical learning goal is, utilizing Bloom's Taxonomy, it should focus more broadly on creating mastery goals within a growth mindset [33]. Evidence suggests that resident learning goals are not of optimal quality, so training clinical teachers to help them develop these could be key to rotation satisfaction, motivation, and achievement [34]. By supporting residents in developing SMART (specific, measurable, achievable, relevant, timely) goals for the rotation, clinical teachers not only support their growth mindset, but they become aware of key areas for observation and feedback.

In addition, the learning environment can be enhanced by utilizing best practices for orienting your learners. This should include addressing inclusive teaching, psychological safety, and creating an environment where they feel supported, know what is expected and feel like they can achieve their highest goals [35]. Expectation setting is key for learners to know what is required of them, and supporting clinical teachers in creating their own expectations is an important first step before they can share those expectations with the learners.

These topics are all adaptable to large and small group settings, virtual or in person. Teaching these skills may require sessions designed to allow personal reflection and discussion around approaches to getting learners to write goals, creating your own expectations, and nurturing a growth mindset. Often, the discussion between individuals in the session (sharing their expectations, experiences that have worked) fosters more discussion and offers significant gains to individuals in creating their own process.

Observation

Direct observation is a key skill in a coach's toolbox and an essential component of competency-based medical education. Despite its importance (as described by the LCME and ACGME), the logistics of direct observation are often challenging, to say nothing of the motivation and skills of clinical teachers. Prior studies have revealed that clinical teachers can lack the time, comfort, and exposure to provide adequate observation, while residents have variable degrees of satisfaction with the experience. A 2024 study by Alex et al. offered a model for direct observation that can overcome some of the challenges, and while the study involved medical students, the model is easily transferable to residents [36].

While observation itself is an active skill, teaching the framework often is more about providing a framework and enhancing clinical teacher comfort. In the article noted above, many of the elements in the model are included in other parts of this chapter—goal setting, expectation setting, feedback, etc. Direct observation could be included in any of the discussions on those topics or this could be delivered as a stand-alone session, which could be virtual or hybrid, and can use active audience participation. A small group breakout is not necessary, but it could be used.

Autonomy and Supervision

The clinical learning environment offers a dynamic and robust experience for trainees to expand their skillset through experience, though that experience must be balanced with patient safety. This leads to the challenge of creating an environment with the ideal balance of supervision with autonomy. Clinical teachers have a wide range of comfort with that balance, despite it being an essential tension for development. Early studies, mostly in medicine, have shown that increased supervision enhances perception of patient care, clinical value of rotations, and education-related outcomes [37, 38], though more recent studies have shown that the pendulum may have swung too far in the direction of supervision [39, 40]. Entrustment assessment is key to the progression of trainees in their clinical skills, and faculty development can focus on best practices for entrustment decisions at various levels of training.

Teaching in the Clinical Environment

Once the clinical teacher sets the stage for learning, builds a safe learning environment, puts themselves in the coaching role, and ensures goal setting and observation, it is time to teach. Teaching in the clinical setting faces numerous challenges, including lack of time, patient care responsibilities, lack of learner engagement, and teacher discomfort.

There are many approaches that have been developed to optimize teaching in a time-limited environment that actively involves the learners. Both the SNAPPS [41] and One-Minute Preceptor models [42], which were created for teaching clinical reasoning in the outpatient setting, but can be adapted for the inpatient setting, have been shown to be impactful for learning. Either of these can be a strong foundational skill for clinical teachers. To increase the confidence of clinical teachers, the development of teaching scripts may be helpful. While exemplary teachers often create teaching scripts over time and experience, any clinical teacher can create teaching scripts for commonly encountered clinical scenarios. Lang and colleagues demonstrated the utility of collaborative development of teaching scripts that can then be shared, while the American Academy of Pediatrics Section on Hospital Medicine has a shared resource of previously developed scripts for inpatient pediatric topics [43]. In addition, clinical teachers can create their own using the templates as provided in this article or on this site. No matter what clinical setting, teaching with the patient is key to resident mastery of patient care and communication. Numerous articles have explored the best practices for clinical teaching, with Ramani giving 12 tips as far back as 2003 [44]. Working with clinical teachers to develop their own frameworks and commitment to bedside teaching is essential. Beyond what has been mentioned, there are numerous resources for clinical teaching from articles to apps, and all can be leveraged for faculty development [45].

An ideal way to teach this topic is, much like feedback, through role play, including the use of Objective Structured Teaching Encounters. While there are existing cases, it is not difficult to create cases for use. While you can address these topics in a virtual large group format, to include the largest number of participants, these skills are best learned and practiced in simulated settings and with ample feedback.

Summative Evaluations

While we have discussed the importance of formative feedback, which is essential for practice-based learning and improvement, summative feedback (or evaluations in the parlance of trainees) is essential in the competency-based model of graduate medical education. According to the ACGME, "evaluation must be documented at the completion of the [resident] assignment" [2]. This process allows for documentation of the achievement of competencies, data that can then be used by the Clinical Competency Committees. Despite the requirement for this, there are significant challenges with summative feedback. Evaluations are often delayed from when the events occurred, lacking specifics for change. They also can have information in them that was not discussed during the rotation, leading to frustration by residents who did not have a chance to address the behaviors and improve. Additionally, there are often significant concerns regarding bias based on gender and race/ethnicity [46–48]. One study in neurosurgery found that trainees "perceived a lack of timeliness, vague categories misaligned with experiences, erroneous data, and rater variability," as well as gender differences [49]. Due to the importance of these within residency assessment and the challenges they pose, it is essential to train clinical teachers to create summative evaluations that are formative and helpful to the trainee.

While the literature to support best practices is sparse, with most focusing on the development of the actual tools for assessment, there are basic principles that should be considered in any faculty development in this area. First, it is essential to address how bias may impact summative assessment, and a discussion of bias should be incorporated into every discussion on this topic. While broader programs on bias are important, intentional focus on summative assessment is unique, and it should be incorporated accordingly. Building off that foundation, it is important to train clinical teachers on how to use specific tools. Tools can include end-of-rotation and real-time app-based evaluations among other models. Attention should be paid to the setting of the clinical encounter. Clinical teachers may only see the learner for one shift or they may work with them for a week of service. It is important to help clinical teachers appreciate the value of completing evaluations regardless of time spent with the learner. The interactions and observations may differ by practice location (e.g., outpatient, inpatient, emergency room), and thus, the clinical teachers should be trained with a lens toward their experience.

Much like other topics for clinical teachers, writing summative evaluations can be taught in a large group. However, we have seen the best success when faculty work through cases, utilizing formative feedback to complete an evaluation based on that scenario. Frameworks are key in teaching, but going through the exercise of writing the summative evaluation and then getting feedback on it is ideal. This can be done virtually or in person, and larger groups could work if there are enough facilitators.

Finally, we strongly encourage programs to utilize the expertise and experience of others. While a review of MedEdPORTAL and PubMed did not reveal many examples of best practices, the topic of summative assessment is often presented at national meetings such as the Association of Pediatric Program Directors, the Council on Medical Student Education in Pediatrics, and the Pediatric Academic Societies. Members of the residency program leadership can attend and bring what they learn back to their program. In addition, the broader institution outside of pediatrics may have resources for faculty development in this area. Regardless of where the training starts, it is essential to provide it to all clinical teachers so that the content of the summative evaluations is useful to help the residents grow while providing the program with the information needed for the broader assessment of the residents.

Additional Topics

While we have discussed some of the core teaching skills that clinical teachers need, there are additional topics that could be useful. These can include role modeling as a teaching tool, professionalism, and graduated autonomy. Resources for these topics (and many others) can be found on MedEdPORTAL and in apps like the Just in Time Teaching App.

Medical Educators

Apart from clinical teachers, medical educators have role modeling and educational responsibilities beyond the day-to-day teaching of learners in the clinical environment. These individuals, including core faculty, associate program directors, and designated coaches, typically have chosen a career path that involves medical education and can have greater success in their roles when equipped with training in key topic areas. Foundational knowledge of topics such as mentorship, leadership, coaching, curriculum development, and scholarship can help prepare medical educators for their roles as leaders within the residency program.

Coaching

Formal coaching programs are an increasingly prominent tool within medical education that offer a unique approach to helping residents achieve their fullest potential [50, 51]. A coach works with a learner by asking nonjudgmental questions to help set goals and probes the learner to identify ways of overcoming barriers to their goals [50, 51]. Coaching can be used to promote clinical performance, support professional or career development, promote well-being, and support a struggling learner. While many intensive longitudinal coaching training programs exist, a single faculty development session can introduce the concept of coaching and can expose faculty to some of the frameworks used by academic coaches. The primary focus of an introductory session should be to provide an opportunity for faculty to practice the use of coaching frameworks and questioning. This focus is particularly important because the coaching model differs from the mentor or advisor relationship in that it relies on asking probing questions under the assumption that the trainee holds the answer to the problem [50]. WOOP, R2C2, appreciative inquiry, and the 5Ds are easy models to introduce and use in role play during coaching workshops. Resources to learn more about these frameworks can be found on the AMA's Academic Coaching in Medical Education website [51].

This topic area is one of the few that is difficult to teach in a virtual or hybrid setting. Because incorporating coaching language requires practice, the ideal setting is one in which faculty members can be paired off and have dedicated time to practice coaching one another. The opportunity to implement those skills and sit on the receiving end of being coached helps emphasize the ways in which the skills differ from mentoring. Additionally, the debrief that occurs after practice helps bring awareness to the ways in which coaching is unique from other relationships. Program directors who are interested in establishing a new coaching program can use an introductory session to lay the groundwork; however, PDs should consider inviting an expert to do an extensive training program for their coaches prior to launching a nascent program. More can be learned about establishing a new coaching program in the AMA's *Coaching in Graduate Medical Education Handbook* [50].

Mentorship

Mentorship is a key component of graduate medical education training and is essential to fostering the growth of a pediatrician. A mentoring relationship is one in which someone with experience (mentor) helps someone else (mentee) in their academic, personal, and/or career development [52]. Mentorship typically occurs between a faculty member and a trainee; however, the relationship is not exclusive to that hierarchy and can occur between peers, colleagues, and interprofessional team members. The role of equity and inclusivity within mentorship has gained increasing attention in recent years. When strategizing mentorship programs and relationships, it is important to ensure that issues of equity, belonging, and inclusivity are prioritized, as mentorship can have lasting impacts on an individual's sense of belonging and attrition within the field.

The ACGME requires core faculty to have dedicated time to perform the activities necessary to train residents [2]. Among those activities is the responsibility of mentoring residents. Mentors are responsible for monitoring growth, providing support to those who struggle, and fostering career development [2]. While the ACGME mandates that mentors are provided to trainees, program directors are left with the ability to implement a mentorship system that best suits the needs of the program [53]. Best practices for designing mentorship programs within pediatrics GME do not exist; however, research confirms that most residencies have formal mentoring programs with very few providing training to the faculty on how to be an effective mentor [53].

Mentorship is a vital aspect of fostering trainee development; therefore, mentors should be prepared for the role by undergoing training. A faculty development workshop on mentoring should prepare core faculty with an understanding of the role that a mentor plays in a trainees' experience, the tools needed to serve as a strong mentor, and ways of overcoming common challenges faced by mentors. A faculty development session on mentorship should also focus on the role that bias can play in a mentorship relationship, particularly when working with a struggling learner [54].

While FD sessions can be tailored to meet the needs of individual programs, a plethora of resources exist to support program directors as they develop FD sessions to help empower their faculty members to be effective mentors. Sessions about mentorship can be held in person or virtually and are effectively taught in a typical didactic format. Tactics to engage learners include probing them to share examples of positive and negative mentorship.

Curriculum Development

Curriculum development is an essential skill for core faculty members, rotation directors, program directors, and other medical faculty who plan educational experiences and didactics. The ACGME mandates that program directors assign faculty member roles that allow them to plan, implement, and oversee the residents' educational experiences; however, faculty are often left without the training, skills, or resources needed to develop curricula in a systematic and effective way. Kern's six-step approach to curriculum development is a broadly embraced, systematic approach to curriculum development [55]. This framework is unique to medical education because medical educators have an obligation to the patient and society to translate knowledge to their learners. Using Kern's six steps, educators can identify learning needs, develop goals and aims to meet those needs, implement educational strategies, and then test the outcomes of their interventions. Empowering medical educators with the skills to develop curricula using Kern's six steps will both ensure that learning needs are met and will allow faculty who are investing time and energy into curriculum development to have a scholarly outcome from their investment.

Kern's steps involve the following: Step 1, problem identification and general needs assessment. During this step, a health problem or learning problem that needs to be addressed is identified. This step should be focused on finding the gap between what is currently happening and should ideally be happening. The next, Step 2, is the targeted needs assessment during which a deeper understanding is gained of why the gap exists at a local level. This step is focused on understanding the needs of the group of learners that are being targeted, and information gleaned during this step will help establish goals and objectives that address the identified problem. Step 3 is writing goals and objectives for the curriculum. Goals are the desired outcome of the curriculum, and objectives are specific and measurable things you want your learners to accomplish. This step is critical as it ensures that content needs are met. Step 4 is focused on identifying the educational strategies that will allow the identified objectives to be met. This step is focused on resources, content, and delivery methods. Step 5 is implementation. During this step, the curriculum is introduced. This step includes procuring resources, piloting the curriculum, engaging learners, addressing barriers, and often including refining the curriculum. The final step (6) is evaluation and feedback. The evaluation step allows the educator to ensure that the knowledge gap was closed, and the goals and objectives were met. Additionally, this step provides an outcome that can be used by the faculty should they decide to translate the curriculum into a scholarly project.

Faculty development sessions on curriculum development are best taught in a didactic format, either virtually or in person. It is most effective and helpful to guide attendees through the steps using an example. Attendees can be encouraged to bring an example curriculum they are developing, and the group can brainstorm the steps together. Alternatively, the presenter can use an example of a previously developed curriculum and can share the ways in which the six steps were executed.

Leadership

Leadership skills are essential for physicians and can empower and strengthen the practice of clinical medicine, in addition to preparing people for careers in advocacy, education, research, or administration. Sessions that specifically target leadership skills are key to a professional development curriculum for medical educators, but particularly important when new members are being added to the leadership team. Sessions should focus on defining different leadership styles, providing practical skills, and helping educators develop into strong leaders. Literature and background provided during the session need not come directly from the field of pediatrics or even medicine, but rather can be leveraged from a broad range of fields. In addition to definitions and skills, it is helpful to provide exposure to existing national leadership programs for those interested in gaining additional training in leadership, such as the Association of Pediatric Program Directors Leadership in Educational Academic Development (APPD LEAD) program. Finally, it is important to spend time teaching inclusive leadership skills and the benefits of diversity to the leadership team.

Leadership faculty development sessions can be held in person or remotely. A helpful way to engage faculty is to provide an assessment tool prior to the start of the session that helps attendees identify their leadership style. Distribution prior to the session can help attendees arrive primed and prepared to engage throughout the session.

Scholarship

The ACGME requires core faculty to engage in scholarship and report productivity annually. Additionally, faculty members are expected to mentor residents and fellows through research projects during training, and thus, it is imperative to have a baseline level of comfort with research. Even though these requirements exist, medical educators often have not received the training needed to engage in their own research or mentor others through a scholarly project. Faculty development sessions that focus on scholarship should have clear objectives and a realistic plan for what they hope to attain. Introducing attendees to the broad view of scholarship and providing information about institutional resources can be a helpful way of introducing the subject matter. Follow-up sessions can cover the general concepts more in depth, including a session dedicated to the skills needed to be a productive mentor to trainees engaging in scholarship. Finally, it is important to expose medical educators to existing faculty development programs that happen longitudinally, should they desire to learn more or enhance their training. Examples of such programs are outlined in Table 30.1.

Although this topic can be taught in the traditional didactic format, an alternative approach is to establish a scholarship group that is led by senior medical educators. These groups should be centered around similar topic areas (medical education, quality improvement, clinical research, medical ethics) and should be scheduled to meet at regular intervals. Group leaders can provide a brief topic overview at the start of the session, and the remaining time can be spent with attendees presenting works in progress and seeking support with questions or challenges they are facing. This format has proven to be helpful to not only create a community of practice but also in creating accountability checks and moving projects forward [56]. These groups also provide a safe and supportive venue where information can be shared about upcoming calls for submissions and topic-relevant conferences.

Table 30.1 Collaborators in pediatrics. These organizations are excellent sources of national priorities, general needs assessment data, and opportunities for collaboration (through listservs, subcommittees, and meetings)

Organization	Curriculum content	Assessment data	Examples of collaboration opportunities
Accreditation Council for Graduate Medical Education (ACGME)	Requirements for curricular content Asynchronous material such as Equity Matters	EPAS/milestones	Sponsored opportunities for residents and fellows such as *back to bedside*
American Board of Pediatrics (ABP)	Board content specification outline	Board pass rates Interactive pediatric workforce data	Resources for implementation of EPAs
American Academy of Pediatrics (AAP)	Pedialink Equipp	Policy statements and associated references	Sections related to subspecialties and interest groups
Association of Pediatric Program Directors (APPD)	APPD LESSON: curriculum content APPD LEARN: scholarship in medical education	National surveys can provide general needs assessment	Listserve with ability to ask questions
Council of Pediatric Subspecialties (COPS)	Webinars and descriptions of different subspecialties	Subspecialty EPAs and milestones	Committees and action teams
Council on medical student education in pediatrics (COMSEP)	Curricula transitioning from UME to GME	COMSEP clerkship competencies	Pathway to pediatric residency
FuturePedsRes	Curricular structure and initiatives of peds residency programs	Data on program sizes and highlights by program and region	Pathway to pediatric residency
Association of Medical School Pediatric Department Chairs (AMSPDC)	Resources for new chairs	Statements on the pediatric workforce	Committees and programs

Format and Delivery Methods

Format

Once the content areas have been selected, the next step is to determine what format to use and how you will ensure successful delivery of the content. The pandemic upended the traditional faculty development model that often utilized in-person, 1 h, or half-day workshops, but that often saw variable attendance. During the pandemic, these programs were shifted online, which made them more easily available to larger groups, but they also faced challenges of attendance due to the pandemic itself [57, 58]. Since the pandemic, faculty development has seen a shift from in-person to virtual or hybrid models, with each having different benefits. As faculty development is being planned, it is important to consider multiple aspects of delivery, including target audience, duration of session, timing of session, as well as the format of the delivery.

Before we consider the specifics of all these elements, it is worth discussing the value of communities of practice in teacher and educator development. The theory of communities of practice, first described by Lave and Wegner in 1991, recognizes the social context of learning for development [59]. The theory was being applied to medicine by the early 2000s and has since been discussed with regard to faculty development [56]. Leveraging these communities of practice when designing programming can result in faculty development options that are experiential, utilize mentorship and role modeling, and create an engaging and inclusive program. As format and delivery are considered, attention should be paid to the social context and community of practice for teachers and educators [60, 61].

Once the community of practice is considered, it is necessary to review the objectives of the session and the intended audience. Does the topic require small group discussion? Is it around a sensitive topic where trust is essential in the group? Will it benefit from skills practice, with or without a formal simulation center? Is the audience spread out across numerous sites? What are the clinical hours of the audience and when will they have time to attend a session? Are they 100% clinical or do they have protected time for a formal role that can be used for faculty development? Is it a topic that is essential for all clinical teachers or is it something that is for a smaller group? The answers to these questions impact the choices around format and delivery.

While we often start with a discussion of the most robust sessions, such as formal programs and retreats, the time limitations of clinical work for clinical teachers often necessitates creativity in the delivery of content. To address the time constraints, in 2007 educators at the University of Nevada developed Snippets. This innovation offers brief, structured sessions to teach specific skills. The sessions are 20 min and no more than 10 slides. Some topics stand alone, while other larger topics are divided into a series of snippets that can be incorporated into other larger meetings [62]. A train-the-trainer model is available through MedEdPORTAL [63, p. 15]

Often, it is easiest to fit faculty development into existing one-hour sessions. These fit neatly during lunch hours or at the end of the day, and depending on the size of the audience, can be didactics or focused workshops. Didactics offer the opportunity to address large groups to disseminate content to the most people possible, often due to a need in the program. If a didactic is the chosen approach, we highly encourage the use of interactive elements [64]. These can include case-based discussion, think–pair–share exercises, and team-based learning [65]. While interactivity can add time to a session, it also offers audience members a chance to interact with the material more and consider application to their practice.

The traditional workshop is still a highly regarded method for faculty development, and it can easily be incorporated into programming. Workshops can be anywhere from 1 to 3 h, though a common length is 1.5 h. These can fit nicely at the end of the day or midday, and they can accommodate a wide range of audience size depending on the activities and need for facilitators. Workshops should lean heavily on active learning when participants can learn new frameworks or approaches and either practice them or plan on how they might incorporate them into their practice. Small group activities and role plays are two common devices used to engage the audience and have them interact more with the material. An excellent guide to workshop development can be found on MedEdPORTAL [66].

When time is available, a half- or full–day retreat can be a highly successful method for delivering content in an interactive manner, while also enhancing the community of practice of clinical teachers and medical educators. While this approach depends on participants being able to secure a half or full day off from clinical duties, it allows for dedicated time to deeply engage in a broader program while building community with colleagues. This is a great option for a department when all members need to have training in multiple areas or if attendance cannot be guaranteed. The proposed date should be provided well in advance so that clinicians can request time off from clinical responsibilities.

There are several other strategies to provide more active learning and engagement, and these are often focused on smaller groups of participants at a time. Objective Structured Teaching Encounters (OSTEs) allow for structured, high-fidelity simulated teaching encounters to provide formative feedback on teaching skills [67, 68]. Clinical teachers practice their teaching skills with standardized learners (who can be trained medical students and residents), with feedback facilitated by trained faculty. The resources required can be reasonable if you train faculty to be facilitators and utilize current students or residents as standardized learners. For a more "in vivo" experience, peer observation of teaching or peer coaching in teaching skills capitalizes on the peer coaching model, improves morale and motivation, increases self-awareness, and decreases anxiety [69, 70]. While David Irby first referenced the concept in 1983, more recent studies have demonstrated the feasibility and impact of a peer-to-peer model [71, 72]. Several models exist including peer observation programs and exemplary programs, with each offering the ability to have teaching observed in a real environment with immediate, structured feedback. These have been shown to be effective and engaging methods for faculty development.

A few other models exist for faculty development that deserve a brief mention. Over the past decades, some institutions have developed certificate programs for clinical teachers and medical educators. These take the form of a longitudinal series of didactics, workshops, and discussion sessions, with some having capstone projects. While there are national versions of these, such as the Advancing Pediatric Educator eXcellence (APEX) Teaching Program and the Educational Scholars Program (ESP), these can be created at individual sites. If they are developed in pediatrics, they can be offered to the broader institution as well. They offer the opportunity for progressing the content, more active participation and investment by the participants, and a consistent community of practice. While these programs are not necessary, their frequent use merits mentioning.

Faculty development sessions have traditionally been taught in a lecture format; however, hybrid learning is an educational innovation that became mainstream during the COVID-19 pandemic and has remained prevalent [73]. Although virtual learning has several limitations, hosting faculty development sessions remotely offers the opportunity for faculty with varying schedules and located at different sites to attend. Table 30.1 outlines the suggested format for each topic area and describes the reasoning behind the choice for in person, which is usually to facilitate role play, team development, or discussion.

One of the largest challenges with faculty development sessions is motivating faculty to attend. The concept of educational RVUs (eRVUs) has emerged as a way of placing value on the educational mission of academic centers [74]. At institutions where eRVUs exist or can be established, assigning eRVUs to faculty development sessions can be a very powerful way to motivate faculty to attend. Similarly, providing continuing medical education (CME) credits can serve as a carrot to encourage attendance. Other models that have been successful at engaging faculty in sessions include financial incentives for participation or linking participation to bonus structures [43, 75]. Finally, it is important to remember the principles of adult learning theory when building faculty development sessions. Harnessing the adult learners' intrinsic motivation and their desire for experiential learning can empower the session creators to incorporate active and relevant learning that will inspire educators to attend. Advertising for faculty development sessions should highlight the opportunities for career success and advancement that can result from participation in the sessions.

Counting Twice

While the immediate goal of faculty development is to improve the skills of departmental clinical teachers and medical educators, it is important to consider, even briefly, how the work can be made to "count twice." The topics we have listed are the foundational ones, but they are by no means the only ones. As graduate medical education evolves, there will be other important topics for faculty development, while there also may be institution-specific needs. Program directors should feel empowered to introduce new topic areas, especially when new areas of need emerge within the department and program. Program directors should also trial innovative educational approaches to faculty development.

Novel topics or formats can be introduced locally or in collaboration with educators at other institutions. The multi-institution approach is particularly appealing when seeking to create a scholarly product. As these faculty development sessions are developed, medical educators should consider how they can disseminate the work they are doing to enhance their own scholarship. To do so, faculty development leaders should consider how to measure outcomes for their individual sessions or broader programs, as well as what is innovative about their topic or approach. Keeping the work grounded in Kern's six steps can be impactful for creating a scholarly product. Using the approach of conducting a needs assessment, establishing objectives, and collecting data with an evaluation tool will provide the framework for successful scholarship.

Several journals have opportunities to publish educational innovations, including the *Journal of Graduate Medical Education* (JGME) and *Academic Pediatrics*. JGME welcomes Educational Innovations and Brief Reports, both of which allow for the sharing of new curriculum that may not have the multisite outcomes of traditional research. *Academic Pediatrics* invites submissions as Brief Reports and Articles on Educational Research. MedEdPORTAL, referenced several times in this chapter, is an open-access journal for educational resources in the health professions. It is MEDLINE-indexed and peer reviewed. Beyond being an area to publish work, it is also a phenomenal resource for existing workshops that can be used, especially when your program does not have many faculty development leaders. If publication seems too daunting, posters and workshops at national meetings are another way to share what you are doing, while also attracting collaborators who can create a multisite use of the innovation (Table 30.2).

We highly encourage programs who are doing the work to develop unique and successful programs to disseminate them so that others can benefit from the efforts they took to build them.

Table 30.2 Faculty development topic areas with recommended content and format for clinical teachers and medical educators

Topic	Recommended content	Resources	Suggested format
For clinical teachers			
Feedback	Differentiate formative and summative feedback Describe elements of effective feedback Discuss and address challenges of feedback Introduce a framework for feedback (e.g., ATA, R2C2) Emphasize the importance of culture and feedback	Ende [15] Watling [17] Dolan [18] French [76] Sargeant [77]	Didactic for general overview and reaching large numbers of faculty Small group with role plan for practice Objective Structured Teaching Encounters
Learning climate and coaching	Describe the learning climate Identify elements that influence it Describe coaching in the clinical realm Introduce a framework for coaching in the clinical setting	Krupat [27] Jacobsen [78] Lombarts [28]	Interactive didactic—Interactive worksheet to develop own approaches to learning climate
Goals and expectations/Growth mindset	Introduce the value of goal writing to learner achievement Define effective goals through SMART goals Discuss expectation setting and orientation	Cook [33] https://bloomstaxonomy.net Gifford [35] Dweck [79]	Large group with individual work
Clinical teaching approaches	Offer a framework for on-the-fly teaching (e.g., one-minute preceptor, SNAPPS, teaching scripts)	Wolpaw [41] Neder [42] Lang 2012 Ramani [44] Fornari [80]	Large group with small group breakout OSTEs Apps
Summative assessment	Provide a framework for effective learner evaluations Describe bias mitigation for learner evaluations Introduce best practices in learner assessment		Large group with individual work and report back
For medical educators			
Coaching	Define coaching in medical education Share frameworks used in coaching Using role play, practice different coaching frameworks (WOOP, R2C2, appreciative inquiry, 5Ds)		Didactic Review of frameworks Role play practicing coach language and frameworks Debrief *Ideally in person to optimize roleplay*

(continued)

Table 30.2 (continued)

Topic	Recommended content	Resources	Suggested format
Mentorship	Define mentorship Share benefits, challenges, of mentorship programs Provide tips for being a good mentor and mentee Provide examples of successful mentorship models	Aylor [52] AAMC Tips for Finding and Working with a Mentor [81] Saint 2014 [82] Gustafson [53]	Traditional didactic *Can be done in person or* via *zoom*
Curriculum development	Describe the six steps of curriculum development and relevant components of each step 1. Problem identification/general needs assessment 2. Targeted needs assessment 3. Goals and objectives 4. Educational strategies 5. Implementation 6. Evaluation and feedback Describe FINER criteria for evaluating a scholarly question Writing goals and objectives	Thomas [55] Martin [83] Navigating the Research Landscape: A Deep Dive into the FINER method [84] https://bloomstaxonomy.net	Traditional didactic Attendees can be encouraged to bring a curricular idea that they want to develop and can use a worksheet to workshop the steps for their idea *Can be done in person or* via *zoom*
Leadership	Practical and theoretical knowledge Leadership styles Leadership skills Exposure to local and national longitudinal leadership training programs (APEX, APPD LEAD, ELAM)	AAMC Leadership Training [85] Steinert [61] Oza [86]	Traditional didactic Incorporation of leadership tests Longitudinal development of skills, rather than a single session Can include peer coaching *Ideally in person to optimize conversation, cohort development, and group work*
Scholarship	Personal scholarship Types of scholarship Asking a scholarly question Finding a community of practice Mentoring trainees through scholarship Setting expectations Benefits and challenges of mentoring trainees Communicating with trainees	APA'S educational scholars program (ESP) https://www.academicpeds.org/program/educational-scholars-program/ Ryan [87] Beattie [88]	Traditional didactic Scholarship groups or communities of practice *Can be done in person or* via *zoom*

References

1. McLean M, Cilliers F, Van Wyk JM. Faculty development: yesterday, today and tomorrow. Med Teach. 2008;30(6):555–84. https://doi.org/10.1080/01421590802109834.
2. ACGME. Common Program Requirements. https://www.acgme.org/Specialties/Program-Requirements-and-FAQs-and-Applications/pfcatid/16/Pediatrics/. Accessed 27 May 2021.
3. Common Program Requirements – Fellowship.
4. Schultz KW, Kolomitro K, Koppula S, Bethune CH. Competency-based faculty development: applying transformations from lessons learned in competency-based medical education. Can Med Educ J. 2023;14(5):95–102. https://doi.org/10.36834/cmej.75768.
5. Orr C, Sonnadara R. Coaching by design: exploring a new approach to faculty development in a competency-based medical education curriculum. Adv Med Educ Pract. 2019;10:229–44. https://doi.org/10.2147/AMEP.S191470.
6. Glossary. https://www.acgme-i.org/accreditation-process/glossary/. Accessed 7 Aug 2024.
7. Sherbino J, Snell L, Dath D, Dojeiji S, Abbott C, Frank JR. A national clinician-educator program: a model of an effective community of practice. Med Educ Online. 2010;15 https://doi.org/10.3402/meo.v15i0.5356.
8. Alexandraki I, Baker R, Kern A, Beck Dallaghan GL, Seegmiller J. Faculty Development for community preceptors: a narrative review of the literature. J Gen Intern Med. 2023;38(6):1501–15. https://doi.org/10.1007/s11606-023-08026-5.
9. Taylor DCM, Hamdy H. Adult learning theories: implications for learning and teaching in medical education: AMEE guide no. 83. Med Teach. 2013;35(11):e1561–72. https://doi.org/10.3109/0142159X.2013.828153.
10. Knowles M. Adult learning processes: pedagogy and andragogy. Relig Educ. 1977;72(2):202–11. https://doi.org/10.1080/0034408770720210.
11. Armstrong E, Parsa-Parsi R. How can physicians' learning styles drive educational planning? Acad Med J Assoc Am Med Coll. 2005;80(7):680–4. https://doi.org/10.1097/00001888-200507000-00013.
12. The Academy of Medical Educators Professional Standards. https://www.medicaleducators.org/Professional-Standards. Accessed 7 Aug 2024.
13. Mahan JD, Kaczmarczyk JM, Miller Juve AK, et al. Clinician educator milestones: assessing and improving educators' skills. Acad Med. 2024;99(6):592. https://doi.org/10.1097/ACM.0000000000005684.
14. Simpson D, Marcdante K, Souza KH. The power of peers: faculty Development for medical educators of the future. J Grad Med Educ. 2019;11(5):509–12. https://doi.org/10.4300/JGME-D-19-00613.1.
15. Ende J. Feedback in clinical medical education. JAMA. 1983;250(6):777–81.
16. Lockyer J, Carraccio C, Chan MK, et al. Core principles of assessment in competency-based medical education. Med Teach. 2017;39(6):609–16. https://doi.org/10.1080/0142159X.2017.1315082.
17. Watling C, Driessen E, van der Vleuten CPM, Lingard L. Learning culture and feedback: an international study of medical athletes and musicians. Med Educ. 2014;48(7):713–23. https://doi.org/10.1111/medu.12407.
18. Dolan BM, Arnold J, Green MM. Establishing trust when assessing learners: barriers and opportunities. Acad Med J Assoc Am Med Coll. 2019;94(12):1851–3. https://doi.org/10.1097/ACM.0000000000002982.
19. Baker K, Haydar B, Mankad S. A feedback and evaluation system that provokes minimal retaliation by trainees. Anesthesiology. 2017;126(2):327–37. https://doi.org/10.1097/ALN.0000000000001471.
20. Ramani S, Post SE, Könings K, Mann K, Katz JT, van der Vleuten C. "It's just not the culture": A qualitative study exploring residents' perceptions of the impact of institutional culture on feedback. Teach Learn Med. 2017;29(2):153–61. https://doi.org/10.1080/10401334.2016.1244014.
21. Bing-You R, Varaklis K, Hayes V, Trowbridge R, Kemp H, McKelvy D. The feedback tango: an integrative review and analysis of the content of the teacher-learner feedback exchange. Acad Med J Assoc Am Med Coll. 2018;93(4):657–63. https://doi.org/10.1097/ACM.0000000000001927.
22. Balmer DF, Tenney-Soeiro R, Mejia E, Rezet B. Positive change in feedback perceptions and behavior: A 10-year follow-up study. Pediatrics. 2018;141(1):e20172950. https://doi.org/10.1542/peds.2017-2950.
23. Fainstad T, McClintock AA, Van der Ridder MJ, Johnston SS, Patton KK. Feedback can be less stressful: medical trainee perceptions of using the prepare to ADAPT (ask-discuss-ask-plan together) framework. Cureus. 2018;10(12):e3718. https://doi.org/10.7759/cureus.3718. PMID: 30906679; PMCID: PMC6428363.
24. Sargeant J, Lockyer J, Mann K, et al. Facilitated reflective performance feedback: developing an evidence- and theory-based model that builds relationship, explores reactions and content, and coaches for performance change (R2C2). Acad Med J Assoc Am Med Coll. 2015;90(12):1698–706. https://doi.org/10.1097/ACM.0000000000000809.
25. Cantillon P, Sargeant J. Giving feedback in clinical settings. BMJ. 2008;337:a1961. https://doi.org/10.1136/bmj.a1961.
26. Fromme HB, Ryan MS, Gray K, et al. A script for what ails your learners: feedback scripts to promote effective learning. Acad Pediatr. 2020;20(5):721–3. https://doi.org/10.1016/j.acap.2020.02.005.
27. Krupat E, Borges NJ, Brower RD, et al. The educational climate inventory: measuring students' perceptions of the Preclerkship and clerkship settings. Acad Med J Assoc Am Med Coll. 2017;92(12):1757–64. https://doi.org/10.1097/ACM.0000000000001730.

28. Lombarts KMJMH, Heineman MJ, Scherpbier AJJA, Arah OA. Effect of the learning climate of residency programs on faculty's teaching performance as evaluated by residents. PLoS One. 2014;9(1):e86512. https://doi.org/10.1371/journal.pone.0086512.
29. The postgraduate medical educational climate assessed by the Danish Residency Educational Climate Test (DK-RECT): a validation and cross-sectional observational study – PubMed. https://pubmed.ncbi.nlm.nih.gov/38087289/. Accessed 9 Aug 2024.
30. Hammoud MM, Dalrymple JL, Christner JG, et al. Medical student documentation in electronic health records: A collaborative statement from the Alliance for clinical education. Teach Learn Med. 2012;24(3):257–66. https://doi.org/10.1080/10401334.2012.692284.
31. Rassbach CE, Blankenburg R. A novel pediatric residency coaching program: outcomes after one year. Acad Med. 2018;93(3):430–4. https://doi.org/10.1097/ACM.0000000000001825.
32. Bannister SL, Wu TF, Keegan DA. The clinical COACH: how to enable your learners to own their learning. Pediatrics. 2018;142(5):e20182601. https://doi.org/10.1542/peds.2018-2601.
33. Cook DA, Artino AR. Motivation to learn: an overview of contemporary theories. Med Educ. 2016;50(10):997–1014. https://doi.org/10.1111/medu.13074.
34. Sawatsky AP, et al. Characteristics and quality of rotation-specific resident learning goals: a prospective study. Med Ed Online. 2020; 25:1. Google Search. https://www.google.com/search?q=Sawatsky+AP+et+al.+Characteristics+and+quality+of+rotation-specific+resident+learning+goals%3A+a+prospective+study.+Med+Ed+Online.+2020%3B+25%3A1.&rlz=1C5GCEM_en&oq=Sawatsky+AP+et+al.+Characteristics+and+quality+of+rotation-specific+resident+learning+goals%3A+a+prospective+study.+Med+Ed+Online.+2020%3B+-25%3A1.&gs_lcrp=EgZjaHJvbWUyBggAEEUYOdIBBzI5NWowajSoAgCwAgE&sourceid=chrome&ie=UTF-8. Accessed 9 Aug 2024.
35. Gifford KA, Choi E, Kieffer KA. Resources for clinical learning environment orientation. Med Educ Online. 2022;27(1):2013404. https://doi.org/10.1080/10872981.2021.2013404.
36. Alex CP, Fromme HB, Greenberg L, et al. Exploring medical student experiences with direct observation during the pediatric clerkship. Acad Med. 2024; https://doi.org/10.1097/ACM.0000000000005747.
37. Farnan JM, Petty LA, Georgitis E, Martin S, Chiu E, Prochaska M, Arora VM. A systematic review: the effect of clinical supervision on patient and residency education outcomes. Acad Med. 2012;87(4):428–42. https://doi.org/10.1097/ACM.0b013e31824822cc.
38. Haber LA, Lau CY, Sharpe BA, Arora VM, Farnan JM, Ranji SR. Effects of increased overnight supervision on resident education, decision-making, and autonomy. J Hosp Med. 2012;7(8):606–10. https://doi.org/10.1002/jhm.1959. Epub 2012 Aug 3.
39. Conner SM, Choi N, Fuller J, Daya S, Barish P, Rennke S, Harrison JD, Narayana S. Trainee autonomy and supervision in the inpatient clinical learning environment. Clin Teach. 2025;22(1):e13844. https://doi.org/10.1111/tct.13844. PMID: 39710509; PMCID: PMC11891390.
40. Mieczkowski AE, Gonzaga AMR, Kraemer K, Habicht R, Friedland AR, Rubio D, Van Deusen R. Perceptions of resident autonomy in internal medicine, pediatrics, and internal medicine-pediatrics. Cureus. 2021;13(3):e13805. https://doi.org/10.7759/cureus.13805. PMID: 33842175; PMCID: PMC8027953.
41. Wolpaw TM, Wolpaw DR, Papp KK. SNAPPS: a learner-centered model for outpatient education. Acad Med. 2003;78(9):893–8. https://doi.org/10.1097/00001888-200309000-00010.
42. Neher JO, Gordon KC, Meyer B, Stevens N. A five-step "microskills" model of clinical teaching. J Am Board Fam Pract. 1992;5(4):419–24.
43. Lang VJ, O'Connor AB, Blatt A, Gracey C. Collaborative development of teaching scripts: an efficient faculty development approach for a busy clinical teaching unit. J Hosp Med. 2012;7(8):644–8. https://doi.org/10.1002/jhm.1971.
44. Ramani S. Twelve tips to improve bedside teaching. Med Teach. 2003;25(2):112–5. https://doi.org/10.1080/0142159031000092463.
45. Zessis NR, Dube AR, Sadanand A, Cole JJ, Hrach CM, Daud YN. Teaching scripts via smartphone app facilitate resident-led teaching of medical students. BMC Med Educ. 2021;21(1):331. https://doi.org/10.1186/s12909-021-02782-w.
46. Boatright D, Anderson N, Kim JG, et al. Racial and ethnic differences in internal medicine residency assessments. JAMA Netw Open. 2022;5(12):e2247649. https://doi.org/10.1001/jamanetworkopen.2022.47649.
47. Yaman R, Hagen KM, Ghaith S, Luong H, Almader-Douglas D, Langley NR. Gender bias in medical education: A scoping review. Clin Teach. 2023;20(4):e13592. https://doi.org/10.1111/tct.13592.
48. Kukulski P, Schwartz A, Hirshfield LE, Ahn J, Carter K. Racial bias on the emergency medicine standardized letter of evaluation. J Grad Med Educ. 2022;14(5):542–8. https://doi.org/10.4300/JGME-D-21-01144.1.
49. Clarke MJ, Frimannsdottir K. Assessment of neurosurgical resident milestone evaluation reporting and feedback processes. Neurosurg Focus. 2022;53(2):E5. https://doi.org/10.3171/2022.1.FOCUS21734.
50. Coaching in Graduate Medical Education: A faculty handbook. https://cloud.e.ama-assn.org/24-0066-Coaching-GME. Accessed 9 July 2024.
51. Academic coaching in medical education. American Medical Association. https://www.ama-assn.org/education/accelerating-change-medical-education/academic-coaching-medical-education. Accessed 22 Jan 2023.

52. Aylor M, Cruz M, Narayan A, 2016 et al. Optimizing your mentoring relationship: a toolkit for mentors and mentees. MedEdPORTAL 12:10459. https://doi.org/10.15766/mep_2374-8265.10459.
53. Gustafson S, Shope M, Fromme HB, Orlov N. Need for time and training: pediatric program directors' perceptions about mentorship of residents. Acad Pediatr. 2024;24(2):330–7. https://doi.org/10.1016/j.acap.2023.09.001.
54. Wofford AM, Burton A, Dennin K, Gardner RT. Equity-minded mentoring toolkit. Inclusive Graduate School Network; 2023.
55. Thomas PA, Kern DE, Hughes MT, Chen BY. Curriculum development for medical education: a six-step approach. Johns Hopkins University Press; 2015. https://pure.johnshopkins.edu/en/publications/curriculum-development-for-medical-education-a-six-step-approach. Accessed 22 June 2024.
56. Cruess RL, Cruess SR, Steinert Y. Medicine as a Community of Practice: implications for medical education. Acad Med. 2018;93(2):185. https://doi.org/10.1097/ACM.0000000000001826.
57. Eltayar AN, Eldesoky NI, Khalifa H, Rashed S. Online faculty development using cognitive apprenticeship in response to COVID-19. Med Educ. 2020;54(7):665–6. https://doi.org/10.1111/medu.14190.
58. Buckley H. Faculty development in the COVID-19 pandemic: so close – yet so far. Med Educ. 2020;54(12):1189–90. https://doi.org/10.1111/medu.14250.
59. Lave J, Wenger E. Situated learning: legitimate peripheral participation. Higher Education from Cambridge University Press; 1991. https://doi.org/10.1017/CBO9780511815355.
60. de Carvalho-Filho MA, Tio RA, Steinert Y. Twelve tips for implementing a community of practice for faculty development. Med Teach. 2020;42(2):143–9. https://doi.org/10.1080/0142159X.2018.1552782.
61. Steinert Y. Faculty development: from workshops to communities of practice. Med Teach. 2010;32(5):425–8. https://doi.org/10.3109/01421591003677897.
62. Bar-on ME, Konopasek L. Snippets: an innovative method for efficient, effective faculty Development. J Grad Med Educ. 2014;6(2):207–10. https://doi.org/10.4300/JGME-D-13-00362.1.
63. Bowler C, Foshee C, Haggar F, Simpson D, Schroedl C, Billings H. Got 15? Try faculty development on the fly: a snippets workshop for microlearning. MedEdPORTAL. 2021;17:11161. https://doi.org/10.15766/mep_2374-8265.11161.
64. White G. Interactive lecturing. Clin Teach. 2011;8(4):230–5. https://doi.org/10.1111/j.1743-498X.2011.00457.x.
65. Guenther AR, Abbott CM. Think-pair-share: promoting equitable participation and in-depth discussion. Primer Peer-Rev Rep Med Educ Res. 2024;8:7. https://doi.org/10.22454/PRiMER.2024.444143.
66. Zenni EA, Turner TL. Planning and presenting workshops that work: a faculty Development workshop. MedEdPORTAL. 2021;17:11158. https://doi.org/10.15766/mep_2374-8265.11158.
67. Kay HG, Mahoney MR, Edwards RA. The objective structured teaching encounter (OSTE) in health professions education: a systematic review. Med Teach. 2023;45(8):893–905. https://doi.org/10.1080/0142159X.2023.2189539.
68. Smith MA, Cherazard R, Fornari A, Adelman P, Snopkowski M, Lesser M. A unique approach to faculty development using an Observed Structured Teaching Encounter (OSTE). Med Educ Online. 2018;23(1):1527627. https://doi.org/10.1080/10872981.2018.1527627.
69. Schwellnus H, Carnahan H. Peer-coaching with health care professionals: what is the current status of the literature and what are the key components necessary in peer-coaching? A scoping review. Med Teach. 2014;36(1):38–46. https://doi.org/10.3109/0142159X.2013.836269.
70. Huston T, Weaver CL. Peer coaching: professional development for experienced faculty. Innov High Educ. 2008;33(1):5–20. https://doi.org/10.1007/s10755-007-9061-9.
71. Siddiqui ZS, Jonas-Dwyer D, Carr SE. Twelve tips for peer observation of teaching. Med Teach. 2007;29(4):297–300. https://doi.org/10.1080/01421590701291451.
72. Stockdill M, Hendricks B, Barnett MD, Bakitas M, Harada CN. Peer observation of teaching: a feasible and effective method of physician faculty development. Gerontol Geriatr Educ. 2023;44(2):261–73. https://doi.org/10.1080/02701960.2021.2019030.
73. Wang X, Liu J, Jia S, et al. Hybrid teaching after COVID-19: advantages, challenges and optimization strategies. BMC Med Educ. 2024;24:753. https://doi.org/10.1186/s12909-024-05745-z.
74. Beck Dallaghan GL, Wright ST, Plant J, Butani L, Morgenstern BZ. Educational relative value units as a measure of academic productivity: a systematic review. Cureus. 2023;15(4):e36995. https://doi.org/10.7759/cureus.36995.
75. Federico Martinez G, Giblin CR, Willis BC. Physician-faculty perceptions towards teaching incentives: a case study at a children's hospital. Med Educ. 2021;55(5):604–13. https://doi.org/10.1111/medu.14418.
76. French JC, Colbert CY, Pien LC, Dannefer EF, Taylor CA. Targeted feedback in the milestones era: utilization of the Ask-Tell-Ask Feedback Model to promote reflection and self-assessment. J Surg Educ. 2015;72(6):e274–9. https://doi.org/10.1016/j.jsurg.2015.05.016.
77. Sargeant J, Armson H, Driessen E, et al. Evidence-informed facilitated feedback: the R2C2 feedback model. MedEdPORTAL. 2016;12:10387. https://doi.org/10.15766/mep_2374-8265.10387.
78. Jacobsen RB, Boor K, Christensen KB, et al. The postgraduate medical educational climate assessed by the Danish Residency Educational Climate Test (DK-RECT): a validation and cross-sectional obser-

vational study. BMC Med Educ. 2023;23:943. https://doi.org/10.1186/s12909-023-04909-7.

79. Dweck CS. Mindset: The new psychology of success. Random House. 2006; https://adrvantage.com/wp-content/uploads/2023/02/Mindset-The-New-Psychology-of-Success-Dweck.pdf
80. Orner D, Conlon K, Affa M, Fornari A. Just in Time Teaching (JiTT) Infographics App for teacher development. J Grad Med Educ. 2022;14(3):344–5. https://doi.org/10.4300/JGME-D-21-01011.1. Epub 2022 Jun 13. PMID: 35754631; PMCID: PMC9200240.
81. 5 Tips for Finding and Working With a Mentor. Students & Residents. https://students-residents.aamc.org/choosing-medical-career/5-tips-finding-and-working-mentor. Accessed 9 Aug 2024.
82. Saint S, Chopra V. How doctors can be better mentors. Harvard Business Review. Published online October 4, 2018. https://hbr.org/2018/10/how-doctors-can-be-better-mentors. Accessed 9 Aug 2024.
83. Martin SK, Ahn J, Farnan JM, Fromme HB. Introduction to curriculum development and medical education scholarship for resident trainees: a webinar series. MedEdPORTAL. 2016;12:10454. https://doi.org/10.15766/mep_2374-8265.10454.
84. Services EA. FINER: a Research Framework | Elsevier Language Services. Elsevier Author Services – Articles. May 25, 2020. https://scientific-publishing.webshop.elsevier.com/research-process/finer-research-framework/. Accessed 9 Aug 2024.
85. Leadership Development. AAMC. https://www.aamc.org/career-development/leadership-development. Accessed 9 Aug 2024.
86. Oza SK, van Schaik S, Boscardin CK, et al. Leadership observation and feedback tool: A novel instrument for assessment of clinical leadership skills. J Grad Med Educ. 2018;10(5):573–82. https://doi.org/10.4300/JGME-D-18-00113.1.
87. Ryan MS, Quigley PD, Lee CC, et al. Innovation to Dissemination Workshop: Selecting Outcome Measures to Translate Educational Innovations Into Scholarship. MedEdPORTAL. 2018;14:10759. https://doi.org/10.15766/mep_2374-8265.10759.
88. Beattie DS, Scholarship GETCOASTFO. Expanding the view of scholarship: introduction. Acad Med. 2000;75(9):871.

Part VIII

Innovation and the Future of Pediatric Education

The Future of Pediatric Education: Challenges, Opportunities and Innovation

31

Megan E. Aylor, Aisha Barber, and Mike Weisgerber

Challenges in Pediatric Medical Education

Pediatric Workforce: NASEM Report and Future Directions

Pediatricians are at the forefront of delivering and advancing high-quality, evidence-based care for children. Both general pediatricians and pediatric subspecialists play crucial roles in preventing, diagnosing, and treating childhood diseases through direct patient care and innovative research. Their work is essential in driving scientific and clinical advancements within the field. Improving care for children not only leads to healthier adults but also has the potential to reduce overall healthcare costs and societal burdens. However, challenges such as poverty, structural and institutional racism, and inadequately managed chronic medical and mental health conditions continue to threaten the health of youth. Given the increasing complexity of these issues, the role of pediatricians is more critical than ever for the health of our nation. Building a robust pediatric workforce is essential to meet the needs of today's children and the adults of tomorrow [1, 2].

Despite this pressing need, the US healthcare system has historically underinvested in pediatric care. As a result, our pediatric workforce falls short of meeting both current and future demands. Long wait times for appointments lead to delayed diagnoses and treatments, and there are significant disparities in accessing subspecialty care. Moreover, the healthcare system's disincentives further hinder recruitment into pediatrics, disproportionately affecting individuals from underrepresented backgrounds and impeding efforts to create a diverse workforce that reflects the populations we serve. Although overall applications to residency programs have risen, applications for pediatric residency have declined, and many pediatric subspecialty fellowships had more open positions than applicants in the 2024 Match [3, 4].

In response to these challenges, the Pediatrics 2025: AMSPDC Workforce Initiative was launched in 2020. This initiative aims to increase the number and diversity of high-quality students entering pediatric, medicine-pediatric, and combined pediatric subspecialty training programs. It also seeks to enhance the supply and distribution of pediatric subspecialists to meet the diverse

M. E. Aylor
Oregon Health Sciences University, Portland, OR, USA

A. Barber
George Washington University and Children's National Hospital, Washington, DC, USA

M. Weisgerber (✉)
Medical College of Wisconsin – Milwaukee, Milwaukee, WI, USA
e-mail: mweisger@mcw.edu

H. McPhillips et al. (eds.), *Graduate Medical Education in Pediatrics*, Excellence in Medical Education 3, https://doi.org/10.1007/978-3-032-12952-9_31

needs of US children, adolescents, and young adults [5, 6]. To support this goal, AMSPDC partnered with the National Academies of Sciences, Engineering, and Medicine (NASEM) and a coalition of sponsors to establish the Committee on the Pediatric Subspecialty Workforce and Its Impact on Child Health and Well-Being. This committee has outlined several strategies and actions to develop a pediatric physician workforce capable of delivering high-quality clinical care and conducting cutting-edge research [1]. AMSPDC remains committed to this mission through ongoing efforts with the Pediatric Workforce Initiative. Pediatric graduate medical education (GME) leaders play a pivotal role in recruiting and training the next generation of pediatricians and should be well-acquainted with the action plan domains outlined in this initiative.

Economic Strategy

There are significant financial disincentives associated with practicing pediatric medicine, particularly in pediatric subspecialty care. Pediatric providers earn approximately 25% less than their adult medicine counterparts, and pediatric subspecialists experience a lifetime earnings shortfall averaging $1.2 million compared to general pediatricians. This disparity largely stems from differences in funding for child health, an overreliance on relative value units (RVUs) for reimbursement, and a focus on remunerating procedural interventions over preventive or nonprocedural care.

The financial inequity extends to policies surrounding pediatric graduate medical education (GME) funding as well. Children's Hospital GME (CHGME) funding, which supports more than half of pediatric residency positions and the majority of pediatric subspecialty fellowship positions, is less than half of what Medicare GME provides per trainee. Addressing these financial disparities requires substantial reform to ensure equitable reimbursement and eliminate the financial barriers to providing pediatric care and training future pediatric residents and fellows.

Redesigning Medical Education/ Enhance Education, Training, Recruitment, and Retention

As practice models evolve, so too must pediatric medical education. Early exposure to pediatrics and pediatric subspecialties through robust pathway programs and clinical experiences during medical school is crucial for recruiting future pediatricians. Graduate medical education (GME) curricula should be designed with the primary goal of meeting patient needs, incorporating comprehensive exposure to pediatric subspecialties.

As trainees spend more time in ambulatory care settings and benefit from flexible, individualized curricula, it is essential that their roles as residents and fellows are not marginalized, and that graduated autonomy is maintained. The advancements in competency-based and precision medical education make time-variable training increasingly feasible.

To address healthcare disparities and meet patient needs effectively, it is imperative that programs focus on recruiting a diverse workforce that mirrors the populations we serve. Moreover, program and hospital leaders must foster inclusive training and working environments to promote a sense of belonging and enhance the retention of a diverse workforce.

Physician Scientist

Pediatric research is continually advancing our capacity to diagnose and treat pediatric diseases. Conditions once considered incurable are now being effectively managed through innovations such as gene therapy, precision medicine, and bone marrow transplantation. A strong pediatric physician-scientist workforce is essential for sustaining this trajectory of innovation and discovery, which is crucial for optimizing child health.

To support this vital workforce, practical measures are needed, including the expansion of the pediatric subspecialty loan repayment program and the enhancement of career development awards for physician-scientists. These supports are critical for fostering the next generation of researchers and ensuring the continued advancement of our field's scientific frontiers.

Practice Models

Team-based care, integrated care, embedded specialties within primary care, telehealth, and e-consults are innovative models that pediatricians have adopted to integrate general pediatric care with subspecialty services. By expanding and refining these models and advocating for insurers to provide appropriate compensation for these systems, we can enhance the effectiveness and reach of both general pediatric and subspecialty care. These efforts will be crucial in optimizing the capacities of our workforce and improving patient outcomes.

Diversification of the Workforce

A core focus of all NASEM domains is the development of a diverse pediatric workforce that mirrors the populations we serve. Building this diverse workforce requires not only targeted efforts to recruit trainees from underrepresented backgrounds but also a commitment to fostering inclusive learning and work environments that promote a sense of belonging for all trainees.

As the workforce initiative progresses, pediatric medical educators will be pivotal in driving the recruitment, innovative training, and retention of future pediatricians. Their role will be essential in shaping a workforce that is both diverse and well-equipped to meet the evolving needs of our patients.

Finance and Medical Education

The financing of graduate medical education (GME) in pediatrics is a multifaceted issue that intersects with national loan repayment programs and initiatives, institutional resources, trainee educational debt, and racial/ethnic disparities, shaping the career trajectories of aspiring pediatricians.

GME Financing

GME is an essential public investment in the future physician workforce; however, less than 1% of the $1.4 trillion in federal and state expenditures on healthcare is allocated to GME [7]. For most teaching hospitals in the United States, the largest source of GME funding is from the Centers for Medicare and Medicaid Services (CMS), but for pediatric training programs that are based at a children's hospital the major sources of GME funding are the Children's Hospital Graduate Medical Education (CHGME) Payment Program and Medicaid [8]. There are shortages in pediatric subspecialists in many fields, with insufficient recruitment of new fellows. The current system of funding GME is inadequate for the needs of the pediatric workforce. A cross-sectional study of 519 fellowship directors in 14 pediatric subspecialties revealed that funding limitations restricted program size (22% of programs) and educational resources (36% of programs). Nineteen percent of programs felt their funding was insecure. Perceived financial insecurity of fellowship programs was strongly associated with smaller program size, nonhospital-based funding sources, and unfilled positions [9]. Potential future directions for increased financial support of pediatric fellowships from an invited commentary from the Council for Pediatric Subspecialties (COPS) for AMPSDC are described in Table 31.1 [9, 10].

Table 31.1 Expenses associated with pediatric fellowship programs and potential strategies for support from Heyman et al. [2]

Expense	Potential strategies
Fellowship program director administrative time	Fund from clinical revenues Negotiate additional support from the hospital Shift funding from other areas in department Centralize departmental administrative support
Funding for fellows	Collaborate with adult T32-supported programs Recruit trainees who are funded by military or foreign government agency Obtain grants from subspecialty or disease-specific organizations, philanthropy, government agencies, pharmaceutical companies, community organizations Fellow personal expenses Provide housing supplement to fellows Support loan repayment programs Establish national repository of resources for fellows

Trainee Debt: Implications for Career Choice and Satisfaction

The impact of trainee debt on career choices and job satisfaction of pediatricians has been a subject of growing concern. Cull et al. studied the impact of trainee debt on the career trajectories of pediatricians a decade after completing residency and found that pediatricians burdened with higher levels of debt are more likely to gravitate toward higher-paying subspecialties or practice settings to alleviate their financial burdens [11]. A cross-sectional study of data obtained during the ABP subspecialty in-training examination (included 15 different subspecialties) post-examination survey in 2018, 2019, and 2021 showed that individuals with $200,000 to <$300,000 of educational debt were 1.4 times more likely than those with no educational debt to be in a positive lifetime earnings potential subspecialty [12]. A recent analysis titled "Comparison of Calculations of the Financial Impact of Fellowship Training by Data Source" published in *JAMA*, 2023, showed the wide variation in lifetime relative net present values by pediatric subspecialty (Figs. 31.1 and 31.2), with the lowest values corresponding to the most undersubscribed pediatric subspecialties [13].

The burden of educational debt disproportionately affects individuals from underrepresented racial and ethnic groups, influencing their decision-making regarding career paths in pediatrics [12]. When stratified by educational debt, there was an interaction between trainee race/ethnicity and mentorship. The higher the educational debt, the less important mentorship was ranked in importance of factors influencing career decisions, with the largest effect noted among Black/African American physicians [12]. For some pediatric trainees, having to focus on debt management may create a misalignment between career aspirations and personal interests, potentially affecting job satisfaction and overall career

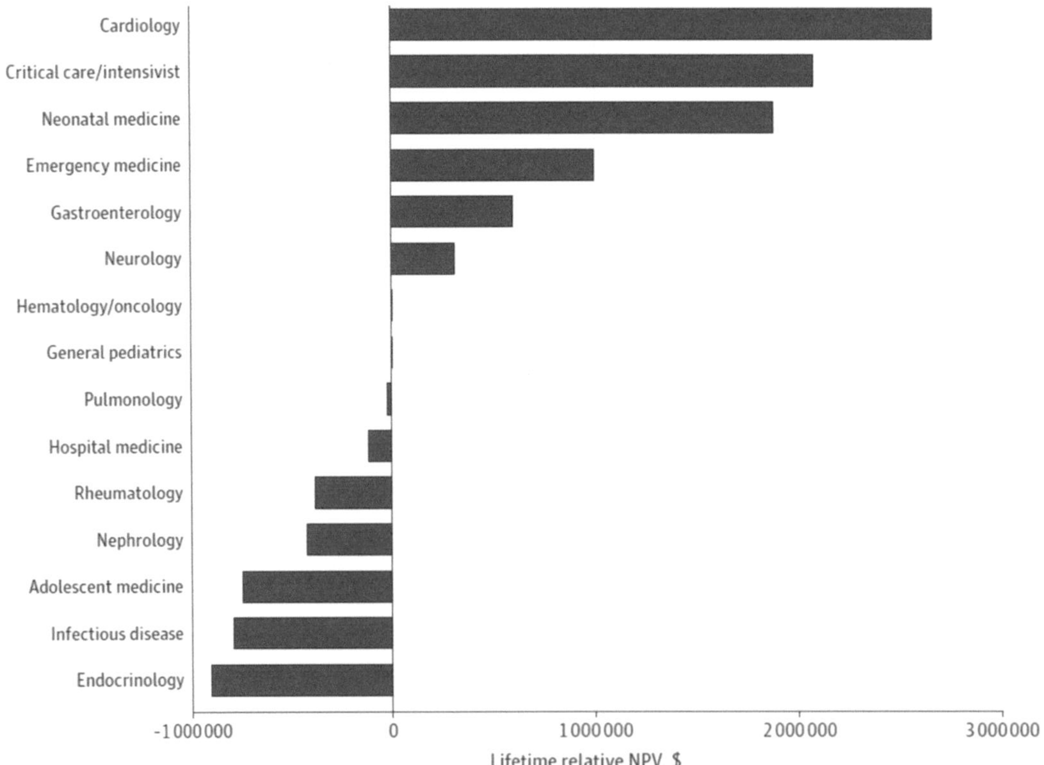

Fig. 31.1 Lifetime relative net present values (NPVs) by subspecialty according to the Association of American Medical Colleges

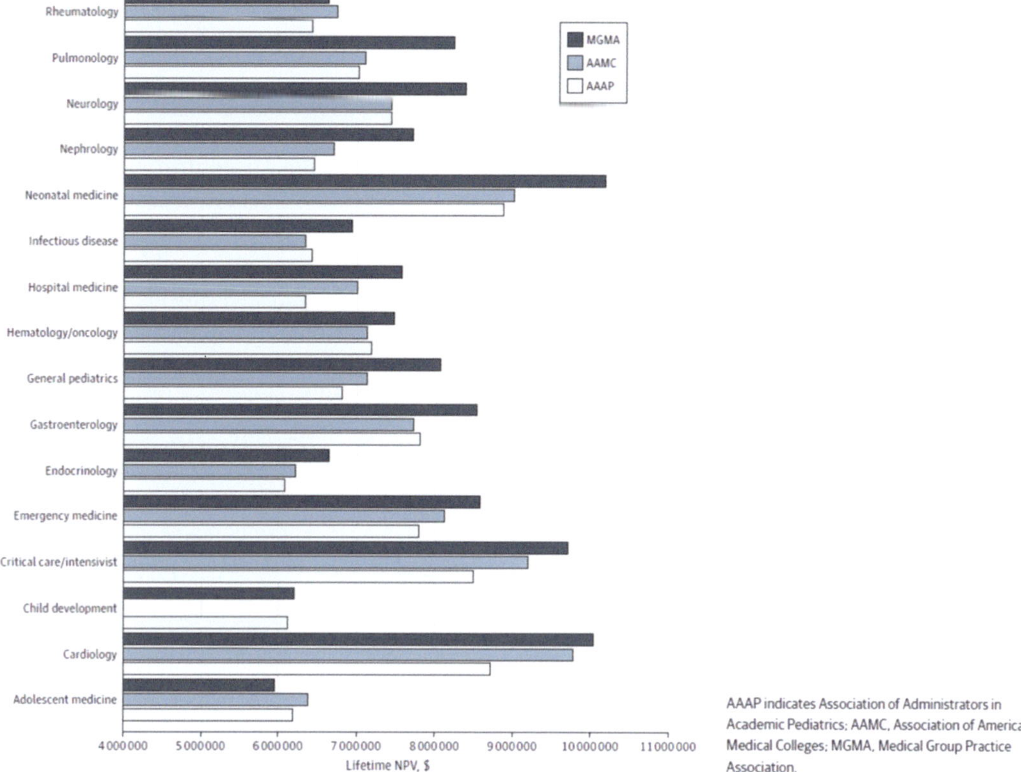

Fig. 31.2 Subspecialties with the greatest and least lifetime NPV for each data source

fulfillment. Understanding the lasting effects of trainee debt is essential to support the financial well-being and professional satisfaction of pediatric practitioners, ensuring that career choices are guided by passion and purpose rather than financial constraints. There is an urgent need to address disparities in educational debt to ensure equitable access to pediatric training opportunities for all aspiring healthcare professionals.

Loan Repayment Programs: A Vital Tool for Growing the Pediatric Specialist Workforce

Recognizing the challenges posed by educational debt and its impact on career decisions, loan repayment programs have emerged as a vital tool to expand the pediatric specialist workforce. There are new loan repayment initiatives to promote pediatricians in pursuing careers practicing in underserved areas and subspecialties. By offering financial assistance in exchange for a commitment to practice in communities with limited access to care, loan repayment programs have the potential to alleviate the financial burden on pediatric trainees, promote workforce diversity, and address healthcare disparities in pediatric practice [14]. Through targeted interventions that support pediatricians in areas of need, loan repayment programs play a pivotal role in shaping the composition and distribution of the pediatric specialist workforce with the goal of enhancing access to quality care for all children.

Addressing Mental Health and Well-Being of Pediatric Trainees, Faculty, and Educational Leaders

Concerns about the well-being of faculty and trainees and increased rates of burnout and challenges with mental health are increasing in pediatrics.

Well-Being of Faculty and Educational Leaders Pediatricians identified three key barriers to well-being: collective pressures, including increasing and competing academic and clinical responsibilities; low-value tasks that consume their time; and erosion of personal life [15]. Faculty reporting a good global fit of their career activities experienced the most personal fulfillment, least burnout, and least intent to leave academic medicine. Having dedicated administrative time in meaningful nonclinical areas contributed to less intent to leave academic medicine while having increased clinical time even if clinical work was described as fulfilling was associated with increased burnout and intent to leave academic medicine [16].

Well-Being of Trainees

Burnout is a significant concern among pediatric residents, and early intervention is needed to prevent negative outcomes [17]. Residents have identified several barriers to pursuing mental health services, including inflexible schedules (82%), guilt about burdening colleagues (65%), fear of confidentiality breach (46%), and difficulty identifying services (44%) [18]. Around half of the pediatric fellows experience burnout, and many believe program directors, faculty, and their patients hold negative attitudes toward mental health problems and a need for treatment. Most fellows fear knowledge of their engagement in counseling could result in not being selected for employment [19].

The Pediatric Residency Burnout-Resilience Study Consortium (PRBRSC) created in 2016 involved more than 60 training programs in order to describe the epidemiology and relationships between burnout, resilience, empathy, and confidence in pediatric and medicine-pediatric residents over time while identifying modifiable factors and interventions that decrease burnout and promote wellness [20]. They discovered that burnout, including depersonalization and a low sense of personal accomplishment, can adversely affect patient care performance as assessed by pediatric milestones among PGY1 residents [21]. They further noted that interventions such as practicing mindfulness and self-compassion were longitudinally associated with lower stress and greater confidence in providing compassionate care [22].

A multisite study focused on creating a concept map for resident well-being was conducted by Babal et al., which identified eight domains aligning with four resident roles that were identified: (1) positive, safe, and diverse culture; (2) unity and connection; (3) professional fulfillment and mindset; (4) personal health and life satisfaction; (5) professional development and recognition; (6) schedule protections and downtime; (7) work systems and benefits; and (8) proactive and compassionate leadership. The eight domains aligned with the following roles: (1) individual, (2) colleague, (3) employee, and (4) emerging pediatrician [23]. These domains provide insight into valuable areas to target for programs striving to improve the well-being of their trainees. Pediatric senior residents and residency program leaders rated the importance of several domain ideas. Figure 31.3 shows both areas of agreement in priority and some notable mismatches. The greatest mismatch was "schedule protections and downtime" rated highest by residents at 4.12 and lowest by program leaders at 3.61 (Fig. 31.3) [23].

Pediatric training program leaders spend a significant amount of time supporting trainee wellness despite receiving little training in this area [24]. Addressing mental health and well-being in pediatric medical education is essential for creating a thriving community of healthcare professionals dedicated to pediatric care. By identifying risk factors for burnout, promoting support systems, and enhancing leadership practices, institutions could better foster a culture of well-being and resilience among pediatric trainees, faculty, and educational leaders.

Climate Health

Climate change is a significant threat to health worldwide, increasing the risk of heat-related illness, asthma, mental health disorders, infections, poor perinatal outcomes, trauma, and displace-

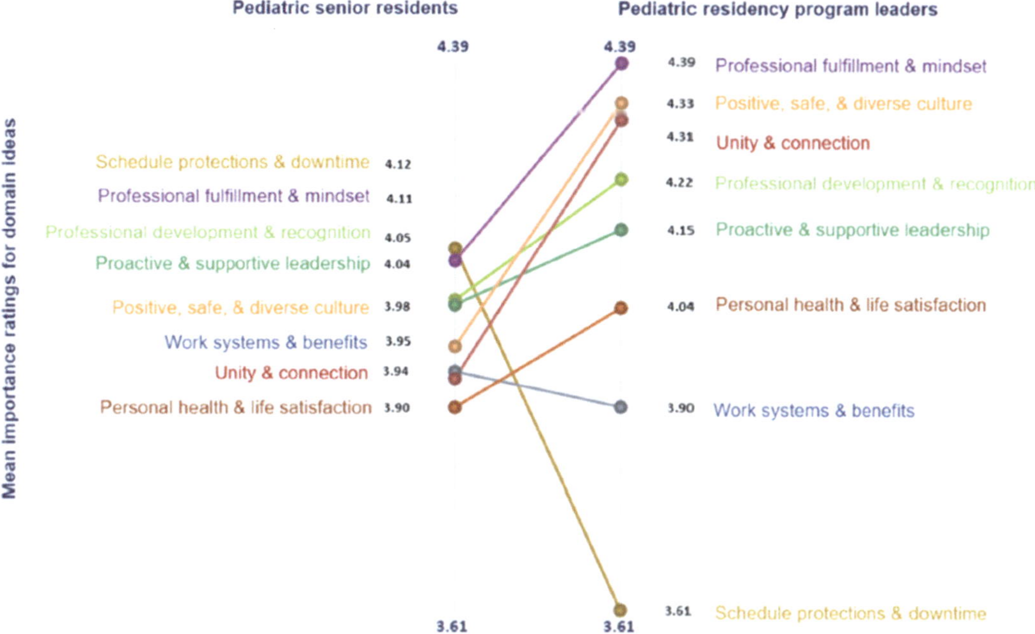

Fig. 31.3 Agreement in priority of well-being targets between senior residents and program leaders. (Figure taken from Babal et al. 2024) [23]

ment, among other harms [25]. In 2019, the American Medical Association created a resolution that was adopted as policy supporting climate change teaching throughout the continuum of medical education. The purpose of this policy was for trainees to have sufficient background knowledge in the science of climate change to "describe the risks that climate change poses to human health, and can counsel patients on how to protect themselves from the health risks posed by climate change." [26–29]

In studies, physicians largely understand that climate change is a human health risk and feel that physicians have a responsibility to advocate for policies that address the health effects of climate change. However, the importance of incorporating climate change into medical education is evident. In a large study of physicians worldwide, 41% of the 4000 physicians surveyed identified their own lack of knowledge about climate change as a factor limiting their communication about this topic. Physicians requested education and prompts about when to take advocacy action to overcome this barrier.

To guide the necessary education, between 2019 and 2021, the Planetary Health Alliance convened a task force to create a guiding framework. Created for practical application, the Planetary Health Education Framework [30, 31] provides an approach to their five climate health education domains: interconnection within nature, Anthropocene and health, systems thinking and complexity, equity and justice, and movement building and systems change. More specific to resident education, Philipsborn and colleagues propose a framework that focuses on how climate change "harms health, necessitates adaptation in clinical practice and undermines health care delivery." [25]

While all physicians require climate change knowledge, the specific impact of climate change varies by specialty. Pediatricians are uniquely poised to promote lifestyles that impact individual and community health via the socioecological model proposed for preventive care in pediatrics [32]. Hellden and co-authors created a conceptual framework for the intersection of climate change and child health based upon their 2021 scoping review [33]. This framework highlights both the causes of climate change and the specific health risks to children. It is inclusive of factors that increase the risk of disease, such as food insecurity, educational attainment, forced migration, toxicant exposure, and in utero exposure. The framework also highlights the specific health effects on child health, including the impact of extreme weather events, infectious diseases, respiratory diseases, and influence on mental health. Many of these areas would benefit from additional research, heightening the importance of early exposure to trainees who may opt to pursue scholarly work in climate health-related topics in the future.

Restrictive Laws Preventing Education and the Practice of Evidence-Based Medicine

Increasingly, the legislature has threatened the ability of academic medicine to enact the systematic change necessary to counteract a history of inequity. In recent years, awareness has grown in medical education prompting consideration of how we can better meet the needs of an increasingly diverse population, many of whom are minoritized and experiencing inequitable health outcomes. However, increasingly, state and national legal decisions restrict aspects of healthcare and healthcare education required to ensure that physicians are best prepared to address the needs of a diverse population. This legislature has a significant impact on populations for whom our healthcare system already marginalizes. Antidiversity, equity, and inclusion, the reversal of *Roe* versus *Wade*, and anti-transgender legislation have impacted healthcare delivery and medical education on state and national levels with significant negative outcomes.

EDI and Addressing Healthcare Disparities

Workforce diversity has been an area of focus for academic medicine given its link with equitable health outcomes. The argument in favor [34] of diversity has grown to recognize that the systemic challenges that inhibit diversity can also inhibit equity in healthcare for diverse or marginalized patient populations. Increasingly, there has been the recognition that the most effective way to improve workforce diversity in healthcare is to look at our systems [35, 36]. While medical education has been making efforts to improve workforce diversity and equity in graduate medical education, legislation has been passed to slow, pause, or prohibit these efforts, including race-conscious admission practices that pursue equitable admissions with intentionality.

Affirmative action is one of the strategies for [37] workforce diversity that is under scrutiny. Affirmative action is defined as "a set of procedures designed to; eliminate unlawful discrimination among applicants, remedy the results of such prior discrimination, and prevent such discrimination in the future." In 1961, President John F. Kennedy issued an executive order for equal opportunity that was considered the first official policy regarding affirmative action in the United States. This has been challenged a number of times since. In 1978, the Supreme Court issued a mixed decision in the case raised by Allan Bakke against [38, 39] the University of California at Davis after his admission was denied in the setting of 16% of the class acceptances being reserved for races and ethnicities considered minorities proposing that it violated Title VI of the Civil Rights Act of 1964 and the Fourteenth Amendment's Equity Protection Clause. The mixed decision indicated that the use of race-based quotas was not constitutional. However, they also noted that it is important to address past discrimination and that consideration of race, along with other factors, was constitutional in some circumstances where a solid argument and background are provided. In 2003, the Supreme Court ruled in *Grutter* v *Bollinger* [38, 40] that the University of Michigan Law School's race-conscious approach, viewing race as one of many significant factors for admissions, was constitutional, noting that all students benefit from a diverse study body. However, on the same day they ruled in *Gratz* v *Bollinger* [41] that it was not constitutional for the University of Michigan's undergraduate affirmative action program to utilize a point system based on race/ethnicity.

The 2023 decision of the US Supreme Court on cases brought by *Students for Fair Admissions* versus *University of North Carolina and Harvard College* is important because it overturned these decades of decisions. Despite being ruled against in lower courts over the preceding decade, the 2023 decision essentially overruled both the 1978 and 2003 cases, which had validated some race-conscious practices for the purposes of intentional action to correct the impact of discrimination.

Since then, numerous other bills have been proposed seeking to limit or prohibit diversity, equity, and inclusion initiatives. In Texas, for example, SB17 [42] requires "color-blind" hiring practices and prohibits the presence of offices or officers in higher education focused on diversity, equity, and inclusion. These bills have already significantly impacted the operations of state-funded GME programs or programs affiliated with a medical school in the impacted states. A currently proposed national bill, the Embracing Anti-Discrimination, Unbiased Curriculum, and Advancing Truth in Education (EDUCATE) Act (H.R. 7725 [43]), was introduced by numerous representatives in March 2024, proposing to amend the Higher Education Act of 1965 (P.L. 89–329) [44], no longer allowing schools to receive federal funding if they have certain diversity, equity, and inclusion policies and practices with provisions to undermine balancing by medical education regulatory bodies who currently require attention to diversity.

The impact of these policy changes is estimated to be profound. Of the 2023 Supreme Court decision, it has been noted that "the mandate provides little discussion, suggesting a lack of understanding of the downstream public health consequences to patients if medical school applicants are denied the benefits of race-conscious admissions policies." [45] In 2024, following the Supreme Court decision, the number of matriculants in US MD-granting medical schools from all groups that are historically underrepresented in medicine declined compared to 2023 data. Black or African American matriculants declined 11.6%; Hispanic, Latino, or of Spanish Origin matriculants fell 10.8%; and American Indian or Alaska Native matriculants declined 22.1% [46]. Continued vigilance and intentionality will be required to address the impact on healthcare workforce diversity important to the care of patients through both individual connections and the impact a diverse workforce has on the design of our systems that serve children [47].

Reproductive Health

After the Mississippi Gestational Age Act limited access to abortion care, Jackson Women's Health Center challenged this act on the grounds that it violated the decision in *Roe* versus *Wade* and *Planned Parenthood of Southeast Pennsylvania* versus *Casey* decades prior. After district and circuit courts affirmed that the Mississippi Act was a violation of the previous rulings, permitting abortion care, the case was brought to the Supreme Court on the grounds that the precedent-setting cases, including *Roe* versus *Wade*, were unconstitutional.

The June 24, 2022 [48–50], Supreme Court decision in the case of *Dobbs* versus *Jackson Women's Health Organization* overturned the long-standing decision in the *Roe* versus *Wade* case that had protected abortion rights. They now granted individual states the power to regulate abortion services [51]. In 2023, restrictions were also proposed for the US Food and Drug Administration's prior approval of mifepristone for use in medical abortions. The US Supreme Court rejected a case to restrict access to the mifepristone based on technicalities of the submission, leaving this case in the appellate courts [52].

Some clinician actions related to abortion are protected including evacuation of fetuses showing no signs of life or who are not expected to survive to full term and for the sake of the mother's health. As well, family planning should not be included in laws restricting abortion services. However, it is unclear how impacted these adjacent domains may become as state laws evolve. Currently, many of these actions are protected by legal language, but the interpretation of that language may vary, leading to a concern that some clinicians may hesitate to take action in life-threatening circumstances like ectopic pregnancies.

While some states already had laws restricting abortion prior to the Dobbs decision, within 10 months of the Dobbs decision, there were laws in 26 states restricting access to abortion, some of which included "abortion trafficking laws" or travel bans to receive abortions in other jurisdictions, particularly for minors . This impacts physicians, pharmacists, faculty, and other healthcare providers based on criminal liability that could ensue. After the Dobbs decision, 75 organizations came together to share their strong concern about the potential impact on patients and clinicians [53].

These laws impact medical education substantially. Shubkin et al. describe the impact of the Dobbs decision on all ACGME domains of residency training. For both professional and personal reasons, residents, fellows, and faculty may preferentially select training programs and jobs in states that have similar views as their own on abortion. Since the Dobbs decision, there was a notable reduction in applications to obstetrics and gynecology residencies in states where there were restrictive laws regarding abortion [54, 55]. This could have long-term consequences for patients in these areas if the climate discourages the recruitment and retention of physicians who would balance the legislative actions with advocacy, research, and clinical initiatives. Even in states without restrictive legislation, pediatric trainees may be impacted as there could be an influx of trainees across specialties from other states seeking opportunities to learn [56]. These collective challenges could lead to reductions in competency performing these abortions and related procedures and counseling, which could worsen patient outcomes.

Pediatricians are well positioned to help mitigate some of the health challenges resulting from these laws if their unique skill sets are more broadly applied or expanded. Pediatricians are trained to take a psychosocial history. Reproductive health could be improved if pediatricians are trained to ask about reproductive health and family planning even outside of the primary care setting, and expand their role to more consistently provide counseling about and prescribe contraception [57]. Further, it has been recommended that comprehensive reproductive health education for all general pediatrics trainees should include the topics of reproductive justice and community-based and policy-level advocacy. It is also important to provide training regarding ethical and legal considerations for when physicians do and do not agree with local and national laws, including conscientious objection and conscientious provision [58, 59]. It is critical to address the moral distress expected when physicians must deny access to care they feel strongly is necessary, but providing that care is now a felony. Finally, faculty development is recommended, so faculty are to mentor our trainees in these topics.

Gender-Affirming Care

Transgender and gender-diverse (TGD) youth face inordinate healthcare challenges. However, failure to provide affirming care is associated with healthcare avoidance, inequitable health outcomes, and healthcare avoidance [60]. Conversely, gender-affirming care models can not only begin to address healthcare inequities but improve mental health outcomes and save lives [61, 62]. The American Academy of Pediatrics has noted the need for "more formal training, standardized treatment, and research" to optimize gender-affirming care [63].

Increasingly, states have passed legislation restricting or banning the provision of gender-affirming care, which impacts the opportunities for trainees to learn to provide gender-affirming care. Gender-affirming care has been significantly impacted by a growing number of jurisdictions that further threaten their access to equitable care, making it extremely important for this to be a component of pediatric training.

In 2023, the American Academy of Pediatrics affirmed their 2018 policy statement "Ensuring Comprehensive Care and Support for Transgender and Gender-Diverse Children and Adolescents." [63] Key aspects of care that facilitate improved outcomes for TGD children and adolescents include adopting a gender-affirmative care model where it is made clear that TGD identities are not disorders but normal variations, are influenced by "biology, development, socialization, and culture," and that if a mental health issue exists, it may be due to the experiences of gender-diverse child in a society that is not gender affirmative. Further, pediatricians competent in social, legal, and medical affirmation as well as facilitating surgical affirmation could improve care. Education in family acceptance, healthcare inequities, and creating safe school environments are key educational topics for pediatricians.

It is important to take advantage of the opportunities existing in medical education to integrate this education. As medical education has been noted to tend toward affirmation of cisgendered norms, training programs are encouraged to incorporate both dedicated curricula and opportunities to learn about and practice gender-affirming care in core clinical experiences and routine educational modalities [64]. For example, Greene and colleagues describe the impact of including standardized patient cases focused on TGD patient care into an objective structured clinical examination (OSCE) [65]. This approach enabled them to identify that their residents underperformed in communicating about gender affirmation but appreciated the opportunity to practice improving their approach.

Opportunities

Though many challenges face the field of pediatric medical education, there are many opportunities in place to enhance and improve education for future pediatricians.

Inclusive Learning Environments

A diverse workforce is important to optimizing health outcomes for all, and a subsequent chapter will be dedicated to this subject. Often, diversity efforts focus on recruiting for a diverse workforce. However, inclusivity that fosters a sense of belonging and allows people from diverse backgrounds to optimally bring their attributes and skills to an environment is an essential concept to achieve the goal of a diverse physician workforce. Often, groups that are seen as "other" are expected to conform to the dominant culture [66]. However, inclusive learning environments do not require this conformity but respect and appreciate differences. Inclusive learning and work environments are important because they are thought to allow people from the nondominant culture to bring their best selves to the table, maximizing their well-being and contributions.

Cultivating Inclusive Learning Environments

Environments that are not inclusive negatively impact both well-being and job performance, harming both the individual and the system's functioning, and therefore patient care. Further, many of the characteristics of the system that have historically led to the exclusion of minoritized groups in academic medicine continue today. To address this, an intentional approach is necessary. Environmental factors that impact inclusivity include discrimination, failure to respond to microaggressions, leadership effectiveness, support for work–life balance, and being inclusive when designing efforts.

Assessing Learning Environment

While regulatory bodies require that programs attend to diversity and inclusion, there is little guidance in the regulatory requirements of what outcomes are necessary and how to achieve them. Assessing the learning environment for the inclusivity required to foster diversity is an important step. This can lead to a thoughtful critique of the traditional approach to medical education and provide a guide for moving forward [36].

On an individual level, when evaluating trainees' experiences, they can also be queried about their experiences that can facilitate or challenge inclusivity in the learning environment. Models such as the inclusion of learning environment questions in end-of-experience evaluations can be helpful to obtain perspective about residents' experiences in the clinical learning environment [67, 68].

The learning environment should also be evaluated on a systems level for the presence of best practices in policies and procedures that drive deep and sustained change. One example is the White Coats 4 Black Lives Racial Justice Report card, which was first released in 2017 to assess medical schools and academic medical centers promoting antiracism, facilitating efforts for change, and ensuring public accountability in promoting antiracist medical practices [35]. Metrics like these could lead to meaningful change, shining a light on structures of oppression and encouraging new approaches to inclusivity [36]. The Racial Justice Report Card has been adapted for graduate medical education.

Mitigating Bias in Assessment

Biases are natural shortcuts to human assessment of situations. However, biases can be damaging. Trainees from underrepresented or historically marginalized backgrounds experience bias in multiple spaces, including in their assessment [69, 70]. A 2024 scoping review notes that bias was often noted by gender and race, while there is a dearth of literature on the topic, particularly when considering the impact of gender diversity, religion, and disability [69].

An example of this bias was found in students' applications for residency. Letters of recommendation and clinical evaluations were noted to be more likely to highlight communal traits for female, Black and Latinx applicants than agentic traits. While in this it did not have the same results in studies of pediatrics applications, the use of different terms demonstrating confidence and competence has been described for residents based on gender and race [71].

Approaches are suggested to mitigate bias in assessments of learners. Strategies include indicating the values that guide assessments, being intentional about the design of the assessment system to focus on less biased approaches to assessment, monitoring your assessment data for biases, and taking measures to optimize your learning environment. Measures such as utilizing multiple evaluation opportunities with scoring rubrics known to evaluator and resident and using a group to make high-stakes decisions based on evaluation data are recommended.

Cultivating Psychological Safety in Training Programs

Psychological safety has been defined as the belief that a person can be and show who they are without fear of negative consequences to themselves or their goal attainment. It is thought to be important to facilitate the personal risk-taking that is necessary to share thoughts, ideas, and concerns, and take actions that will positively impact patients, the team, and the organization as psychological safety is thought to improve team function and reduce patient-facing errors [72].

Grailey et al. propose that multiple factors contribute to psychological safety, including system characteristics like infrastructure, safety curriculum, culture, and teamwork. They also describe personal factors that contribute to psychological safety, including ability, motivation, and confidence. To address psychological safety, programs and faculty are urged to provide clear expectations and feedback to trainees and encourage self-efficacy and appropriate autonomy, and teamwork [73].

Supporting International Medical Graduates in Transition to US Residencies

International Medical Graduate (IMG) residents have an important role in medical education. They are thought to represent 25% of the US physician workforce, increase racial and ethnic diversity of the workforce, and are more likely than US grads to practice in underserved areas [74]. In addition, in the clinical environment, IMG residents bring alternate perspectives and experiences.

IMG physicians encounter barriers as well since many require visa sponsorship. This can be a barrier to being selected by a residency program. After starting training, IMG residents can encounter additional barriers such as adapting to a new healthcare system, electronic medical records, and ineligibility for NIH funding.

Onboarding is an area for focus for training program directors. A specific/tailored curriculum can be useful for fostering an understanding of medical culture in the United States and prompting reflection. In addition, some IMG residents would benefit from additional support early in training to ease their transition as they move to a new country.

Advocacy/Creating Brave Spaces

In medical education, we often refer to safe spaces where trainees can feel free to be themselves without judgment or harsh ridicule for failure. Brave spaces contrast safe spaces in that they are venues for talking through sensitive and challenging questions [75, 76] together. Discomfort and disagreement are expected in brave spaces; however, it is important to hold these challenging conversations to provide a better training experience and improve patient care.

However, these conversations must be trauma responsive, which means to consider the potential for past traumas to impact residents throughout their training experience. Approaches proposed to promote trauma-responsive environments include ensuring safety, establishing trustworthiness, maximizing choice, maximizing collaboration, and prioritizing empowerment [77].

Teaching and Learning Across Generational Differences

As the landscape of medical education continues to evolve, the intersection of generational differences among educators and learners has become increasingly apparent. The dynamics between different age groups within the pediatric workforce have been a subject of interest and exploration in recent research studies.

Many generations with typical learning attributes, characteristics, and effective teaching methods have been described from the Baby Boomers to Generation Z (Table 31.2) [78].

While understanding some characteristics and learning style preferences that may affect many trainees and faculty in a given generation, it is important to recognize every individual is different and many factors, including but not limited to generational influences, affect individual learning styles and preferences. Bracken et al. advocate for adopting an approach of *generational situatedness* rather than one of *generationalism*. Generationalism is a simplified, exaggerated view of generations that uses generational stereotypes and perpetuates cognitive bias similar to racism, classism, sexism, and ableism.

Table 31.2 Generational differences and learning strategies

Generation	Synopsis	Learning strategies to use when working with this generation
Baby Boomers	Born between 1946 and 1964, value hard work, loyalty, and respect for authority. Experienced significant social changes	Provide opportunities for leadership roles and recognition Acknowledge their experience and expertise Offer flexibility in work arrangements to accommodate work–life balance
Generation X	Born between 1965 and 1980, independent, resourceful, and value work–life balance. Experienced rapid technological advancements	Provide opportunities for autonomy and decision-making Offer diverse learning opportunities and feedback mechanisms Embrace technology in teaching and communication
Millennials	Born between 1981 and 1996, tech-savvy, collaborative, and seek purpose in their work. Grew up in the digital age	Foster a collaborative and team-oriented work environment Provide regular feedback and opportunities for skill development Utilize technology for interaction and engagement
Generation Z	Born between 1997 and 2012, diverse, entrepreneurial, and value authenticity. Digital natives who prioritize social causes	Create a diverse and inclusive learning environment Incorporate real-world applications and experiential learning Encourage creativity, innovation, and independent thinking

Note: A brief synopsis of generational attributes and learning strategies [78–82]

Generational situatedness is an approach to generational theory that more comprehensively situates generational differences within larger patterns of sociocultural, economic, technological, and institutional change [79]. Many other factors can interact with generational influences such as gender and other factors [80].

One example of an innovative approach to stimulate learning for current medical education learners and promote creativity and innovative thinking is the Journal Club for the Millennial Resident, which uses an interactive, no-prep approach, with teams first designing a new study approach for a given problem prior to then reading about an actual study on the topic learning from the comparison of their theoretical design and the one chosen by the authors [81]. This approach engages millennial residents in a meaningful and relevant way, recognizing and leveraging their distinct learning preferences and digital fluency.

Rather than fear or be critical of emerging generations of medical education learners, they are to be celebrated for the additional perspectives they bring [82]. By fostering understanding and collaboration across generations, embracing generational situatedness, and acknowledging the strengths that each generation brings to the table, educators can cultivate a rich and dynamic learning environment that benefits learners of all ages.

Transitions Across the Continuum

The transition from medical school to residency, and from residency to fellowship, presents several challenges that can negatively impact both learners and programs. These challenges include the disproportionate focus on securing positions rather than on training, misalignment between applicant goals and program missions, mistrust between medical schools and residency program directors, overreliance on licensure exam scores, significant financial costs, individual and systemic biases, exacerbation of inequities, and high levels of stress for both learners and program directors.

In 2021, the Coalition for Physician Accountability's Undergraduate Medical Education-Graduate Medical Education Review Committee (UGRC) issued comprehensive recommendations to improve these transitions [83]. Thirty-four recommendations were organized into nine themes:

- Collaboration and Continuous Quality Improvement
- Diversity, Equity, and Inclusion
- Trustworthy Advising and Definitive Resources
- Outcome Framework and Assessment Process
- Away Rotations
- Equitable Mission-Driven Application Review
- Optimization of Application, Interview, and Selection Processes
- Educational Continuity and Resident Readiness
- Health and Wellness

These recommendations provide a roadmap for the UME and GME communities to support trainees throughout the continuum of medical education. While the recommendations focus on the transition from medical school to residency, many principles also apply to the transition from residency to fellowship or independent practice.

In pediatric graduate medical education, two action teams have been addressing various aspects of the UGRC recommendations. The Pediatric Residency Recruitment Action Team and Fellowship Recruitment Action Team, comprising leadership from the Association of Pediatric Program Directors (APPD), Council on Medical Student Education in Pediatrics (COMSEP), Council of Pediatric Subspecialties (CoPS), Association of Medical School Pediatric Department Chairs (AMSPDC), the American Academy of Pediatrics Section on Pediatric Trainees (AAP SOPT), FuturePedsRes, and NextGenPediatricians, with input from trainee stakeholders, are working to optimize the recruitment process for residency and fellowship programs. These teams focus on effective assessment, equity, and cost savings, minimizing time away from clinical duties, and reducing environmental impact. This collaborative model has advanced many of the UGRC recommendations and set the stage for ongoing efforts to support UME-GME transitions and beyond.

While many pediatric residency and fellowship programs have developed thoughtful orientation activities, such as subspecialty-specific intensive training sessions (e.g., fellow "boot camps"), there is currently no standardized curriculum to support learner transitions in pediatric GME. Other specialties have implemented national curricula that include self-directed learning, group workshops, and coaching [84], which could serve as a model for standardizing transition support in pediatrics.

Finally, as trainees move through these critical transitions, it is important to address how program and institutional practices can exacerbate stress with competing obligations. For instance, the Council on Pediatric Subspecialties convened a multispecialty action team to address the timing of pediatric fellowship start dates. Recognizing the overlap between residency end dates (typically June 30) and fellowship orientation activities (often before July 1), the action team found that this scheduling creates undue stress, particularly for those relocating to new institutions. Based on feedback from residency and fellowship program directors, Designated Institutional Officials (DIOs), and residents, the team recommended that fellowship programs begin no earlier than July 7, with orientation activities starting no earlier than July 5. Adhering to these recommendations helps support trainee well-being during these high-stress periods of transition [85].

Unionization

Residents and fellows serve in a dichotomous role of trainee and employee [86, 87]. While the Accreditation Council on Graduate Medical Education (ACGME) regulates activities of residents as trainees, resident unions often aim to address the needs of residents through the lens of the resident as an employee. Through these methods, there is the potential for unionization to have an impact on physicians and the care that they provide to patients [88, 89]. While resident unionization is not well studied, particularly in pediatrics, at times unions have been perceived as agents of positive change, while at other times barriers to the traditional perspective on professional identity formation and educational alliance [90].

Unions representing the specific interests of resident physicians have been reported since 1934 to advocate for the initiation of pay for residents. There have been spikes in unionization periodically, most recently beginning in 2020. There have been challenges to residents unionizing over the years, including in 1976 when it was ruled that residents were students who were not protected by the National Labor Relations Board (NLRB); however, in 1999, that ruling was overturned and residents were again permitted to unionize [88, 91].

Twenty percent of all residents in 2024 were estimated to be represented by unions [91]. Of 1909 family medicine, internal medicine, pediatrics, and psychiatry residency programs in the United States, 67 were documented as being unionized in 2023 [92]. There has been a rise in the rate of trainee unionization in recent years. While most training programs are not currently unionized, 18 groups of physicians in training voted to unionize between 2011 and 2023, with the majority occurring in 2023 [92]. Notably, in nearly every instance of a union vote in recent years, it passed. This suggests that unionization is expected to increase, perhaps due in part to the profound impact of the COVID-19 pandemic on healthcare.

The limited research available about resident unionization portrays a mixed picture of the benefits and challenges. Physician, and specifically resident, unionization can be beneficial. Many times, bargaining collectively can be advantageous, particularly for salary. The financial opportunities realized by the bargaining unit can extend to those around them, positively impacting those beyond the bargaining unit. In a secondary analysis of data collected through the Surgical Education Culture Optimization Through Targeted Interventions Based on National Comparative Data (SECOND) trial, it was found that surgical residents valued the agency in their own well-being. The most commonly noted benefits were financial. In a larger study, over 5000 surgical residents were surveyed, with 10.5% working in unionized programs. This study found that while unionized programs were more likely to offer more vacation and housing stipends, there was no difference between unionized and nonunionized groups with respect to burnout index, suicidality, job satisfaction, duty hour violations, mistreatment, educational environment, and salary. While the other domains were not impacted in this case, the feeling of agency in decisions about residents' own well-being could be a powerful factor for resilience.

A concern related to physician unionization that is specific to the unique duality of a resident is its impact on the resident–program director alliance. In the qualitative study of surgical trainees and faculty, "framing of resident-faculty relationships as adversarial" was a noted concern. This becomes particularly problematic when it weakens the educational alliance. The educational alliance framework indicates that between the resident and program director, there must be mutual understanding, an agreement about how to work toward the goals of training, and respect, trust, and value of the program director by the resident [94]. The residents' value of the program director is influenced by the resident's perception of their credibility and ability to help them achieve their goals, which is often judged through observations of the director's to assist in their development. Often, this is best demonstrated through the advocacy program directors do for their residents, an aspect many program directors report as fulfilling. When programs are unionized, there could be a loss of the program director's power to advocate for the needs of their residents and program, particularly when the bargaining unit includes multiple programs [95]. In addition, it can be challenging to determine where unions' influences begin and end, with some noting that the complexity introduced by unions' influence on remediation could reduce educators' likelihood of intervening when performance is inadequate [93].

Despite the above concerns, participation of residents in the union was noted to allow for a better understanding of the needs of trainees. Resident unions offer representation to resident physicians. In studies, residents feel that resident unions can benefit them by providing a voice, agency, and financial benefits [91]. During a critical and challenging time for professional identity formation, unionization's benefits and ways to mitigate the challenges should be explored. In addition, perhaps there are lessons in the unionized programs that will benefit nonunionized programs and that will help to mitigate the impact of having or not having a union in place.

LEARN Research Network for Education Scholarship

The Association of Pediatric Program Directors Longitudinal Educational Assessment Research Network (APPD LEARN) is a pioneering research network dedicated to advancing pediatric training through collaborative and meaningful educational research. Established in 2009, APPD LEARN aims to address limitations in medical education research, such as small sample sizes, lack of generalizability, and unequal access to research resources [96]. The network's mission is to "conduct meaningful educational research that advances the training of future pediatricians by developing and promoting participation and collaboration in research by program directors for the purpose of improving the health and wellbeing of children."

Since its inception, APPD LEARN has distinguished itself as a productive and influential research network. It boasts high levels of program and program director engagement, robust collaboration within the APPD and with partner organizations [including the American Board of Pediatrics (ABP), Accreditation Council for Graduate Medical Education (ACGME), and the Council on Medical Student Education in Pediatrics (COMSEP)], and a strong record of educational scholarship. The network has produced numerous high-quality published articles, reflecting rigorous research and relevant outcomes.

APPD LEARN's mission-driven strategic activities include [96]

- Conducting network research studies
- Maintaining a study repository with shareable data
- Providing professional development for program directors as education researchers
- Offering consultation on study design and analysis
- Communicating and disseminating network activities within the organization and with partner organizations
- Coordinating research activities with other organizations

Since its creation, APPD LEARN has developed three subnetworks: Pediatric Residency Investigators in Medical Education (PRIME), Subspecialty Pediatrics Investigator Network (SPIN), and Surveys Enhancing Educator Knowledge (SEEK). These subnetworks enhance the network's capacity for pediatric education scholarship and present significant opportunities for pediatric GME leaders to advance evidence-based training practices, ultimately improving the health and well-being of children.

Opportunities to Collaborate Across Organizations

Pediatric GME leaders have a strong tradition of collaboration across organizations, and various structures within pediatric medical education and pediatric GME foster intentional partnerships within the community. One notable example is the APPD Confronting Racism Action Team (CRAT), established in 2020. The CRAT is dedicated to taking actionable steps to dismantle racism within pediatric residency and fellowship programs. It brings together pediatric leaders from multiple partner organizations to address critical issues such as organizational role modeling, developing pathways for underrepresented individuals in medicine, creating inclusive training environments, and establishing equitable systems of care for patients.

The APPD Pediatric Medical Education Conference serves as another important platform, gathering pediatric educators across the continuum. This conference brings together established and emerging content experts and leaders in pediatric medical education from various organizations, facilitating knowledge sharing and collaborative problem-solving on the challenges facing the field.

GME leaders play a crucial role in the AMSPDC workforce initiative, which focuses on advancing workforce development and addressing critical issues in pediatric medical education. The Organization of Program Directors Associations (OPDA) is committed to promoting the role of residency and fellowship program directors and in supporting program director societies in achieving excellence in graduate medical education. This collaborative group shares best practices and strategies to tackle common challenges in graduate medical education.

As we continue to address complex problems in pediatrics and medical education, these deliberate partnerships and collaborative efforts to share ideas and unite toward common goals will be instrumental in advancing the pediatric GME community.

Educating Lifelong Learners Who Can Remain Competent in the Face of Rapidly Evolving Science

In the rapidly evolving landscape of pediatric medicine, it is imperative to educate future physicians who are not only competent but also equipped with the skills and mindset to engage in lifelong learning, adapt to new scientific discoveries throughout their careers, and provide state-of-the-art high-quality care to their young patients.

Self-directed learning, critical thinking, and reflective practice are key components of lifelong learning and the foundation for cultivating pediatricians who are capable of interpreting and applying new information effectively in their clinical practice [97]. *Self-directed learning* in medical education merges the elements of the

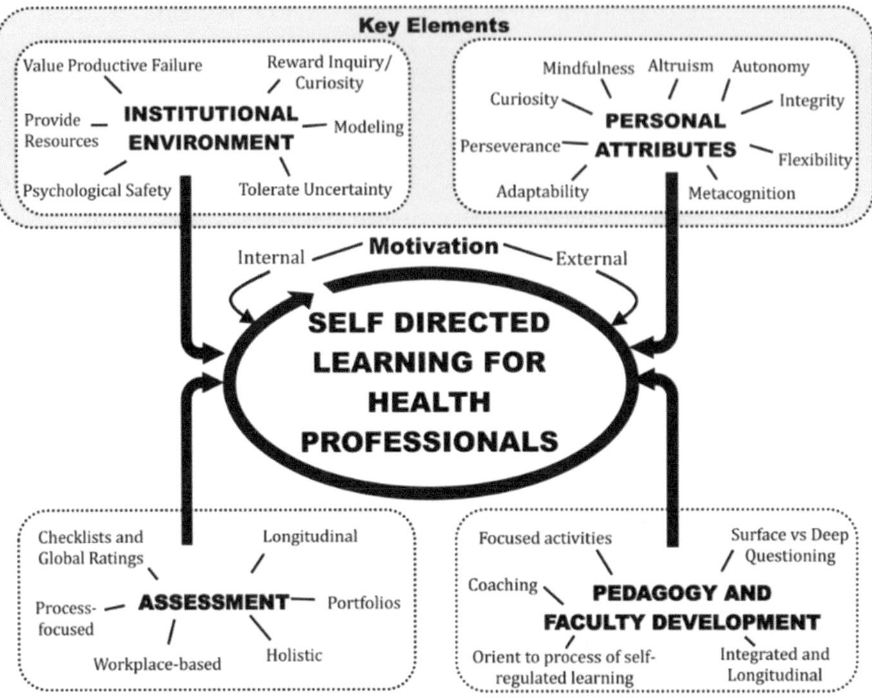

Fig. 31.4 Self-directed learning for health professionals [98]

institutional environment, learner attributes, assessment processes, and faculty development to promote a culture that prepares learners for a lifetime of discovery (Fig. 31.4) [98].

Reflective learning can help pediatricians deepen their understanding of complex clinical scenarios, identify areas for improvement, and integrate new knowledge into their existing practice. By encouraging regular reflection on their experiences, pediatric educators can foster a culture of continuous learning and growth among trainees [99]. Promoting a *growth mindset* in competency-based medical education both at UME and GME levels can further enhance learners' ability to embrace challenges, persist in the face of setbacks, and view feedback as an opportunity for growth [100].

Faculty development programs play a crucial role in providing educators with the necessary skills, knowledge, and resources to facilitate effective learning experiences for trainees [101].

By embracing the principles of lifelong learning, fostering a growth mindset, promoting self-directed learning, facilitating reflective practice, and investing in faculty development, pediatric medical education can prepare future pediatricians to navigate the complexities of modern healthcare and remain competent in the face of rapidly evolving science.

Innovations in Pediatric Medical Education

Competency-Based Medical Education

Medical education has traditionally operated on a time-based model, where trainees progress to the next stage based on the completion of educational experiences within a set timeframe. Summative decisions are made at predetermined intervals, and most learners advance assuming competence unless there is substantial evidence to the contrary. Only a small percentage of learners with identified concerns are "held back" from progression [102].

Competency-based medical education (CBME) disrupts this traditional paradigm by placing patient and family needs at the heart of curriculum development. CBME recognizes that learners acquire knowledge and skills at varying rates and times. This approach challenges educators to identify patient-centered skills essential for independent practice and assess competence using direct observation and reliable assessment tools. Entrustable professional activities (EPAs), informally known as "Everyday Pediatrician Activities," offer a framework for defining the patient-focused skills that physicians should be able to perform independently [103, 104].

Although CBME has been part of the medical lexicon for nearly 25 years, the practical application of its principles and tools continues to evolve. The potential for CBME to revolutionize medical education is substantial, and a later chapter of this book will delve deeper into the subject of CBME.

Time-Variable Education/Accelerated Learning

Shifting the focus toward patient needs and competence achievement allows for a time-variable approach to trainee advancement. In 2017, the Josiah Macy Foundation assembled a diverse group of experts in medicine, nursing, pharmacy, education, learners, and accreditors to address the challenges of implementing competency-based, time-variable health professions education [105]. The resulting report calls for a transformation in educational practices to ensure that patients receive the right care at the right place, at the right time, and at the right cost. The consensus vision outlined by the leaders is

> With the achievement of competency-based, time-variable health professions education, we envision a health care system in which all learners and practitioners are actively engaged in their own education and continuing professional development to improve the health of the public. In this system, learners and faculty partner to co-produce learning, all practitioners are lifelong learners, and all health care environments place a high value on learning. (Macy Report, 2017)

The Education in Pediatrics Across the Continuum (EPAC) Study Group exemplifies an innovative pilot for pediatric competency-based medical education (CBME). The EPAC Study Group aims to "establish a model for true competency based medical education through variable-time, meaningfully assessed demonstration of competence across the UME-GME continuum." [106, 107] This initiative involves a collaboration among five medical schools and their affiliated pediatric residency programs. These programs utilize predetermined competencies, including core entrustable professional activities (EPAs) for entering residency, to facilitate advancement from undergraduate medical education (UME) to graduate medical education (GME) [108]. With two of the participating programs implementing time-variable advancement, this pilot project lays the foundation for further exploration of competency-based, time-variable education.

Workplace-Based Assessments

Multimodal assessments are a fundamental component of competency-based medical education (CBME), with direct observation of activities playing a crucial role in informing entrustment decisions and assessing competence for independent practice. Workplace-based assessments (WBAs) are particularly valuable, allowing faculty to provide real-time feedback and assessment during daily patient care, which supports ongoing learning.

A scoping review of WBA implementation highlights several key themes [109]:

- Numerous WBA tools and programs have been introduced, but common barriers to successful implementation persist across various fields and specialties.
- Theoretical perspectives consistently underscore the importance of data-driven strategies for effective implementation.
- User perceptions of WBAs vary and are often influenced by specific implementation factors.
- Technological solutions hold potential for enhancing WBA tools and processes.
- Significant opportunities for future research and innovation remain in this area.

WBAs will be explored in greater detail in a subsequent chapter. As the use of WBAs continues to expand, there is ample opportunity for the development of evidence-based best practices in this evolving field.

Coaching

As competency-based, learner-driven medical education continues to evolve, coaching has emerged as a powerful tool for supporting trainee self-reflection and self-monitoring [110]. Once a mainstay in sports and business, coaching has gained traction over the past decade as a valuable asset in medical education. Beyond enhancing trainees' knowledge and technical skills, coaching programs have been shown to foster professional identity formation [111] and improve residents' appreciation of patient feedback [112].

Effective coaching hinges on several key components [110]:

- *A trusting and engaged relationship*: establishing clear expectations and maintaining credibility are essential.
- *Skilled faculty coaches*: coaches should possess mature inquiry and listening skills, be capable of developing a shared agenda, guiding goal setting, identifying problems, and referring to appropriate resources.
- *Reflective and humble learners*: trainees should be self-reflective, seek information to achieve their goals, and be able to solve problems effectively.

The expansion of coaching programs within pediatric graduate medical education (GME) presents valuable opportunities for mentors to provide direct observation, prompt reflection, and help pediatrics residents and fellows develop and create tailored learning plans for pediatric trainees. Coaching is covered comprehensively in a later chapter.

New ACGME Requirements Allow for Flexibility and Program Innovation

In July 2025, the implementation of new ACGME Pediatric Residency Requirements ushered in a period of greater flexibility for pediatric trainees and programs. The ACGME envisions pediatricians as physicians who provide "comprehensive patient-centered preventive, acute, and chronic care for the growing and developing child from birth through the transition to adult care." [113] The revised Pediatric Review Committee requirements emphasize that pediatricians should be well-equipped to address medical, psychosocial, and behavioral issues common in childhood and adolescence. Furthermore, these requirements underscore the importance of cultivating adaptability, advocacy, lifelong learning, and collaborative partnership skills throughout pediatric training.

The new requirements introduce a significant shift by evenly dividing required experiences among inpatient, outpatient, and individualized curriculum time. This new structure designates several weeks of unprescribed time, offering pediatric residency program leaders the opportunity to innovate within their curricula and tailor educational experiences to align with the mission and values of their programs. This flexibility enables programs to ensure that core content is thoroughly covered while integrating novel educational approaches and experiences that meet the unique needs of their trainees.

Additionally, these changes support the integration of new pedagogical methods and the adaptation of training to emerging healthcare needs and practices. The increased autonomy granted to program directors allows for the incorporation of cutting-edge practices, interdisciplinary collaboration, and enhanced focus on areas such as advocacy and mental health, thereby enriching the overall training experience and better preparing pediatricians for the evolving landscape of child healthcare.

As pediatric residency programs adapt to these new requirements, they will be better positioned to offer comprehensive, individualized training that not only meets but exceeds current standards, ultimately fostering a more dynamic and responsive educational environment for future pediatricians.

Alternate Models of Care

As pediatricians work to provide high-value, accessible care for their patients with complex needs, alternate models of care can be utilized to align the skill of the primary care pediatrician with the expertise of specialists. Children and youth visit their primary care provider frequently; therefore, aligning services helps to remove barriers to access for patients and families. Integrated and collocated behavioral health in primary care clinics is a sample of this effort to increase access to pediatric mental and behavioral health services for pediatric patients [114]. Hoff et al. describe several models for behavioral health in the primary care setting:

- Coordinated care, where primary care pediatricians and specialists share information frequently, but practice separately
- Collocated care, in which specialty services are available at the primary pediatrician's office to facilitate referrals
- Integrated care, in which primary care pediatricians and specialty providers work together as a care team
- Collaborative care, in which specialists and primary care pediatricians provide care to patients using a shared treatment plan

As pediatricians work to provide high-value, accessible care through these innovative models, integrating these approaches into medical education ensures that future pediatricians are equipped with the skills and collaborative mindset necessary to effectively navigate and implement such models in their practice.

Value-Conscious Medicine

In the realm of pediatric medicine, the integration of value-conscious medicine principles into medical education is essential for developing a new generation of pediatricians who are not only clinically skilled but also adept at navigating the economic complexities of healthcare delivery. The Association of American Medical Colleges has recognized the importance of cost-conscious care and created two of its core entrustable professional activities with this focus (AAMC). Medical schools have therefore incorporated formal didactics into their curricula [115]. Similarly, pediatric residents must "demonstrate competence in incorporating considerations of value, equity, cost awareness, delivery and payment, and risk-benefit analysis in patient and/or population-based care as appropriate" (ACGME 2023 pediatric program requirements) [116]. Pediatric residents' experience with high-value care occurs in a complex medical environment where multiple factors influence their decision-making toward higher or lower value-conscious care, including fear of missing diagnoses, the impact of autonomy influencing care in both directions of high and low value in different circumstances, patient and family experiences, and collaboration with health team members [116]. Role modeling can be an effective way to promote value-conscious practices among learners [115, 117, 118].

Enhancing Interprofessional Education (IPE)

A hierarchical and siloed approach to clinical care can hinder collaboration and effective communication, potentially contributing to medical errors. Similarly, operational teams that work in parallel rather than collaboratively can perpetuate power imbalances, marginalize the voices of patients, families, and team members, and obstruct system improvement efforts.

Interprofessional care and interprofessional education (IPE) offer solutions by fostering collaboration among families and healthcare team members. This approach encourages teams to work together, challenging traditional power structures and incorporating diverse perspectives. By engaging the expertise and leadership of all team members, regardless of their discipline, interprofessional care ensures that patients and families are actively involved in decision-making [119].

Interprofessional education promotes learning across disciplines, allowing students to "learn about, from, and with each other to enable effective collaboration and improve health outcomes." [120] Many medical schools have integrated IPE into their curricula, and graduate medical education (GME) programs can further enhance IPE through shared educational conferences, simulations, and case discussions.

Incorporating family voices into residency and fellowship training activities is also crucial. Trainees benefit from hearing the diverse perspectives of patients and families as part of their education. In order to optimize the ability for families to engage in training events, program leaders should make deliberate efforts to support their involvement. Scheduling meetings or trainings at times that are convenient for families and compensating families for their time can improve family participation. Using family-friendly language during meeting and training times and actively welcoming family input will ensure that families feel their voices and perspectives are valued [119]. This inclusive approach ensures that the voices of patients and families are integral to the educational process, ultimately leading to improved care and system performance.

Utilizing Technology to Optimize Patient Care and Trainee Education

In recent years, the field of pediatrics has witnessed a transformative shift with the integration of cutting-edge technologies aimed at optimizing patient care and enhancing trainee education. These include but are not limited to the use of artificial intelligence and machine learning applications, telehealth, tools for asynchronous learning, augmented and virtual reality, and simulation.

Precision Medical Education

As medical educators strive to train a diverse pediatric workforce capable of addressing the complexities of a varied patient population, individualizing training experiences to the needs of each learner becomes paramount. Precision medical education (PE) emerges as a powerful approach to this challenge, leveraging a continuous improvement model that utilizes multisource data to transform lifelong learning.

Desai et al. (2024) describe a conceptual framework and fundamental principles for precision education [121]. At its core, PE integrates various data sources, including workplace-based assessments, clinical evaluations, ACGME milestones assessments, and patient-level data such as procedure logs, patient types, diagnoses, and prescribing behaviors as *inputs* into the system. This data provides a comprehensive view of each learner's experiences and performance. Programs can *analyze* this data to identify patterns and gaps, such as frequently encountered clinical diagnoses and areas of limited exposure. Based on these *insights*, learners and program leaders can set tailored learning goals and plan individualized educational *interventions*.

Effective learning interventions must be assessed using trustworthy, equitable, valid, and scalable methods. The ultimate goal is to ensure high-quality, equitable patient care. As *outcomes* are measured and compared to the learner's goals—with the support of a trusted coach—ongoing *adjustments* can be made, and the data informs the subsequent learning cycle. This iterative process ensures that learning is continuously aligned with both learner needs and evolving clinical demands.

For precision education to be implemented effectively and equitably, several key principles and standards must be established. First, it is crucial to promote equity in the structures and processes of PE systems to mitigate, rather than perpetuate, biases and structural racism present in current systems. Ensuring that multisource data is used to address these issues is essential. Additionally, learner engagement is a critical component of successful PE systems; learners should be actively involved in designing and refining these systems to ensure they meet their needs.

Another vital principle is alignment with clinical workflow. Given the administrative burdens often placed on trainees and faculty, PE systems must be seamlessly integrated into existing workflows to avoid adding unnecessary strain.

Precision education holds significant promise as a tool for lifelong, self-directed learning. By continuing to refine and apply PE principles, pediatricians can manage the ongoing growth and evolution of medical knowledge throughout their careers, ultimately enhancing patient care and supporting professional development.

Utilizing Artificial Intelligence and Machine Learning in Pediatrics

Artificial intelligence (AI) and machine learning (ML) have emerged as powerful tools in pediatric healthcare, offering new possibilities for improving patient and educational outcomes. Artificial intelligence (AI) is a broad term describing the use of machine-based learning algorithms and software [122]. Machine learning (ML) is a specific branch of AI focused on altering programs or algorithms based on exposure to data in order to improve performance over time [123] Natural language processing (NLP) solutions use ML to help computers understand, categorize, and extract insights from natural language data sets [122, 123]. In the field of medicine, by harnessing AI algorithms, healthcare providers can leverage predictive analytics, clinical decision support systems, and automated note writing to enhance diagnostic accuracy and treatment planning. Large language models (LLMs) are deep learning algorithms that can perform a variety of NLP tasks and represent a subset of NLP [124].

Clinical Decision Support: AI has been used for clinical decision support in a variety of conditions and circumstances to enhance efforts in the areas of risk prediction, diagnosis, therapy and response monitoring, and clinical workflow efficiency [123, 125]. One example is the care of pediatric asthma where AI and MLM have been used to enhance care in many domains. These have included the ability to predict hospitalization [126, 127], and asthma persistence [128], monitoring disease state and advising medication management. A novel cell phone app combines inputs from smart sensors from home spirometry, inhaler use, and local weather conditions to provide real-time early notification of the need for medication management adjustments to prevent asthma exacerbations [129, 130]. Other examples include the use of AI to improve the care of children with severe sepsis [131] and rare conditions in critically ill patients in the NICU and PICU [132]. While innovations in AI have shown clinical benefits, there are risks and challenges also. Complex patient care situations commonly exist where human values may conflict among patient, parent, payer, and pediatrician [133]. This can result in varying conclusions from LLM algorithms depending on whose perspective is taken with the risk of suboptimal decision-making. Understanding the benefit and limitations of AI in combination with the contributions of physician, patient, and family insights and values will be crucial as AI is incorporated more and more into clinical practice.

Recruitment: Natural language processing and machine learning can be utilized to help recruitment efforts including screening. Performing holistic reviews of a large number of applications is time and resource intensive. NLP and MLM can be utilized to create a model based on desired attributes and experiences that may be described in free-text elements of an application to help programs to identify applicants for further review and potential invitation. An example of this is the University of Utah med-peds program [134] that developed a 10-attribute model with moderate sensitivity and high specificity for identifying applicants to invite for interviews.

Letter Writing: AI can be used in letter writing as a part of medical school, residency, and fellowship applications by both applicants and those writing letters of support for applicants. Applicants are increasingly utilizing AI as part of personal statement writing and other elements of the application. This is a controversial area where many experts have urged the focus be on how to responsibly use AI rather than attempt to prevent its use. Guidance for students and educators with regard to applicant AI use exists focused on using AI to enhance applications while preserving creativity, accuracy, and ownership of the accuracy of information shared [135].

Educating Learners to Work with Augmented Intelligence (AI)

Augmented intelligence (AI) is increasingly used in society, healthcare, and many aspects of medical education [136, 137]. AI has proven to be effective in enhancing trainees' and physicians' practical skills, assisting in disease diagnosis and treatment, and providing support in clinical applications. AI offers the potential to offer personalized and adaptive learning experiences [136].

While many programs are finding ways to utilize AI to educate trainees, few training programs have educated future doctors and pediatricians in how to effectively use AI in their own practice. It will be important for training programs to develop strategies to train effective pediatric consumers and users of AI given its strengths, limitations, and potential to enhance or diminish the effectiveness of clinical decision-making and educational decision-making by pediatricians and pediatric educators [138]. One study described a novel use of AI to help medical students learn about AI using an application exercise where students compared the use of AI and more traditional methods, including textbooks and online searches, and found students demonstrated high interest, engagement, and high-level reflection recognizing some of the bias and risks associated with the AI-generated results [139]. Ehrman et al. highlighted the need for a curriculum to train critical care physicians in machine learning to help them practice in a field with ever-increasing myriad data to develop meaningful discriminative machine learning (ML) use, knowing future best practices can be neither ML-free nor blindly trust it [140].

Augmented Reality/Virtual Reality in Education

The integration of virtual reality (VR) technologies into pediatric medical education shows great promise in enhancing learning outcomes, improving efficiency, and providing immersive training experiences for medical trainees. Several distinct themes have emerged with many benefits of integrating VR into pediatric medical education.

Enhanced Experiential Learning: VR technologies offer immersive and interactive experiences that enhance the understanding of complex medical concepts and procedures. Trainees can engage in realistic scenarios, improving their practical skills and decision-making abilities. VR can occur with different types of (1) immersion [low (2D), medium (rooms with projections on walls), or highly immersive (3D) environments], (2) displays (standalone, mobile, console, computer based), and (3) content [141] (see table from Pallavicini below). VR has been used for medical education training in several areas, including emergency medicine, nursing, pediatrics, radiology, and cardiology [141] This technology has been successfully used for teaching various topics, including complex anatomy and three-dimensional spacing constructs [142].

Immersive Learning Experiences: VR can be used as a part of trainee assessment as trainees engage with realistic patient cases, improving their diagnostic and treatment skills. VR has been utilized to assess trainee performance in areas of communication, including counseling and conflict management, achieving performance standards in clinical activities, and procedural competency [143].

Personalized Learning Pathways: The integration of AI with VR in asynchronous learning tools allows for the customization of learning pathways based on individual trainee performance metrics. This personalized approach enhances the educational experience by providing targeted feedback and adaptive learning opportunities [143].

Telehealth Innovations in Pediatric Practice

Telehealth has emerged as a vital component of pediatric healthcare, enabling remote consultations, monitoring, and care delivery. Telehealth plays a crucial role in enhancing clinical exposure and facilitating virtual learning experiences for trainees. The COVID-19 pandemic greatly accelerated the adoption of pediatric telehealth that provided an opportunity for lessons learned during a time of increased telehealth utilization. Some of these lessons included (1) a better understanding of the education and training needed for participating effectively in telehealth such as toolkits, webinars, and learning modules; (2) development and adaptation of clinical workflows needed for telehealth including triage systems, video visit technology, schedule support, virtual rooming, and virtual care team formation and use; (3) patient assessment and treatment, including training providers in virtual history taking and virtual physical exam techniques; and (4) family-centered care with methods developed to include and even expand access to families in both ambulatory, inpatient, and ICU settings using video visits and telerounding [144–146]. Telehealth has the potential to enhance both pediatric primary care practice [147] and public health by improving access to care and addressing healthcare disparities [148].

The use of telemedicine in pediatric training programs has increased substantially. A 2022 needs assessment conducted by Fitzgerald et al. surveyed pediatric residency and fellowship directors and showed 12% of programs used telemedicine in the training program pre-pandemic and 71% during the pandemic. Despite its growth and increased use, 69% of programs either had no formal curriculum or were unsure if they did [149]. Seventeen essential telemedicine skills for pediatric residents were identified to inform future development of structured training programs in pediatric telehealth [150]. The UCLA internal medicine residency successfully developed and implemented a telehealth curriculum focused on virtual physical examination techniques and teleconsultation skills, which resulted in increased trainee confidence in delivering virtual healthcare [151].

Enhancing Trainee Education Through Asynchronous Learning Tools

Asynchronous learning tools, encompassing a wide array of digital platforms such as podcasts, webinars, virtual simulations, mobile applications, learning management systems (LMS), and social media channels, offer pediatric trainees the flexibility and convenience to engage in self-directed learning experiences tailored to their individual needs and preferences. The COVID-19 pandemic accelerated the need and use of blended and e-learning in pediatric education in many forms [152].

Podcasts as educational resources in medical training have increased utilization and are increasingly incorporated into existing medical curricula. Podcast educational outcomes showed favorable reaction data, increased engagement, equal to increased learning effectiveness compared to other formats, and behavior change with improvement in documentation skills and self-reported practice change in residents after listening to podcasts [153, 154]. Numerous mobile applications are currently utilized in pediatric training. One example is a mobile application for pediatric procedural skills training that resulted in increased confidence and competency among pediatric trainees [155]. Social media platforms have emerged as valuable tools for physician engagement and knowledge sharing [156, 157].

Success Stories from Pediatric Training Programs

This chapter has examined selected aspects of the future of pediatric medical education highlighting selected challenges, opportunities, and innovations. We would like to conclude the chapter with a success story of an exemplary educational innovation that incorporates all of these. A common *challenge* that has faced residency programs is the dual mission to optimize pediatric residents' longitudinal outpatient experience (continuity clinic) while they simultaneously care for patients in a variety of core inpatient and outpatient settings. A key principle in education and business is "be here now"; however, sometimes trainees struggled with feeling they needed to be in two places at once (i.e., be present for their ICU patients in the morning, handoff their patients with many pending tasks, get to continuity clinic on time to see a full schedule and somehow find time to do notes on the patients seen in both settings). This challenge sometimes diluted the educational experience in both settings while raising trainee stress levels. In 2018, five programs saw an *opportunity* to adapt a novel internal medicine scheduling system for pediatric use [158, 159]. X + Y schedules first developed in internal medicine [160] contain X rotations (often inpatient-based rotations without continuity clinic) and Y rotations (contain bursts of continuity clinic, longitudinal experiences, and other ambulatory rotations). These five programs received an ACGME waiver under the Advancing *Innovation* in Resident Education (AIRE) pilot (AIRE reference) allowing residents to attend 36 or more continuity clinics in fewer than the required

26 weeks. This X + Y schedule pilot yielded several improved outcomes, including improved resident and faculty perceptions of patient continuity, inpatient workflow and handoff quality, and increased time for teaching during inpatient blocks and continuity clinic (Fig. 31.5) [158, 159]. The pilot was later expanded to include additional programs with continued success. In response to the continued educational improvements achieved by X + Y pilot programs, the updated ACGME pediatric program requirements will allow continuity clinic to be scheduled at least every 8 weeks instead of the previous requirement of 26 or more weeks, allowing any program the option to utilize X + Y scheduling [113]. This story is a good example of an approach that will be crucial as we head into the future of pediatric medical education to turn today's challenges into tomorrow's successful innovations.

a Outpatient General Pediatrics

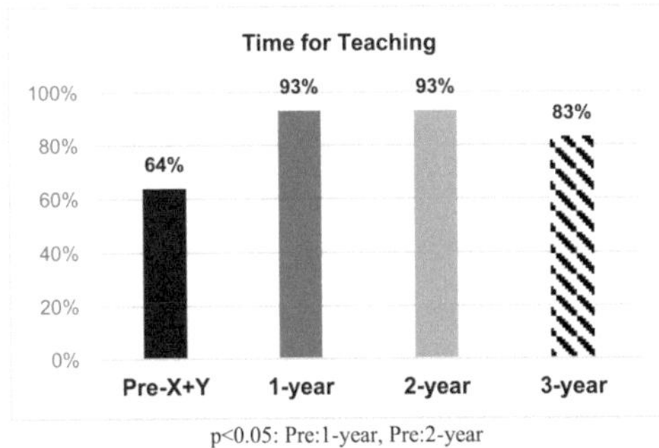

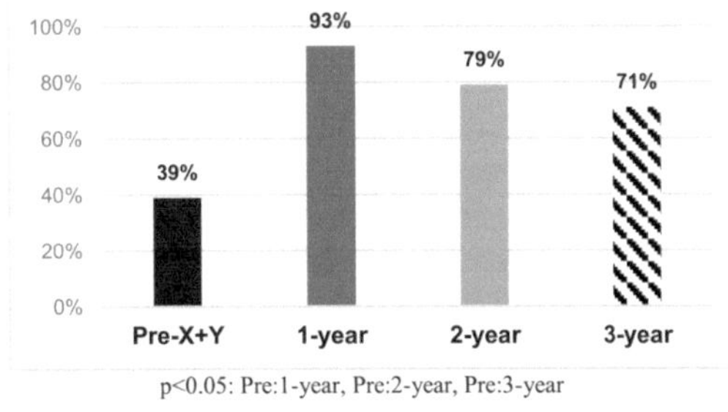

b Hospital Medicine

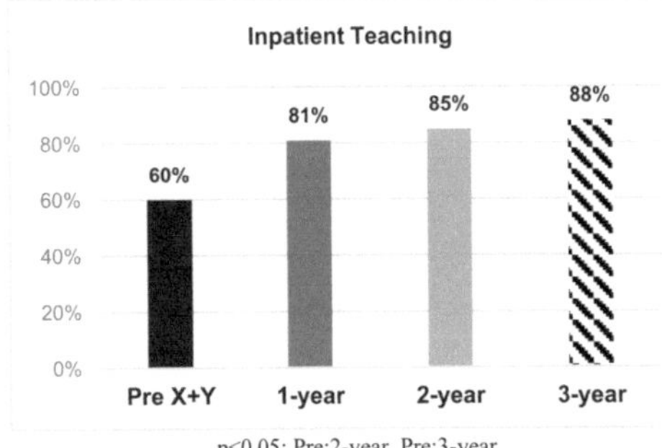

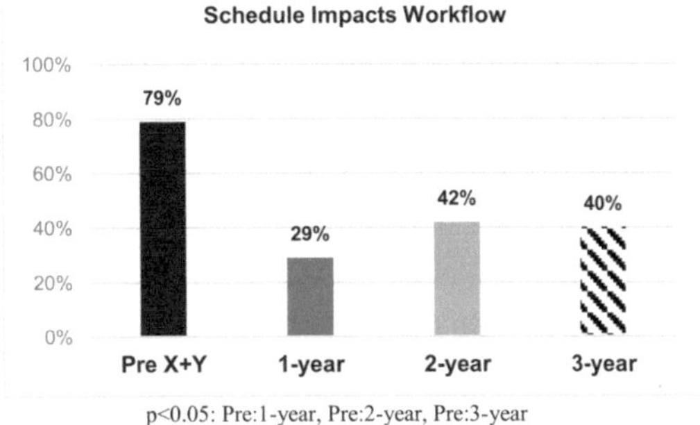

c Subspecialty

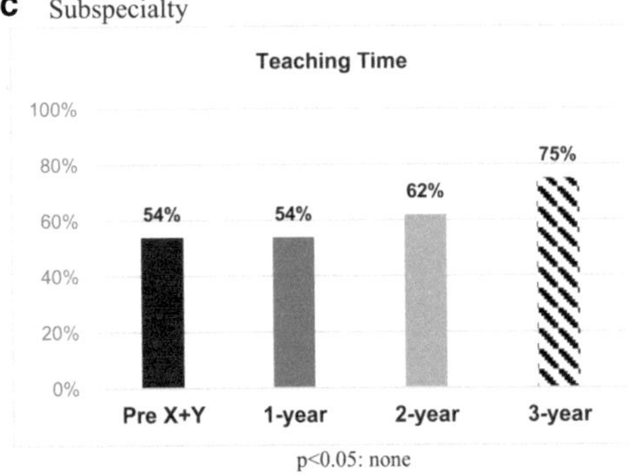

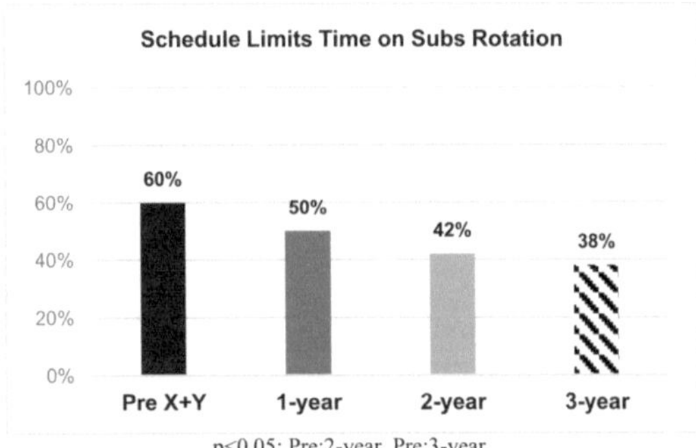

Fig. 31.5 X + Y faculty outcomes. (Figure taken from Myers et al.) [158]

Future Directions and Conclusion

Pediatricians hold the unique privilege of nurturing the health and development of today's children, who will become the adults of tomorrow, and pediatric educators are entrusted with the vital role of shaping the future pediatric workforce. Despite the challenges and hurdles inherent in our field, we stand on the brink of an exciting era, brimming with transformative opportunities. The advent of artificial intelligence, machine learning, and the growth of competence-based and precision medical education promise to revolutionize our approach to both clinical care and training. Our path forward is illuminated by a dynamic and supportive network of educational leaders, collaborative pediatric organizations, and a thriving research community dedicated to advancing medical education. As we navigate this promising horizon, we are well-positioned to harness these innovations and continue to excel in our mission to educate and prepare the pediatricians of the future, ensuring that they are equipped with the knowledge, skills, and compassion needed to meet the evolving needs of our patients and the healthcare landscape.

References

1. Committee on the Pediatric Subspecialty Workforce and Its Impact on Child Health and Well-Being, Board on Health Care Services, Board on Children, Youth, and Families, Health and Medicine Division, Division of Behavioral and Social Sciences and Education, National Academies of Sciences, Engineering, and Medicine. The future pediatric subspecialty physician workforce: meeting the needs of infants, children, and adolescents. National Academies Press; 2023. p. 27207. https://doi.org/10.17226/27207.
2. Szilagyi MA, Szilagyi PG. A vision for children in America. Acad Pediatr. 2024;24(6):879–82. https://doi.org/10.1016/j.acap.2024.06.004.
3. Results and Data: 2024 Main Residency Match | NRMP. Accessed 21 May 2025. https://www.nrmp.org/match-data/2024/06/results-and-data-2024-main-residency-match/.
4. ERAS® Statistics | AAMC. Accessed 21 May 2025. https://www.aamc.org/data-reports/data/eras-statistics-data.
5. Pediatrics 2025 Workforce Initiative Sponsored by AMSPDC. Accessed 21 May 2025. https://amspdc.org/workforce/.
6. Vinci RJ, Degnon L, Gillooly M, Gigante J, Buchanan A, Blankenburg R. The match, the workforce, the future: the key role for medical educators. Acad Pediatr. 2025;25(4):102794. https://doi.org/10.1016/j.acap.2025.102794.
7. Hartman M, Martin AB, Benson J, Catlin A, National Health Expenditure Accounts Team. National health spending in 2011: overall growth remains low, but some payers and services show signs of acceleration. Health Aff Proj Hope. 2013;32(1):87–99. https://doi.org/10.1377/hlthaff.2012.1206.
8. Committee on Pediatric Workforce, Rimsza ME, Hotaling AJ, et al. Financing graduate medical education to meet the needs of children and the future pediatrician workforce. Pediatrics. 2016;137(4):e20160211. https://doi.org/10.1542/peds.2016-0211.
9. Weiss P, Myers AL, McGann KA, et al. Current fellowship funding limitations and their threat to the pediatric subspecialty workforce. Acad Pediatr. 2021;21(8):1328–30. https://doi.org/10.1016/j.acap.2021.08.006.
10. Heyman MB, Weiss P, Boyer D, et al. Challenges of funding pediatric fellowship programs-invited commentary from the Council of Pediatric Subspecialties. J Pediatr. 2019;204:4–6.e1. https://doi.org/10.1016/j.jpeds.2018.10.006.
11. Cull WL, Katakam SK, Starmer AJ, Gottschlich EA, Miller AA, Frintner MP. A study of pediatricians' debt repayment a decade after completing residency. Acad Med. 2017;92(11):1595–600. https://doi.org/10.1097/ACM.0000000000001721.
12. Orr CJ, Turner AL, Ritter VS, Gutierrez-Wu J, Leslie LK. Pursuing a career in pediatrics: intersection of educational debt and race/ethnicity. J Pediatr. 2023;252:162–70. https://doi.org/10.1016/j.jpeds.2022.08.014.
13. Freed GL, Wickham K. Comparison of calculations of the financial impact of fellowship training by data source. JAMA Netw Open. 2023;6(7):e2326639. https://doi.org/10.1001/jamanetworkopen.2023.26639.
14. Harris E. Loan repayment program aims to grow US pediatric specialist workforce. JAMA. 2023;330(2):111. https://doi.org/10.1001/jama.2023.10737.
15. Webber S, Babal JC, Shadman KA, Coller RJ, Moreno MA. Exploring academic pediatrician perspectives of factors impacting physician well-being. Acad Pediatr. 2020;20(6):833–9. https://doi.org/10.1016/j.acap.2020.02.018.
16. Slovin A, Bora S, Barber JR, et al. Meaningful work, career fit, and professional well-being of pediatric academicians in the United States. Hosp Pediatr. 2024;14(5):364–73. https://doi.org/10.1542/hpeds.2022-007080.

17. Dahmash AB, Alajmi MF, Aldayel AY, et al. Burnout and associated risk factors in pediatric residents. Ochsner J. 2021;21(2):152–7. https://doi.org/10.31486/toj.20.0037.
18. Cellini MM, Serwint JR, Chaudron LH, Baldwin CD, Blumkin AK, Szilagyi PG. Availability of emotional support and mental health care for pediatric residents. Acad Pediatr. 2017;17(4):424–30. https://doi.org/10.1016/j.acap.2017.01.011.
19. Weiss AK, Quinn SM, Danley AL, Wiens KJ, Mehta JJ. Burnout and perceptions of stigma and help-seeking behavior among pediatric fellows. Pediatrics. 2021;148(4):e2021050393. https://doi.org/10.1542/peds.2021-050393.
20. Pediatric Resident Burnout-Resilience Study Consortium. Accessed 23 May 2025. https://pedsresresilience.com/objectives-rationale/.
21. Staples BB, Burke AE, Batra M, et al. Burnout and association with resident performance as assessed by pediatric milestones: an exploratory study. Acad Pediatr. 2021;21(2):358–65. https://doi.org/10.1016/j.acap.2020.08.006.
22. Kemper KJ, McClafferty H, Wilson PM, et al. Do mindfulness and self-compassion predict burnout in pediatric residents? Acad Med. 2019;94(6):876–84. https://doi.org/10.1097/ACM.0000000000002546.
23. Babal JC, Lelkes E, Kloster H, et al. Pediatric resident well-being: a group concept mapping study. Acad Pediatr. 2024;24(3):535–43. https://doi.org/10.1016/j.acap.2024.01.004.
24. Reilly MR, Perkins K, Carson SL, Li STT. Pediatric program leadership's contribution toward resident wellness. Acad Pediatr. 2020;20(4):440–1. https://doi.org/10.1016/j.acap.2019.12.012.
25. Philipsborn RP, Sheffield P, White A, Osta A, Anderson MS, Bernstein A. Climate change and the practice of medicine: essentials for resident education. Acad Med. 2021;96(3):355–67. https://doi.org/10.1097/ACM.0000000000003719.
26. Mallone WT, Cox N. Climate action in academic medicine an overview of how medical schools and teaching hospitals and health systems are responding to climate change. AAMC. https://www.aamc.org/media/64106/download.
27. American Medical Association. Resolution #A19-302. Climate change education across the medical education. Continuum. 2019. Accessed 27 July 2024. https://www.psr.org/wp-content/uploads/2019/07/ama-climate-change-education-policy-2019.pdf.
28. World Health Organization. Climate change and health. Accessed 3 Jan 2023. https://www.who.int/news-room/fact-sheets/detail/climate-change-and-health.
29. Centers for Disease Control and Prevention. Justice, equity, diversity, and inclusion in climate adaptation planning. Accessed 13 Jan 2023. https://urlisolation.com/browser?clickId=CB263209-2BDA-4ECF-B2F9-9C83880BE1B1&traceToken=1747873945%3Bcnmc_hosted%3Bhttps%3A%2Fdocs.google.com%2Fdocument%2F&url=https%3A%2F%2Fwww.cdc.gov%2Fclimate-health%2Fphp%2Fbrace%2Fjedi.html%3FCDC_AAref_Val%3Dhttps%3A%2F%2Fwww.cdc.gov%2Fclimateandhealth%2FJEDI.htm.
30. Guzman, CAF, Potter T. The Planetary Health Education Framework. Planetary Health Alliance. https://urlisolation.com/browser?clickId=CB263209-2BDA-4ECF-B2F9-9C83880BE1B1&traceToken=1747873945%3Bcnmc_hosted%3Bhttps%3A%2Fdocs.google.com%2Fdocument%2F&url=https%3A%2F%2Fd1wqtxts1xzle7.cloudfront.net%2F96173855%2FEd_Framework_Web.pdf__filename_UTF-8Ed_Framework_Web-libre.pdf%3F1671658138%3D%26response-content-disposition%3Dinline%253B%2Bfilename%253DThe_Planetary_Health_Education_Framework.pdf%26Expires%3D1747883879%26Signature%3DBfb3GqCKmye31-DTi~dxiW2gVYa7dIhZpJ1dlhhQQSqt33S33CkfUsbCaOh4EIX5gpIgeB0CPYtwGJqlXaFjwaowJ2inY5bBjHQtMBwK7zApSShyjBl8CbYDU~j2W4bJx1k4fJzi3KdTqlVPbwQhcxvP8GRx6p1LXSbg-hFAS5NxGCvQRpMuTGl2sHqXa9IfLGHbq0cdyWd27sQUNIPLWne~9qpoKPGsTJLWVTb3kScFtW5YbkWxhbUuE1fIlI1m2-F2JCSm0Gmfo51eYL3jd1C0S9eMtNQ1iglIQSVwZaPcokamFDaSopZtmLHsFQd07IcwUO6w7lCyb4uBZdNBxw__%26Key-Pair-Id%3DAPKAJLOHF5GGSLRBV4ZA.
31. Guzmán CAF, Aguirre AA, Astle B, et al. A framework to guide planetary health education. Lancet Planet Health. 2021;5(5):e253–5. https://doi.org/10.1016/S2542-5196(21)00110-8.
32. Muth ND, Bolling C, Hannon T, et al. The role of the pediatrician in the promotion of healthy, active living. Pediatrics. 2024;153(3):e2023065480. https://doi.org/10.1542/peds.2023-065480.
33. Helldén D, Andersson C, Nilsson M, Ebi KL, Friberg P, Alfvén T. Climate change and child health: a scoping review and an expanded conceptual framework. Lancet Planet Health. 2021;5(3):e164–75. https://doi.org/10.1016/S2542-5196(20)30274-6.
34. Poitevien P, Blankenburg R. It's not you, it's us. Pediatrics. 2021;148(1):e2021050884. https://doi.org/10.1542/peds.2021-050884.
35. WC4BL. Racial Justice Report Card. https://whitecoats4blacklives.org/rjrc/.
36. Garg PS, Barber A. Developing antiracism metrics: steps forward to drive change in medical education. Acad Pediatr. 2023;23(8):1522–3. https://doi.org/10.1016/j.acap.2023.08.001.
37. Cornell Law School. Affirmative action. Legal Information Institute - Cornell Law School. Accessed 28 July 2024. https://www.law.cornell.edu/wex/affirmative_action.
38. PBS. Regents of University of California v. Bakke (1978). The Supreme Court. Accessed 28 July 2024. https://www.thirteen.org/wnet/supremecourt/rights/landmark_regents.html.

39. Cornell Law School. Regents of the University of California v. Bakke. 1978. Legal Information Institute - Cornell Law School. Accessed 13 April 2025. https://www.law.cornell.edu/wex/regents_of_the_university_of_california_v_bakke_(1978).
40. Cornell Law School. Grutter v. Bollinger. 2003. Legal Information Institute - Cornell Law School. Accessed 13 April 2025. https://www.law.cornell.edu/wex/grutter_v_bollinger_%282003%29.
41. Cornell Law School. GRATZ v. BOLLINGER. Legal Information Institute - Cornell Law School. Accessed 13 April 2025. https://www.law.cornell.edu/supremecourt/text/02-516.
42. Creighton et al. A bill to be entitled an act. https://capitol.texas.gov/tlodocs/88R/billtext/pdf/SB00017I.pdf.
43. H.R.7725 - 118th Congress (2023–2024). To amend the Higher Education Act of 1965 to prohibit graduate medical schools from receiving Federal financial assistance if such schools adopt certain policies and requirements relating to diversity, equity, and inclusion. Congress.gov. March 19, 2024. https://www.congress.gov/bill/118th-congress/house-bill/7725?s=1&r=2.
44. AAMC. EDUCATE Act Introduced by Rep. Greg Murphy, M.D. AAMC. March 22, 2024. https://www.aamc.org/advocacy-policy/washington-highlights/educate-act-introduced-rep-greg-murphy-md.
45. Boumil MM, Beninger P, Curfman GD. The US supreme court and affirmative action: the negative impact on the physician workforce. Clin Ther. 2023;45(10):1004–7. https://doi.org/10.1016/j.clinthera.2023.08.008.
46. Press Release New AAMC Data on Medical School Applicants and Enrollment in 2024. Accessed 23 May 2025. https://www.aamc.org/news/press--releases/new-aamc-data-medical-school-applicants-and-enrollment-2024.
47. Yancy CW, Barabino G, Bright C, Laurencin CT, Montgomery RV. The supreme court and the importance of diversity in medicine. N Engl J Med. 2023;389(8):677–9. https://doi.org/10.1056/NEJMp2306195.
48. What Does the Dobbs Decision Mean for Medical Professionals?; 2022. https://www.youtube.com/watch?v=_tQejqpF2E8.
49. Shubkin CD, Sieplinga K, Hunter RJ, Crichton KG. Transforming pediatric education in response to Dobbs v. Jackson: empowering adolescents to manage their reproductive choices. Acad Pediatr. 2024;24(3):381–4. https://doi.org/10.1016/j.acap.2023.08.010.
50. U.S., 142 S.Ct. 2228. Dobbs v. Jackson Women's Health. Supreme Court of the United States. 2022. Accessed 19 Sept 2023. https://www.supremecourt.gov/opinions/21pdf/19-1392_6j37.pdf.
51. Cornell Law School. Abortion. Legal Information Institute - Cornell Law School. https://www.law.cornell.edu/wex/abortion.
52. Tanne JH. Mifepristone: US Supreme Court rejects ban on abortion drug. BMJ. Published online June 14, 2024:q1321. https://doi.org/10.1136/bmj.q1321.
53. American College of Obstetricians and Gynecologists. More than 75 health care organizations release joint statement in opposition to legislative interference. The American College of Obstetricians and Gynecologists July 7, 2022. https://www.acog.org/news/news-releases/2022/07/more-than-75-health-care-organizations-release-joint-statement-in-opposition-to-legislative-interference.
54. AAMC. Training location preferences of U.S Medical School graduates post Dobbs v. Jackson Women's Health Organization Decision. AAMC. Accessed 16 May 2023. https://www.aamc.org/advocacy--policy/aamc-research-and-action-institute/training-location-preferences.
55. Klingensmith ME, Gosman GG, Khabele D, Brinkmann BS. Roe v Wade, Dobbs, and the future of graduate medical education. J Grad Med Educ. 2023;15(3):407–10. https://doi.org/10.4300/JGME-D-23-00279.1.
56. Stephenson-Famy A, Sonn T, Baecher-Lind L, et al. The Dobbs decision and undergraduate medical education: the unintended consequences and strategies to optimize reproductive health and a competent workforce for the future. Acad Med. 2023;98(4):431–5. https://doi.org/10.1097/ACM.0000000000005083.
57. Goldstein RL, Carlson JL, Tyson NA. Dobbs v. Jackson decision: it's time to get uncomfortable. Hosp Pediatr. 2022;12(10):e364–6. https://doi.org/10.1542/hpeds.2022-006829.
58. Chen R, Gordon M, Chervenak F, Coverdale J. Addressing moral distress after Dobbs v. Jackson women's health organization: a professional virtues-based approach. Acad Med. 2024;99(1):12–5. https://doi.org/10.1097/ACM.0000000000005476.
59. Why the Post- *Roe* era requires protecting conscientious provision as we protect conscientious refusal in health care. AMA J Ethics. 2022;24(9):E906–12. https://doi.org/10.1001/amajethics.2022.906.
60. Dhar CP, Dixon SV, Michelson C. Protecting graduate medical education and gender-diverse youth. J Grad Med Educ. 2024;16(3):264–6. https://doi.org/10.4300/JGME-D-23-00910.1.
61. Inwards-Breland D, Tordoff D, Wanta J, Stepney C. Mental health outcomes and receipt of gender-affirming care. Pediatrics. 2022;149(1 Meeting Abstracts February 2022):590.
62. Tordoff DM, Wanta JW, Collin A, Stepney C, Inwards-Breland DJ, Ahrens K. Mental health outcomes in transgender and nonbinary youths receiving gender-affirming care. JAMA Netw Open. 2022;5(2):e220978. https://doi.org/10.1001/jamanetworkopen.2022.0978.
63. Rafferty J, Committee on Psychosocial Aspects of Child and Family Health, Committee on Adolescence, et al. Ensuring comprehensive care and support for transgender and gender-diverse children and adoles-

cents. Pediatrics. 2018;142(4):e20182162. https://doi.org/10.1542/peds.2018-2162.
64. Kelley AD. Medical schools as cisgendered organizations. Soc Sci Med. 2024;350:116913. https://doi.org/10.1016/j.socscimed.2024.116913.
65. Greene RE, Blasdel G, Cook TE, Gillespie C. How do OSCE cases activate learners about transgender health? Acad Med. 2020;95(12S):S156–62. https://doi.org/10.1097/ACM.0000000000003704.
66. Youmans QR, Maldonado M, Essien UR, Lupton K. Building inclusion and belonging in training environments. J Grad Med Educ. 2022;14(3):333–4. https://doi.org/10.4300/JGME-D-22-00307.1.
67. Slovin A, Hippolyte J, Gelin D, Barber A. From the residents' perspectives: health equity and bias in the clinical learning environment. Poster #522 presented at: Pediatric Academic Societies; April 28, 2023; Washington, D.C. Accessed 25 May 2025. https://2023.pas-meeting.org/fsPopup.asp?efp=WFJFTkxUVUcxNzk2Mw&PosterID=562383&rnd=6.585103E-02&mode=posterinfo.
68. Boatright D, Nguyen M, Hill K, et al. Development of a tool to measure student perceptions of equity and inclusion in medical schools. JAMA Netw Open. 2024;7(2):e240001. https://doi.org/10.1001/jamanetworkopen.2024.0001.
69. Ismaeel R, Pusic L, Gottlieb M, Chan TM, Oyedokun TO, Thoma B. Bias in observed assessments in medical education: a scoping review. Acad Med. 2024;99(12):1438–50. https://doi.org/10.1097/ACM.0000000000005794.
70. Karani R, Varpio L, May W, et al. Commentary: racism and bias in health professions education: how educators, faculty developers, and researchers can make a difference. Acad Med. 2017;92(11S):S1–6. https://doi.org/10.1097/ACM.0000000000001928.
71. Boolchandani H, Osborn R, Tiyyagura G, et al. Words used in letters of recommendation for pediatric residency applicants: demographic differences and impact on interviews. Acad Pediatr. 2023;23(8):1614–9. https://doi.org/10.1016/j.acap.2023.02.012.
72. Grailey KE, Murray E, Reader T, Brett SJ. The presence and potential impact of psychological safety in the healthcare setting: an evidence synthesis. BMC Health Serv Res. 2021;21(1):773. https://doi.org/10.1186/s12913-021-06740-6.
73. McClintock AH, Fainstad TL, Jauregui J. Creating psychological safety in the learning environment: straightforward answers to a longstanding challenge. Acad Med. 2021;96(11S):S208–9. https://doi.org/10.1097/ACM.0000000000004319.
74. David YN, Issaka RB. Advancing diversity: the role of international medical graduates. Lancet Gastroenterol Hepatol. 2021;6(12):980–1. https://doi.org/10.1016/S2468-1253(21)00376-9.
75. Winks L. Erratum to: discomfort, challenge and brave spaces in higher education. In: Leal Filho W, editor. Implementing sustainability in the curriculum of universities. Springer International Publishing; 2018. p. E1. https://doi.org/10.1007/978-3-319-70281-0_21.
76. Wasserman JA, Browne BJ. On triggering and being triggered: civil society and building brave spaces in medical education. Teach Learn Med. 2021;33(5):561–7. https://doi.org/10.1080/10401334.2021.1887740.
77. Carello J, Butler LD. Practicing what we teach: trauma-informed educational practice. J Teach Soc Work. 2015;35(3):262–78. https://doi.org/10.1080/08841233.2015.1030059.
78. Evans KH, Ozdalga E, Ahuja N. The medical education of generation Y. Acad Psychiatry. 2016;40(2):382–5. https://doi.org/10.1007/s40596-015-0399-5.
79. Bracken RC, Fredrickson ME, Fredrickson LA, Appleman M. Generational situatedness: challenging generational stereotypes in health professions education. Med Teach. 2023;45(4):380–7. https://doi.org/10.1080/0142159X.2022.2135428.
80. Spector ND, Cull W, Daniels SR, et al. Gender and generational influences on the pediatric workforce and practice. Pediatrics. 2014;133(6):1112–21. https://doi.org/10.1542/peds.2013-3016.
81. Dzara K, Frey-Vogel AS. Medical Education Journal Club for the Millennial Resident: an interactive, no-prep approach. Acad Pediatr. 2019;19(6):603–7. https://doi.org/10.1016/j.acap.2019.05.004.
82. Barak G, Carroll MR, Dean A. The kids are alright: a new generation of educators. Med Sci Educ. 2022;32(5):1189–94. https://doi.org/10.1007/s40670-022-01618-6.
83. The Coalition for Physician Accountability's Undergraduate Medical Education-Graduate Medical Education Review Committee (UGRC): Recommendations for Comprehensive Improvement of the UME-GME Transition. Accessed 3 Aug 2024. https://physicianaccountability.org/.
84. Winkel AF, George K, Wagner S, et al. Facilitating an optimal transition to residency in obstetrics and gynecology. Obstet Gynecol. 2022;140(6):931–8. https://doi.org/10.1097/AOG.0000000000004987.
85. Mink RB, Wininger DA, Turner A, et al. Reducing trainee stress by delaying the pediatric fellowship start date. Pediatrics. 2020;146(3) https://doi.org/10.1542/peds.2019-3500.
86. Weiner S. Thousands of medical residents are unionizing. Here's what that means for doctors, hospitals, and the patients they serve. AAMC. June 7, 2022. https://www.aamc.org/news/thousands-medical-residents-are-unionizing-here-s-what-means-doctors-hospitals-and-patients-they.
87. Harmon R. Intern and Resident Organizations in the United States: 1934–1977. Sch Public Health Community Med Univ Wash Seattle. 1978;56(4). https://www.milbank.org/wp-content/uploads/mq/volume-56/issue-04/56-4-Intern-and-Resident-Organizations-in-the-United-States.pdf.

88. Bowling D, Richman BD, Schulman KA. The rise and potential of physician unions. JAMA. 2022;328(7):617. https://doi.org/10.1001/jama.2022.12835.
89. Lin GL, Ge TJ, Pal R. Resident and fellow unions: collective activism to promote well-being for physicians in training. JAMA. 2022;328(7):619. https://doi.org/10.1001/jama.2022.12838.
90. Physician Unionization: might physician unions be a useful solution to help restore physician autonomy?; 2024. https://edhub.ama-assn.org/ama-education/video-player/18859963
91. Mikolajczyk AE, Goodman C. Resident labor unions—learning as we go. JAMA Netw Open. 2024;7(7):e2421634. https://doi.org/10.1001/jamanetworkopen.2024.21634.
92. Ahmed A, Li X. Labor unionization among physicians in training. JAMA. 2023;330(19):1905. https://doi.org/10.1001/jama.2023.17494.
93. Foote DC, Rosenblatt AE, Amortegui D, et al. Experiences with unionization among general surgery resident physicians, faculty, and staff. JAMA Netw Open. 2024;7(7):e2421676. https://doi.org/10.1001/jamanetworkopen.2024.21676.
94. Krzyzaniak SM, Sebok-Syer SS, Akhtar S, Gallahue F. Exploring How Housestaff Unions Impact the Program Director–Resident Educational Alliance. Acad Med. 2024;99(10):1073–7. https://doi.org/10.1097/ACM.0000000000005649.
95. Yager J, Anzia JM, Bernstein CA, et al. What sustains residency program directors: social and interpersonal factors that foster recruitment and support retention. Acad Med. 2022;97(12):1742–5. https://doi.org/10.1097/ACM.0000000000004887.
96. Schwartz A, King B, Mink R, et al. The APPD longitudinal educational assessment research network's first decade. Pediatrics. 2023;151(5):e2022059113. https://doi.org/10.1542/peds.2022-059113.
97. Opipari VP, Daniels SR, Wilmott RW, Jacobs RF. Association of Medical School Pediatric Department Chairs Principles of lifelong learning in pediatric medicine. JAMA Pediatr. 2016;170(11):1087. https://doi.org/10.1001/jamapediatrics.2016.2258.
98. Ricotta DN, Richards JB, Atkins KM, et al. Self-directed learning in medical education: training for a lifetime of discovery. Teach Learn Med. 2022;34(5):530–40. https://doi.org/10.1080/10401334.2021.1938074.
99. Gathu C. Facilitators and barriers of reflective learning in postgraduate medical education: a narrative review. J Med Educat Curri Develop. 2022;9:23821205221096106. https://doi.org/10.1177/23821205221096106.
100. Richardson D, Kinnear B, Hauer KE, et al. Growth mindset in competency-based medical education. Med Teach. 2021;43(7):751–7. https://doi.org/10.1080/0142159X.2021.1928036.
101. Carlson ER, McGowan E. Faculty development for the twenty-first century. Oral Maxillofac Surg Clin North Am. 2022;34(4):555–70. https://doi.org/10.1016/j.coms.2022.02.004.
102. Carraccio C, Lentz A, Schumacher DJ. Dismantling fixed time, variable outcome education: abandoning 'ready or not, here they come' is overdue. Perspect Med Educ. 2023;12(1):68–75. https://doi.org/10.5334/pme.10.
103. Competency-Based Medical Education (CBME) | The American Board of Pediatrics. Accessed 21 May 2025. https://www.abp.org/content/competency-based-medical-education-cbme.
104. Competency-Based Medical Education (CBME) | AAMC. Accessed 21 May 2025. https://www.aamc.org/about-us/mission-areas/medical-education/cbme.
105. Lucey CR. Achieving competency-based, time-variable health professions education. Proceedings of a conference sponsored by Josiah Macy Jr. Foundation in June 2017. New York: Josiah Macy Jr. Foundation; 2018.
106. Andrews JS, Bale JF, Soep JB, et al. Education in Pediatrics Across the Continuum (EPAC): first steps toward realizing the dream of competency-based education. Acad Med. 2018;93(3):414–20. https://doi.org/10.1097/ACM.0000000000002020.
107. Education in Pediatrics Across the Continuum (The EPAC Project) | AAMC. Accessed 21 May 2025. https://www.aamc.org/what-we-do/mission-areas/medical-education/cbme/epac.
108. Murray KE, Lane JL, Carraccio C, et al. Crossing the gap: using competency-based assessment to determine whether learners are ready for the undergraduate-to-graduate transition. Acad Med. 2019;94(3):338–45. https://doi.org/10.1097/ACM.0000000000002535.
109. Anderson HL, Kurtz J, West DC. Implementation and use of workplace-based assessment in clinical learning environments: a scoping review. Acad Med J Assoc Am Med Coll. 2021;96(11S):S164–74. https://doi.org/10.1097/ACM.0000000000004366.
110. Deiorio NM, Carney PA, Kahl LE, Bonura EM, Juve AM. Coaching: a new model for academic and career achievement. Med Educ Online. 2016;21(1):33480. https://doi.org/10.3402/meo.v21.33480.
111. Hoang K, Grow HM, Rooholamini SN, et al. Impact of longitudinal coaching on pediatric residents' professional identity formation: a multi-institution qualitative study. Acad Pediatr. 2024;24(5):866–74. https://doi.org/10.1016/j.acap.2024.04.012.
112. Rassbach CE, Bogetz AL, Orlov N, et al. The effect of faculty coaching on resident attitudes, confidence, and patient-rated communication: a multi-institutional randomized controlled trial. Acad Pediatr. 2019;19(2):186–94. https://doi.org/10.1016/j.acap.2018.10.004.
113. ACGME Program Requirements for Graduate Medical Education in Pediatrics. Accessed 22 May 2025. https://www.acgme.org/globalassets/pfassets/programrequirements/2025-reformatted-requirements/320_pediatrics_2025_reformatted.pdf.

114. Hoff A, Hughes-Reid C, Sood E, Lines M. Utilization of integrated and Colocated behavioral health models in pediatric primary care. Clin Pediatr (Phila). 2020;59(14):1225–32. https://doi.org/10.1177/0009922820942157.
115. Makhoul AE, Kertai MD, Powers J, Dahlman KB, Suojanen K. Training tomorrow's physicians in value conscious medicine. Acad Med. 2023;98(7):795–9. https://doi.org/10.1097/ACM.0000000000005160.
116. Seltz LB, Nathaniel E, Ball A, Jimenez S, Tchou M. Pediatric residents' experiences with high-value care at an Academic Children's hospital. J Grad Med Educ. 2022;14(1):80–8. https://doi.org/10.4300/JGME-D-21-00665.1.
117. Tan E, Ng WM, Soh PC, Tan D, Cleland J. 'But what if you miss something …?': Factors that influence medical student consideration of cost in decision making. BMC Med Educ. 2023;23(1):437. https://doi.org/10.1186/s12909-023-04349-3.
118. Moleman M, Van Den Braak GL, Zuiderent-Jerak T, Schuitmaker-Warnaar TJ. Toward high-value, cost-conscious care—supporting future doctors to adopt a role as stewards of a sustainable healthcare system. Teach Learn Med. 2021;33(5):483–97. https://doi.org/10.1080/10401334.2021.1877710.
119. Baird J, Ashland M, Rosenbluth G. Interprofessional teams. Pediatr Clin N Am. 2019;66(4):739–50. https://doi.org/10.1016/j.pcl.2019.03.003.
120. WHO (World Health Organization). Framework for action on interprofessional education and collaborative practice. 2010. Accessed 22 May 2025. https://www.who.int/publications/i/item/framework-for-action-on-interprofessional-education-collaborative-practice.
121. Desai SV, Burk-Rafel J, Lomis KD, et al. Precision education: the future of lifelong learning in medicine. Acad Med. 2024;99(4S):S14–20. https://doi.org/10.1097/ACM.0000000000005601.
122. Chang AC. Intelligence-based medicine: artificial intelligence and human cognition in clinical medicine and healthcare. Academic Press is an imprint of Elsevier; 2020.
123. Bhargava H, Salomon C, Suresh S, et al. Promises, pitfalls, and clinical applications of artificial intelligence in pediatrics. J Med Internet Res. 2024;26:e49022. https://doi.org/10.2196/49022.
124. Shahab O, El Kurdi B, Shaukat A, Nadkarni G, Soroush A. Large language models: a primer and gastroenterology applications. Ther Adv Gastroenterol. 2024;17:17562848241227031. https://doi.org/10.1177/17562848241227031.
125. Haug CJ, Drazen JM. Artificial intelligence and machine learning in clinical medicine, 2023. Drazen JM, Kohane IS, Leong TY, eds. N Engl J Med. 2023;388(13):1201–8. https://doi.org/10.1056/NEJMra2302038.
126. Luo G, He S, Stone BL, Nkoy FL, Johnson MD. Developing a model to predict hospital encounters for asthma in asthmatic patients: secondary analysis. JMIR Med Inform. 2020;8(1):e16080. https://doi.org/10.2196/16080.
127. Patel SJ, Chamberlain DB, Chamberlain JM. A machine learning approach to predicting need for hospitalization for pediatric asthma exacerbation at the time of emergency department triage. Cloutier R, ed. Acad Emerg Med. 2018;25(12):1463–70. https://doi.org/10.1111/acem.13655.
128. Bose S, Kenyon CC, Masino AJ. Personalized prediction of early childhood asthma persistence: a machine learning approach. Roy S, ed. PLoS One. 2021;16(3):e0247784. https://doi.org/10.1371/journal.pone.0247784.
129. Larson EC, Goel M, Boriello G, Heltshe S, Rosenfeld M, Patel SN. SpiroSmart: using a microphone to measure lung function on a mobile phone. In: Proceedings of the 2012 ACM conference on ubiquitous computing. ACM; 2012. p. 280–9. https://doi.org/10.1145/2370216.2370261.
130. Van Sickle D, Barrett M, Humblet O, Henderson K, Hogg C. Randomized, controlled study of the impact of a mobile health tool on asthma SABA use, control and adherence. In: 5.2 Monitoring Airway Disease. European Respiratory Society; 2016. p. PA1018. https://doi.org/10.1183/13993003.congress-2016.PA1018.
131. Kamaleswaran R, Akbilgic O, Hallman MA, West AN, Davis RL, Shah SH. Applying artificial intelligence to identify physiomarkers predicting severe sepsis in the PICU*. Pediatr Crit Care Med. 2018;19(10):e495–503. https://doi.org/10.1097/PCC.0000000000001666.
132. Clark MM, Hildreth A, Batalov S, et al. Diagnosis of genetic diseases in seriously ill children by rapid whole-genome sequencing and automated phenotyping and interpretation. Sci Transl Med. 2019;11(489):eaat6177. https://doi.org/10.1126/scitranslmed.aat6177.
133. Yu KH, Healey E, Leong TY, Kohane IS, Manrai AK. Medical artificial intelligence and human values. Drazen JM, ed. N Engl J Med. 2024;390(20):1895–904. https://doi.org/10.1056/NEJMra2214183.
134. Drum B, Shi J, Peterson B, Lamb S, Hurdle JF, Gradick C. Using natural language processing and machine learning to identify internal medicine–pediatrics residency values in applications. Acad Med. 2023;98(11):1278–82. https://doi.org/10.1097/ACM.0000000000005352.
135. Chen JX, Bowe S, Deng F. Residency applications in the era of generative artificial intelligence. J Grad Med Educ. 2024;16(3):254–6. https://doi.org/10.4300/JGME-D-23-00629.1.
136. Nagi F, Salih R, Alzubaidi M, et al. Applications of artificial intelligence (AI) in medical education: a scoping review. In: Mantas J, Gallos P, Zoulias E, et al., editors. Studies in health technology and informatics. IOS Press; 2023. https://doi.org/10.3233/SHTI230581.

137. Tozsin A, Ucmak H, Soyturk S, et al. The role of artificial intelligence in medical education: a systematic review. Surg Innov. 2024;31(4):415–23. https://doi.org/10.1177/15533506241248239.
138. Younis HA, TAE E, Nasser M, et al. A systematic review and meta-analysis of artificial intelligence tools in medicine and healthcare: applications, considerations, limitations, motivation and challenges. Diagnostics. 2024;14(1):109. https://doi.org/10.3390/diagnostics14010109.
139. Müller MEB, Laupichler MC. Medical students learning about AI – with AI? Med Educ. 2023;57(11):1156. https://doi.org/10.1111/medu.15211.
140. Ehrmann D, Harish V, Morgado F, et al. Ignorance isn't bliss: we must close the machine learning knowledge gap in pediatric critical care. Front Pediatr. 2022;10:864755. https://doi.org/10.3389/fped.2022.864755.
141. Pallavicini F, Pepe A, Clerici M, Mantovani F. Virtual reality applications in medicine during the COVID-19 pandemic: systematic review. JMIR Serious Games. 2022;10(4):e35000. https://doi.org/10.2196/35000.
142. Stanford Children's Health. Stanford pioneers use of VR for patient care, education and experience. 2017. http://www.stanfordchildrens.org/en/about/news/releases/2017/virtual-reality-programStanford WEW.
143. Zackoff MW, Klein M, Real FJ. Virtual reality to inform and facilitate trainee assessment. Acad Pediatr. 2024;24(5):716–8. https://doi.org/10.1016/j.acap.2024.01.016.
144. Curfman A, McSwain SD, Chuo J, et al. Pediatric telehealth in the COVID-19 pandemic era and beyond. Pediatrics. 2021;148(3):e2020047795. https://doi.org/10.1542/peds.2020-047795.
145. Haynes SC, Marcin JP. Pediatric telemedicine. Adv Pediatr Infect Dis. 2022;69(1):1–11. https://doi.org/10.1016/j.yapd.2022.04.002.
146. Rogers A, Lynch K, Toth H, Weisgerber M. Patient and family centered (tele)rounds: the use of video conferencing to maintain family and resident involvement in rounds. Acad Pediatr. 2020;20(6):765–6. https://doi.org/10.1016/j.acap.2020.05.026.
147. Wasserman RC, Fiks AG. The future(s) of pediatric primary care. Acad Pediatr. 2021;21(3):414–24. https://doi.org/10.1016/j.acap.2020.10.015.
148. Wang CJ, Ma J, Zuckerman B, Car J. The opportunities for telehealth in pediatric practice and public health. Pediatr Clin N Am. 2020;67(4):603–11. https://doi.org/10.1016/j.pcl.2020.03.001.
149. Fitzgerald M, Bhatt A, Thompson LA, et al. Telemedicine in pediatric training: a National Needs Assessment of the current state of telemedicine education in pediatric training. Acad Pediatr. 2022;22(5):713–7. https://doi.org/10.1016/j.acap.2021.10.009.
150. Scott TE, Costich M, Fiorino EK, Paradise BN. Using a modified Delphi methodology to identify essential telemedicine skills for pediatric residents. Acad Pediatr. 2023;23(3):511–7. https://doi.org/10.1016/j.acap.2022.08.014.
151. McConnell M, Kumar P, Mullur R. The virtual visit: a telehealth curriculum for internal medicine residents featuring a virtual physical examination. J Grad Med Educ. 2023;15(5):582–6. https://doi.org/10.4300/JGME-D-22-00635.1.
152. Fitzgerald DA, Scott KM, Ryan MS. Blended and e-learning in pediatric education: harnessing lessons learned from the COVID-19 pandemic. Eur J Pediatr. 2022;181(2):447–52. https://doi.org/10.1007/s00431-021-04149-1.
153. Kelly JM, Perseghin A, Dow AW, Trivedi SP, Rodman A, Berk J. Learning through listening: a scoping review of podcast use in medical education. Acad Med. 2022;97(7):1079–85. https://doi.org/10.1097/ACM.0000000000004565.
154. Smith A. The impact of podcasts on knowledge retention in pediatric residents. Pediatrics. Published online 2020.
155. Jones B. Mobile application for pediatric procedural skills training: a randomized controlled trial. Pediatrics. Published online 2021.
156. Perez MJ, Omurtag K, Aagaard E, Klingensmith M, Bhayani RK. Innovative social media summit: providing a path for physicians on social media. Acad Med. 2022;97(7):1009–11. https://doi.org/10.1097/ACM.0000000000004633.
157. Maldonado G, Smart J, Wiechmann W, et al. Frequency of social media and digital scholarship keywords in U.S. medical schools' promotion and tenure guidelines. Acad Med. 2022;97(1):105–10. https://doi.org/10.1097/ACM.0000000000004324.
158. Myers RE, Thoreson L, Howell HB, et al. Three years of X + Y scheduling: longitudinal assessment of resident and faculty perceptions. Acad Pediatr. 2022;22(7):1097–104. https://doi.org/10.1016/j.acap.2022.01.014.
159. Myers RE, Thoreson L, Howell HB, et al. Impact of X+Y scheduling on pediatric resident and faculty perceptions of education and patient care. Acad Pediatr. 2021;21(7):1273–80. https://doi.org/10.1016/j.acap.2021.02.018.
160. Mariotti JL, Shalaby M, Fitzgibbons JP. The 4:1 schedule: a novel template for internal medicine residencies. J Grad Med Educ. 2010;2(4):541–7. https://doi.org/10.4300/JGME-D-10-00044.1.

Concluding Remarks

32

Heather McPhillips, Patricia Poitevien, Rebecca Blankenburg, and Joanna Lewis

Throughout the book, we have highlighted the essential structures that sustain strong residency programs: accreditation standards, curriculum development, assessment strategies, and well-being initiatives. We have also shared emerging practices and innovations that reflect the dynamic landscape of pediatric education: reimagined training models, competency-based frameworks, inclusive learning environments, and new approaches to mentoring and advising.

What unites all of these efforts is a shared commitment to improving child health through excellence in education. Our trainees enter the workforce at a time of growing complexity—medically, socially, and systemically. The responsibility to prepare them has never been greater. It requires collaboration, adaptability, creativity, and an unwavering dedication to equity and belonging.

The community of pediatric medical educators is one of resilience, generosity, and vision. We hope this book has served not only as a practical resource but also as a source of inspiration. Whether you are just beginning your journey as a program leader or are guiding transformative change in an established institution, we invite you to return to these pages as your work evolves.

The future of pediatric education will be shaped by those willing to question assumptions, embrace new models, and place learners—and their future patients—at the center of every decision. We are confident that, with the collective wisdom and courage of this community, the future is bright.

Suggested Reading and Listening

1. Vinci RJ, et al. Pediatrics 2025: the AMSPDC workforce initiative. J Pediatr. 2021;237:5–8.e1.
2. The Future of Pediatrics in the US. https://edhub.ama-assn.org/jn-learning/audio-player/18892878.

H. McPhillips (✉)
University of Washington School of Medicine, Seattle, WA, USA
e-mail: hmcphil@uw.edu

P. Poitevien
The Warren Alpert Medical School of Brown University, Providence, RI, USA
e-mail: patricia_poitevien@brown.edu

R. Blankenburg
Stanford School of Medicine, Stanford, CA, USA
e-mail: rblanke@stanford.edu

J. Lewis
Advocate Children's Hospital, Park Ridge, IL, USA
e-mail: joanna.lewis@aah.org

H. McPhillips et al. (eds.), *Graduate Medical Education in Pediatrics*, Excellence in Medical Education 3, https://doi.org/10.1007/978-3-032-12952-9_32

Index

A
AAMC Residency Explorer, 96
AAP CPTI AP, 213
ABP entrustable professional activity, 191
ABP Program Portal, 35
Abstract conceptualization, 223
Academic Pediatric Association (APA), 7, 88, 200, 362–363
Academic Pediatrics Association (APA) Task Force on Child Poverty, 202
Academic/planned curriculum
  academic half days *vs.* morning reports *vs.* noon conferences, 171, 172
  active learning strategies, 166
  curriculum development, 167
  definition, 161, 162
  evaluation and feedback, 172, 173
  game-based learning, 168, 169
  GME, teaching strategies, 168
  harness peer expertise, 166, 167
  key objectives, 164, 165
  learners control, 167
  pacing, 165, 166
  structure education, content themes in, 162
    board preparation, 163
    case-based learning and diagnostic uncertainty, 163
    DEI and health equity, 164
    procedural training, 164
    quality improvement and patient safety, 163, 164
  structured education faculty and staff, roles for, 169, 170
  Team-based learning, 168
Accelerated Research Pathway (ARP), 48
Acceptability, 271
Accreditation, 41
Accreditation Council for Graduate Medical Education (ACGME), 5, 6, 11, 19, 20, 33, 41–43, 69, 89, 175, 176, 193, 279, 282–286, 288, 360
  clinical curriculum, 149, 150
  CPR, 185
  financial impact of, 11–12
  outcomes-based accreditation, 24
  resources, 29, 30
  rotation, 46–47
Accreditation cycle, 24–25
Accreditation data system (ADS), 25, 284, 285, 288
Accreditation feedback, 28–29
Accreditation site visits, 57–58
  accreditation cycle, timeline for, 24, 25
  documentation and data collection, 25
  organizing site visit logistics, strategies for, 25
  self-study report, developing, 25
Accreditation standards
  common program requirements, 22
  purpose of, 21
ACGME Pediatric Review Committee, 6
ACGME Accreditation Data System (ADS), 24
ACGME-accredited pediatric residency training program, 5
ACGME Clinical Learning Environment Review (CLER) program, 186
ACGME International (ACGME-I) programs, 34
ACGME Well-being Survey data, 341
Active experimentation, 223
Active learning strategies, 166
Adequate pediatric subspecialty disciplines, 46–47
Administrative support, 12
Administrative team, 72
Adolescent medicine, 46–47
Adult learning, 389
Advance practice providers (APPs), 46
Advanced practice practitioners (APPs), 12
Advising
  definition, 317
  faculty and learner development, 321–322
  framework, 319
  program development, 321
  structures, 321

H. McPhillips et al. (eds.), *Graduate Medical Education in Pediatrics*, Excellence in Medical Education 3, https://doi.org/10.1007/978-3-032-12952-9

Advocacy, 49
community level, 207–209
curriculum, learner assessment, and program evaluation, 200–203
educators, scholarship for, 212–214
individual level
screening for social drivers, 205, 206
screening special populations, 206
social drivers of health, 206, 207
pediatricians as, 199, 200
policy level, 211–212
socio-ecological framework, 203
community level, 204
individual level, 203
legislative level, 205
structural level, 204, 205
structural level
healthcare systems and communities, 209, 210
media advocacy, 210, 211
training, 200
Advocacy portfolio (AP), 213
Advocacy-related pediatric medical education, 214
Affinity matching, 363
Affirmative action, 416
Agency for Health Care Administration (AHCA), 56–57
AI-driven assistive technology, 195
Ambulatory curriculum, 153–154
American Academy of Pediatrics (AAP), 7, 89, 360, 362–363
American Academy of Pediatrics National Conference and the Pediatric Academic Societies Conference, 96
American Board of Medical Specialties (ABMS), 5
American Board of Osteopathic Pediatrics (AOBP), 5
American Board of Pediatrics (ABP), 5, 6, 51, 74, 89, 150, 190, 200
certification assessments, 35, 36
initial certification examination, 36
in-training examination, 36
maintenance of certification, 37
prerequisites for, 34
program directors, 35
time-limited eligibility, 36
trainee responsibilities, 35
training pathways, 33, 34
American Osteopathic Association (AOA), 5, 6
American Osteopathic Board of Pediatrics (AOBP), 5, 6, 89
American Pediatric Society (APS), 200
American Physician Scientists Association, 96
Americans with Disabilities Act (ADA), 54
AMSPDC Workforce Initiative, 409
Annual faculty evaluations, 387
Anonymous reporting tools, 366
APPD Residency Recruitment Action Team (APPD RRAT), 99, 101
Applicant Criteria Identification and Prioritization, 99
Artificial intelligence (AI), 100, 170, 248, 257–260, 431, 432
Assistant program directors (APDs), 59, 69
Association of American Medical Colleges (AAMC), 6, 9, 82, 94
Association of Medical School Pediatric Department Chairs (AMSPDC), 7
Association of Pediatric Program Directors (APPD), 6, 30, 70, 72, 85, 95, 136, 221, 226, 362–363
Association of Pediatric Program Directors Longitudinal Educational Assessment Research Network (APPD LEARN), 424, 425
Association of Pediatric Program Directors (APPD) mission, 87
Asynchronous learning tools, 433
Audience, 3
Audio presentations, 252
Augmented intelligence (AI), 431–432

B
Backwards design, 165
Bag-mask ventilation, 237, 238
Behavioral/mental health (BMH)
educational strategies
experiential learning, 223–224
observation of experts with shared reflection, 224
situated learning theory, 224–225
faculty development, 225
financial barrier, 226
future aspects, 227
growing needs, 217–218
hidden curriculum, 225
for pediatricians, 218–220
for pediatric trainees
curricula, 221
dedicated mental health rotation/block, 222
integrating mental health services, 221–222
Mental Health Track, 221
program evaluation and assessment, 226–227
resources, 226
Big Gear, 133, 134
Block and longitudinal curriculum, 156
Block system scheduling, 158
Board preparation, 163

C
Capacity building, 42–43
Capital cost/expenses, 13
Cardiopulmonary resuscitation (CPR), 165
Career advancement, 81–83
Career exploration, 180
Career focus, 182
Career guidance, 118
Case-based learning, 163, 360
Case conferences, 189
Centers for Medicare and Medicaid Services (CMS), 47
Change management, 61, 80
ChatGPT, 170, 287
Chief resident, 72, 73
compensation models, 382
definition, 371

division of labor, 377, 378
job description
clinical responsibilities, 377
education, 374–375
intern orientation, 374
program representation, 373
residency recruitment, 374
resident support, 375–376
scheduling, 373
transition planning and chief resident handoff, 376–377
professional development
advancing chief residents' goals, 378–380
advancing programmatic goals, 380–381
chief resident year, 381, 382
middle management, 381
training for the chief role, 378
selection of, 372
types of, 371–372
Chief resident year, 376, 377, 379, 382
Child poverty, 202
Children's Hospital Association (CHA), 10
Children's hospitals GME (CHGME) program, 10
Children's National Hospital (CNH), 362
Chronic medical condition management, 154
Classical mentorship model, 363
Climate change, 415
Climate health, 414–416
Climate surveys, 365
Clinical Competency Committees (CCCs), 159, 267, 270–272, 276
membership, 279–283
processes, 283
during-CCC meeting group, 283–285, 287–288
post-CCC meeting feedback, 283–285, 288–289
pre-CCC meeting preparation, 283–287
Clinical curriculum
ABP content, 152
ACGME requirements, 149, 150
arrangement of each clinical year, 158
block and longitudinal curriculum, 156
clinical experiences, 150
ambulatory curriculum, 153, 154
ICU, 153
individualized curriculum, 154
inpatient curriculum, 150, 151, 153
program discretionary time, 154, 155
clinical skill assessment, 158, 159
Clinical environment, 116–119
faculty role, 118
OSCEs, 119
role-play, 118
senior peers, 117, 118
simulation, 119
support networks, 117
Clinical experiences, 150
ambulatory curriculum, 153, 154
ICU, 153
individualized curriculum, 154
inpatient curriculum, 150, 151, 153
program discretionary time, 154, 155
Clinical learning environment (CLE), 274, 359–360, 367
equitable feedback, assessment, and evaluation, 361–362
formal education, 360
multimodal education, 360–361
Clinical skill assessment, 158, 159
Clinical supervision, 117
Clinical teachers, 388
autonomy and supervision, 392
clinical environment, 392–393
feedback, 390
goals, expectations, and growth mindset, 391–392
learning climate, 390, 391
observation, 392
summative evaluations, 393–394
Coaching, 308, 391, 392, 394, 395, 399, 401, 402, 423, 428
definition, 318
faculty and learner development, 321
framework, 319, 320
program development, 321
structures, 320
Coalition for Physician Accountability (CoPA), 109
Collaboration, 443
Collecting clinical learning environment climate data, 365
Commission on Osteopathic Accreditation (COCA), 86
Common program requirements, 22
Communication channel establishment, 111
Communication skills, program director, 80
Community Access to Child Health (CATCH) program, 208
Community-based advocacy, 209
Community-based participatory research (CBPR), 209
Community level, advocacy at, 207–209
Community partnerships, 209
Community Pediatrics Training Initiative (CPTI), 201, 213
Competency, 190–192
Competency-based faculty development (CBFD), 387, 388
Competency-based medical education (CBME), 35, 175, 355, 426–428
assessment
collecting data, 269–272
desired outcomes, 266–269
interpreting data, 272
CLEs, 274, 275
coaching, 428
components, 265, 266, 271, 274, 276
feedback, 266, 270–275
programmatic assessment, 276
time variable education/accelerated learning, 427
workplace based assessments, 427–428
Conceptual fidelity, 232
Concrete experience, 223
Conflict management, program director, 81
Congress, 14
Constructive criticism, 292

Council of Pediatric Subspecialties (CoPS), 7
Council on Medical Student Education in Pediatrics (COMSEP), 7
COVID-19 pandemic, 95, 247, 252–254
Creative expression, 333
Credentialing, 112
C-suite, 42
Cultivating psychological safety, 420
Culture of accountability, 366, 368
Culture of professional responsibilities, 26, 27
Curricular development, 27
Curriculum assessment, advocacy, 200–203
Curriculum development, 131, 167, 395, 396
  curriculum mapping, 143
  curriculum-specific general needs assessment, 138
  dissemination, 147
  educational methods, 132, 142
  evaluation and feedback, 133, 144, 145
  goals and objectives, 132, 141, 142
  implementation, 132, 133, 143, 144
  journey, 147
  little gears, zooming in, 134, 135
  ongoing curriculum maintenance and enhancement, 146
  problem identification and general needs assessment, 131, 135–137
  6-step approach, 133, 134
  systematic approach, 138
  targeted needs assessment, 132, 139–141
Curriculum evaluation, 172, 173
Curriculum mapping, 143

D
Dean of Graduate Medical Education, 87
Debriefing, 232, 234, 235, 239, 334, 335
Deep learning, 248
DEI, *see* Diversity, equity, and inclusion
Delivering feedback training, 390
Designated Institutional Officer (DIO), 69, 86, 289, 297, 299, 300
Design-based learning, 255
Developmental and Behavioral Pediatrics, 46–47
Direct GME (DGME), 10
Disability services management, 74
Diverse workforce, 409–411, 417, 419
Diversity, 124
Diversity, equity, and inclusion (DEI), 164, 326

E
Education Commission of Foreign Graduate Medical Education (ECFMG) certification, 56
Educational excellence, 301
Educational methods, curriculum development, 132, 142
Educational strategies
  experiential learning, 223–224
  observation of experts with shared reflection, 224
  situated learning theory, 224–225
Educational support, 118
Effective onboarding, 110
E-learning modules, 119
Electronic health record, 114
Electronic Residency Application Service (ERAS), 94, 95
Emotional support, 118
Entrustable Professional Activities (EPAs), 24, 35, 89, 141, 157, 159, 190, 265–270, 272, 282, 287
Equity impact assessments, 366
Ethical decision making, 123
Experiential learning cycle model, 223
Experiential learning theory, 223, 255, 257

F
Faculty assessment, 308
Faculty development (FD), 52–53, 225, 362–363
  adult learning, 389
  annual faculty evaluations, 387
  CBFD, 388
  clinical teachers, 388
    autonomy and supervision, 392
    clinical environment, 392–393
    feedback, 390
    goals, expectations, and growth mindset, 391–392
    learning climate, 390, 391
    observation, 392
    summative evaluations, 393–394
  counting twice, 400
  definition, 388
  format and delivery methods, 398–400
  medical educators, 388
    coaching, 394
    curriculum development, 395, 396
    leadership, 396
    mentorship, 395
    scholarship, 396, 397
  programs, 426
Faculty performance
  in academic advancement, 308–309
  assessments, 306
  effective mentorship skills, 308
  evaluation of, 306
  frameworks and models, 309–310
  mentorship relationship, 310
  peer evaluation, 306
  professional identity, 308
  program leadership, 311
  reflective practice, 306
  role models, 308
  student and trainee evaluations, 310
  teaching style, 305
  team building, 308
Faculty, role of, 118
Family Medical Leave Act (FMLA), 351, 353
Federation of Pediatric Organizations (FOPO), 7
Feedback, 28, 117, 172, 390, 401, 402
Fellowship and Residency Electronic Interactive Database (FREIDA), 96
Fidelity, 232

Finance and medical education
  career choices and job satisfaction, 412–413
  GME, 411–412
  loan repayment programs, 413
Financial barrier, 226
Finding meaning in medicine, 325
Flexible learning, 248
Flipped classroom approach, 252
Focused individualized learning plan (FILP), 295, 297–303
Formal supervision, 118
Fostering UIM Education Leadership (FUEL) Program, 85
Full-time equivalent (FTE), 43–45, 69, 70
Funding, pediatric education, 9
  ACGME changes, financial impact of, 11, 12
  advocacy, 15
  core faculty time, 12
  department and hospital funding, 11
  Federal Medicaid and Children's Hospital Funding, 9, 10
  industry, 11
    pediatric workforce, finances on, 13–15
    philanthropy, 11
    program leadership and administrative support, 12
    residency budget considerations, 13
    resident unions, influence of, 13
    stimulating access to research in residency, 10

G
Game-based learning, 168, 169
Gamification, 166
Gender-affirming care, 418–419
Generationalism, 421
Geographic preference, 97
GME-based interprofessional education
  case conferences and safety event reviews, 189
  in-situ improvement work within the healthcare system, 190
  interprofessional simulations, 189, 190
  patient- and family-centered rounds, 188, 189
Graduate degrees, program director, 83, 84
Graduate education committee (GMEC), 30
Graduate medical education (GME), 3, 41, 109, 185, 366
  due process policy, 297
  office, 74
  program director, 81
Graduate Medical Education Committee (GMEC), 50–51, 82, 86

H
Harness peer expertise, 166, 167
Health disparities, 206
Health equity, 164
Health Insurance Portability and Accountability Act (HIPAA), 114
Health systems, 194
Hidden curriculum, 225
Human resources, 74

I
Imposter phenomenon, 330
Imposter syndrome, 121
Inclusion initiatives, 124
Inclusive learning environments, 419–422
Individualized curriculum (IC), 154, 175–177
  career, 182
  curricular structure, 177, 178
  evaluation, 180
  future directions, 182
  program leadership, 179, 180
  rotation structure, 177–179
  trainee assessment, 180
  training year, 180–182
Individualized learning plans (ILPs), 110, 116, 295
Innovation, 443
Inpatient curriculum, 150–153
In-situ improvement work, 190
Institute for Healthcare Improvement (IHI), 49
Institute for Patient- and Family-Centered Care (IPFCC), 189
Institutional and individual program, 109
Institutional buy-in, 60, 61
Institutional policy changes, 366
Integrating mental health services, 221
Intelligent tutoring systems, 257
Interactive learning modules, 252, 253
International medical graduates (IMGs), 112, 420
Interprofessional case conferences (ICC), 189
Interprofessional education (IPE), 185–188, 429–430
  AI-driven assistive technology, 195
  assessing competency, 190–192
  challenges, 192–194
  CLE, learning, and collaborative practice in, 186–188
  evolving technology, 195
  GME-based interprofessional education
    case conferences and safety event reviews, 189
    in-situ improvement work within the healthcare system, 190
    interprofessional simulations, 189, 190
    patient- and family-centered rounds, 188, 189
Interprofessional learning, 185
Interprofessional simulation, 189, 190
Interprofessional team members, 53
In-training examinations (ITE), 35
I-PASS, 114

J
Job demands-resource model, 339
Joint Commission, 56–57

K
Kern and Thomas model, 131
Key personnel, 115
Kolb's cycle, 255

L

Labor & Employee Relations, 74
Leadership, 78, 79, 87, 396
Learners, 247–256, 258, 259, 261
  assessment, 158, 200–203
  certification, American Board of Pediatrics, 33
    assessments, 35, 36
    initial certification examination, 36
    in-training examination, 36
    maintenance of certification, 37
    prerequisites for, 34
    program directors, 35
    time-limited eligibility, 36
    trainee responsibilities, 35
    training pathways, 33, 34
  control, 167
Learning climate, 390–391, 401
Learning communities (LC), 87
Learning (instructional) design, 254–256
  design thinking, 255
  educator's skills and knowledge, 255–256
  learner engagement and centering, 255–256
Learning management systems (LMS), 253, 254, 256–257
LEARN Research Network, 424–425
Legislative advocacy, 211–212
Legitimate participation, 224
Liaison Committee on Medical Education (LCME), 86
Licensure, 112
Logistic planning, 170
Lumbar puncture, 238

M

Machine learning (ML), 248, 258–260, 431, 432
Manikins, 229–231, 237, 239, 240
Master Adaptive Learner (MAL) framework, 319
Master of Business Administration (MBA), 83
Master of Education (MEd), 83
Master of Healthcare Administration (MHA), 84
Master of Health Management (MHM), 84
Master of Health Professions Education (MHPE), 83
Master of Science in Health Professions Education (MS-HPE), 83
Meal cards, 50–52
MedEdPortal.org, 153
MedHub, 141
Media advocacy, 210, 211
Media engagement, 43
Medicaid, 9
Medical Assistance Programs, 56
Medical educators, 388, 389, 396, 397, 399, 400
  coaching, 394
  curriculum development, 395, 396
  leadership, 396
  mentorship, 395
  scholarship, 396
Medicare, 9, 10, 15
Medicare GME funding, 9
Mental health, 46–47, 154
Mental Health Track, 221
Mentoring
  benefits of, 318
  definition, 318
  faculty and learner development, 321
  framework, 320
  program development, 321
  structures, 320
Mentorship, 77, 118
  affinity matching, 363
  classical mentorship, 363
  families, 363
  mentoring across differences, 363
  peer mentorship, 363
  programs, 124
Metrics, 99
Mimics, 166
Mindfulness techniques, 332
Mini-CEX, 120
Mission and vision integration, 359
Mitigating bias, 420
Mock codes, 189
Moral distress, 329
Moral injury, 329
MyERAS application, 97

N

National Academy of Distinguished Educators in Pediatrics (NADEP), 88
National Institutes of Health (NIH), 209
National Resident Matching Program (NRMP), 6, 44, 64, 94–95
National service, 87
Natural advocates, 199
Natural language processing, 258
Negotiation skills, program director, 81
Neonatal Intensive Care Unit (NICU), 55
Neonatal Resuscitation Program (NRP), 115
New ACGME Pediatric Residency Requirements, 428
  alternate models of care, 428–429
  IPE, 429
  value-conscious medicine, 429
New innovations, 141
New Jersey Pediatric Residency Advocacy Collaborative (NJPRAC), 203
New program, data requirements, 55–56
New training track
  determination rationale, 59, 60
  educational content determination, 62, 63
  evaluation, 66, 67
  funding positions for, 63–65
  identifying champions for, 60
  obtaining institutional buy-in, 60, 61
  postgraduate/non-residency tracks, 65, 66
  recruit leaders for, 61, 62
NRMP Match® Code of Conduct, 103

O

Observed Structured Clinical Encounters (OSCEs), 119
Onboarding process, 110, 125
Onboarding residents, 111
Organizational tools, 141
Orientation, 109, 110
  continued learning and growth, resources for, 122
  diversity and inclusion initiatives, 124
  ethical and professional considerations, 122
  imposter syndrome and self-doubt, 121, 122
  pediatric residency programs, program evaluation and improvement in, 125
  planning, purpose and objectives of, 113
  professionalism issues, 123
  programs, 110
    electronic health record and technology training, 114
    Healthcare Facility and Training Institutions, 113
    key personnel, 115
    policies, procedures, and protocols, 114
    residents as educators, 115
    socialization, 116
    special certifications, 115
    specific patient populations, 113, 114
    wellness and self-care, 115
  seeking support and guidance, 122
  supportive environment, 123
  time management and workload prioritization, 121

P

Paid time off (PTO), 54
Parental leave
  duration, 350, 351
  planning, 350
  policies, 351–353
  well-being, 351
Patient- and family-centered rounds, 188–189
Patient safety, 49, 163, 229, 235
Pediatric Academic Societies (PAS), 89
Pediatric Advanced Life Support (PALS), 115
Pediatric advocacy, 213
Pediatric education, funding, 9
  ACGME changes, financial impact of, 11, 12
  advocacy, 15
  core faculty time, 12
  department and hospital funding, 11
  Federal Medicaid and Children's Hospital Funding, 9, 10
  industry, 11
  pediatric workforce, finances on, 13–15
  philanthropy, 11
  program leadership and administrative support, 12
  residency budget considerations, 13
  resident unions, influence of, 13
  stimulating access to research in residency, 10
Pediatric-focused training, 15
Pediatric hospital closures, 14–15
Pediatric Intensive Care Unit (PICU), 55
Pediatric interns, 120
  challenges and concerns during training, 121
  feedback and guidance, 120
Pediatric medical education, 443
  advocacy/creating brave spaces, 421
  climate health, 414–416
  collaboration across organizations, 425
  competency-based medical education, 426–428
    coaching, 428
    time variable education/accelerated learning, 427
    workplace based assessments, 427–428
  evidence-based medicine, EDI and healthcare disparities, 416–417
  faculty development programs, 426
  finance and medical education
    career choices and job satisfaction, 412–413
    GME, 411–412
    loan repayment programs, 413
  gender-affirming care, 418–419
  generational differences and learning strategies, 421–422
  inclusive learning environments, 419–422
    assessing learning environment, 419–420
    cultivating psychological safety, 420
    IMG residents, 420
    mitigating bias, 420
  LEARN Research Network, 424–425
  new ACGME Pediatric Residency Requirements, 428
    alternate models of care, 428–429
    IPE, 429
    value-conscious medicine, 429
  pediatric workforce, 409–411
    diversification, 411
    economic strategy, 410
    physician scientist, 410
    practice models, 411
    redesigning medical education/enhance education, training, recruitment and retention, 410
  reflective learning, 426
  reproductive health, 417–418
  self-directed learning, 425, 426
  technology
    artificial intelligence, 431
    asynchronous learning tools, 433
    augmented intelligence, 431–432
    augmented reality/virtual reality, 432
    machine learning, 431
    precision medical education, 430
    telehealth, 432, 433
  transition, 422, 423
  unionization, 423–424
  well-being trainees, 414
  X+Y faculty outcomes, 434
Pediatric organizations, 5–7
Pediatric partner organizations, 7
Pediatric program requirements, 212
Pediatric residency programs, 10, 41, 45–46
  program evaluation and improvement in, 125
  Specialty-specific requirements for, 23, 24
Pediatric training programs, 292

Pediatric workforce, 409–411
  diversification, 411
  economic strategy, 410
  finances, 13
    pediatric interest, drivers of decline in, 15
    primary care pediatricians, demand for, 14
    volatile pediatric funding and pediatric hospital closures, 14, 15
  physician scientist, 410
  practice models, 411
  redesigning medical education/enhance education, training, recruitment and retention, 410
Pediatricians, 292
Peer evaluation, 306
Peer mentorship, 363
Peer PDs, 74
Peer support groups, 122
Periodic external program audits, 366
Personalized learning, 248–250
Personnel management, 79
Philanthropy, 11
Physical fidelity, 233
Physician task load (PTL) index, 339
Policymakers, 212
Positive psychology, 333
Postgraduate/faculty tracks, 65
Postgraduate/non-residency tracks, 65, 66
Postgraduate training tracks, 65
Postgraduate year (PGY), 43
Post-match review, 105
Precision medical education (PE), 430
Primary care pediatricians, 14
Procedural competency, 48
Procedural training, 164
Professional development, 53
Professional identity formation (PIF), 175, 326, 365
Professionalism, 122
Professional responsibilities, 26–27
Professional support, 118
Program accreditation, 3
Program coordinators, 72
Program director (PD) career, 46, 59, 77
  department, 77
  extra-mural, 78
  institutional, 77, 78
  service and leadership opportunities, 85–87
  skill building
    career advancement, 81–83
    change management, 80
    communication skills, 80
    conflict management, 81
    GME finance, 81
    graduate degrees, 83, 84
    leadership skills, 78, 79
    leading from middle, 80
    negotiation skills, 81
    personnel management and team building, 79
    program management, 79
    resources, 84, 85
    running meetings, 80
Program discretionary time, 154–155
Program enhancement, quality improvement and accreditation strategies, 27
  faculty and resident survey, program quality improvement projects, 28
  feedback, 28, 29
  long-term planning, 29
  program outcomes, continuous improvement in, 28
Program launch, 43
Program leaders, 336, 338, 339, 341
Program leadership, 12, 44–45, 59, 170, 179, 180, 311, 312
Program letter of agreement (PLA), 30, 54
Program management, 79
Program outcomes, continuous improvement, 28
Program requirements, 149
Proximal development and scaffolding theory, 257
Psychological fidelity, 233
Psychological flexibility, 331, 332
Psychological supports, 52
Push learning vs. retrieval learning, 248–249

Q

Quality improvement (QI), 28, 49, 114, 163, 164, 379

R

R2C2 model, 320
Rank order list (ROL), 104
Recruitment
  application review
    artificial intelligence, 100
    holistic review, 98–100
    materials and components, 97, 98
    process establishment, 98
    underrepresented in medicine, 100, 101
  categorical tracks and combined programs, 105, 106
  ERAS, thalamus, and NRMP, 94, 95
  interview techniques and assessment, 102, 103
  match week, 104, 105
  navigating interview day, 102
  planning, preparing team, invitations, 101, 102
  post-interview communication and second looks, 103, 104
  post-match review, 105
  rank order list, 104
  recruitment cycle, 95
  seeking out applicants, 95–97
  team establishment, 93, 94
  transfers between programs, 106
Recruitment cycle, 95
Reddit and Student Doctor Network, 96
Reflective learning, 426
Reflective practice, 306, 310, 311
Relational practices, 333–334
Reliability, 270–272
Remediation
  components, 295
  FILP *vs.* formal, 297–299

individualized learning plan, 295
interventions, 295, 296
leaders and learners, 300–301
legal considerations, 299–300
narrative evaluations, 295
outcomes, 299
SOAP framework, 296
Reproductive health, 417–418
Research and scholarly activity, 48–49
Residency budget, 13
Residency leadership team, 69–74
Residency Management Software (RMS), 50
Residency navigator, 96
Residency programs, 19, 51, 72
accreditation site visits, preparing for
documentation and data collection, 25
organizing site visit logistics, strategies for, 25
self-study report, developing, 25
timeline for, 24, 25
accreditation standards, 21
common program requirements, 22
purpose of, 21
accrediting body, 20
ACGME outcomes-based accreditation, 24
ACGME resources, 29, 30
challenges, 26
culture of professional responsibilities, 26, 27
curricular development, 27
evaluations, 27
faculty qualifications, 26
responsibilities of faculty, 27
core requirements, 22, 23
definition and process, 19, 20
detail requirements, 23
importance of, 21
outcome requirements, 23
pediatric residency programs, specialty-specific requirements for, 23, 24
program enhancement, quality improvement and accreditation strategies, 27
accreditation feedback, 28, 29
faculty and resident survey, program quality improvement projects, 28
feedback mechanisms, 28
long-term planning, 29
program outcomes, continuous improvement in, 28
Review Committee, structure and role of, 20, 21
tracks, 47–48
Resident Continuity Clinic, 46–47
Resident onboarding
communication channel establishment, 111
coordination with other departments, 112, 113
licensure and credentialing, 112
practical considerations, 111, 112
setting onboarding expectations, 110, 111
special considerations, 112
Resident performance challenges, 293–295
Resident remediation, 44
Resident unions, influence of, 13
Resilience, 326–328, 331, 333, 334, 336, 341
Return to work
childcare considerations, 355
lactation considerations, 354
parenting electives, 353
part-time and flexible time, 353–354
Review Committee (RC), 5, 20, 21
Review Committee for Pediatrics, 20
Role modeling, 117
Role-play, 118
Rome Visiting Professorships, 202
Rotation-embedded education, 162
Rotation structure, 177–179
Running meetings, 80

S

Safety event reviews, 189
Sage on the stage model, 167
Scholarship, 212–214, 396
Seeking out applicants, 95–97
Self-care, 115
Self-compassion, 332, 333
Self-directed learning, 425, 426
Self-directed learning in medical education (SDL-ME), 176
Self-doubt, 121
Self-study report, 25–26
Senior peers, 117, 118
Simulation, 119
Simulation-based learning, 361
Simulation-based medical education (SBME)
benefits/efficacy, 230
debriefing, 234, 235
history, 229
interpersonal and communication skills, 241–242
learner behaviors and patient outcomes and comparative studies, 242
limitations/overcoming challenges, 230–232
for medical knowledge and clinical decision-making, 239–241
assessment of residents' clinical progress, 241
clinical management and skills, 240–241
resuscitation, 239–240
patient safety, 229
for procedures
ACGME-mandated procedures, 238
bag-mask ventilation, 237, 238
lumbar puncture, 238
non-mandated procedures, 238–239
simulation-based procedural training, 236–237
simulation education for procedures, 236–239
simulation formats, 232–234
fidelity, 232, 233
locations, 233
modalities, 232
simulation societies/networks/collaborations, 235–236

Simulation-based procedural training, 236–237
Simulation formats
  fidelity, 232, 233
  locations, 233
  modalities, 232
Site visits, 24–26
Situated learning theory, 224–225
Social drivers of health, 204, 206, 207
Socialization, 116
Socio-ecological framework, advocacy, 203
  community level, 204
  individual level, 203
  legislative level, 205
  structural level, 204, 205
Space and technology needs, 49–50
Sponsoring Institution (SI), 41, 42
Stake, 328
Stanford Faculty Development Program (SFDP) framework, 310
Stanford Professional Fulfillment Index, 341
Stimulating Access to Research in Residency (StARR), 10–11
Structural level, advocacy, 209–211
  healthcare systems and communities, 209, 210
  media advocacy, 210, 211
Structured education, 162
  faculty and staff, roles for, 169, 170
Supporting residents/planning families
  CBME, 355
  parental leave
    duration, 350, 351
    planning, 350
    policies, 351–353
    well-being, 351
  pregnancy and delivery considerations, 350
  residents as parents, 349–350
  return to work
    childcare considerations, 355
    lactation considerations, 354
    parenting electives, 353
    part-time and flexible time, 353–354
Support networks, 117
Supportive institutional culture, 190
Supportive remediation, 291

T
Targeted needs assessment, curriculum development, 132, 139–141
Teaching style, 305
Team-based learning, 168
Team culture, 336–337
Teaming domain, 186
Technology
  AI/machine learning/deep learning, 248
  for asynchronous learning, 252–254
  economic trends, 250
  educational resources, 250
  enhance in-person learning, 250–252
  experiential learning, 255
  flexible learning, 248
  learners, 247
  learning (instructional) design, 254–256
    design thinking, 255
    educator's skills and knowledge, 255–256
    learner engagement and centering, 255–256
  in pediatric resident learner assessment, 256–260
    clinical learning environment, 259
    content and text analysis, 258
    feedback, personalization of, 257–258
    generation of education materials, 258–259
    generative AI, 257
    GME recruitment, 259–260
    LMS analytics, 256–257
  personalized learning, 249–250
  proximal development and scaffolding theory, 257
  push learning *vs.* retrieval learning, 248–249
  safety/quality experience, 247–248
  teleconferencing, 254
Teleconferencing technology, 252–254
Telehealth, 432–433
Thalamus, 94–95
Total parenteral nutrition (TPN), 181–182
Track-specific lectures, 63
Traditional faculty clinical teacher, 388
Trainee assessment, 180
Trainee Education in Advocacy and Community Health (TEACH), 202
Training Administrators for Graduate Medical Education (TAGME) certification, 72
Training year, 180–182

U
Undergraduate medical education (UME), 109
Undergraduate Medical Education to Graduate Medical Education Review Committee (UGRC), 109
Underrepresented in medicine (URiM), 96, 100, 101, 326, 359, 363, 364, 366, 367
Unionization, 423, 424
Unionized programs, 13
United States Medical Licensing Examination (USMLE), 51

V
Validity, 271
Value-conscious medicine, 429
Vice Chair of Education, 86
Video/recorded presentations, 253
Virtual reality (VR), 432
Virtual therapy, 247
Volatile pediatric funding, 14, 15
Voluntary Withdrawal of Accreditation/Recognition, 30

W
Well-being
  ACGME requirements, 328
  assessing outcomes, 340–341

barriers, 326–327
vs. burnout, 327–328
burnout, mental health, substance use and fatigue, 330
centered leadership, 341–342
characteristics, 328–329
communication, transparency, and setting expectations, 338
creative expression, 333
debriefing, 334, 335
exercise, 331
finding meaning in medicine, 325
fostering competence, 339
grief and loss, 329–330
imposter phenomenon, 330
meaningful self-care, 330–331
mental health programming and resources, 335–336
mindfulness techniques, 332
mistreatment, 337–338
monitoring, 340
moral distress and injury, 329
nutrition, 331
positive psychology, 333
psychological flexibility, 332
relational practices, 333–334
schedules and attention to workload, 339
self-compassion, 332, 333
sleep, 331
stake, 328
team culture, 336–337
trainees, 414
workload, 339
Well-being initiatives, 52
Wellness, 115
Women Infants and Children (WIC), 153
Workforce, 177
Workforce diversity, 416
Workload, 339
Workplace-based assessment (WBA), 269, 270, 274, 427, 428

X
X+Y scheduling model, 3, 158, 339

Z
Zone of proximal development, 167

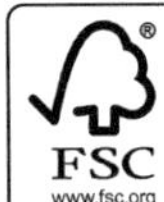

MIX
Papier aus verantwortungsvollen Quellen
Paper from responsible sources
FSC® C105338

If you have any concerns about our products,
you can contact us on
ProductSafety@springernature.com

In case Publisher is established outside the EU,
the EU authorized representative is:
Springer Nature Customer Service Center GmbH
Europaplatz 3, 69115 Heidelberg, Germany

Printed by Libri Plureos GmbH
in Hamburg, Germany